McCRACKEN'S

REMOVABLE PARTIAL
PROSTHODONTICS

Victor L. Steffel, D.D.S.

May 11, 1897   May 22, 1978

An excellent clinician, a highly motivated teacher,
an energetic contributor to the dental profession,
a respected gentleman, and a close personal friend.

DAVIS HENDERSON

McCRACKEN'S
REMOVABLE PARTIAL PROSTHODONTICS

DAVIS HENDERSON, B.S., D.D.S., F.A.C.D.

Professor, Department of Removable Prosthodontics, University of Florida
College of Dentistry, Gainesville, Florida; formerly Chairman,
Department of Prosthodontics, University of Kentucky College of Dentistry,
Lexington, Kentucky; Fellow, Academy of Denture Prosthetics;
Member, American Prosthodontic Society; Member and Past President,
Southeastern Academy of Prosthodontics; Charter Member, American College of
Prosthodontists; Charter Member and Past President, Carl O. Boucher
Prosthodontic Conference; Diplomate and Past President, American Board of Prosthodontics;
Captain, DC, United States Navy (Ret.)

VICTOR L. STEFFEL, D.D.S., F.A.C.D., F.A.D.P., F.I.C.D.

Late Professor Emeritus and former Chairman, Division of Removable Partial
Prosthodontics, The Ohio State University College of Dentistry, Columbus, Ohio;
Past President: The Ohio Dental Association, Academy of Denture Prosthetics,
American Prosthodontic Society, and The Federation of Prosthodontic
Organizations; Executive Director-Treasurer, The American Prosthodontic
Society; Honorary Sponsoring Fellow, Carl O. Boucher Prosthodontic Conference;
Recipient, The Ohio State University Centennial Achievement Award (1970);
Past Supreme Grand Master, Psi Omega Fraternity; Honored Recipient,
The Annual Steffel Lectures in Dentistry, founded February, 1974

SIXTH EDITION

with **765** illustrations

The C. V. Mosby Company

ST. LOUIS • TORONTO • LONDON   1981

MOSBY
1906 75 1981
YEARS

A TRADITION OF PUBLISHING EXCELLENCE

SIXTH EDITION

The C. V. Mosby Company
11830 Westline Industrial Drive, St. Louis, Missouri 63141

Library of Congress Cataloging in Publication Data

McCracken, William L
McCracken's Removable partial prosthodontics.

Bibliography: p.
Includes index.
1. Partial dentures, Removable.   I.   Henderson,
Davis.   II.   Steffel, Victor L., 1897-1978.
III.   Title.   IV.   Title: Removable partial prostho-
dontics.   [DNLM: 1.   Denture, Partial, Removable.
WU 515 M132p]
RK665.M33   1981   617.6′92   80-28701
ISBN 0-8016-2146-1

GW/CB/B   9 8 7 6 5 4 3 2 1   03/B/367

To those dentists
who have so unselfishly shared
their knowledge and experience
that others may learn

PREFACE
to sixth edition

The rapid rate of development in scientific endeavor makes it necessary that a textbook covering any discipline be revised regularly. With the present-day emphasis on prevention in dentistry and the results being achieved in the saving of many teeth that would otherwise have been lost, the demand for removable partial dentures is the greatest ever, which is justification for this sixth edition of *Removable Partial Prosthodontics*. A critical perusal of this edition will disclose our continuing efforts to present an up-to-date philosophy of mouth reconstruction through the medium of removable partial dentures (using predominantly extracoronal retainers). The contents of the book extend from initial diagnosis to postplacement service, including relining procedures and repairs. Steps are progressively covered in normal sequence. When we could simplify, we have done so. Redundant and obsolete materials and references have been eliminated as far as feasible. We have striven for clarity in all aspects and have standardized terminology throughout to encourage unanimity in the usage of terms for clearer communication.

The greatest possible number of clinical skills and related factors are involved in treating patients with removable partial dentures. With all due respect for the importance of the other disciplines in dentistry, it may be stated that the science of removable partial prosthodontics involves *all* the basic sciences—the laws and effects of leverages, consideration of supports, occlusal contacts, direction of forces, and relative health of all oral structures (to name only a few)—to a far greater extent than does any other oral health service. (Note: Specifically involved in function are soft tissues, supporting bone, circulation, periodontal ligaments, occlusion of both natural and artificial teeth, individ-

ual restorations, crowns, fixed partial dentures, and biomechanics.)

We have continued to emphasize that *fundamentals* do not change; only materials, methods, and technical procedures change, always—it is hoped—to better complement those things which are basic. Thus the science of removable partial prosthodontics cannot ever be considered static. Constant revising and updating are necessary to keep the study dynamic.

We have endeavored to uphold the original objectives of the late Dr. William L. McCracken. It was his intention that the book, although encompassing both *clinical* and *laboratory* aspects, should distinctly and understandingly supply undergraduate, postgraduate, and graduate students, as well as practicing dentists, with basic principles and practical, time-tested procedures, thereby helping all to avoid pitfalls in providing therapeutic and functional removable restorations.

An important plus for this edition is the continued contribution of Drs. Sharry, Costich, White, and Low in revising their material contained in the fifth edition.

In summary, *The Glossary of Prosthodontic Terms* has been accepted as a reasonable guide throughout this sixth edition. Different techniques and broad references to the works of others provide the dentist with alternative routes to accomplish the same end. Again, chapters are arranged in an orderly sequence of learning; that is, components and their biomechanical characteristics, denture bases, surveying, and principles of design precede diagnosis and treatment planning. The bibliography has been revised, especially to include contemporary references. Self-assessment aids have been included in this edition, appearing at the end of Chapters 2 through 22.

We gratefully acknowledge those who
offered constructive criticism of the fifth
edition. Many of the changes made in this
edition resulted from their suggestions. We
have been most appreciative of, and flattered
by, the general acceptance of this textbook.

Davis Henderson

PREFACE
to first edition

Although I welcomed the invitation to author a textbook on the subject of partial denture construction, I realized from the outset that such a book would follow closely in the wake of several excellent textbooks on this subject. I therefore approached the task with a sense of great responsibility. However, I would not have accepted the challenge had I not felt sincerely that I could add something to what had already been written and thus produce a text in this field which is sorely needed and which provides the dental student, the dental practitioner, and the dental laboratory technician with the information necessary to produce a partial denture that is in itself a definitive restorative entity. It is my sincere hope that this textbook will be used not only by teachers of prosthetic dentistry but also by practicing dentists and dental technicians, and that in this book the dentist and dental technician may find a common meeting ground for better solution of the problems associated with the partially edentulous patient.

I am deeply grateful for the opportunities that I have had to combine private practice with teaching and for the knowledge that has evolved from this experience. Although I have attempted to present various philosophies and techniques in order that the reader may select that which to him seems most applicable, it is inevitable that certain preferences will be obvious. These are based upon convictions evolved through experience both in private practice and in the teaching of clinical prosthodontics. It is only logical, then, that I should therefore state my own personal beliefs, which are as follows:

1. I believe that the practice of prosthetic dentistry must forever remain in the hands of the dentist and that he must therefore be totally competent to render this service.

In the fabrication of a partial denture restoration, the dentist must be competent to render a comprehensive diagnosis of the partially edentulous mouth and, utilizing all of the mechanical aids necessary, plan every detail of treatment. He must either personally accomplish whatever mouth preparations are necessary or delegate to his colleagues such specialized services as surgical, periodontal, and endodontic treatment. In any case, primary responsibility for adequate mouth preparations remains his alone. He must undertake whatever impression procedures are necessary and must be primarily responsible for the accuracy of any casts of the mouth upon which work is to be fabricated. He must provide the laboratory technician with an adequate prescription in the form of diagrams and written instructions and with a master cast which has been completely surveyed with a specific design outlined upon it. He must be solely responsible for the accuracy and adequacy of any jaw relation records and must specify all materials and, in many instances, the exact method by which occlusion is to be established on the finished restoration. Finally, he must be competent to judge the excellence of the finished restoration or recognize its inadequacies and must assume the responsibility for demanding a degree of excellence from the technician that will continually raise rather than lower the standards of dental laboratory service.

2. I believe that the dental laboratory technician has a responsibility to his profession to demand a quality of leadership from the dentist which he can respect and follow without question. The responsibility for providing adequate prosthetic dentistry service to the patient must be shared by both dentist and technician, and each has not only a right to expect that the other do

his part competently but also an obligation to demand a quality of service from the other that will not jeopardize the finished product. The technician therefore would do dentistry a great service if he would reject inadequate material from the dentist and respectfully suggest whatever improvements are necessary for him to produce an acceptable piece of work. As long as the technician accepts inadequate material from the dentist and the dentist is willing to place an inadequate product in the patient's mouth, the quality of removable prosthetic appliances will continue to be, as it all too frequently is, a far poorer service than the dentist and technician together are capable of rendering.

I believe also that dental laboratories should always be willing to adopt newer techniques and philosophies developed by the dental profession and being taught to dental graduates. Too often the commercial dental laboratory insists upon using stereotyped techniques that suit its production methods and actively attempts to discourage the recent graduate from putting into practice modern methods and techniques that were painstakingly taught to him in dental school by instructors whose knowledge of the subject far exceeds that of the laboratory technician who depreciates it.

3. I believe that any free-end partial denture must have the best possible support from the underlying edentulous ridge and that the design of the abutment retainers must apply a minimum of torque to the adjacent abutment teeth. I believe that some kind of secondary impression is necessary to obtain adequate support for the denture base, both through tissue placement and from the broadest possible coverage compatible with biologic requirements and limitations.

4. I believe in the functional, or dynamic, registration of occlusal relationships rather than in relying upon intraoral adjustment of an established centric occlusion or upon the ability of an instrument to simulate articulatory movements. I believe that the occlusion on a partial denture, be it fixed or removable, should be made to harmonize with the existing adjusted natural occlusion, and that this can best be accomplished by the registration of functional occlusal paths. For this to be done adequately, occlusion on the partial denture must be established upon either the final denture base(s) or upon an accurate substitute for the final base(s). The practice of attempting to submit jaw relation records to the technician prior to the fabrication of the denture framework is therefore, with few exceptions, strongly condemned.

5. I believe that a partial denture, when properly designed, carefully made, and serviced when needed, can be an entirely satisfactory restoration and can serve as a means of preserving remaining oral structures as well as restoring missing dentition. Unless a partial denture is made with adequate abutment support, with optimal base support, and with harmonious and functional occlusion, it should be clear to all concerned that such a denture should be considered only a temporary treatment, or interim denture rather than a restoration representative of the best that modern prosthetic dentistry has to offer.

W. L. McCracken

CONTENTS

1 **Terminology,** 1

2 **Clasp-retained partial denture,** 6

Six phases of partial denture service, 6
  Patient education, 7
  Treatment planning and design, 8
  Support for distal extension denture
    bases, 9
  Establishment of occlusal relations, 10
  Initial placement procedures, 11
  Periodic recall, 11
Reasons for failure of clasp partial
  denture, 11

3 **Classification of partially
edentulous arches,** 13

Requirements of an acceptable method of
  classification, 13
Kennedy's classification, 13
  Applegate's rules for applying the
    Kennedy classification, 16

4 **Major and minor connectors,** 18

Major connectors, 18
  Mandibular major connectors, 21
    Indications for the use of a
      linguoplate, 25
  Maxillary major connectors, 26
    Single palatal bar or strap, 26
    U-shaped palatal connector, 27
    Combination anterior and posterior
      palatal strap-type connectors, 28
    Palatal plate–type connector, 30
    Design, 32
  Minor connectors, 34
    Functions of the minor connectors, 34
    Form and location of minor
      connectors, 34
  Reaction of tissues to metallic
    coverage, 38
  Major connectors in review, 39
    Lingual bar, 39
    Mandibular linguoplate, 39
    Single strap–type palatal major
      connectors, 40
    Single broad palatal major
      connector, 40
    Anterior-posterior strap–type major
      connectors, 41

Full palatal coverage major
  connectors, 41
U-shaped palatal major connector, 41

5 **Rests and rest seats,** 44

Form of the occlusal rest and rest
  seat, 44
Interproximal occlusal rest seats, 46
Internal occlusal rests, 49
Possible movements of partial
  denture, 49
Support for rests, 53
Rest seat preparations in sound
  enamel, 54
Lingual rests on canines and incisor
  teeth, 56
Incisal rests and rest seats, 58

6 **Direct retainers,** 62

Internal attachments, 64
Extracoronal direct retainers, 64
  Relative uniformity of retention, 67
  Flexibility of clasp arm, 67
  Reciprocal-stabilizing cast clasp
    arm, 69
  Advantages and disadvantages of any
    given clasp design, 70
  Basic principles of clasp design, 72
  Circumferential clasp arms, 74
  Bar clasp arms, 81
  Combination clasp, 83
  Lingual retention in conjunction with
    internal rests, 85
  Other types of clasps, 86
  Hart-Dunn attachment for unilateral
    distal extension partial dentures, 87
Other types of retainers, 89
  Neurohr spring-lock attachment, 89
  Dowel rest attachment, 91

7 **Indirect retainers,** 97

Denture rotation about an axis, 97
Factors influencing effectiveness of
  indirect retainers, 100
Auxiliary functions of indirect
  retainers, 101
Forms of indirect retainers, 101

8   Denture bases and stressbreakers (stress equalizers), 105

Denture bases, 105
    Functions of tooth-supported partial
        denture base, 105
    Functions of distal extension partial
        denture base, 105
    Ideal denture base, 108
    Advantages of metal bases, 108
    Attaching artificial teeth to metal
        bases, 109
    Need for relining, 112
Stressbreakers (stress equalizers), 113
    Types of stressbreakers, 114
    Advantages of stressbreakers, 117
    Disadvantages of stressbreakers, 117
    Advantages of a rigid design, 118
    Disadvantages of a rigid design, 118

9   Principles of removable partial denture design, 120

Biomechanical considerations, 120
Other factors influencing the design of
    removable partial dentures, 125
Differentiation between two main
    types, 126
    Differences in support, 126
    Impression registration, 127
    Differences in clasp design, 127
Essentials of partial denture
    design, 128
    Class III removable partial
        denture, 128
    Class I, bilateral, distal extension
        partial dentures, 129
    Class II partial dentures, 131
Components of partial denture, 132
    Major connectors, 133
    Direct retainers for tooth-borne
        partial dentures, 133
    Direct retainers for distal extension
        partial dentures, 134
    Stabilizing components, 134
    Guiding planes, 134
    Ridge support, 136
    Indirect retainers, 137
Other considerations influencing
    design, 137
    Use of a splint bar for denture
        support, 137
    Internal clip attachment, 139
    Overlay abutment as support for a
        denture base, 139

10   Surveying, 143

Description of dental surveyor, 143
Purposes of surveyor, 148
    Surveying the diagnostic cast, 148
    Contouring wax patterns, 150
    Surveying ceramic veneer crowns, 150
    Placement of intracoronal retainers
        (internal attachments), 150
    Placement of internal rests, 150
    Machining cast restorations, 151
    Surveying the master cast, 151
Factors that determine path of placement
    and removal, 152
    Guiding planes, 152
    Retentive areas, 152
    Interference, 153
    Esthetics, 153
Step-by-step procedures in surveying a
    diagnostic cast, 153
    Guiding planes, 153
    Retentive areas, 155
    Interference, 155
    Esthetics, 156
Final path of placement, 157
Recording relation of cast to
    surveyor, 158
Surveying the master cast, 158
Measuring retention, 159
Blocking out the master cast, 161
Relieving the master cast, 162
Paralleled blockout, shaped blockout,
    arbitrary blockout, and relief, 165

11   Diagnosis and treatment planning, 168

Visual examination, 168
    Need for determining type of
        mandibular major connector, 169
    Need for reshaping remaining
        teeth, 169
    Reduction of unfavorable tooth
        contours, 170
Dental cast surveyor, 170
    Recording the path of placement, 171
Oral examination, 172
    Objectives of prosthodontic
        treatment, 172
    Sequence for oral examination, 172
Roentgenographic interpretation, 175
    Value of interpreting bone
        density, 176
    Index areas, 177
    Alveolar lamina dura, 178
    Root morphology, 178
    Third molars, 179
Diagnostic casts, 179
    Purposes for which diagnostic casts
        are used, 179
    Mounting diagnostic casts, 181

Mounting maxillary cast to axis-
orbital plane, 181
Jaw relationship records for
diagnostic casts, 185
Materials and methods for recording
centric relation, 190
Factors involved in occlusal
analysis, 192
Examination data, 193
Differential diagnosis: fixed or
removable partial dentures, 195
Indications for use of fixed
restorations, 195
Tooth-bounded edentulous regions, 195
Modification spaces, 195
Anterior modification spaces, 195
Nonreplacement of missing molars, 196
Indications for removable partial
dentures, 196
Distal extension situations, 196
After recent extractions, 196
Long span, 197
Need for effect of bilateral
stabilization, 197
Esthetics in anterior region, 197
Excessive loss of residual bone, 197
Unusually sound abutment teeth, 198
Economic considerations, 198
The choice between complete dentures and
removable partial dentures, 198
Factors in selecting metal alloys for
removable partial denture frameworks, 200
Comparative physical properties, 200
Wrought wire: selection and quality
control, 202

**12 Preparation of mouth for removable
partial dentures,** 210

Oral surgical preparation, 210
Extractions, 211
Removal of residual roots, 211
Impacted teeth, 212
Malposed teeth, 212
Cysts and odontogenic tumors, 212
Exostoses and tori, 212
Hyperplastic tissue, 214
Muscle attachments and freni, 214
Bony spines and knife-edge
ridges, 215
Polyps, papilloma, and traumatic
hemangiomas, 215
Hyperkeratoses, erythroplasia, and
ulcerations, 215
Dentofacial deformity, 215
Periodontal preparation, 215
Objectives of periodontal
therapy, 216
Periodontal diagnosis and treatment
planning, 217

Diagnosis, 217
Treatment planning, 218
Initial disease control therapy
(phase 1), 218
Oral hygiene instruction, 218
Scaling and root planing, 218
Elimination of local irritating
factors other than calculus, 220
Elimination of gross occlusal
interferences, 220
Guide to occlusal adjustment, 220
Temporary splinting, 221
Use of nightguard, 222
Minor tooth movement, 222
General therapy (phase 2), 223
Periodontal surgery, 223
Recall maintenance (phase 3), 226
Advantages of periodontal therapy, 226
Abutment teeth, 227
Abutment restorations, 227
Contouring wax patterns, 228
Rest seats, 228

13 Preparation of abutment teeth, 231

Classification of abutment teeth, 231
Sequence of abutment preparations on
sound enamel or existing restorations, 232
Abutment preparations using cast
inlays, 233
Abutment preparations using cast
crowns, 236
Ledges on abutment crowns, 237
Veneer crowns for support of clasp
arms, 241
Splinting of abutment teeth, 242
Use of isolated teeth as abutments, 243
Missing anterior teeth, 244
Temporary crowns and temporary fixed
partial dentures, 245
Temporary crowns when a partial denture
is being worn, 248
Cementation of temporary crowns, 249
The making of crowns and inlays to fit
existing denture retainers, 250
Cementations for fixed restorations, 252
Advantages of semipermanent
cementation of fixed restorations, 253

**14 Impression materials and procedures
for removable partial dentures,** 255

Rigid materials, 255
Plaster of paris, 255
Metallic oxide pastes, 256
Thermoplastic materials, 256
Modeling plastic, 256
Impression waxes and resins, 257

Elastic materials, 258
  Reversible hydrocolloids, 258
  Irreversible hydrocolloids, 258
  Mercaptan rubber-base impression
    materials, 258
  Silicone impression materials, 259
Impressions of the partially edentulous
  arch, 259
  Important precautions to be observed
    in the handling of hydrocolloid, 261
  Step-by-step procedure for making a
    hydrocolloid impression, 261
  Step-by-step procedure for making a
    stone cast from a hydrocolloid impression, 262
  Possible causes of an inaccurate cast
    of a dental arch, 263
  Pouring of working casts upon which
    abutment restorations are to be
    fabricated, 265
Individual impression trays, 266
  Technique for making individual
    acrylic resin impression trays, 267

15 **Support for the distal extension
denture base,** 274

Distal extension removable partial
  denture, 274
Factors influencing the support of a
  distal extension base, 274
  Quality of the residual ridge, 275
  Extent of residual ridge coverage by
    the denture base, 275
  Type of the impression
    registration, 276
  Accuracy of the denture base, 280
  Design of the partial denture
    framework, 280
  Total occlusal load applied, 280
Methods for obtaining functional support
  for the distal extension base, 282
Functional relining method, 282
Selective tissue placement impression
  method, 285
Fluid-wax functional impression
  method, 289
  Objectives in the making of a fluid-
    wax impression, 291
Assembled metal bases, 293
  Adding metal bases to the partial
    denture, 295

16 **Occlusal relationships for
removable partial dentures,** 298

Desirable contact relationships for
  removable partial dentures, 299
Methods for establishing occlusal
  relationships, 300
  Direct apposition of casts, 301
  Interocclusal records with posterior
    teeth remaining, 301
  Occlusal relations using occlusion
    rims on record bases, 302
  Jaw relation records made entirely on
    occlusion rims, 303
  Establishing occlusion by the
    recording of occlusal pathways, 303
  Materials for artificial posterior
    teeth, 309
  Arranging teeth to an occluding
    template, 311
  Functional registration of occlusal
    surfaces for fixed partial dentures
    and single crowns, 316
  Establishing jaw relations for a
    mandibular removable partial denture
    opposing a maxillary complete denture, 322

17 **Laboratory procedures,** 325

Duplicating a stone cast, 325
  Duplicating materials and flasks, 326
  Duplicating procedure, 328
Waxing the partial denture framework, 333
  Forming the wax pattern for a lower
    Class II removable partial denture
    framework, 336
  Waxing metal bases, 346
Anatomic replica patterns, 349
  Procedure for making an anatomic
    replica pattern, 350
Spruing, investing, burnout, casting,
  and finishing the partial denture
  framework, 351
  Spruing, 352
  Investing the sprued pattern, 354
  Burnout, 357
  Casting, 359
  Removing the casting from the
    investment, 359
  Finishing and polishing, 360
Making of impression trays and record
  bases, 361
  Technique for making a sprinkled
    acrylic resin record base or impression
    tray, 362
  Technique for making an impression
    tray attached to a framework, 367
Occlusion rims, 367
Making a stone occlusal template from a
  functional occlusal record, 370

Arranging posterior teeth to an opposing
cast or template, 372
Posterior tooth forms, 372
Arranging teeth to an occluding
surface, 373
Types of anterior teeth, 375
Waxing and investing the partial denture
prior to processing resin bases or
attachments, 376
Waxing the partial denture base, 376
Investing the partial denture, 378
Processing the denture, 381
Layered silicone rubber flasking, 381
Remounting and occlusal correction to an
occlusal template, 382
Precautions to be taken in
remounting, 383
Polishing the denture, 384
Denture borders, 384
Facial surfaces, 385
Finishing gingival and interproximal
areas, 385

18   Work authorizations for removable partial dentures, 389

Work authorization, 389
Content, 389
Function, 389
Characteristics, 389
Definitive instructions by work
authorizations, 392
Legal aspects of work
authorizations, 392
Delineation of responsibilities by work
authorizations, 393

19   Initial placement, adjustment, and servicing of the removable partial denture, 395

Occlusal interference from denture
framework, 396
Adjustments to bearing surfaces of
denture bases, 396
Adjustment of occlusion in harmony
with natural and artificial
dentition, 397
Instructions to the patient, 402
Follow-up services, 403

20   Relining and rebasing the removable partial denture, 406

Relining tooth-borne denture bases, 406
Relining distal extension partial
denture bases, 408
Methods of reestablishing occlusion on a
relined partial denture, 409
Tissue conditioning prior to relining
a partial denture base, 410

21   Repairs and additions to removable partial dentures, 412

Classification of repairs and
additions, 412
Broken clasp arms, 412
Fractured occlusal rests, 413
Distortion or breakage of other
components, such as major and minor
connectors, 413
Loss of an additional tooth or teeth
not involved in the support or
retention of the restoration, 414
Loss of an abutment tooth
necessitating not only its replacement
but also the substitution of a new
clasp assembly on another
abutment, 414
Other types of repairs, 414
Procedures for making repairs and
additions, 414
Replacing a broken clasp arm with a
wrought-wire retentive arm, 415
Repairing by soldering, 415

22   Interim, transitional, and treatment removable partial dentures, 418

Interim partial dentures, 418
Transitional partial dentures, 419
Treatment partial dentures, 419

23   Miscellaneous partial prosthodontics, 423

John J. Sharry, B.S., D.M.D.

Cleft palate prostheses, 423
Classification, 423
Etiology, 423
Personality evaluation, 423
Anatomy, 424
Pathology, 427
Physiology of speech, 427
Surgical treatment, 427
Prosthetic treatment, 429
Impressions with alginate
hydrocolloid impression materials, 429
Psychologic aspects, 435
Maxillofacial prosthesis, 435

Selected references, 438

McCRACKEN'S
REMOVABLE PARTIAL
PROSTHODONTICS

1 TERMINOLOGY

Significant strides have been made in prosthodontic terminology in recent years, eliminating much confusion created by conflicting terms. An updated *Glossary of Prosthodontic Terms* is available to the profession through the continuing efforts of the Academy of Denture Prosthetics.* Then, too, the second edition of a glossary of accepted terms in all disciplines of dentistry, *Current Clinical Dental Terminology*, is also available.† Both these glossaries provide excellent bases for dignified, spoken and written communication in prosthetic dentistry.

The conflicting or indefinite terms in common usage in prosthodontics require definition and clarification. Many of these are used synonymously; even today others are used incorrectly. Whereas the following is not meant to be a complete glossary of removable partial prosthodontic terminology, some definitions will be given, based on available reference material. The discussion type format does not lend itself to alphabetical arrangement of defined words or terms, hopefully creating only a minor inconvenience to students.

A *prosthesis* is the replacement of an absent part of the human body by some artificial part such as an eye, a leg, or a denture. *Prosthetics*, then, is the art or science of supplying missing parts of the human body.

When applied to dentistry, the term *prosthetics* becomes *prosthodontics* and denotes the branch of dental art or science that treats specifically with the replacement of missing dental and oral tissues. The term *prosthodontics* is somewhat preferable to the term *prosthetic dentistry*. The former may be defined as "that branch of dentistry pertaining to the restoration and maintenance of oral functions, comfort, appearance, and health of the patient by the replacement of missing teeth and contiguous tissues with artificial substitutes."

The replacement of missing teeth in a partially edentulous arch may be accomplished by a fixed, or cemented, prosthesis or by a removable prosthesis. The fixed prosthesis may be in two pieces, with a locking joint between, or all in one piece and is not designed to be removed by the patient. This type of restoration is a *fixed partial denture*. On the other hand, a *removable partial denture* is designed so that it can be removed conveniently from the mouth and replaced by the patient.

A *complete denture prosthesis* is entirely supported by the tissues (mucous membrane, connective tissues, and underlying bone) to which it is attached. A *removable partial denture* may be entirely tooth supported or may derive its support from both the teeth and the tissues of the residual ridge. The denture base of a tooth-borne removable partial denture derives its support from abutment teeth at each end of the edentulous area. The tissue it covers is not used for support. A tooth-tissue–supported removable partial denture has at least one denture base that extends anteriorly or posteriorly, terminating in a denture base portion that is not tooth supported. Such a base extending posteriorly on a removable partial denture qualifies the restoration as a *distal extension denture*.

Sufficient differences exist between the tooth-supported and the tooth-tissue–supported removable restorations to justify a distinction between them. Principles of design and techniques employed in construction

---

*This glossary first appeared in the March, 1956, issue of *The Journal of Prosthetic Dentistry* (published by The C. V. Mosby Co., St. Louis, Mo.) The lastest reprint (fourth edition), published in 1977, may be obtained from the Education and Research Foundation of Prosthodontics, Dr. Charles C. Swoope, Secretary-Treasurer, Dentistry (SM-52), University of Washington, Seattle, Wash. 98195.

†Boucher, C. O., editor: Current clinical dental terminology, a glossary of accepted terms in all disciplines of dentistry, ed. 2, St. Louis, 1974, The C. V. Mosby Co.

may be completely dissimilar. The points of difference are as follows:

1. Manner in which the prosthesis is supported
2. Impression methods required for each
3. Types of direct retainers best suited for each
4. Denture base material best suited for each
5. Need for indirect retention

A distinction between these two types of removable restorations is adequately made by an acceptable classification of removable partial dentures.

The term *appliance* is correctly applied only to a device worn by the patient in the course of treatment, such as splints, orthodontic appliances, and space maintainers. A denture, an obturator, a fixed partial denture, or a crown is properly called a *prosthesis*. The terms *prosthesis*, *restoration*, and *denture* generally will be used synonymously in this book to avoid tiresome repetition of the single word *prosthesis*.

An *interim denture* is a dental prosthesis to be used for a short time for reasons of esthetics, mastication, occlusal support, and convenience until more definite prosthetic dental treatment can be provided or for conditioning the patient to accept an artificial substitute for missing natural teeth.

A *transitional denture* is a removable partial denture that serves as a temporary prosthesis to which teeth will be added as more teeth are lost and that will be replaced after postextraction tissue changes have occurred. A transitional denture may become an interim denture when all the teeth have been removed from the dental arch.

A *treatment denture* is a dental prosthesis used for treating or conditioning the tissues that are called on to support and retain a denture base.

Use of the term *acrylic* as a noun will be avoided. Instead it will be used only as an adjective, such as *acrylic* resin. The word *plastic* may be used either as an adjective or a noun; in the latter sense it refers to any of various substances that harden and retain their shape after being molded. The term *resin* will be used broadly for substances named according to their chemical composition, physical structure, and means for activation or curing, such as acrylic *resin*.

The term *denture base* will be used to designate the part of a denture, whether of metal or of a resinous material, that holds the artificial teeth and that receives support from the abutment teeth, the residual ridge, or both. The word *saddle* is considered objectionable terminology when used to designate the base of a removable partial denture.

The structures underlying the denture base will be mentioned as the *residual ridge* or *edentulous ridge*, referring to the residual bone with its soft tissue covering. The exact character of this soft tissue covering may vary, and it includes the mucous membrane and the underlying fibrous connective tissue.

Resurfacing of a denture base with new material to make it fit the underlying tissues more accurately will be spoken of as *relining*. *Rebasing* refers to a process that goes beyond relining and involves the refitting of a denture by the replacement of the denture base with new material without changing the occlusal relations of the teeth.

Perhaps no other terms in prosthodontics have been associated with more controversy than have *centric jaw relation* and *centric occlusion*. All confusion could be terminated by acceptance of one definition of centric relation and one definition of centric occlusion and then using these respective positions as references for other horizontal locations of the mandible or other relationships of opposing teeth. The following definitions, which are given in the *Glossary of Prosthodontic Terms*, are selected as meaningful.

centric jaw relation the most posterior relation of the mandible to the maxillae at the established vertical dimension.

centric occlusion the centered contact position of the occlusal surfaces of the mandibular teeth against the occlusal surfaces of the maxillary teeth.

For complete dentures, centric occlusion should be made to coincide with centric relation for that patient. In an adjustment of natural occlusion the objective may be to establish harmony between centric relation and centric occlusion. With removable partial dentures the objective is to make the artificial occlusion coincide and be in harmony with the remaining natural occlusion. Ideally the natural occlusion has been adjusted to harmonious contact in centric relation and is free of eccentric interference before a similar occlusion is established on the partial denture.

In a description of the various components of the partial denture, conflicting terminology must be recognized and the preferred terms defined. A *retainer* is defined as "any type of clasp, attachment, or device used for the fixation or stabilization of a prosthesis."* Thus the attachment may be either intracoronal or extracoronal and may be used as a means of retaining either a removable or a fixed restoration. The term *internal attachment* will be used in preference to precision attachment, frictional attachment, and other terms to describe any mechanical retaining device that depends on frictional resistance between parallel walls of male and female (key and keyway) parts. Precision attachment is discarded because its usage implies that all other types of retainers are less precise in their design and fabrication.

Clasp (direct retainer) will be used in conjunction with the words *retainer, arm,* or *assembly* whenever possible. The clasp assembly will consist of a *retentive clasp arm* and a *reciprocal* or *stabilizing clasp arm,* plus any minor connectors and rests from which they originate or with which they are associated. *Bar clasp arm* will be used in preference to Roach's name to designate this type of extracoronal retainer and is defined as a clasp arm that originates from the base of framework, traverses soft tissue, and approaches the tooth undercut area from a gingival direction. In contrast, the term *circumferential clasp arm* will be used to designate a clasp arm that originates above the height of contour, traverses part of the suprabulge portion of the tooth, and approaches the tooth undercut from an occlusal direction. Both types of clasp arms terminate in a retentive undercut lying gingival to the height of contour, and both provide retention by the resistance of metal to deformation rather than frictional resistance of parallel walls.

A *major connector* is the part of a removable partial denture that connects the components on one side of the arch to the components on the opposite side of the arch.

The term *indirect retainer* denotes a part of a removable partial denture that assists the direct retainers in preventing displacement of distal extension denture bases by functioning through lever action on the opposite side of the fulcrum line.

A *continuous bar retainer* is a component of the partial denture framework that augments the major connector and lies on the lingual or facial surface of several teeth. It is most frequently used on the middle third of the lingual slope of lower anterior teeth. If attached to the lingual bar major connector by a thin, contoured apron, the major connector is then designated as a *linguoplate.*

Any thin, broad palatal coverage used as a major connector is called a *palatal major connector* or if of lesser width, a *palatal bar.* A palatal major connector may be further described according to its anteroposterior location on the palatal surface, for example, an anterior palatal major connector or a posterior palatal bar. The term *anatomic replica* will be used to designate cast metal palatal major connectors that duplicate the topography of that portion of the patient's mouth. This is in keeping with a desire to use descriptive terminology whenever possible.

The term *rest* will be used to designate any component of the partial denture that is placed on an abutment tooth, preferably in a seat prepared to receive it, so that it limits movement of the denture in a gingival direction. When a rest is placed on the occlusal surface of a posterior tooth, it is designated as an *occlusal rest.* If the rest occupies a position on the lingual surface of an anterior tooth, it is referred to as a *lingual rest.* A rest placed on the incisal edge of an anterior abutment tooth is called an *incisal rest.* All these rests function to prevent movement of the denture toward the soft tissues and to assist in providing occlusal support for the prosthesis.

An *abutment* is a tooth used for the support of a fixed or removable prosthesis.

The term *height of contour* is defined as a line encircling a tooth designating its greatest circumference at a selected position.

The term *undercut* when used in reference to an abutment is that portion of a tooth that lies between the height of contour and the gingivae; when it is used in reference to other oral structures, undercut means the contour or cross section of a residual ridge or dental arch that would prevent the placement of a denture.

Two or more parallel axial surfaces of abut-

---

*From Academy of Denture Prosthetics, Nomenclature Committee: Glossary of prosthodontic terms, ed. 4, St. Louis, 1977, The C. V. Mosby Co.

ment teeth so shaped as to direct a prosthesis during placement and removal are called *guiding planes*. Guiding plane surfaces are parallel to the path of the placement; however, they may or may not face each other.

The term *canine* (tooth) and *premolar* (tooth) will be used to designate those teeth commonly called cuspid and bicuspid teeth. Denton gives the chief arguments for the use of the word *canine* as "(1) it is the term used in other sciences, and (2) other terms in standard usage can be understood only in relation to *canine* tooth: canine eminence, canine muscle, canine fossa." For the use of *premolar* he gives the following arguments: "(1) the term bicuspid is not descriptive of all teeth of that class, and (2) the acceptance of premolar makes uniform the terminology of dentistry and comparative dental anatomy."*

To describe an impression and the resulting cast of the supporting form of the edentulous ridge, *functional impression* and *functional ridge form* will be used in the absence of a more descriptive terminology. These terms have become accepted as meaning the form of the edentulous ridge when it is supporting a denture base. It is artificially created by means of a specially molded (individualized) tray or an impression material, or both, that displaces those tissues that can be readily displaced and that would be incapable of rendering support to the denture base. Firm areas are not displaced due to the flow characteristics of the impression material. Thus the tissues are recorded more nearly in the form they will assume when supporting a functional load. In contrast, the static form of the edentulous ridge, as often recorded in a soft impression material such as hydrocolloid, rubber-base material, or metallic oxide impression paste, is referred to as the *anatomic ridge form* and results when an impression tray is uniformly relieved. This is the surface form of the edentulous ridge when at rest or when not supporting a functional load.

Functional occlusal registration is sufficiently descriptive and is used to designate a dynamic registration of opposing dentition rather than the recording of a static relationship of one jaw to another. While centric position is found somewhere in a functional occlusal registration, eccentric positions are also recorded, and the created occlusion is made to harmonize with all gliding and chewing movements the patient is capable of making.

The word *cast* may be used as a verb (to cast) or as an adjective (cast framework or cast metal base). It is used most frequently in this text as a noun to designate a positive reproduction of a maxillary or mandibular dental arch made from an impression of that arch. Such an objective is further designated according to the purpose for which it is made, such as *diagnostic cast*, *master cast*, or *investment cast*. An investment cast also may be referred to as a *refractory cast*, since it is compounded to withstand high temperatures without disintegrating and, incidentally, to perform certain functions relative to the burnout and expansion of the mold. A *refractory investment* is an investment material that can withstand the high temperatures of casting or soldering. Plaster of paris and artificial stone also may be considered *investment* if either is used to invest any part of a dental restoration for processing it.

A *wax pattern* is coverted to a *casting* by the elimination of the pattern by heat, leaving a mold into which the molten metal is forced by centrifugal force or other means. *Casting* is therefore used most frequently as a noun, meaning "a metal object shaped by being poured into a mold to harden." It is used primarily to designate the cast metal framework of a partial denture but also may be used to describe a molded denture base, which is also actually cast into a mold.

Cast in dentistry should always imply that it is an accurate reproduction of the tissues being studied or on which a restoration may be fabricated. Any cast that is admittedly inaccurate is unpardonable and unacceptable in modern dentistry because of the excellence of impression and cast materials available today.

The word *cast* is preferable to the term *model*, which should be used only to designate a reproduction for display or demonstration purposes. A model of a dental arch or any portion thereof may be made of durable and attractive material. It need not be an accurate reproduction but should be a reasonable facsimile of the original. It is fre-

---

*From Denton, G. B.: The vocabulary of dentistry and oral science, Chicago, 1958, American Dental Association.

quently made of tooth- and tissue-colored acrylic resin.

Mold is also incorrect when applied to a reproduction of a dental arch or a portion thereof. It is used to indicate either the cavity into which a casting is made or the shape of an artificial tooth.

Dental stones are used to make an artificial stone reproduction from an impression, and they are used as an investment or for mounting purposes. All dental stones are gypsum products. Use of the word *stone* in dentistry should be applied only to those gypsum materials that are employed for their hardness, accuracy, or abrasion resistance.

Some controversy exists over the use of the terms *x-ray*, *radiograph*, and *roentgenogram* in dentistry. The American Academy of Oral Roentgenology has indicated its preference for the use of roentgenogram, at the same time admitting that it may leave much to be desired as descriptive terminology. Examination of several recent textbooks on dental subjects finds usage divided between all three terms. However, in deference to the terminology preferred by the American Academy of Oral Roentgenology, the terms *roentgenogram, roentgenographic survey*, and *roentgenographic interpretation* are used herein.

Stability is defined as the quality of a denture to be firm, that is, not subject to change of position, when forces are applied. Stability becomes more meaningful when thought of as a denture base to supporting bone relationship.

Retention is spoken of as that quality inherent in the denture that resists the force of gravity, the adhesiveness of foods, and the forces associated with opening the jaws. Retention, considered in terms of complete dentures, should be considered a denture base to soft tissue relationship. In removable partial prosthodontics we speak in terms of direct retention. *Direct retention* is the retention obtained in a removable partial denture by the use of attachments or direct retainers (clasps) that resist their removal from the abutment teeth.

Balanced occlusion is a term that describes the contact of opposing teeth. It is defined as the simultaneous contacting of maxillary and mandibular teeth on the right and left in the anterior and posterior occlusal areas in centric or any eccentric position.

A *dental cast surveyor* is an instrument used to determine the relative parallelism of two or more axial surfaces of teeth or other parts of a cast of a dental arch.

The word *wrought*, when used to describe an alloy, means worked into shape by artistry or effort. Mechanical treatment of an alloy has two primary objectives. One objective is to obtain a desired form for use, for example, wires, bands, bars, and sheets. Another objective is to enhance certain mechanical properties that are unsatisfactory in a cast alloy.

Many other terms used in prosthodontics might be defined in this chapter, but such an undertaking is worthy of the efforts of those who again have recently directed their thoughts to that end. The Nomenclature Committee of the Academy of Denture Prosthetics is to be commended for their continuing efforts in compiling a current glossary that may be used for guidance in prosthodontic terminology.

Familiarity with accepted prosthodontic terminology should be acquired by the predoctoral student-dentist because once a vocabulary is established, it is difficult to change.

2 CLASP-RETAINED PARTIAL DENTURE

The clasp-retained partial denture utilizing the extracoronal direct retainer is probably used a hundred times more frequently than is the intracoronal, or internal attachment, partial denture (Fig. 2-1). Although the clasp-retained partial denture has disadvantages, for reasons of economy and time involved, it will probably continue to be employed because it is capable of providing physiologically sound treatment for the greatest number of patients needing partial denture restorations in keeping with their ability to pay for such treatment. Some of the possible disadvantages of a clasp partial denture are as follows:

1. Caries may develop beneath clasp components, especially if the abutments are not protected with cast restorations and if the patient fails to keep the prosthesis and the abutments clean.

2. Strain too often is placed on the abutment teeth by improper clasp designs.

3. Clasps are often unesthetic, particularly when placed on visible tooth surfaces.

Despite these disadvantages the use of removable prostheses may be preferred whenever there are tooth-bounded edentulous spaces of greater magnitude than can be restored safely with fixed prostheses or when cross-arch stabilization and wider distribution of forces is desirable. The removable partial denture retained by internal attachments eliminates some of the disadvantages of clasps, but it has other disadvantages, one of which is too great a cost for a large percentage of patients needing partial dentures. *Fixed partial dentures should always be used whenever indicated.*

When the alignment of the abutment teeth is favorable, the clinical crown is of sufficient length, the pulp size is diminished by tooth maturity, and the economic status of the patient permits, an internal attachment prosthesis is unquestionably preferable for esthetic reasons. In most instances, if the internal attachment denture is designed properly, this is its only advantage, since abutment protection and stabilizing components should be used with both internal and external retainers. However, economics permitting, esthetics alone may justify the use of an internal attachment denture.

We do not believe in the routine use of hinges or other types of stressbreakers for distal extension partial dentures. It is not that they are ineffective but they they are more frequently misused and substituted for adequate support for the partial denture base. Particularly in the mandibular arch, in the absence of the cross-arch stabilization inherent in a rigid denture design, a stressbroken distal extension denture frequently subjects the edentulous ridge to excessive trauma from horizontal forces.

Because it must be used in conjunction with some form of stressbreaker, the locking or dovetail-type internal attachment is not indicated when one or more distal extension edentulous spaces exist. A rigid design is preferred, and therefore some type of extracoronal retainer must be used. Of these retainers, the clasp retainer is still the most frequently used, and it seems likely that its use will continue until a more widely acceptable retainer is devised.

SIX PHASES OF PARTIAL DENTURE SERVICE

Partial denture service logically may be divided into six phases. The first phase is related to *patient education.* Included in the second phase are *treatment planning, design of the partial denture framework,* and *execution of mouth preparations.* The third phase is *provision of adequate support for the distal extension denture base.* The fourth phase is *establishment of harmonious occlusal relationships with opposing and remaining natural teeth.* The fifth phase involves *initial placement procedures* including adjustments to the bearing surfaces of denture bases, adjustments to assure occlusal harmony, and a review of instructions given the patient to optimally maintain oral structures and the provided restorations. The sixth and final phase of partial denture service is *follow-up services by the dentist* through recall appointments for periodic evaluation of the responses of oral tissues to restorations and of the acceptance of the restorations by the patient.

Patient education

The term patient education is described in Boucher's *Current Clinical Dental Terminology,* ed. 2, 1974, as "Effective communication between the dentist and/or his auxiliaries and the patient concerning dentistry and the principles of treatment and prevention. The procedure of increasing the patient's knowledge of the oral cavity and its care to the point where he can understand the reasons for proposed dental services."

Responsibility for the ultimate success of a removable partial denture is shared by the dentist and the patient. It is folly to assume that a patient will have an understanding of the benefits of a removable partial denture unless he is so informed. It is also unlikely that he will have the knowledge to avoid misuse of the restoration or be able to provide the required oral care and maintenance procedures to ensure the success of the partial denture unless he is adequately advised.

The finest biologically oriented removable partial denture is often doomed to extremely limited success if the patient relaxes proper oral hygiene habits or fails to respond to recall appointments. One of the primary objectives for a partial denture, *preservation,* will most likely not be achieved with only token cooperation on the part of the patient.

Patient education should begin at the initial contact with the patient and continue throughout his treatment. This educational procedure is especially important when the treatment plan and prognosis are discussed with the patient. The limitations imposed on the success of treatment through failure of

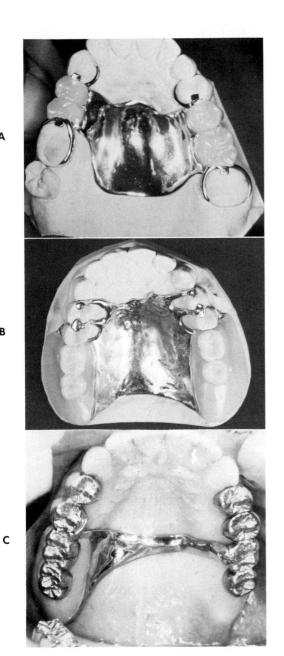

Fig. 2-1. A, Maxillary removable partial denture entirely supported by teeth abutting edentulous areas. **B,** Maxillary bilateral distal extension denture supported by both the natural teeth and the residual ridges. **C,** Maxillary unilateral distal extension denture supported by natural teeth and residual ridge but utilizing internal attachments rather than extracoronal retainers. (**C** courtesy Dr. P. K. Thomas.)

the patient to accept his responsibility must be explained before definitive treatment is undertaken. A patient will not usually retain all the information presented in the oral educational instructions. For this reason, patients should be presented with written suggestions to reinforce the oral presentations.

Treatment planning and design

After a health history and a history of past dental experiences have been obtained and after a complete oral examination has been made including interpretation of roentgenograms, evaluation of the occlusal relations of the remaining natural teeth, and survey of diagnostic casts, a treatment plan is evolved that is based on the support available for the partial denture. Distal extension situations in which no posterior abutments remain and in which extension bases must derive their principal support from the underlying residual ridge require an entirely different partial denture design than does one in which total abutment support is available. This is apparent from visual examination, but roentgenographic interpretation and the surveying of abutments and soft tissue contours must take into consideration the greater torque and tipping leverages of the distal extension partial denture.

Basically, the same principles apply to the unilateral distal extension denture as to the bilateral distal extension denture. On the other hand, entirely different principles of design apply to a prosthesis that is totally tooth supported. Each type must be designed according to the manner of support.

The dental cast *surveyor* is necessary in any dental office in which patients are being treated with removable partial dentures. There is no more reason to justify its omission from a dentist's armamentarium than to ignore the need for roentgenographic equipment or the mouth mirror and explorer or the periodontal probe used for diagnostic purposes.

Several moderately priced surveyors that will adequately accomplish the diagnostic procedures necessary for designing the partial denture are on the market. And yet in many dental offices today this most important phase of dental diagnosis is delegated to the commercial dental laboratory because of the absence of a single necessary piece of equipment or apathy on the part of the dentist who does include removable partial prosth-

odontics in his practice. This is a deplorable and degrading situation, which makes no more sense than relying on the technician to interpret roentgenograms and to render a diagnosis therefrom.

After treatment planning, mouth preparations may be performed with a definite goal in mind. Through the aid of diagnostic casts upon which the tentative design of the partial denture has been outlined and the mouth changes have been indicated in colored pencil, occlusal adjustments, abutment restorations, and abutment modifications can be accomplished, providing for adequate support and retention and a harmonious occlusion for the partial denture.

Selected proximal tooth surfaces should be made parallel to provide guiding planes during placement and removal of the prosthesis. Occlusal rest seats that will direct occlusal forces along the long axis of the supporting teeth as nearly as possible should be established so that neither the tooth nor the denture will be displaced under occlusal loading. This dictates that the floor of the rest preparation be made to incline apically from the marginal ridge and be spoon shaped, with the marginal ridge lowered to permit sufficient bulk without occlusal interference from the rest.

Retentive areas must be identified or created that will provide, as far as is feasible, for relatively equal and uniform retention on all abutment teeth, sufficient only to resist reasonable dislodging forces. *Tooth surfaces upon which reciprocal and stabilizing clasp arms may be placed also must be identified or created.*

After mouth preparations are believed completed, an impression should be made in irreversible hydrocolloid and a cast poured in quick-setting stone. This cast can then be surveyed, with the patient still present, to ascertain whether the planned abutment contours have been accomplished or if additional recontouring is necessary. When mouth preparations have been completed, the impression for the master cast should be made and the cast poured immediately. The master cast must then be surveyed so that the design of the denture framework can be drawn upon it.

The final design of the denture framework should be outlined with colored pencils on the master cast, including the location of clasp arms. It must be remembered that the location of the clasp arms will be determined by the height of contour of the abutment teeth and that this exists for a given path of placement only; hence proximal guiding planes and accurate blockout of proximal tooth surfaces are desirable. The position of the cast in relation to the surveyor must be recorded so that the technician may similarly place the cast on his surveyor to parallel the blockout material. This is easily done by scoring the base of the cast on three sides parallel to the path of placement or by tripoding the cast, but this must be done before the cast is removed from the surveyor.

It is necessary that a specific design be planned carefully in advance of mouth preparations and that these mouth preparations be carried out with care, as outlined on the diagnostic cast. Then specific and exact mouth preparations, including abutment restorations, will dictate the final form of the denture framework to be outlined on the master cast. This should be drawn accurately onto the master cast after surveying so that there will be no doubt in the mind of the technician as to the exact design of the partial denture framework that he is to construct under guidance and supervision of a dentist.

Surveying the master cast, recording the relationship of the cast to the surveyor, and drawing a definite outline on the master cast are still not enough. It is difficult to draw all the details of the denture design upon the master cast. This should be done by labeling a colored pencil drawing upon a chart, which provides the technician with an outline of the partial denture framework and allows for instructions for the technician to follow in fabricating the denture. From this information it is possible for the technician to return a casting *that the dentist can superimpose* upon the outline as drawn on the master cast. From any lesser instructions the technician cannot be criticized for returning a more stereotyped partial denture design.

The dentist should be responsible for the design of the partial denture framework from the beginning to the finish; therefore he is accountable for providing the technician with all the information needed. It is the responsibility of the technician to follow the written instructions given him by the dentist, but at the same time it is his prerogative to demand that these instructions be so informative that he can follow them without question.

Up to this point the treatment planning and preliminary design of the partial denture, the mouth preparation procedures, and the design of the denture framework have been accomplished by the dentist. Given thorough written instructions and the master cast upon which the dentist has drawn precisely the denture design, the technician then may fabricate the metal framework. The finished framework should be returned to the dentist so that he can evaluate its fit in the mouth and make any necessary occlusal adjustments on the framework.

When laboratory procedures are correctly executed, the framework should fit the master cast as planned. If the framework does not fit the mouth as planned, the dentist then can determine whether the error is due to a faulty impression on his part, to an inaccurate master cast, or to a laboratory procedure. In any event adequate support for distal extension denture bases and the need for exacting occlusal records make it necessary for the denture framework to be returned to the dentist for further records before completion of the restoration.

Support for distal extension denture bases

The third of the six phases in the treatment of a patient with a partial denture is obtaining adequate support for distal extension bases; therefore it does not apply to toothborne removable partial dentures. In the latter, support comes entirely from the abutment teeth through the use of rests.

For the distal extension partial denture, however, a base made to fit the anatomic ridge form does not provide adequate support under occlusal loading. Neither does it provide for maximum border extension nor accurate border detail. Therefore some type of correction impression is necessary. This may be accomplished by several means, all of which satisfy the requirements for support of any distal extension partial denture base.

Foremost is the requirement that certain soft tissues should be recorded or related under some loading so that the base may be made to fit the form of the ridge when under function, thereby providing support and assuring a maintenance of that support for the longest possible time. This requirement makes the distal extension partial denture unique in that the support from the tissues underlying the distal extension base must be made as equal to and compatible with the tooth support as is possible.

A complete denture is entirely tissue supported, and the entire denture can move tissueward under function. In contrast, any movement of a partial denture base is inevitably a rotational movement, which may result in a loss of planned occlusal contacts and the application of undesirable forces to the abutment teeth. Therefore every effort must be made to provide the best possible support for the distal extension base to minimize these forces.

Usually no single impression technique will adequately record the anatomic form of the teeth and adjacent structures and at the same time record the supporting form of the lower edentulous ridge. However, the same relative results can be accomplished, provided an individualized acrylic resin tray is used and is so prepared that placement of the soft tissue on the buccal shelf (the primary stress-bearing area) is accomplished. Some method should be used that will record these tissues either in their supporting *form* or in a supporting *relationship* to the rest of the denture. This may be accomplished by one of several methods. One method is to reline the finished denture to provide adequate support. Another is to make a combination impression by finger loading a previously made anatomic impression at the time that it is related to the rest of the arch in an overall elastic impression. The latter method does not attempt to record a different surface form of the ridge but instead records the relationship of the ridge to the rigid parts of the denture in the same manner that it will be related to the rest of the arch when an occlusal load is applied. This method presumes that there will be some rebound of the tissues when an occlusal load is released.

A third method records the supporting form of the ridge with a secondary impression through the use of a mouth-temperature wax. Although there are minor variations in this technique, the one most commonly used is the making of the wax impression in a resin base attached to the denture framework. Anatomic ridges are cut away and discarded, and that portion of the master cast is repoured to conform to the new wax impression. This provides a corrected master cast upon which the denture base will be processed.

A fourth method of recording also involves the correction of the edentulous areas of the master cast. Special acrylic resin trays that cover the edentulous areas are attached to the metal framework. The trays are modified with modeling plastic placed on the tissue surface to stabilize the trays during border molding procedures. Then borders are molded in modeling plastic to obtain their correct contour and extension. The modeling plastic inside the tray is relieved in selected areas, and a secondary impression is made with a free-flowing impression material. We prefer this latter method for the mandibular distal extension removable partial denture.

The *corrected master cast* impression procedures are usually related to the lower distal extension removable partial denture. The same procedures are applicable to the maxillary arch. However, adequate support for the distal extension maxillary denture base can be obtained by the use of a specially prepared individual acrylic resin impression tray that will record the teeth and basal surfaces in a one-piece impression. Larger support areas are available on the maxillary arch than exist on the lower edentulous ridge. It is important that those tissues in either arch that can better bear additional stress be made to do so. The tissues that are easily displaced cannot adequately support a denture base.

Establishment of occlusal relations

Whether the partial denture is tooth borne or has one or more distal extension bases, the recording of occlusal relationships comprises the final step in the construction of a partial denture. For the tooth-borne partial denture, ridge form is of less significance than the tooth- and tissue-supported prosthesis, since it is not called on to support the prosthesis. For the distal extension base, however, jaw relation records should be made only after obtaining the best possible support for the denture base. This necessitates the making of a base or bases that will provide the same support as the finished denture. Therefore jaw relations cannot be recorded until after the denture framework has been returned to the dentist and a secondary impression has been made. Then either a new resin base or a corrected base must be used to record jaw relations.

Occlusal records for a removable partial denture may be made by several methods. The one most frequently used is the recording of static jaw relationships with the opposing teeth. This method involves the use of a face-bow to correctly orient the maxillary cast to an adjustable articulator, a centric relation record to mount the lower cast, and protrusive and lateral eccentric records to program the articulator.

A second method, a graphic one, may be used to record centric jaw relation, but only where the opposing teeth and the remaining natural teeth are noninterfering. This is because a graphic record is usually made on one plane and does not allow for cuspal inclinations. Therefore this method is generally used only where a removable partial denture is being constructed to an opposing complete denture.

A third method is the registration of functional paths. This records the opposing teeth in function and allows the occlusion on the partial denture to conform to the cuspal influence of the remaining natural teeth. Such a wax record is converted to a stone template, and the prosthetically supplied teeth are modified to occlude with the template. When there are natural teeth remaining in contact, they will influence jaw movements by cuspal guidance, rather than by condylar guidance. Registration of functional paths permits seating of the denture under a functional relationship with the opposing teeth and in cuspal harmony with the remaining natural teeth.

Initial placement procedures

The fifth phase of treatment occurs when the patient is given possession of the removable restoration(s). Inevitably it seems that minute changes in the planned occlusal relationships occur during processing of the dentures. Not only must occlusal harmony be assured before the patient is given possession of the dentures, but additionally the processed bases must be reasonably perfected to basal seats. It must also be assured that the patient understands the suggestions and recommendations given by the dentist for care of the dentures and oral structures, as well as expectations in the adjustment phases and use of the restorations. These facets of treatment are discussed in detail in Chapter 19.

Periodic recall

Initial placement and adjustment of the restoration(s) are certainly not the end of treatment for the partially edentulous patient. Periodic recall of the patient to evaluate the oral tissues, their response to the restorations, and the restorations themselves is a part of total treatment responsibility. Changes in the oral structures or the dentures must be ascertained rather soon to avoid compromised oral health. This can be accomplished by periodic recall. Although a six months' recall period is adequate for most patients, a more frequent evaluation may be required for some patients. Chapter 19 contains some suggestions concerning this phase of treatment.

REASONS FOR FAILURE OF CLASP PARTIAL DENTURE

Experience with the clasp-retained partial denture made by the methods outlined has proved its merit and justifies its continued use. The occasional objection to the visibility of retentive clasps can be minimized through the use of wrought-wire clasp arms. There are few contraindications for use of a properly designed clasp partial denture. Practically all objections to this type of denture can be disposed of by pointing to deficiencies in its design and fabrication and to deficiencies related to patient education. These are as follows:

1. Inadequate diagnosis and treatment planning
2. Failure to either use the surveyor or to use it properly during diagnosis and treatment planning
3. Inadequate mouth preparations, usually due to insufficient planning of the design of the partial denture
4. Failure to provide the technician with a specific design and the necessary information for executing it
5. Failure of the technician to follow the design and instructions outlined (This is either due to disagreement as to the wisdom of the dentist's design or to resistance on the part of the dental laboratory to follow other than stereotyped designs, which may be mass produced. Either of these causes can and must be eliminated or rectified through closer cooperation between the dentist and the technician.)
6. Incorrect use of clasp designs and use of cast clasps that have too little flexibility, too broad tooth coverage, and too little consideration for esthetics
7. Failure to provide for adequate tissue

support for distal extension denture bases

8. Failure to provide for posterior occlusal forms that are in harmony with the cuspal relationships of the remaining natural teeth
9. Failure on the part of the dentist to carry out necessary patient education procedures
10. Failure on the part of the patient to accept his responsibility in treatment

A removable partial denture designed and fabricated so that it avoids the errors and deficiencies listed previously is one that proves the clasp-type partial denture can be made functional, esthetically pleasing, and long lasting without damage to the supporting structures. The proof of the merit of this type of restoration lies in the knowledge that (1) it permits treatment for the largest number of patients as the need for this service increases with advances in other phases of dentistry and is made economically possible by the avoidance of elaborate mechanical devices and high laboratory costs; (2) it provides restorations that are comfortable and efficient over a long period of time, with adequate support and maintenance of occlusal contact relations; (3) it provides for healthy abutments, free of caries and periodontal disease; (4) it provides for the continued health of restored, healthy tissues of the basal seats; and (5) it makes possible a partial denture service that is definitive and not merely an interim treatment.

Removable partial dentures thus made contribute to a concept of prosthetic dentistry that has as its goal the preservation of remaining oral structures, the restoration of partially edentulous mouths, and *an elimination of the ultimate need for complete dentures.*

SELF-ASSESSMENT AIDS

1. In chronological order of accomplishment give the six sequential, correlated phases in treating a partially edentulous patient with removable restorations.
2. If responsibility for the success of treatment is shared by the dentist and the patient, what must be undertaken to prepare the patient to accept his or her responsibility?
3. Since treatment planning is the sole responsibility of the dentist, which of the following may be omitted as noncontributory to total treatment: (1) a complete health history, (2) a history of past dental experiences, (3) an oral examination, (4) a roentgenographic examination, (5) an evaluation of occlusal relations of remaining teeth, and (6) a survey of diagnostic casts?
4. A specific design of the removable restoration must be planned prior to mouth preparation procedures. The dentist (can) (should not) delegate the responsibility for the design to a dental laboratory technician.
5. Stability in a removable restoration is desirable to help maintain the health of oral structures. A tooth-borne restoration usually (can) (cannot) be made more stable than a restoration supported by teeth and residual ridges.
6. When a removable partial denture is supported both by teeth and residual ridges, support by the residual ridge should be made as equal as possible to the support given by the teeth. This may be accomplished by recording which form of the residual ridge in making impressions—anatomic or functional?
7. Development of occlusal harmony is a most important aspect of treating patients with removable restorations. Horizontal relationship of the mandible to the maxillae in both centric and eccentric positions provide the opportunity to obtain adequate occlusion. Can you recall three methods by which maxillomandibular relations may be obtained?
8. In the fifth phase of treatment (initial placement of the restoration(s)) three things are done before the patient is given possession of the denture(s). Two of these are correction of occlusal discrepancies as a result of processing, and review of patient education including adjustment expectations. What other step must be accomplished during the appointment?
9. What is the purpose of periodic recall of patients treated with removable partial dentures?
10. What is the one predominant reason why the clasp-type partial denture is used much more frequently in most practices than is the internal attachment–type restoration?
11. Deficiencies in design and fabrication and those related to patient education are the culprits of limited success in treatment with removable restorations. Avoiding these deficiencies will make the goal of prosthetic dentistry obtainable. This goal is _____, _____, and _____.

3 CLASSIFICATION OF PARTIALLY EDENTULOUS ARCHES

Several methods of classification of partially edentulous arches have been proposed and are in use today. This has led to much confusion and disagreement concerning which method should be adopted and which best classifies all possible combinations.

It has been estimated that there are over 65,000 possible combinations of teeth and edentulous spaces in a single arch. It is obvious that no single method of classification can be descriptive of any except the most basic types. Therefore a basic classification should be sufficient. It is unfortunate that no single method has been universally adopted by the profession. This fact probably has done more to prevent a comprehensive approach to the principles of partial denture design than has any other single factor.

Although classifications are actually descriptive of the partially edentulous arches, the removable partial denture restoring a particular class arch is described as a denture of that class. For example, we speak of a Class III or Class I removable partial denture. Certainly this is acceptable and promotes an economy of words. It is simpler to say "a Class II partial denture" than to say "a partial denture restoring a Class II partially edentulous arch."

The most familiar classifications are those originally proposed by Kennedy, Cummer, and Bailyn. Classifications have also been proposed by Beckett, Godfrey, Swenson, Friedman, Wilson, Skinner, Applegate, Avant, Miller, and others. It is evident that an attempt should be made to combine the best features of all classifications so that a universal classification can be adopted in the future.

Kennedy's method of classification is probably the most widely accepted classification of partially edentulous arches today. Any method that will satisfy the requirements of a classification is acceptable. In an attempt to simplify the problem and encourage more universal usage of a classification and in the interest of adequate communication, the Kennedy classification will be used in this textbook. The student is referred to the Selected References for sources of information relative to other classifications.

REQUIREMENTS OF AN ACCEPTABLE METHOD OF CLASSIFICATION

The classification of a partially edentulous arch should satisfy the following requirements:

1. It should permit immediate visualization of the type of partially edentulous arch being considered.
2. It should permit immediate differentiation between the tooth-borne and the tooth- and tissue-supported removable partial denture.
3. It should be universally acceptable.

KENNEDY'S CLASSIFICATION

The Kennedy method of classification was originally proposed by Dr. Edward Kennedy in 1925. Like the Bailyn classification and also the Skinner classification, it attempts to classify the partially edentulous arch in a manner that will suggest certain principles of design for a given situation (Fig. 3-1).

Kennedy divided all partially edentulous arches into four main types. Edentulous areas other than those determining the main types were designated as *modification spaces* (Fig. 3-2).

The Kennedy classification is as follows:

CLASS I. Bilateral edentulous areas located posterior to the remaining natural teeth
CLASS II. A unilateral edentulous area located posterior to the remaining natural teeth

13

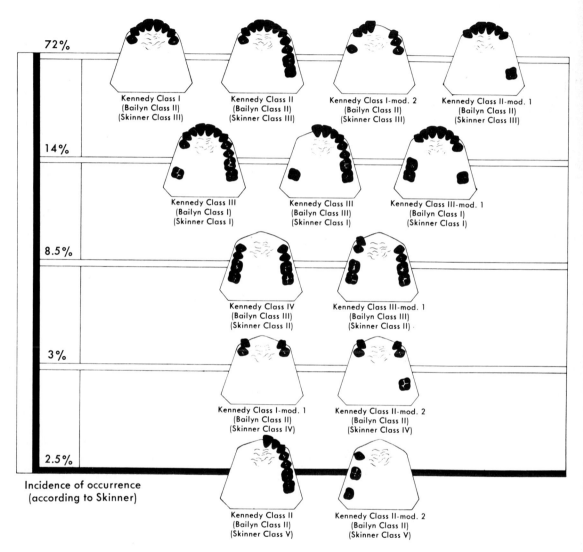

Fig. 3-1. Representative examples of partially edentulous arches classified by the Kennedy, Bailyn, and Skinner methods of classification.

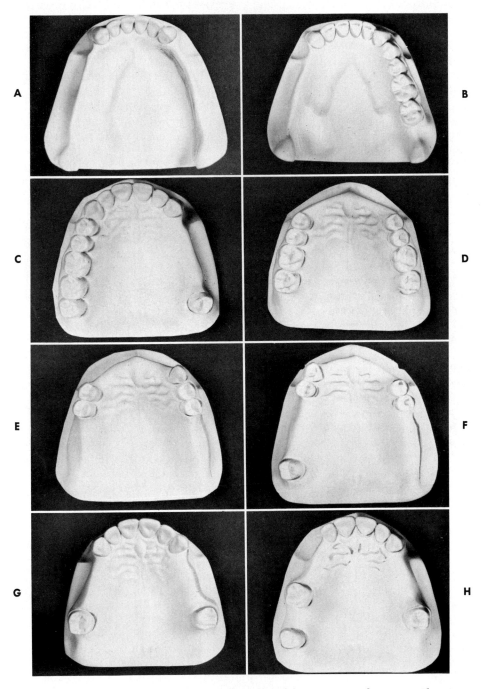

Fig. 3-2. Kennedy classification with examples of modifications. **A,** Class I; **B,** Class II; **C,** Class III; **D,** Class IV; **E,** Class I, modification 1; **F,** Class II, modification 2; **G,** Class III, modification 1; **H,** Class III, modification 2.

CLASS III. A unilateral edentulous area with natural teeth remaining both anterior and posterior to it.

CLASS IV. A single, but bilateral (crossing the midline), edentulous area located anterior to the remaining natural teeth

One of the principal advantages of the Kennedy method is that it permits immediate visualization of the partially edentulous arch. Those schooled in its use and in the principles of partial denture design may immediately compartmentalize their thinking concerning the basic partial denture design that will be employed. It permits a logical approach to the problems of design. It makes possible the application of sound principles of partial denture design and is therefore a logical method of classification.

Applegate's rules for applying the Kennedy classification

The Kennedy classification would be difficult to apply to every situation without certain rules for application. Applegate has provided the following eight rules governing the application of the Kennedy method:

RULE 1. Classification should follow rather than precede any extractions of teeth that might alter the original classification.

RULE 2. If the third molar is missing and not to be replaced, *it is not considered in the classification.*

RULE 3. If a third molar is present and is to be used as an abutment, *it is considered in the classification.*

RULE 4. If a second molar is missing and is not to be replaced, *it is not considered in the classification* (for example, if the opposing second molar is likewise missing and is not to be replaced).

RULE 5. The *most posterior edentulous area* (or areas) always determines the classification.

RULE 6. Edentulous areas other than those determining the classification are referred to as *modifications* and are designated by their number.

RULE 7. The *extent* of the modification is not considered, only the *number* of additional edentulous areas.

RULE 8. There can be no modification areas in Class IV arches. (Another edentulous area lying posterior to the "single bilateral area crossing the midline" would instead determine the classification.)

One suggested change in the order of the Kennedy classification is an attempt to correlate the Class I and Class II partially edentulous arches with the number of edentulous areas involved. Thus Class I would be a unilateral edentulous area posterior to the remaining teeth, and Class II would be a bilateral edentulous area posterior to the remaining teeth.

Whereas it is true that there is some confusion in the mind of the student initially as to why Class I should refer to two edentulous areas and Class II should refer to one, the principles of design make this position logical. Either by design or by accident, presumably the former, Kennedy placed the Class II unilateral distal extension type between the Class I bilateral distal extension type and the Class III toothbounded classification. Any change in this order would be illogical for the following reasons. The Class I partial denture is designed as a tooth-*and* tissue-supported denture. Three of the features necessary for the success of such a denture are adequate support for the distal extension bases, flexible direct retention, and some provision for indirect retention. The Class III partial denture is designed as a toothborne denture, without need generally (but not always) for indirect retention, without base support from the ridge tissues, and with direct retention, the only function of which is to retain the prosthesis. An entirely different design is therefore common to each class because of the difference in support.

However, the Class II partial denture must embody features of both, especially when tooth-borne modifications are present. Having a tissue-supported extension base, it must be designed similarly to a Class I denture, but frequently there is a tooth-supported, or Class III, component elsewhere in the arch. Thus the Class II partial denture rightly falls between the Class I and the Class III because it embodies design features common to both. In keeping with the principle that design is based upon the classification, the application of such principles of design is simplified by retaining the original classification of Kennedy.

Another proposed alteration of the Kennedy method is to add the letters *A* and *P* to designate modifications. Thus an additional edentulous space is identified specifically as being anterior or posterior. It is doubtful that this change in the original classification adds

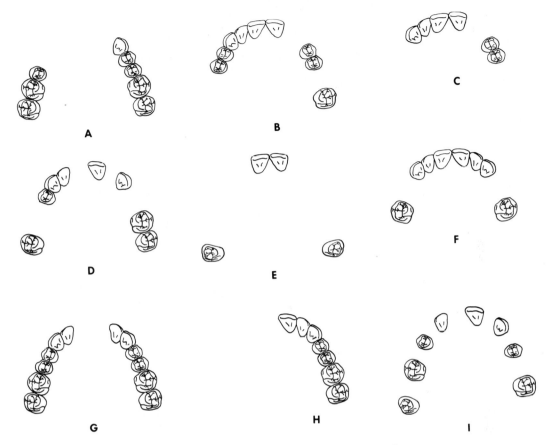

Fig. 3-3. Nine types of partially edentulous arches.

little, if any, clarification to it. However, if it is used only to supplement the original classification rather than to replace it, there can be little objection to the use of the *A* and *P* designations. They cannot be applied to the Class IV arch, however, since a Class IV arch has no modifications.

SELF-ASSESSMENT AIDS

1. Would you agree that the primary purpose of a classification is to enhance communication among dentists?
2. Many classification systems have been proposed; however, the most widely accepted system in the United States is the one proposed by _____ in 1925.
3. A classification of partially edentulous arches should satisfy at least three requirements. Can you recall these three requirements?
4. Kennedy divided all partially edentulous arches into _____ main types.
5. What is meant by a modification space?
6. Which two classes of partially edentulous arches have the greatest incidence?
7. Dr. O. C. Applegate contributed greatly to the application of the original Kennedy classification system. What was this contribution?
8. Classify the partially edentulous arches illustrated in Fig. 3-3.

4 MAJOR AND MINOR CONNECTORS

A typical removable partial denture will have the following components (Fig. 4-1, A).

1. Major connector
2. Minor connectors
3. Rests
4. Direct retainers
5. Reciprocal or stabilizing components (as parts of a direct retainer assembly)
6. Indirect retainers (if the prosthesis has one or more distal extension bases)
7. One or more bases, each supporting one to several replacement teeth (Fig. 4-1, B and C)

Major and minor connectors will now be considered separately as to their function, their location, and their acceptability of design, keeping in mind both biologic and mechanical considerations. Rests, direct retainers, indirect retainers, and denture bases are presented in Chapters 6 to 8.

MAJOR CONNECTORS

A major connector is the unit of the partial denture that connects the parts of the prosthesis located on one side of the arch with those on the opposite side. It is that unit of the partial denture to which all other parts are directly or indirectly attached (Fig. 4-2).

The major connector may be compared to the frame of an automobile, and in the construction of a removable partial denture it is just as essential. It might also be compared to the foundation of a building for the same reason. It must be rigid so that stresses applied to any one portion of the denture may be effectively distributed over the entire and supporting subjacent tissue areas. Being rigid, the major connector resists torque that would otherwise be transmitted to the abutment teeth as leverage.

It is only through the rigidity of the major connector that all other component parts of the partial denture may be effective. If they

are attached to, or originate from, a flexible major connector, the effectiveness of these components is jeopardized to the detriment of the oral structures and the discomfort of the patient. Many removable partial dentures have failed to serve comfortably and effectively only because the major connector failed to provide rigid support to the rest of the prosthesis. Any removable partial denture design utilizing a nonrigid major connector is doomed to failure, either by causing discomfort to the patient or by subjecting the remaining structures to trauma. Trauma may be mainfested by damage to the periodontal support of the abutment teeth, injury to the supporting ridge areas, or impingement of underlying tissues because of flexing of the major connector.

The major connector should be located in a favorable relation to moving tissues and at the same time should avoid impingement of gingival tissues. It also should be located so that areas of bony and tissue prominence are not encountered during placement and removal of the denture. Sufficient relief must be provided beneath a major connector to avoid its settling into hard areas such as an inoperable manidbular torus, a palatal torus, or the elevated palatal median suture line. Location and relief must also take into consideration possible impingement of gingival tissues and other areas as the extension denture rotates from applied forces. Relief is covered at the end of this chapter and expanded upon in Chapter 10 under Relieving the Master Cast.

Planned relief beneath the major connector, when indicated, avoids the need for later adjustments to provide relief of the prosthesis after tissue damage has occurred. Adjustments are not simply time consuming: frequently the grinding involved so weakens the connector that flexibility and sometimes frac-

Fig. 4-1. A, Framework for mandibular removable partial denture with following components: *1,* lingual bar major connector; *2,* minor connector by which the acrylic resin denture bases will be attached; *3,* occlusal rests; *4,* direct retainer arm, which is part of the total clasp assembly; *5,* reciprocal and stabilizing components of the clasp assembly; and *6,* an indirect retainer consisting of a minor connector and an occlusal rest. **B,** Maxillary removable partial denture with acrylic resin denture bases supporting artificial posterior teeth. Bases are attached to metal framework by ladderlike minor connectors. **C,** Mandibular bilateral distal extension removable partial denture with acrylic resin denture bases supporting artificial posterior teeth. Anterior segment of the denture is supported by a splint bar.

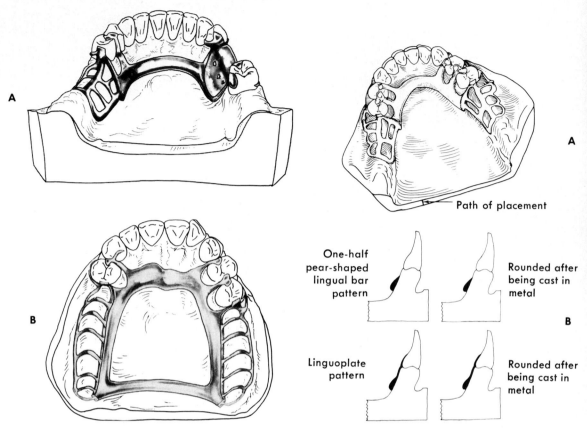

Fig. 4-2. **A,** Lingual bar major connector for mandibular removable partial denture framework. It rigidly joins cast base on right side to other elements of the framework on left side. **B,** Anterior-posterior bar-type maxillary major connector for a Class I partially edentulous arch. This is a rigid type of major connector and covers only a small portion of palatal tissue.

Fig. 4-3. **A,** Lingual bar major connector should be located at least 4 mm below gingival margins and more if possible. **B,** The inferior border of both a lingual bar and a linguoplate must be gently rounded after the framework has been cast. Such a configuration is infinitely more kind to the sensitive tissues in the floor of the mouth than is a sharp edge in this area.

ture result. It seems that tissues once impinged by the connector require more relief than would have been required originally. The adjustment necessary to provide this additional relief seriously weakens the connector because the original bulk did not provide for the possibility of future reduction.

Margins of major connectors adjacent to gingival tissues should be located far enough from those tissues to avoid any possible impingement. The upper border of a lingual bar connector should be located at least 4 mm below the gingival margin(s) and more if possible (Fig., 4-3). The limiting factor, inferiorly, is the height of the moving tissues in the floor of the mouth. Since the connector

must have sufficient width and bulk to provide rigidity, a linguoplate must be used in lieu of a lingual bar in many instances.

In the maxillary arch, since there are no moving tissues in the palate as in the floor of the mouth, the borders of the major connector may be placed well away from gingival tissues. Impingement of gingival tissues is not justifiable because adequate support for the connector is almost always available elsewhere. Structurally the tissues covering the palate are well suited for placement of the connector and have adequate deep blood supply. However, when soft tissue covering the median portion of the palate is less displaceable than the tissue covering the residual ridge, varying amounts of relief under the connectors must be provided to avoid impingement of tissue with its resulting sequelae. The amount of relief required is directly proportional to the difference in displaceability of tissues covering the medial palatal raphe and tissues covering the residual ridges. The gingival tissues, on the other hand, must have an unrestricted superficial blood supply to remain healthy. The borders of the palatal connector should be placed a minimum of 6 mm away from gingival margins and should be located parallel to their mean curve. Minor connectors that must cross gingival tissues should do so abruptly, joining the major connector at nearly a right angle (Fig., 4-4). In this way the maximum freedom of gingival tissues is assured.

Except for a palatal torus or elevated median suture line, palatal connectors ordinarily require no relief, nor is relief desirable. Intimate contact between the connector and the supporting tissues adds much to the retention and stability of the denture. Except for gingival areas, intimacy of contact elsewhere in the palate is not of itself detrimental to the health of the tissues, if supported against settling by rests on abutment teeth.

An anterior palatal bar or the anterior border of a palatal plate also should be located as far posteriorly as possible to avoid interference with the tongue in the rugae area. It should be *flat* or *straplike* rather than half-oval and should be located so that its anterior border follows existing valleys between crests of the rugae. The anterior border of such palatal major connectors will therefore be irregular in outline as it follows the valleys between the rugae. The tongue may then pass from one rugae prominence to another without encountering the border of the denture lying between. When a rugae crest must be crossed by the connector border, it should be done abruptly, avoiding the crest as much as possible.

A rule to be used throughout partial denture design is as follows: *Try to avoid adding any part of the denture framework to an already convex surface. Rather, try to utilize existing valleys and embrasures for the location of component parts of the framework. All components should be tapered where they join convex surfaces.*

The characteristics of major connectors

Fig. 4-4. Palatal major connector should be located at least 6 mm away from gingival margins and parallel to their mean curvature. All adjoining minor connectors should cross gingival tissues abruptly and should join major connectors at nearly a right angle.

contributing to the maintenance of health of the oral environment and the well-being of the patient may be listed as follows:
1. Is made from an alloy compatible with oral tissues
2. Is rigid—employs the broad distribution of stress principle
3. Does not interfere with and is not irritating to the tongue
4. Does not substantially alter the natural contour of the lingual surface of the mandibular alveolar ridge or of the palatal vault
5. Does not impinge on oral tissues when the restoration is placed, removed, or rotates in function
6. Covers no more tissue than is absolutely necessary
7. Does not contribute to retention or trapping of food particles
8. Has support from other elements of the framework to minimize rotation tendencies in function.

Mandibular major connectors

The basic form of a mandibular major connector is the *half-pear–shaped lingual bar*, located above moving tissues but as far below the gingival tissues as possible. It is usually made of a reinforced, 6-gauge, half-pear–shaped wax or a similar plastic pattern (Fig. 4-5).

The major connector must be contoured so that it does not present sharp margins to the

Fig. 4-5. Sagittal section showing half-pear shape of a lingual bar. The inferior border of the bar was rounded after the framework was cast to avoid impingement of lingual tissues when the denture rotates even slightly in function. A taper of the superior border of the bar to soft tissues above will minimize interference to the tongue and will be more acceptable to the patient than would a dissimilar contour.

tongue and cause irritation or annoyance by its angular form. The superior border of a lingual bar connector should be tapered to the tissues above, with its greatest bulk at the lower border. This results in a contour that is known as a half-pear shape, being flat on the tissue side, tapered superiorly, and having the greatest bulk in the inferior third. Lingual bar patterns, both wax and plastic, are made in this conventional shape. However, the inferior border of the lingual bar should be slightly rounded when the framework is polished. A rounded border will not impinge on the lingual tissue when the denture bases rotate inferiorly under occlusal loads. Frequently additional bulk is necessary to provide rigidity, particularly when the bar is long or an alloy of lesser rigidity is used. This is accomplished by underlying the ready-made form with a sheet of 24-gauge casting wax rather than altering the original half-pear shape.

The inferior border of a lingual mandibular major connector must be so located that it does not impinge on the tissues in the floor of the mouth as they change elevations during normal activity, that is, swallowing, speech, licking the lips, and so forth. Yet at the same time, it seems logical to locate the inferior border of these connectors as far inferiorly as possible to avoid interference to the resting tongue and trapping of food substances when they are introduced into the mouth. Additionally, the more inferiorly a lingual bar can be located, the farther the superior border of the bar can be placed from the lingual gingival crevices of adjacent teeth, which in

itself will avoid impingement on the gingival tissue.

There are at least two clinically acceptable methods to determine the relative height of the floor of the mouth to locate the inferior border of a lingual mandibular major connector. The first method is to measure the height of the floor of the mouth with a periodontal probe in relation to the lingual gingival margins of adjacent teeth (Fig. 4-6). During these measurements the tip of the patient's tongue should be just lightly touching the vermilion border of the upper lip. Recording of these measurements permits their transfer to both diagnostic and master casts, thus assuring a rather advantageous location of the inferior border of the major connector. The second method is to use an individualized impression tray having its lingual borders about 3 mm short of the elevated floor of the mouth and then to use an impression material that will permit the impression to be accurately molded as the patient licks his lips (Fig. 4-7). The inferior border of the planned major connector can then be located at the height of the lingual sulcus of the cast resulting from such an impression. Of the two methods, we have found the measuring of the height of the floor of the mouth to be less variable and more clinically acceptable.

Fortunately there are few situations in which extreme lingual inclination of the remaining lower premolar and incisor teeth prevents the use of a lingual bar connector. By conservative mouth preparations in the form of disking and by blockout, a lingual connector can almost always be used. Lingually inclined teeth may sometimes have to be reshaped by means of crowns. Although the use of a labial major connector may be necessary in rare instances, this should be avoided by resorting to necessary mouth preparations, rather than accepting a condition that is otherwise correctable. The same applies to the use of a labial bar when a mandibular torus interferes with the placement of a lingual bar. *Unless surgery is definitely contraindicated, interfering mandibular tori should be removed rather than a labial bar connector used.*

A continuous bar retainer located on or slightly above the cingula of the anterior teeth may be added to the lingual bar for one reason or another, but this should never be done without good reason (Fig. 4-8).

Fig. 4-6. A, Height of floor of mouth (tongue elevated) in relation to lingual gingival sulci measured with a periodontal probe. **B,** Recorded measurements are transferred to the diagnostic cast and then to the master cast after mouth preparations are completed. **C,** Line connecting marks is indicative of the location of the inferior border of a major connector. If periodontal surgery is performed, the line on the cast can be related to incisal edges of the teeth and the measurements recorded for subsequent use.

Fig. 4-7. Individualized acrylic resin impression tray. Lingual flanges should be so trimmed that elevated position of alveolar lingual sulcus can be accurately recorded in an impression material when patient touches vermilion border of upper lip with tip of tongue. Tray was constructed as illustrated in Fig. 14-10.

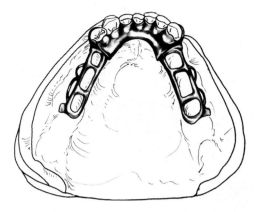

Fig. 4-8. Lingual bar and continuous bar retainer major connector. Upper portion of this major connector is located on cingula of anterior teeth and is extended superiorly to interproximal contact points. Requirement of positive support by rest seats, at least as far anteriorly as the canines, is critical. Note that superior border of bar portion must be placed objectionably close to gingival margins if sufficient rigidity is to be obtained. This type of major connector is definitely a food trap and is often much more objectionable to patient than a linguoplate from the standpoint of annoyance.

Fig. 4-9. Linguoplate is used when space between bounding connectors is better filled in than left open. Such an apron does not serve to replace those connectors but, instead, is added to fundamental denture design to make major connector rigid.

Fig. 4-10. View of mandibular Class II design with contoured linguoplate. Linguoplate is made as thin as possible and follows contours of teeth contacted, resulting in a scalloped shape.

When a linguoplate is otherwise indicated and the axial alignment of the anterior teeth is such that excessive blockout of interproximal undercuts must be made, a continuous bar retainer may be indicated. Additionally, when wide diastemas exist between the lower anterior teeth, a continuous bar retainer may be more esthetically acceptable than a linguoplate.

If the rectangular space bounded by the lingual bar, the continuous bar retainer, and the bounding minor connectors is filled in, a linguoplate results (Figs. 4-9 and 4-10). Again, this should only be done for good reason. The following rule applies: *No component of a partial denture should be added arbitrarily or conventionally. Each component should be added for a good reason and to serve a definite purpose.* The reason for adding a component may be for stabilization against horizontal rotation, retention, support, patient comfort, preservation of the health of the tissues, esthetics, or any one of several other reasons, *but the dentist alone should be responsible for the choice of design used and he should have good reasons, both biologic and mechanical, for doing so.*

A linguoplate should be made as thin as is technically feasible and should be contoured to follow the contours of the teeth and the embrasures. The patient should be made as little aware of added bulk and altered contours in this area as is possible. The upper border should follow the natural curvature of the supracingular surface of the teeth and should not be located above the middle third of the lingual surface except to cover interproximal spaces to the contact points. All gingival crevices and deep embrasures must be blocked out parallel to the path of placement to avoid gingival irritation and any wedging effect between the teeth. In many

Fig. 4-11. If a linguoplate major connector was indicated for this patient with overlapped anterior teeth, judicious recontouring of lingual proximal surfaces of right lateral, right central, and left lateral incisors would eliminate some gross undercuts, thereby permitting a closer adaptation of lingual apron of major connector.

Fig. 4-12. Apron of a linguoplate is closely adapted to the teeth extending into nonundercut interproximal embrasures, resulting in a scalloped form. This form will utilize some of the anterior teeth in group function to help resist horizontal rotation tendencies of the restoration.

instances the judicious recontouring of lingual proximal surfaces of overlapped anterior teeth permits a closer adaptation of the linguoplate major connector, eliminating otherwise deep interproximal embrasures to be covered (Fig. 4-11).

The linguoplate should be something that is added to, not something replacing, the conventional lingual bar. The half-pear shape of a lingual bar should still be present, with the greatest bulk and rigidity at the inferior border. The linguoplate does not in itself serve as an indirect retainer. When indirect retention is required, definite rests must be provided for this purpose. Both the linguoplate and the continuous bar retainer should ideally have a terminal rest at each end regardless of the need for indirect retention. But when indirect retainers are necessary, it is incidental that these rests may serve also as terminal rests for the linguoplate or continuous bar retainer. In such instances it is the rests—not the linguoplate or continuous bar retainer—that function as indirect retainers.

Indications for the use of a linguoplate. The indications for the use of a linguoplate may be listed as follows:

1. *For stabilizing periodontally weakened lower teeth.* Although not as effective as fixed splinting and not as effective as the addition of a labial bar, lingual splinting can be of definite value when used in conjunction with definite rests on sound adjacent teeth.

A continuous bar retainer may be used to accomplish the same purpose, since it is actually the upper border of a linguoplate without the gingival apron. The continuous bar retainer accomplishes stabilization along with the other advantages of a linguoplate. However, it is frequently more objectionable to the patient's tongue and is certainly more of a food trap than is the contoured apron.

2. *In Class I situations in which the residual ridges have undergone excessive vertical resorption.* Flat residual ridges offer little resistance to horizontal rotational tendencies of a denture. The remaining teeth must be depended on to resist such rotation. A correctly designed linguoplate will utilize remaining teeth to resist horizontal rotations (Fig. 4-12).

3. *When the lingual frenum is high or the space available for a lingual bar is slight.* In either instance the superior border of a lingual bar would have to be placed objectionably close to gingival tissues. Irritation could be avoided only by generous relief, which would not only be annoying to the tongue but would also create an undesirable food trap. Use of a linguoplate permits the gingivae to be bridged and the superior border to be tapered to tooth contact, permitting its inferior border to be placed higher without tongue and gingival irritation and without compromise of rigidity.

4. *When the future replacement of one or more incisor teeth will be facilitated by the*

Fig. 4-13. Sagittal section through a linguoplate demonstrating basic half-pear-shaped inferior border with a metallic apron extending superiorly. Note that gingival crevice is "bridged" by linguoplate to avoid impingement of gingival tissue. The linguoplate receives positive support from a lingual rest (in a properly prepared rest seat) on the canine and a mesioocclusal rest on the first premolar. Extension of the linguoplate to height of contour on premolar was accomplished to enclose a rather large triangular interproximal space inferior to contact point between canine and premolar. Such spaces may often be bridged to eliminate obvious food traps and to provide a more hygienic oral environment.

addition of retention loops to an existing linguoplate. Mandibular incisors that are periodontally weak may thus be retained, with the knowledge that future additions to the partial denture are possible.

The same reasons for use of a linguoplate anteriorly apply also to its use elsewhere in the lower arch. If a lingual bar alone is to be used anteriorly, there is no reason for adding an apron elsewhere. However, when auxiliary splinting is used for stabilization of the remaining teeth or for horizontal stabilizing of the prosthesis, or for both, small rectangular spaces sometimes remain. Tissue response to such small spaces is better when bridged with an apron than when left open. Generally this is done to avoid gingival irritation or the entrapment of food debris or to cover generously relieved areas that would be irritating to the tongue (Fig. 4-13). Sometimes a dentist is faced with a clinical situation wherein a linguoplate is indicated as the major connector of choice even though the anterior teeth are quite spaced and the patient strenuously objects to metal showing through the spaces. The linguoplate can then be so constructed that metal will not appreciably show through the spaced anterior teeth (Fig. 4-14). Rigidity of the major connector is not greatly altered; however, such a design may be as much of a food trap as

Fig. 4-14. Diastemas are not bridged by the major connector. Framework must be supported by rests on canines placed in properly prepared rest seats. Rigidity of major connector is not necessarily compromised, but such a contour definitely lends itself to food being retained around teeth and under apron extensions.

the continuous bar retainer type of major connector.

Maxillary major connectors

Four basic types of maxillary major connectors will be considered: (1) single palatal bar or strap, (2) U-shaped palatal connector, (3) combination anterior and posterior palatal strap-type connectors, and (4) palatal plate–type connectors.

Single palatal bar or strap. The single palatal bar is perhaps the most widely used and yet the least logical of all palatal major connectors (Fig. 4-15). It is difficult to say whether this or the U-shaped palatal connector is the more objectionable of palatal connectors.

For a single palatal bar to have the necessary rigidity, it must have concentrated bulk. The latter may be avoided only by ignoring the need for rigidity, which unfortunately is too frequently done. For a single palatal bar to be rigid enough to be effective, it must be centrally located between the two halves of the denture. This means that a single palatal bar always must be centrally located with concentrated bulk. Mechanically this practice may be sound enough, but from the standpoint of patient comfort and alteration of palatal contours, it is highly objectionable.

A partial denture made with a single palatal bar is frequently either too flexible or too objectionable to the patient's tongue, or

Fig. 4-15. Half-round palatal bar must be bulky to obtain rigidity required for cross-arch distribution of stress. Its bulk may make it objectionable to patient's tongue.

both. The decision to use a single palatal bar should be based on the size of the denture areas being connected and on whether a single connector located between them would be rigid without objectionable bulk. Bilateral tooth-borne restorations of short spans may be effectively connected with a single, broad palatal strap connector, particularly when the edentulous areas are located posteriorly (Fig. 4-16). Such a connector can be made rigid, without objectionable bulk and interference to the tongue, provided its surface lies in three planes.

For reasons of torque and leverage, a single palatal connector should not be used to connect anterior replacements with distal extension bases. To be rigid enough to resist torque and to provide adequate horizontal and vertical support as well, a single strap would have to be objectionably bulky. When placed anteriorly, this bulk becomes even more objectionable to the patient, since it interferes with speech formation.

U-shaped palatal connector. From both the patient's standpoint and a mechanical standpoint the U-shaped palatal connector is the least desirable of maxillary major connectors. It should never be used arbitrarily. When a large inoperable palatal torus exists and occasionally when several anterior teeth are to be replaced, the U-shaped palatal connector may have to be used (Fig. 4-17). In most instances, however, other designs will serve more effectively.

Fig. 4-16. This single palatal strap-type major connector may be used for tooth-borne restorations of bilateral edentulous areas of short span. It may also be used in a tooth-borne unilateral edentulous situation with provision for cross-arch attachment by either extracoronal retainers or internal attachments. Width of palatal strap should be confined within the boundaries of supporting rests. **B,** Sagittal section through **A.** Midportion of major connector is slightly elevated to provide rigidity. Thinness of major connector does not appreciably alter palatal contours.

Fig. 4-17. U-shaped palatal connector is probably the least rigid type of maxillary major connector and should be used only when a large inoperable palatal torus prevents use of palatal coverage or a combination anterior-posterior palatal strap-type designed framework.

Fig. 4-18. Common partial denture design utilizing an objectionable U-shaped palatal major connector. Such a connector lacks necessary rigidity, places bulk where it is most objectionable to patient, and impinges on gingival tissues lingual to remaining teeth, resulting in chronic inflammation. This denture failed primarily because it lacked rigidity in the major connector, provision for indirect retention, occlusal support, and consideration of gingival health in the location of anterior border of major connector.

To be rigid the U-shaped palatal connector must have bulk where the tongue needs the most freedom, which is in the rugae area. Without sufficient bulk the U-shaped design leads to increased flexibility and movement at the open ends. In distal extension dentures when posterior tooth support is non-existent, movement is particularly noticeable and is traumatic to the residual ridge. Many maxillary partial dentures have failed for no other reason except the flexibility of a U-shaped major connector (Fig. 4-18). No matter how well the extension base is supported or how harmonious the occlusion, when horizontal movement under function is not resisted by a rigid major connector, the residual ridge suffers.

The wider the coverage of a U-shaped major connector, the more it resembles a palatal plate with its several advantages. But when used as a narrow U design, the necessary rigidity is usually lacking. A U-shaped connector may be made more rigid by providing multiple tooth support through definite rests. A common error in the design of a U-shaped connector, however, is its proximity to, or actual contact with, gingival tissues. The

principle that the borders of major connectors should either be supported by rests in prepared rest seats or be located well away from gingival tissues has been given previously. The majority of U-shaped connectors fail to do either, with resulting gingival irritation and periodontal damage to the tissues adjacent to the remaining teeth.

Combination anterior and posterior palatal strap-type connectors. Structurally the most rigid of palatal major connectors, the anterior and posterior palatal bar combination, may be used in almost any maxillary partial denture design (Figs. 4-19 and 4-20).

Whenever it is necessary for the palatal connector to make contact with the teeth for reasons of support, definite tooth support must be provided. Anterior tooth support is sometimes necessary, particularly when the denture includes anterior replacements. This is best accomplished by establishing definite rest seats on gold restorations, using veneer crowns, three-quarter crowns, or pin-ledge restorations. These should be located far enough above the gingival attachment to provide for bridging the gingival crevice with blockout. At the same time, they should be low enough on the tooth to avoid unfavorable leverage, and low enough on maxillary incisors and canine teeth to avoid incisal interference at the cingulum of the tooth.

Connector borders resting on unprepared tooth surfaces can lead only to slippage of the denture along inclines, or to orthodontic movement of the tooth, or to both. In any case, settling into gingival tissues is inevitable. When the needed vertical support ceases to exist, the health of the surrounding tissues is usually impaired. Similarly, interproximal projections resting upon the gingival third of the tooth and upon gingival tissues that are structurally unable to render support can only cause impingement to the detriment of the health of those tissues.

A cardinal rule, then, for the location of the major connector in relation to the remaining teeth and their surrounding gingivae is this: *Either support the connector by definite rests on the teeth contacted, bridging the gingivae with adequate relief, or locate the connector far enough away from the gingivae to avoid any possible restriction of blood supply and entrapment of food debris.* All gingival crossings should be abrupt and at right angles to the major connector,

Fig. 4-19. Anterior and posterior palatal bar combination is the most rigid of palatal major connectors and, when properly designed, is neither objectionable to patient nor harmful to adjacent tissues.

Fig. 4-20. Anterior and posterior palatal bar-type major connectors. Anterior bar is a flat strap located as far posteriorly as possible to avoid rugae coverage and tongue interference. Anterior border of this bar should be located just posterior to a rugae crest or in the valley between two crests. Posterior bar is half-oval (approximately 6 gauge) and is located as far posteriorly as possible, yet entirely on hard palate. It should be located at right angles to midline rather than on a diagonal.

Fig. 4-21. Anterior-posterior bar-type major connector for a Class IV partially edentulous arch. Positive support for anterior portion of major connector is furnished by a "splint bar" joining the four crowned premolars. Notice that lateral portions of major connector are placed at least 6 mm from lingual gingival crevices.

and these should bridge the gingivae with adequate relief.

Creating a sharp, angular form of any portion of a palatal connector should be avoided, and all borders should be tapered slightly toward the tissues. A posterior palatal bar should be half-oval in shape and located as far posteriorly as possible to avoid interference with the tongue. A posterior bar or the posterior border of any palatal connector should never be placed on moving tissues and should be located on the hard palate anterior to the line of flexure formed by the junction of the hard and soft palates. The only condition preventing its use is when there is an inoperable maxillary torus that extends posteriorly to the soft palate. In this situation a broad U-shaped major connector must be used.

The strength of this major connector design lies in the fact that the half-oval posterior strap and the flat anterior strap are joined together by longitudinal connectors on either side, forming a square or rectangular frame. Each component braces the other against possible torque and flexure. Flexure is practically nonexistent in such a design.

Ordinarily both the anterior and posterior connectors should be placed as far posteriorly as possible to avoid interference with the tongue. The anterior connector may be extended anteriorly to support anterior tooth replacements, or it may be widened to form a thin palatal plate with a posterior brace

(Fig. 4-21). In this form a U-shaped connector is made rigid because of the added horizontal brace posteriorly. Frequently a maxillary torus may thus be encircled by the major connector without sacrificing rigidity.

Fig. 4-22. Palatal major connector covering two thirds of palate. Anterior border follows valleys between rugae and does not extend anterior to indirect retainers on first premolars. Posterior border is located at junction of hard and soft palates but does not extend onto soft palate. In a bilateral distal extension situation as illustrated, indirect retainers are a must to aid in resisting horizontal rotation of the restoration. Note that provisions have been made for a butt-type joint joining the denture bases and framework as denture base on each side passes through pterygomaxillary notch.

Fig. 4-23. Maxillary Class I partial denture framework with anatomic replica palatal major connector. Although retention is increased by using a broad major connector, the need for indirect retainers still exists, and they are placed on mesiocclusal surfaces of first premolars. Direct retention is furnished by bar-type clasps engaging distobuccal undercuts on second premolars. A metal extension from the framework contacts prepared guiding planes on distal surfaces of second premolars to complete clasp assembly.

The combination anterior-posterior connector design may be used with any Kennedy class of partially edentulous arch. It is used most frequently in Classes II and IV, whereas the single wide palatal bar or strap is more frequently used in Class III situations and the palatal plate or full coverage most frequently in Class I situations for reasons to be explained subsequently.

Both anterior and posterior connectors, and also the anterior and posterior borders of a palatal plate, should cross the midline at a right angle rather than on a diagonal. This is for reasons of symmetry. The tongue, being a bilateral organ, will accept symmetrically placed components far more readily than those placed without regard for bilateral symmetry. Therefore any curves in the connector should be placed to one side of the midline so that the connector may pass from one side to the other at right angles to the sagittal plane.

Palatal plate–type connector. For lack of better terminology, the words *palatal plate* are used to designate any thin, broad, contoured palatal coverage used as a maxillary major connector covering one half or more of the hard palate (Fig. 4-22). The older types

of thin castings, usually made of 26-gauge wax, were of indefinite thickness. This was due both to the wax's being thinned during adaptation to the cast and to polishing with abrasive wheels. Newer techniques have resulted in the production of anatomic replica palatal castings that have uniform thickness and strength by reason of their corrugated contours. Thinner castings possessing greater rigidity are possible by this method. Through the use of electrolytic polishing, uniformity of thickness can be maintained and the anatomic contours of the palate faithfully reproduced in the finished denture.

The anatomic replica palatal major connector has several advantages over other types of palatal major connectors. Some of these follow:

1. It permits the making of a uniformly thin metal plate that reproduces faithfully the anatomic contours of the patient's own palate. Because of its uniform thinness, its familiar feel to the patient's tongue, and the thermal conductivity of the metal, the palatal plate is probably accepted more readily by the tongue and underlying tissues than any other type of connector.

2. The corrugation in the anatomic replica

Fig. 4-24. Anatomic replica palatal major connector for a Class II, modification 1, partial denture. Anterior border avoids coverage of anterior rugae; posterior border lies well back on immovable hard palate, crossing midline at a right angle. Total contact provides excellent auxiliary retention without objectionable bulk.

Fig. 4-25. Full palatal major connector. Posterior border terminates at junction of hard and soft palates. Anterior portion is in the form of a palatal linguoplate and is supported by positive lingual rest seats on canines. Location of finishing lines is most important in this type of major connector. Unless they relatively follow the line of the arch and are located just lingual to an imaginary line contacting the lingual surfaces of the lost natural teeth, alteration of natural palatal contour should be anticipated with its attendant detrimental effect on speech.

adds strength to the casting; a thinner casting with adequate rigidity can thus be made than could formerly be constructed with adapted sheet wax.

3. Surface irregularities are intentional rather than accidental; therefore electrolytic polishing is all that is needed. The original uniform thickness of the plastic pattern is thus maintained.

4. Interfacial surface tension between metal and tissues provides the prosthesis with greater retention. Retention must be adequate to resist the pull of sticky foods, the action of moving border tissues against the denture, the forces of gravity, and the more violent forces of coughing and sneezing. These are all resisted to some extent by the

retention of the base itself in proportion to the total area of denture contact. The amount of both direct and indirect retention required will depend on the amount of retention provided by the denture base.

The palatal plate may be used in one of three ways. It may be used as a plate of varying width covering the area between two or more edentulous areas (Fig. 4-23), or it may be used as a full or partial cast plate extending posteriorly to the junction of the hard and soft palates (Fig. 4-24 and 4-25), or it also may be used in the form of an anterior palatal connector with a provision for extending an acrylic resin denture base posteriorly (Fig. 4-26).

In most situations the palatal plate will be

Fig. 4-26. A, Maxillary major connector in the form of a palatal linguoplate with provision for attaching a full-coverage acrylic resin denture base. **B,** Completed removable partial denture with acrylic resin base. Palatal linguoplate is supported by rests occupying lingual rest seats prepared in gold restorations on canines. This type of removable partial denture is particularly applicable where (1) residual ridges have undergone extreme vertical resorption and (2) terminal abutments have sufferd some bone loss and splinting cannot be accomplished for some reason.

located anterior to the posterior palatal seal area. Little posterior seal is ever necessary with a metal palate because of the accuracy and stability of the cast metal. This is in contrast to the posterior palatal seal needed with resin complete denture bases. Inevitably the release of inherent strains in a processed acrylic resin base covering the palate and tuberosities requires that some provision be made for intimate contact of the posterior portion of the denture base and the tissue upon which it is resting. This is accomplished

by scoring the master cast to form a groove approximately 1.5 × 1.5 mm through the pterygomaxillary notches and across the junction of the hard and soft palates.

When the last remaining abutment tooth on either side of a Class I arch is the canine or first premolar tooth, full palatal coverage is not only advisable but is also practically mandatory when the residual ridges have undergone excessive vertical resorption. This may be accomplished in one of two ways. One method is to use a casting anteriorly with retention posteriorly for the attachment of a resin denture base, which then extends posteriorly to a palatal seal (Fig. 4-26). The other method is to utilize a full cast palate extending to the posterior palatal seal area (Fig. 4-25). The several advantages of a cast palate over a full resin palate make the full cast palate sufficiently preferable to offset the slight additional cost. However, when the cost and fee must be held to a minimum, the former method may be used satisfactorily. The partial metal palate may also be used when later rebasing is anticipated. In such case the posterior seal can be redone as part of the rebasing procedure.

Whereas the full palatal plate is not a connector that may be used universally, it has become accepted as the most satisfactory palatal connector for many maxillary partial dentures. In all circumstances the portion contacting the teeth must have positive support from adequate rest seats. The dentist should be familiar with its use and, at the same time, with its limitations, so that it may be used intelligently and to fullest advantage.

Design. In 1953 Blatterfein described a systematic approach to designing maxillary major connectors. His method involves five basic steps and is certainly applicable to most of maxillary removable partial denture situations. With a diagnostic cast in hand and a knowledge of the relative displaceability of the tissues covering the median palatal raphe, he recommends the following basic steps:

STEP 1. *Outline of primary bearing areas.* The primary bearing areas are those that will be covered by the denture base(s) (Fig. 4-27, *A* and *B*).

STEP 2. *Outline of nonbearing areas.* The nonbearing areas are the lingual gingival tissues within 5 to 6 mm of the remaining teeth, hard areas of the median palatal raphe (in-

Fig. 4-27. A, Diagnostic cast of partially edentulous maxillary arch. **B,** Denture base areas are outlined. **C,** Nonbearing areas outlined in black, which include lingual soft tissue within 5 to 6 mm of teeth, an unyielding median palatal raphe area, and soft palate. The space bounded by the bearing and nonbearing area outlines is available for placement of a major connector. **D,** Major connector selected will be rigid, noninterfering to tongue, and cover a minimum of the palate.

cluding tori, and palatal tissues posterior to the vibrating line) (Fig. 4-27, *C*).

STEP 3. *Outline of bar areas.* Steps 1 and 2, when completed, provide an outline or designate areas that are available to place components of major connectors (Fig. 4-27, *C*).

STEP 4. *Selection of bar type.* Selection of the type of connecting bar(s) is based on four factors: mouth comfort, rigidity, location of denture bases, and indirect retention. Connecting bars should be of minimum bulk and so positioned that interference to the tongue during speech and mastication is not encountered. Connecting bars must have a maximum of rigidity to distribute stress bilaterally. The double bar type of major connector provides the maximum of rigidity without bulk and total tissue coverage. In many instances the choice of a bar type is limited by the location of the edentulous ridge areas. When edentulous areas are located anteriorly, the use of only a posterior bar is not possible. By the same token, when only posterior edentulous areas are present, the use of only an anterior bar is not a plausible choice. The need for indirect retention influences the outline of the major connector: provision must be made in its location so that indirect retainers may be attached.

STEP 5. *Unification.* After selection of the type bar(s) based on the considerations in Step 4, the denture base areas and connecting bars are joined (Fig. 4-27, *D*).

The indications for the use of full palatal coverage have been previously discussed in this chapter. Although there are many variations in palatal major connectors, a thorough comprehension of all factors influencing their design will lead the dentist to the best design for a particular patient.

MINOR CONNECTORS

Arising from the major connector, the minor connector joins the major connector with other parts of the denture. For example, each direct retainer and each occlusal rest are joined to the major connector by a minor connector. In many instances a minor connector may be identified even though continuous with some other part of the denture. For example, an occlusal rest at one end of a linguoplate is actually the terminus of a minor connector, even though that minor connector is continuous with the linguoplate.

Similarly, the portion of a denture base frame that supports the clasp and the occlusal rest is a minor connector, joining the major connector with the clasp proper. Those portions of a denture framework by which the denture bases are attached are minor connectors.

Functions of the minor connectors. In addition to joining denture parts, the minor connector serves two other purposes. These are diametric in function.

1. *To transfer functional stress to the abutment teeth.* Occlusal forces applied to the artificial teeth are transmitted through the base to the underlying ridge tissues if that base is primarily tissue supported. Occlusal forces applied to the artificial teeth nearer to an abutment are transferred to that tooth through the occlusal rest. Similarly, occlusal forces are transferred to other abutment teeth supporting auxiliary rests and to the abutment teeth supporting a partial denture that is entirely tooth borne. The minor connectors arising from a rigid major connector make possible this transfer of functional stress throughout the dental arch. This, then, is a *prosthesis-to-abutment* function of the minor connector.

2. *To transfer the effect of the retainers, rests, and stabilizing components to the rest of the denture.* This is an *abutment-to-prosthesis* function of the minor connector. The effect of occlusal rests on supporting tooth surfaces, the action of retainers, and the effect of reciprocal clasp arms, guiding planes, and other stabilizing components are transferred to the rest of the denture by the minor connectors and then throughout the dental arch. Thus forces applied on one portion of the denture may be resisted by other components placed elsewhere in the arch for that purpose. A bracing or stabilizing component on one side of the arch may be placed to resist horizontal forces originating on the opposite side. This is possible only because of the transferring effect of the minor connector, which supports that stabilizing component, and the rigidity of the major connector.

Form and location of minor connectors. Like the major connector, the minor connector must have sufficient bulk to be rigid; otherwise the transfer of the stresses and of the effect of other components cannot be effective. At the same time, the bulk of the minor connector must be as unobjectionable as possible.

A minor connector contacting the axial surface of an abutment should not be located on a convex surface but instead should be located in an embrasure in which it will be least noticeable to the tongue. It should conform to the interdental embrasure, passing vertically from the major connector to the other components. It should be thickest toward the lingual surface, tapering toward the contact area. The deepest part of the interdental embrasure should have been blocked out to avoid interference during placement and removal and to avoid any wedging effect on the teeth contacted.

Generally the minor connector should form a right angle with the major connector so that the gingival crossing may be abrupt and cover as little of the gingival tissues as possible. All gingival crossings should be relieved by blockout of the gingival crevice on the master cast before a refractory cast is made.

When a minor connector contacts tooth surfaces on either side of the embrasure in which it lies, it should be tapered to the teeth so that the tongue may encounter a smooth surface (Fig. 4-28). Sharp angles should be avoided, and spaces should not exist for the trapping of food debris.

It is a minor connector that contacts the guiding plane surfaces of the abutment teeth whether as a connected part of a direct retainer assembly or a separate entity (Fig. 4-29). Here the minor connector must be wide enough to utilize the guiding plane to fullest advantage. When it gives rise to a clasp arm, the connector should be tapered to the tooth below the origin of the clasp. If no clasp arm is formed, as when a bar clasp arm originates elsewhere, the connector should be tapered to a knife edge the full length of its buccal aspect.

When an artificial tooth will be placed against a proximal minor connector, the minor connector's greatest bulk should be located toward the lingual aspect of the abutment tooth. In this manner sufficient bulk is assured with the least interference to the placement of the artificial tooth. Ideally the artificial tooth should contact the abutment tooth with only a thin layer of metal intervening buccally. Lingually the bulk of the minor connector should lie in the interdental embrasure the same as between two natural teeth.

Fig. 4-28. Undercuts in lingual embrasure between premolars have been blocked out parallel to path of placement. The minor connector is V shaped to avoid bulk, the greatest depth of the V being at junction with occlusal rests.

Fig. 4-29. Minor connector (arrows) contacting guiding plane surface is as broad as about two thirds the distance between the tips of the adjacent buccal and lingual cusps of the abutment tooth. It extends gingivally contacting an area of the abutment from the marginal ridge to two thirds the length of the enamel crown. Viewed from above, it is triangular in shape, the apex of the triangle being buccally located and the base of the triangle lingual. Less interference with arrangement of adjacent artificial tooth is encountered with minor connector so shaped.

The minor connector, then, should be positioned to pass vertically in an interdental embrasure whenever possible. Its shape should conform to the interdetnal embrasure, with sufficient bulk to be rigid but tapered to the tooth surface when exposed to the tongue, and it should be designed so that it will not interfere with the placement of an artificial tooth.

As stated previously, those portions of a denture framework by which acrylic resin denture bases are attached are minor connectors. This type of minor connector should

Fig. 4-30. Finishing line at junction of ladder-like minor connector and major connector blends smoothly into minor connector, contacting distal guiding plane on second premolar. Framework is "feathered" toward tissue anterior to finishing line to avoid as much bulk in this area as possible—without compromising the strength of the butt-type joint.

Fig. 4-31. Wax pattern for minor connector by which acrylic resin denture base will be attached. It is extended on both lingual and buccal surfaces of residual ridge and is made using 12-gauge half-round forms and 18-gauge round forms. Note that this minor connector is extended at least two thirds of the length of the edentulous span.

be so constructed that it will be completely embedded within the denture base.

The junctions of these mandibular minor connectors with the major connectors should be strong butt-type joints but without appreciable bulk (Fig. 4-30). Angles formed at the junctions of the connectors should not be greater than 90 degrees, thus assuring the most advantageous and strongest connection between the acrylic resin denture base and the major connector.

An open latticework or ladder type of construction is preferable and is conveniently made by using preformed 12-gauge half-round and 18-gauge round wax strips. The minor connector for the lower distal extension base should extend posteriorly about two thirds the length of the edentulous ridge and have elements on both the lingual and buccal surfaces. Not only will such an arrangement add strength to the denture base, but in all probability it will also minimize distortion of the cured base from its inherent strains due to processing. The minor connector must be planned with care so that it will not interfere with the arrangement of artificial teeth (Fig. 4-31). A means to attach acrylic resin individualized trays to the mandibular framework when a secondary impression is planned must be arranged when the framework pattern is being developed. Three "nailhead" minor connectors fabricated as part of the denture base minor connector serve this purpose well (Fig. 4-32). Unless

Fig. 4-32. Three small "nailhead" minor connectors (arrows) by which individualized impression trays may be attached when a secondary impression is utilized. These nailheads are initially made of 18-gauge round wax strips on framework pattern and can be removed from framework, if desired, after an impression for master cast has been made.

some similar arrangement is made, the resin trays may become detached or loosened during impression-making procedures.

Minor connectors for maxillary distal extension denture bases should extend the entire length of the residual ridge and should also be of a ladderlike and loop construction (Fig. 4-33). The finishing line junction with the major connector should take the form of an angle of less than 90 degrees, therefore being somewhat undercut (Fig. 4-34). Of course the medial extent of the minor connector depends on the lateral extent of the major palatal connector. Too little attention is given this finishing line location in many

Fig. 4-33. Extension of finishing line to area of pterygomaxillary notch provides butt-type joint for attachment of border portion of acrylic resin base through pterygomaxillary notch.

Fig. 4-34. Frontal sections through lingual finishing lines of palatal major connectors. Figure on right is through a cast base; figure on left is through an acrylic resin denture base. In both these situations the location of finishing lines minimizes the bulk of acrylic resin attaching the artificial teeth. Palatal contours are restored, enhancing speech and contributing to a feeling of naturalness for the patient.

Fig. 4-35. Note the direct retainer arm tapers from its tip to the finishing line. Without a finishing line (arrow) at junction of direct retainer arm and minor connector for denture base, flexing of direct retainer arm would create minute cracks in anterior border of denture base—often contributing to chipping of borders as well as an unhygienic condition from food particle impaction.

instances. If the finishing line is located too far medially, the natural contour of the palate will be altered by the thickness of resin supporting the artificial teeth. If, on the other hand, the finishing line is located too far buccally, it will be most difficult to create a natural contour of the acrylic resin on the lingual of the artificial teeth. The location of the finishing line at the junction of the major and minor connector should be based on restoring the natural palatal shape, taking into consideration the presumed anteroposterior and lateral alignment of the missing natural posterior teeth.

Just as consideration is given the junction of major and minor connectors attaching the denture base, so must equal consideration be given the junction of minor connectors and bar-type direct retainer arms (Fig. 4-35). These junctions are also butt-type joints and when so made possess the same advantages of the butt-type joint previously discussed.

REACTION OF TISSUES TO METALLIC COVERAGE

The reaction of tissues to metallic coverage has been the subject of some controversy between periodontists and prosthodontists. Particularly areas that the controversy concerns are gingival crossings and broad areas of metal contact with tissues.

From the prosthodontic viewpoint, if oral tissues may not be safely covered with the framework of removable partial dentures, then all parts of the partial denture resting on or crossing soft tissues jeopardize the health of those tissues. If this is true, it is not the fact of coverage alone but several factors that jeopardize the tissues.

First of these is *pressure due to lack of support*. If relief over gingival crossings and other areas of contact with tissues that are incapable of supporting the prosthesis is inadequate, then impingement on those tissues is inevitable. Impingement will likewise occur if the denture settles due to loss of tooth support. This may be due to failure of the rest areas as a result of improper design, caries involvement, or the flow of amalgam alloy restorations, or to intrusion of abutment teeth under occlusal loading. It is the responsibility of the prosthodontist to provide and maintain adequate relief and adequate occlusal support.

Settling of the denture also may produce pressure elsewhere in the arch, such as beneath major connectors. Again, the cause of settling must be prevented or corrected if it becomes manifest. Fisher has shown that pressure alone may have a nonspecific effect on tissues, which has been mistaken for allergic response or the effect of coverage. Pressure, then, must be avoided whenever oral tissues must be covered or crossed by elements of the partial denture.

The second reason is *uncleanliness*. It is known that tissues respond unfavorably to an accumulation of food debris and bacterial enzymes. Coverage of oral tissues with dentures that are not kept clean irritates those tissues, not because they are covered but because of the accumulation of irritating factors. This has lead to a misinterpretation of the effect of tissue coverage by prosthetic restorations.

A third explanation of unfavorable tissue response to coverage is the *amount of time the denture is worn*. It is apparent that mucous membrane reverts to connective tissue if isolated from the oral environment for a long enough period of time. Evidence of this is the appearance of tissue, once mucous membrane, beneath the pontics of fixed partial dentures. A raw, denuded surface is visible on removal of the fixed restoration. The same thing can occur beneath removable prosthetic restorations if they are allowed to remain against the tissue long enough.

Some patients become so accustomed to wearing a removable restoration that they neglect to remove it often enough to give the tissues any respite from constant contact. This is frequently true when anterior teeth are replaced by the partial denture and the individual will not allow the restoration to be out of the mouth at any time except in the privacy of the bathroom during toothbrushing.

The fact remains that living tissue should not be covered all the time or changes in those tissues will occur. *Partial dentures should not be worn upon retiring at night, so that the tissues may rest and be returned to a normal environment at least several hours in the twenty-four hours.*

Clinical experience with the use of linguoplates and palatal plates has shown conclusively that when factors of pressure, cleanliness, and time are controlled, tissue coverage is not in itself detrimental to the health of oral tissues.

MAJOR CONNECTORS IN REVIEW*

It is only through the rigidity of the major connector that all other components of the partial denture may be effective.

Design of major connectors must be determined during diagnostic and treatment planning phases because mouth preparation procedures depend in part on the contemplated design of major connectors.

Major connectors must be located in favorable relation to moving tissues and, at the same time, must avoid impingement of gingival tissues.

No component of a removable partial denture framework may engage undercuts other than the terminal portions of retentive direct retainer arms.

Adequate but not excessive tissue relief beneath major connectors, when indicated, avoids the need for later adjustments to provide relief after tissue damage has occurred. Sufficient relief must be provided beneath major connectors to avoid any settling into hard areas such as inoperable tori, other exostoses, or prominent median palatal suture areas. The amount of such relief is determined by ascertaining the difference in displaceability of the tissues to be covered by the maxillary major connector and those of the primary stress-bearing areas of residual ridges. Additionally, the quality of support anticipated by utilizing other elements of the framework to resist horizontal rotations and displacement toward the tissues is another factor to be considered in the amount of relief to be provided for any type of major connector.

Relief of free gingival margins must be provided for any component of the framework, in addition to denture bases. This support is derived primarily from components terminating in rest seats specifically prepared to receive them.

Anatomic replica patterns for palatal major connectors permit the rather faithful reproduction of palatal contours and are probably more readily accepted by the patient than are other types of construction and may be made thinner without sacrificing rigidity.

---

*A review of factors influencing the choice of design, definitive location, and average pattern specifications of various major connectors is now presented in a rather condensed version. It is hoped that such a presentation coming after a general discussion will be a meaningful guide to student-dentists in their decision-making processes.

Operable tori or other bony exostoses should be removed to avoid compromises in the design and optimum location of major connectors.

LINGUAL BAR

INDICATIONS FOR USE: The lingual bar should be used for mandibular removable partial dentures wherein sufficient space exists between the slightly elevated alveolar lingual sulcus and the lingual gingival tissues to place a rigid bar.

CHARACTERISTICS AND LOCATION: (1) Half-pear shaped with bulkiest portion inferiorly located. (2) Superior border should be tapered to soft tissue. (3) Superior border located at least 4 mm inferior to gingival margins and more if possible. (4) Inferior border located at the ascertained height of the alveolar lingual sulcus when the patient's tongue is slightly elevated.

BLOCKOUT AND RELIEF OF MASTER CAST: (1) All tissue undercuts parallel to path of placement. (2) All tissue undercuts parallel to path of placement, plus an additional thickness of 24-gauge sheet wax when the lingual surface of the alveolar ridge is either undercut or parallel to the path of placement. (3) No relief necessary when the lingual surface of the alveolar ridge slopes inferiorly and posteriorly.

WAXING SPECIFICATIONS: (1) Six-gauge, half-pear-shaped wax form reinforced by 22- to 24-gauge wax sheet or similar plastic pattern adapted to design width. (2) Long bar requires more bulk than short bar; however, the cross-sectional shape remains the same.

FINISHING LINES: Butt-type joint(s) with minor connector(s) for retention of denture base(s).

MANDIBULAR LINGUOPLATE

INDICATIONS FOR USE: (1) Where the alveolar lingual sulcus so closely approximates lingual gingival crevices that adequate width for a rigid lingual bar does not exist. (2) In those instances in which the residual ridges in Class I arch have undergone such vertical resorption that they will offer only minimal resistance to horizontal rotations of the denture though its bases. (3) For utilizing periodontally weakened teeth in "group" function to furnish support to the prosthesis and to help resist horizontal (off-vertical) rotation of the distal extension–type denture. (4) When the future replacement of one or more incisor teeth will be facilitated by the addition of retention loops to an existing linguoplate.

CHARACTERISTICS AND LOCATION: (1) Half-pear shape with bulkiest portion inferiorly located. (2) Thin metal apron extending superiorly to contact cingula of anterior teeth and lingual surfaces of involved posterior teeth at their height of contour. (3) Apron extended interproximally to height of contact points, that is, closing interproximal spaces. (4) Scalloped contour of apron as dictated by interproximal blockout. (5) Superior border finished to continuous plane with contacted teeth. (6) Inferior border at the ascertained height of the alveolar lingual sulcus when the patient's tongue is slightly elevated.

BLOCKOUT AND RELIEF OF MASTER CAST: (1) All involved undercuts of contacted teeth parallel to the path of placement. (2) All involved gingival crevices. (3) Lingual of alveolar ridge the same as for a lingual bar.

WAXING SPECIFICATIONS: (1) Inferior border—6-gauge, half-pear-shaped wax reinforced with 24-gauge sheet wax or similar plastic pattern. (2) Apron—24-gauge sheet wax.

FINISHING LINES: Butt-type joint(s) with minor connector(s) for retention of denture base(s).

SINGLE STRAP–TYPE PALATAL MAJOR CONNECTORS

INDICATIONS FOR USE: Bilateral edentulous spaces of short span in a tooth-borne restoration.

CHARACTERISTICS AND LOCATION: (1) Anatomic replica form. (2) Anteror border follows the valleys between rugae as nearly as possible at right angles to median suture line. (3) Posterior border at right angle to median suture line. (4) Approximately as wide as the combined width of a maxillary premolar and first molar. (5) Confined within an area bounded by the four principal rests.

BLOCKOUT AND RELIEF OF MASTER CAST: Usually none required except slight relief of elevated median palatal raphe or any exostosis crossed by the connector.

WAXING SPECIFICATIONS: (1) Anatomic replica pattern equivalent to 22- to 24-gauge wax depending on arch width. (2) 22- to 24-gauge sheet wax reinforced with "faired" 14-gauge half-round wax form in the center portion when an anatomic replica pattern or matte pattern is not used.

FINISHING LINES: (1) Undercut and slightly elevated. (2) Follow curvature of arch. (3) No farther medially than 2 mm medial to an imaginary line contacting lingual surfaces of principal abutments and teeth to be replaced.

SINGLE BROAD PALATAL MAJOR CONNECTOR

INDICATIONS FOR USE: (1) Class I partially edentulous arches having residual ridges that have undergone little vertical resorption and will lend excellent support. (2) V- or U-shaped palates. (3) Strong abutments (single or made so by splinting). (4) More teeth in arch than six remaining anterior teeth. (5) Direct retention retainers do not offer a problem. (6) No interfering tori.

CHARACTERISTICS AND LOCATION: (1) Anatomic replica form. (2) Anterior border follows valleys of rugae as near right angle to median suture line as possible and does not extend anterior to occlusal rests or indirect retainers. (3) Posterior border located at junction of hard and soft palate but does not extend onto soft palate; at right angle to the median suture line; extended to pterygomaxillary notches.

BLOCKOUT AND RELIEF OF MASTER CAST: Usually none required except relief of elevated median palatal raphe or any small exostosis covered by the connector.

WAXING SPECIFICATIONS: Anatomic replica pattern equivalent to 24-gauge sheet wax thickness.

FINISHING LINES: (1) Provision for butt-type joint at pterygomaxillary notches. (2) Undercut and slightly elevated. (3) No farther medially than 2 mm to an imaginary line that would contact the lingual surfaces of the missing natural teeth. (4) Follow the curvature of the arch.

ANTERIOR-POSTERIOR STRAP–TYPE MAJOR CONNECTORS

INDICATIONS FOR USE: (1) Class I and II arches in which excellent abutment support and residual ridge support exists, and direct retention can be made adequate without the need for direct-indirect retention. (2) Long edentulous spans in Class II, modification 1 arches. (3) Class IV arches in which anterior teeth must be replaced with a removable partial denture. (4) Inoperable palatal tori that do not extend posteriorly to the junction of the hard and soft palates.

CHARACTERISTICS AND LOCATION: (1) Paralelogram shaped and open in center portion. (2) Relatively narrow (6 to 9 mm) anterior and posterior palatal straps. (3) Lateral palatal straps 5 to 6 mm broad and parallel to curve of arch; minimum of 6 mm away from gingival crevices of remaining teeth. (4) Anterior palatal strap: anterior border not placed farther anteriorly than anterior rests and never closer than 6 mm to lingual gingival crevices; follows the valleys of the rugae at right angles to the median palatal suture. Posterior border, if in rugae area, follows valleys of rugae at right angles to median palatal suture. (5) Posterior palatal strap: posterior border located at junction of hard and soft palates and at right angles to median palatal suture; half-oval in cross section o approximately 6-gauge thickness; extended to hamular notch area(s) on distal extension side(s). (6) Anatomic replica or matte surface.

BLOCKOUT AND RELIEF OF MASTER CAST: Usually none required except slight relief of elevated median palatal raphe where anterior or posterior straps cross the palate.

WAXING SPECIFICATIONS: (1) Anatomic replica patterns or matte surface forms of 22-gauge thickness. (2) Posterior palatal strap—half-oval form of approximately 6-gauge thickness and width.

FINISHING LINES: Same as for single broad palatal major connector.

FULL PALATAL COVERAGE MAJOR CONNECTORS

INDICATIONS FOR USE: (1) In most situations where only some or all anterior teeth remain. (2) Class II arch with a posterior modification space and some missing anterior teeth in distal extension edentulous area. (3) Class I arch with one to four premolars and some or all anterior teeth remaining, and abutment support is poor and cannot otherwise be enhanced; residual ridges have undergone extreme vertical resorption; direct retention is difficult to obtain. (4) In the absence of a pedunculated torus.

CHARACTERISTICS AND LOCATION: (1) Anatomic replica form for full palatal metal casting supported anteriorly by positive rest seats. (2) Palatal linguoplate supported anteriorly and designed for the attachment of acrylic resin extension posteriorly. (3) Contacts all or almost all the teeth remaining in the arch. (4) Posterior border: terminates at the junction of the hard and soft palates; extended to hamular notch area(s) on distal extension side(s); at a right angle to median suture line.

BLOCKOUT AND RELIEF OF MASTER CAST: Usually none required except relief of elevated median palatal raphe or any small palatal exostosis.

WAXING SPECIFICATIONS: (1) Anatomic replica pattern equivalent to 22- to 24-gauge sheet wax thickness. (2) Acrylic resin extension from linguoplate the same as for a complete denture.

FINISHING LINES: As illustrated here and previously discussed.

U-SHAPED PALATAL MAJOR CONNECTOR

This connector should be used only in those situations where inoperable tori extend to the posterior limit of the hard palate.

The U-shaped palatal major connector is the least favorable design of all palatal major connectors because it lacks the rigidity of other types of connectors. Where it must be used, any portion of the connector extending anteriorly from the principal occlusal rests must be supported by indirect retainers. Anterior border areas of this type of connector must be kept at least 6 mm away from adjacent teeth. If for any reason the anterior border must contact remaining teeth, the connector must again be supported by rests placed in properly prepared rest seats. It should never be supported even temporarily by inclined lingual surfaces of anterior teeth.

Waxing specifications, finishing lines, and so forth are the same as for full palatal castings or other similar major connectors previously discussed.

SELF-ASSESSMENT AIDS

1. A Class I removable partial denture will or should have six components. Can you name the components?
2. Define the term *major connector* in your own words.
3. Several desirable characteristics of major connectors are listed in the first few pages of chapter 4. Can you recall five of these characteristics?
4. What purposes are served by rigid major connectors as contrasted to a flexible connector?
5. Major connectors should be located in a favorable relation to moving tissues, gingival tissues, and areas of bony and tissue prominences. What difficulties would the patient encounter if the preceding is not carried out?
6. Can you name and draw the cross-sectional form of the basic mandibular connector?
7. Margins of major connectors adjacent to gingival tissues should be located far enough from those tissues to avoid possible impingement when the denture rotates from functional and parafunctional forces. The superior border of a lingual bar should be located at least _____ mm from gingival crevices.
8. The inferior border of a lingual bar is located as far inferiorly as possible without encroaching on the constantly moving tissues in the alveolar lingual sulcus. Can you describe two methods by which the location of the inferior border can be accurately determined?
9. Sufficient *relief* must be provided beneath a major connector to avoid impingement and gross displacement of soft tissues resulting in an inflammatory response. What is meant by the word relief? Can you rationalize planned relief for a lingual bar and give quantitative rules of thumb depending on the contour of the anterior, lingual alveolar ridge.
10. Discuss those clinical observations which indicate the choice of a lingual bar as a major connector.
11. What is the form of a mandibular linguoplate major connector?
12. Give four clinical observations that indicate utilizing a linguoplate rather than a lingual bar as a major connector.
13. Can you draw a sagittal section through a cast showing the basic form of a linguoplate?
14. Is there a difference in determining the location of the inferior borders for lingual bars and linguoplates?
15. Describe the superior extent of the apron portion of a linguoplate in relation to the lingual surfaces of teeth contacted by the major connector.
16. What are the indications for use of a lingual bar–continuous bar retainer type of major connector?
17. Interpret in your own words the rationale of the following statement made by McCracken: "No componet of a partial denture should be added arbitrarily or conventionally. Each component should be added for a good reason and to serve a definite purpose."
18. How may a linguoplate be modified to avoid an overdisplay of metal when used on an arch in which wide diastemas exist between anterior teeth?
19. The dentist alone is responsible for the design of the restoration, which is based on both biologic and mechanical principles. Can you give the dimensional specifications for developing the wax patterns of mandibular major connectors?
20. At what point in treating the partially edentulous patient must the choice of maxillary and mandibular major connectors be made? Rationalize your answer please.
21. There are basically four types of maxillary major connectors. Can you recall these four types of basic connectors?
22. What objections are usually manifested in use of the single bar–type palatal major connector?
23. Which type of palatal major connector is probably the most rigid and at the same time covers the smallest amount of soft tissues?
24. In what situations would you be most likely to use a single palatal strap–type major connector?
25. There are definite rules of thumb for the location of the anterior and posterior borders of all palatal major connectors. Can you relate borders to rugae, junction of hard and soft palates, gingival crevices, pterygomaxillary notches, and palatal tori?
26. Whenever it is necessary for the palatal major connector to make contact with the teeth for reasons of support, can adequate support be

obtained by resting the connector on tooth inclines?

27. Rationalize this statement: "Either support the connector by definite rests on the teeth contracted, bridging the gingivae with adequate relief, or locate the connector far enough away from the gingivae to avoid any possible restriction of blood supply and entrapment of food debris."

28. Why should all gingival crossings by components of a framework be abrupt and at right angles to the major connector and bridge the gingivae with adequate relief?

29. What clinical and diagnostic observations would lead you to select an anterior-posterior bar-type palatal major connector?

30. Under what circumstances is full palatal coverage by the major connector indicated?

31. Describe a palatal linguoplate major connector and tell why you would select such a design.

32. Can you look at a diagnostic cast of a Class I maxillary arch and apply the five steps outlined by Blatterfein for the design of palatal major connectors?

33. What is a *minor* connector?

34. What are the functions of minor connectors?

35. Should minor connectors be structurally rigid or flexible? Why?

36. Can you describe the shape of a minor connector contacting axial surfaces of adjacent abutments at interproximal areas?

37. Point out all minor connectors in this drawing.

38. Minor connectors used to attach acrylic resin denture bases to major connectors should be located on both buccal and lingual sides of the residual ridge. Why?

39. State rules of thumb for the form and length of minor connectors connecting acrylic resin denture bases to major connectors.

40. What advantages accrue to the restoration by having minor connectors for acrylic resin denture bases attached to the major connector in a butt-type joint?

41. Describe the best location for palatal finishing lines at the junction of major and minor connectors. How do you determine this optimal location on a cast? Why is it important that the natural contour of the palatal vault be restored with a removable restoration?

42. The last few pages in Chapter 4 review major connectors in cookbook style. Indications for use, characteristics and location, blockout and relief of master casts, waxing specifications, and finishing lines for major connectors are condensed. Your practice of dentistry will be more rewarding if you assimilate the information presented or at least have it available as reference material.

5 RESTS AND REST SEATS

Occlusal support for the partial denture must be provided by some kind of rests placed on the abutment teeth (Fig. 5-1). These always should be located upon tooth surfaces properly prepared to receive them.

Any unit of a partial denture that rests upon a tooth surface to provide vertical support to the denture is called a *rest*. A rest may be placed upon the occlusal surface of a premolar or molar tooth, upon the prepared lingual surface of an anterior tooth that is capable of withstanding the forces applied, or upon an incisal surface. Occlusal support is sometimes obtained upon a tooth surface inclined occlusally or incisally from its greatest convexity, but any rest so placed on an unprepared surface is subject to slippage along tooth inclines. This violates one of the basic rules for rest design: *a rest should be designed so that transmitted forces are directed along the long axis of the supporting tooth as nearly as possible.* A second rule is that *a rest must be placed so that it will prevent movement of the restoration in a cervical direction.*

In an all-tooth-borne denture the rests should be capable of transferring *all* the vertical occlusal stresses to the abutment teeth. This is one of the principal functions of a rest, in addition to preventing movement of the partial denture in a cervical direction. A tooth-supported denture may therefore function like a fixed partial denture, the rests serving the same purpose as the soldered unions of the pontic with the abutment crowns. For this degree of stability to exist, it is obvious that the rest must be rigid and must receive positive support from the abutment tooth.

In a removable partial denture having one or more distal extension bases, the denture becomes increasingly tissue supported as the distance from the abutment increases. Closer to the abutment, however, the occlusal load is transmitted to the abut-

ment tooth by means of the rest. The load is thereby distributed between the abutment and the supporting residual ridge tissues.

In addition to distributing the occlusal load, the rest serves other purposes. It acts to maintain the occlusal relationship with the opposing teeth by preventing settling of the partial denture. At the same time, settling of the denture against gingival tissues is prevented, thereby avoiding any impingement of the gingival tissues adjacent to the abutment teeth.

By the rest's preventing movement of the denture in a cervical direction, the position of the retentive portion of the clasp arm is maintained in its intended relation to the tooth undercut. Although passive when in its terminal position, the retentive portion of the clasp arm should remain in contact with the tooth, ready to resist a vertical dislodging force. Then when a dislodging force is applied, the clasp arm should immediately become active to resist vertical displacement. If because of settling of the denture the clasp arm is standing away from the tooth, some vertical displacement is possible before the retainer can become functional. The rest serves to prevent such settling and thereby helps to maintain the vertical stability of the partial denture. Rests are designated by the surface of the tooth prepared to receive the rest, that is, *occlusal rest, lingual rest, incisal rest.*

Form of the occlusal rest and rest seat. An occlusal rest is located upon the occlusal surface of a molar or premolar tooth that has been prepared to receive it (Fig. 5-2). The outline form of an occlusal rest seat should be a "rounded" triangular shape with the apex toward the center of the occlusal surface. It should be as long as it is wide, and the base of the triangular shape (at the marginal ridge) should be at least 2.5 mm for both premolars and molars. Rest

Fig. 5-1. A, Framework for tooth-supported removable partial denture. Arrows point to components (rests) located on specifically prepared areas of abutment teeth. Denture will be supported through three occlusal rests and one incisal rest on canine. **B,** Canines have been restored with ceramic-metal crowns on which lingual rest seats have been developed to support a linguoplate major connector. **C,** Tooth support for this framework is provided by rests occupying definite, prepared, lingual rest seats on canines and occlusal surfaces of posterior teeth. **D,** Maxillary bilateral distal extension removable partial denture supported by rests occupying lingual rest seats on canines. Rest seats were placed on three-quarter crowns.

**Deepest part of
rest preparation**

Fig. 5-2. Deepest part of an occlusal rest preparation should be inside lowered marginal ridge at X. Marginal ridge is lowered to accommodate origin of occlusal rest with the least occlusal interference without sacrificing bulk.

Fig. 5-3. Occlusal rest seat preparation on a molar. Preparation is rounded, triangular concavity having smooth margins on occlusal surface and a lowered, rounded marginal ridge.

seats of smaller dimensions do not provide for an adequate bulk of metal for rests, especially if the rest is contoured to restore the occlusal morphology of the abutment tooth. The marginal ridge of the abutment tooth at the site of the rest seat must be lowered to permit a sufficient bulk of metal for strength and rigidity of the rest and minor connector. This then means that a reduction of the marginal ridge of approximately 1.5 mm is usually necessary.

The floor of the occlusal rest seat should be apical to the marginal ridge and occlusal surface and should be concave or *spoon shaped* (Fig. 5-3). Caution should be exercised in preparing a rest seat to avoid creating *sharp edges or line-angles in the preparation.* The angle formed by the occlusal rest and the vertical minor connector from which it originates should be less than a right angle, or less than 90 degrees (Figs. 5-4 and 5-5). Only in this way can the occlusal forces be directed along the long axis of the abutment tooth. An angle greater than 90 degrees fails to transmit occlusal forces along the supporting axis of the abutment tooth. It also permits slippage of the prosthesis away from the abutment and causes orthodontic forces to be applied, which are the result of forces applied to an inclined plane (Fig. 5-6).

When an existing occlusal rest preparation on enamel or on an existing cast restoration cannot be modified or deepened because of fear of perforation of the enamel or gold, yet the existing floor is inclined apically toward the reduced marginal ridge, a secondary occlusal rest must be employed to prevent slippage of the primary rest and

orthodontic movement of the abutment tooth (Fig. 5-7). Such a rest should pass over the lowered marginal ridge on the side of the tooth opposite the primary rest and should, if possible, be inclined slightly apically from the marginal ridge. However, two opposing occlusal rests on diverging tooth inclines will function to prevent unfavorable forces if all related connectors are sufficiently rigid.

In any partly tissue-supported partial denture the relation of the occlusal rest to the abutment should be that of a shallow ball-and-socket joint so shaped to prevent a possible transfer of horizontal stresses to the abutment tooth. The occlusal rest should provide only occlusal support. Stabilization against horizontal movement of the prosthesis must be provided by other components of the partial denture rather than by any locking effect of the occlusal rest, which might cause the application of leverages to the abutment tooth.

Interproximal occlusal rest seats. The design of a direct retainer assembly quite frequently requires that interproximal occlusal rests be utilized (Fig. 5-8). The rest seats are prepared as adjoining occlusal rest seats with the exception that the preparations must be extended farther lingually than is ordinarily accomplished (Fig. 5-9). Adjacent rests rather than a single rest are used to avoid interproximal wedging by the framework. Additionally, the joined rests will shunt food away from contact points.

In preparing such rest seats, care must be exercised to avoid eliminating contact points of abutment teeth. Yet sufficient tooth structure must be removed to allow for adequate bulk of the component for strength and to

Fig. 5-4. Occlusal rest should be spoon shaped and slightly inclined apically from marginal ridge on an occlusal surface properly prepared to receive it. The rest should restore occlusal morphology of the tooth that existed prior to preparation of rest seat.

Fig. 5-5. Floor of occlusal rest seat should be inclined apically from lowered marginal ridge. Any angle less than 90 degrees is acceptable as long as disking of proximal surface and lowering and rounding of marginal ridge precede completion of rest seat itself.

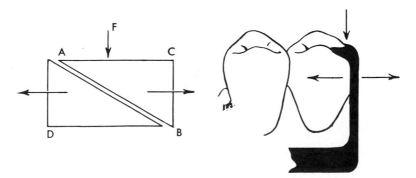

Fig. 5-6. Result of a force applied to an inclined plane when floor of an occlusal rest preparation inclines apically toward marginal ridge of abutment tooth. *F*, Occlusal force applied to abutment tooth. *AB*, Relationship of occlusal rest to abutment tooth when angle is greater than 90 degrees. *ABC*, Partial denture framework. *ABD*, Abutment tooth.

Fig. 5-7. A, An existing gold crown on the molar, having a previous, minimally prepared mesiocclusal rest seat, could be recontoured only on mesial proximal surface, with slight reduction of distal marginal ridge, without fear of penetrating the crown. Mesial and distal occlusal rests (each on an unfavorable inclined plane) were used to direct forces as near axially as possible. **B,** lingual view of **A.** Bar extension from cast base was used to attach direct retainer assembly to molar. Opposing arch was restored with a complete denture. **C,** Anterior tilt of molar precludes preparation of acceptable rest seat on mesiocclusal surface. Patient could not affort either a crown to improve axial alignment or orthodontic treatment to upright the molar. Occlusal rests were utilized on mesiocclusal and distocclusal surfaces to support restoration and direct forces over greatest root mass of abutment.

Fig. 5-8. Design of direct retainer assembly on left premolar abutments consisted of bar-type retainer arm engaging a distobuccal undercut on second premolar, a minor connector contacting guiding plane on distal of second premolar, and a reciprocal, stabilizing, supporting interproximal element. Joined occlusal rests occupy specifically prepared adjoining rest seats.

Fig. 5-9. Rest seat preparations on premolars fulfill requirements of properly prepared rest seats. Preparations are extended lingually to provide strength (through bulk) without overly filling interproximal space with minor connector. This type of preparation is rather difficult, and care must be exercised to avoid violation of contact points—yet marginal ridge of each abutment should be sufficiently lowered (1.5 mm).

permit the component to be so shaped that occlusion will not be altered.

Internal occlusal rests. A partial denture that is totally tooth supported by means of cast retainers on all abutment teeth may utilize internal occlusal rests for both occlusal support and horizontal stabilization (Figs. 5-10 to 5-12).

An internal occlusal rest is not in any way a retainer and therefore should not be confused with an internal attachment. The term *precision* is applied to both, *but any element of a partial denture should possess the accuracy and exactness synonymous with precision.*

Occlusal support is derived from the floor of the rest seat and from an additional occlusal bevel if such is provided. Horizontal stabilization is derived from the near-vertical walls. The form of the rest should be parallel to the path of placement, tapered slightly occlusally, and slightly dovetailed to prevent dislodgement proximally.

The principal advantages of the internal rest are that it facilitates the elimination of a visible clasp arm bucally and permits the location of the rest seat in a more favorable position in relation to the "tipping" axis (horizontal) of the abutment. Retention is provided by a lingual clasp arm, either cast or of wrought wire, lying in a natural or prepared infrabulge area on the abutment tooth.

Technical obstacles to the use of internal rests are gradually being overcome. Such a rest seat usually cannot satisfactorily be carved in wax or machined in gold. Ready-made plastic rest patterns are generally too bulky. Assembly of a ready-made rest similar to an internal attachment necessitates soldering operations and added cost. The best solution seems to be the use of a machined mandrel made of chrome-cobalt alloy,* which can be waxed into the crown or inlay pattern, invested, and cast-to, having been positioned parallel to the path of placement with a dental cast surveyor. The mandrel is easily tapped out, leaving the internal rest formed in the abutment casting. Further developments of this technique promise more widespread use of the internal occlusal rest but only for tooth-supported partial dentures.

Possible movements of partial denture. At least three possible movements of a distal extension partial denture exist. One is rotation about an axis through the most posterior abutments. This axis may be through occlusal

---

*Ticon PRP mandrel and surveyor fixture, Ticonium Division, CMP Industries, Inc., Albany, N.Y.

Fig. 5-10. Mandibular internal rest partial denture. **A,** Abutment crowns with internal rests. Both dovetail design and a gingival well prevent horizontal movement. **B,** Completed partial denture framework with cast lingual retention on all four abutments. A short buccal stabilizing and removal arm is used on molar abutments.

Fig. 5-11. Mandibular internal rest partial denture. **A,** Internal rests in four abutment crowns. **B,** Occlusal view showing proximal guiding planes. **C,** Buccal view showing machined parallelism of proximal surface. **D,** Completed gold alloy casting with wrought-wire lingual retention on all four abutments. Use of a buccal stabilizing arm is optional.

Fig. 5-12. Maxillary internal rest partial denture. **A,** Internal rest seats in four abutment crowns. **B,** Completed partial denture with lingual retentive clasp arms on canine and premolar abutments. **C** and **D,** Buccal views of completed restoration showing abutted resin teeth (upon which gold occlusal surfaces will be fabricated) and absence of visible clasp arms on premolar abutments.

rests or any other rigid portion of a direct retainer assembly located occlusally or incisally to the height of contour of the abutments (Fig. 5-13, A). This axis, known as the *fulcrum line*, is the center of rotation as the distal extension base moves *toward* the supporting tissues when an occlusal load is applied. The axis of rotation shifts to anteriorly placed elements, occlusal or incisal to the height of abutment contour, as the base moves *away* from the supporting tissues when vertical dislodging forces become effective. These dislodging forces are the vertical pull of food between opposing tooth surfaces, the effect of moving border tissues, and the forces of gravity against a maxillary denture. Presuming that the direct retainers are functional and that the supportive anterior elements remain seated, rotation rather than total displacement occurs. Vertical tissueward movement of the denture base is resisted by the tissues of the residual ridge in proportion to the supporting quality of

those tissues, the accuracy of the fit of the denture base, and the total amount of occlusal load applied. Movement of the base in the opposite direction is resisted by the action of the retentive arms of clasps on terminal abutments in conjunction with seated, vertical support elements of the framework anterior to the terminal abutments acting as indirect retainers. Of course, unless supporting elements anterior to the terminal abutments are seated when a dislodging force is initiated, the axis of rotation will run through the retentive tips of direct retainers (clasps) on the terminal abutments.

A second movement is rotation about a longitudinal axis as the distal extension base moves in a rotary direction about the residual ridge (Fig. 5-13, B). This movement is resisted primarily by the rigidity of the major connector and its ability to resist torque. If the major connector is not rigid or if a stressbreaker exists between the distal extension base and the major connector, this rota-

Fig. 5-13. Three possible movements of distal extension partial denture. **A,** Rotation around fulcrum line passing through the two principal occlusal rests when denture base moves toward supporting residual ridges. **B,** Rotation around a longitudinal axis formed by crest of residual ridge. **C,** Rotation around a vertical axis located near center of arch.

tion about a longitudinal axis either applies undue stress to the sides of the supporting ridge or causes horizontal shifting of the denture base.

A third movement is rotation about an imaginary vertical axis located near the center of the dental arch (Fig. 5-13, *C*). This movement occurs under function as diagonal and horizontal occlusal forces are brought to bear upon the partial denture. It is resisted by stabilizing components, such as reciprocal clasp arms and minor connectors that are in contact with vertical tooth surfaces. Such stabilizing components are essential to any partial denture design regardless of the manner of support and the type of direct retention employed. Stabilizing components on one side of the arch act to stabilize the partial denture against horizontal forces applied from the opposite side. It is obvious that rigid connectors must be employed to make this effect possible.

Horizontal forces always will exist to some degree because of lateral stresses occurring during mastication and bruxism. The magnitude of lateral stress may be minimized by fabricating an occlusion that is in harmony with the opposing dentition and free of lateral interference during excursive jaw movements. The amount of horizontal shift occurring in the partial denture will therefore depend upon the magnitude of lateral forces applied and the effectiveness of the stabilizing components.

In a tooth-borne partial denture, movement of the base *toward* the edentulous ridge is prevented primarily by the rests on the abutment teeth and to some degree by any rigid portion of the framework located occlusal to the height of contour. Movement *away* from the edentulous ridge is prevented by the action of direct retainers on the abutments, situated at each end of each edentulous space. Therefore the first of the three possible movements is nonexistent in the tooth-borne denture. The second possible movement, which is about a longitudinal axis, is prevented by the rigid components of the direct retainers on the abutment teeth as well as by the ability of the major connector to resist torque. This movement is much less in the tooth-borne denture because of the presence of posterior abutments. The third possible movement occurs in any partial denture; therefore stabilizing components against horizontal movement must be incorporated into any partial denture design.

The functions of the occlusal rest are not directly involved in either of the latter two movements. Instead the occlusal rest should provide occlusal support only. All movements of the partial denture other than in a gingival direction should be resisted by other components. For the occlusal rest to enter into a stabilizing function would result in a direct transfer of torque to the abutment tooth. Since three movements are possible in a distal extension partial denture, an occlusal rest for such a partial denture should not have steep vertical walls or locking dovetails, which could possibly cause horizontal and torquing forces to be applied intracoronally to the abutment tooth.

In the tooth-borne denture the only movements of any significance are horizontal, and these may be resisted by the stabilizing effect of components placed on the axial surfaces of the several abutments. Therefore, in the tooth-borne denture the use of intracoronal rests is permissible. In such usage the rests provide not only occlusal support but also horizontal stabilization to some degree.

Force distribution in a tooth-supported partial denture is, or should be, such that each abutment tooth is assisted by others in the dental arch, and possible movements of the partial denture under function are held within acceptable physiologic limitations. It is therefore possible and acceptable to utilize an intracoronal type of occlusal rest if desired in any tooth-supported situation. In such a case vertical walls of an internal occlusal rest may be utilized to transfer horizontal forces to the abutment teeth and, by so doing, stabilize the partial denture against horizontal movement. An internal occlusal rest can thus be substituted

for an external stabilizing clasp arm and, by utilizing a retentive clasp arm on the lingual surface of an abutment tooth, can eliminate altogether the necessity for a visible clasp arm buccally or labially.

The use of intracoronal rests and intracoronal direct retainers is optional with the tooth-borne denture. However, with the distal extension denture the ball-and-socket type of rest or the nonlocking internal rest is preferable and should be used whenever possible.

Support for rests. Rests may be placed upon sound enamel, cast restorations, or silver amalgam alloy restorations. The use of a silver amalgam alloy restoration as support for an occlusal rest is the least desirable because of its tendency to flow under pressure and also because of the comparative weakness of a marginal ridge made of this alloy.

Rests placed on sound enamel are not conducive to caries in a mouth with a low caries index, provided good oral hygiene is maintained. Proximal tooth surfaces are much more vulnerable to caries attack than are the occlusal surfaces supporting an occlusal rest. The decision to use abutment coverage is usually based upon proximal and cervical vulnerability of the tooth rather than upon the vulnerability of an occlusal rest area. When precarious fissures are found in the occlusal rest areas in teeth that are otherwise sound, they may be removed and restored, preferably with gold foil, without resorting to more extensive abutment protection.

Whereas it cannot be denied that the best protection from caries for an abutment tooth is full coverage, it must be presumed that such crowns will be contoured properly to provide support and retention for the partial denture and that full coverage restorations will provide subgingival protection to the tooth. Little is accomplished by the placement of full crowns if the more vulnerable cervical areas of an abutment tooth are not fully protected.

In making the decision whether to use unprotected enamel surfaces for rests, future vulnerability must be considered, for it is not easy to fabricate full crowns later to accommodate rests and clasp arms. In many instances sound enamel may be used safely for the support of occlusal rests.

In such situations the patient should be advised that future caries susceptibility is not predictable and that much will depend upon his oral hygiene and possible future changes in his caries susceptibility. Although the decision to use unprotected abutments logically should be left up to the dentist, economic factors may influence the final decision. The patient should be made aware of the risks involved and of his responsibility for maintaining good oral hygiene and for returning periodically for observation.

Rest seat preparations in sound enamel. In most instances, disking of proximal tooth surfaces is necessary to provide proximal guiding planes and to eliminate undesirable undercuts that rigid parts of the framework must pass during its placement and removal. The preparation of occlusal rest seats *always must follow proximal disking*, never precede it. Only after the disking is completed may the location of the occlusal rest seat in relation to the marginal ridge be determined. When disking follows the preparation of the occlusal rest seat, the inevitable consequence is that the marginal ridge is too low and too sharp, with the center of the floor of the rest seat too close to the marginal ridge. Therefore it is often impossible to correct the rest preparation without making it too deep, and then irreparable damage has been done to the tooth.

Occlusal rest seats in sound enamel may be prepared with diamond points of approximately the size of Nos. 6 and 8 round burs or with carbide burs (Fig. 5-14). The larger of the two diamonds is used first to lower the marginal ridge and to establish the outline

Fig. 5-14. Recontouring of axial surfaces and rest seat preparations in enamel may be readily accomplished by selected use of pictured accessories (from top, left to right): round carbide burs, round diamond stones, tapered diamond stone with round end, cylindric diamond stone, inverted cone diamond stone, wet or dry sanding disks, abrasive rubber polishing disks and points, and pointed brush and polishing cup to be used with flour of pumice.

form of the rest seat. The resulting occlusal rest seat is then complete except that the floor is not sufficiently concave. The smaller diamond point is then used to deepen the floor of the occlusal rest seat, at the same time forming the desired spoon shape inside the lowered marginal ridge. Smoothing the enamel rods by the planing action of a round bur of suitable size revolving at moderate speed, followed by the use of an abrasive rubber point, is usually the only polishing needed.

When a small enamel defect is encountered in the preparation of an occlusal rest seat, it is usually best to ignore it until the rest reparation has been completed and then, with small burs, prepare the remaining defect to receive a small gold foil restoration. This then may be finished flush with the floor of the rest preparation previously established.

Occlusal rest seat preparations in existing restorations are treated the same as those in sound enamel. Any proximal disking must be done first, for if the occlusal rest seat is placed first and then the proximal surface is disked, the outline form of the occlusal rest seat is sometimes irreparably altered.

There is always a possibility that an existing restoration may be perforated in the process of preparing an ideal occlusal rest seat. Although some compromise is permissible, the effectiveness of the occlusal rest seat should not be jeopardized for fear of perforating an existing inlay or crown. The rest seat may be widened to compensate for its shallowness, but the floor of the rest seat should still be slightly inclined apically from the marginal ridge. When this is not possible, a secondary occlusal rest should be used on the opposite side of the tooth to prevent slipping of the primary rest.

When perforation does occur, it may be filled with gold foil, but occasionally the making of a new restoration is unavoidable. In such a situation the original crown or inlay preparation should be modified to accommodate the occlusal rest, which is then placed in the wax pattern to avoid risking again the perforation of the completed restoration.

Occlusal rest seats in new restorations always should be placed in the wax pattern. The location of the occlusal rest should be known at the time that the tooth is prepared for a crown or an inlay so that sufficient clearance may be provided in the preparation for the rest. The final step in the preparation of the tooth should be to make sure that such clearance exists and, if not, to make a depression to accommodate the depth of the rest (Fig. 5-15).

Occlusal rest seats in crowns and inlays are generally made somewhat larger and deeper than are those in enamel. Those made in abutment crowns supporting tooth-borne dentures may be made slightly deeper than those in abutments supporting a distal extension base, thus approaching the effectiveness of boxlike internal rests.

Internal rest seats also should be created first in wax, either with suitable burs in a handpiece holder or by waxing around a lubricated mandrel held in the surveyor. In either situation the rest preparation must be finished on the casting with burs in a handpiece holder or with a precision drill press. Plastic and metal shoes that fit over

Fig. 5-15. A, Pattern for full crown on molar has been carved to meet the requirements of occlusion and optimal location of direct retainer components. Occlusal rest seat has been prepared on mesiocclusal surface. **B,** Pattern is removed from the die. Note concavity in prepared abutment to accommodate an adequate depth for occlusal rest seat on finished crown. The need for such a procedure is determined by observation of accurately mounted diagnostic casts before abutment preparation is initiated.

a mandrel are also available for this purpose, thus assuring a smooth casting and eliminating the need for finishing the inside of the internal rest with burs. Sufficient clearance must have been provided in the preparation of the abutment to accommodate the depth of the internal rest.

Lingual rests on canines and incisor teeth. Whereas the preferred site for an external rest is the occlusal surface of a molar or premolar, an anterior tooth may be the only abutment available for occlusal support of the denture. Also, an anterior tooth occasionally must be used to support an indirect retainer or an auxiliary rest. A canine is much preferred over an incisor for this purpose. When a canine is not present, multiple rests spread over several incisor teeth are preferable to the use of a single incisor. Root form, root length, inclination of the tooth, and ratio of the length of the clinical crown to the alveolar support must be considered in determining the site and form of rests placed on incisors.

A lingual rest is preferable to an incisal rest because it is placed nearer the horizontal axis of rotation (tipping) of the abutment and therefore will have less tendency to tip the tooth. In addition, lingual rests are more esthetically acceptable than are incisal rests.

If an anterior tooth is sound and the lingual slope is gradual rather than perpendicular, a lingual rest may sometimes be placed in an enamel seat at or just incisally to the cingulum (Fig. 5-16). *This type of lingual rest is usually confined to maxillary canines having a gradual lingual incline and a prominent cingulum.* In a few instances such a rest also may be placed on maxillary central incisors. The lingual slope of the mandibular canine is usually too steep for an adequate lingual rest seat to be placed in the enamel, and some other provision for rest support must be made. *Lingual rest seat preparations in enamel are rarely satisfactory because of a lack of thickness of enamel in which to prepare a seat of adequate form to be truly supportive.*

The preparation of an anterior tooth to receive a lingual rest may be accomplished in one of two ways. These are as follows:

1. A slightly "rounded" V is prepared on the lingual surface at the junction of the gingival and middle one third of the tooth.

The apex of the V is directed incisally. A preparation may be started by using an inverted cone-shaped diamond stone and progressing to smaller, tapered stones with round ends to complete the preparation. All line angles must be eliminated, and the enamel seat must be highly polished. Shaped, abrasive rubber polishing points, following by flour of pumice, produce an adequately smooth and polished rest seat. A predetermined path of placement for the denture must be kept in mind in preparing the rest seat. The lingual rest seat must not be prepared as though it were going to be approached from a direction perpendicular to the lingual slope. The floor of the rest seat should be toward the cingulum rather than the axial wall (Fig. 5-17). Care must be taken not to create an enamel undercut, which would interfere with placement of the denture.

2. The most satisfactory lingual rest, from the standpoint of support, is one placed on a prepared rest seat in a cast restoration (Fig. 5-18). This is done most effectively by planning and executing a rest seat in the wax pattern rather than by attempting to cut a rest in a cast restoration in the mouth. The contour of the framework may then restore the lingual form of the tooth.

By accentuating the cingulum in the wax pattern, the floor of the rest seat is readily carved to be the most apical portion of the preparation. A saddlelike shape, which provides a positive rest seat located favorably in relation to the long axis of the tooth, is thus formed. The framework of the denture is made to fill out the continuity of the lingual surface so that the tongue contacts a smooth surface without the patient's being conscious of bulk or irregularities.

The lingual rest may be placed on the lingual surface of a cast veneer crown, a three-quarter crown, or some type of inlay (Fig. 5-19). The latter displays less metal than the three-quarter crown, especially on the mandibular canine where the lingual rest placed on a cast restoration is frequently used, and it is a more conservative restoration. The three-quarter crown may be used if the labial surface of the tooth is sound and retentive contours are satisfactory. However, if the labial surface presents inadequate or excessive contours for placement of a retentive clasp arm, or if gingival decalcification

Fig. 5-16. Lingual rest seat placed in enamel just incisally to cingulum. Its preparation requires slight reduction of a portion of cingulum. Rest seat preparation should be confined to maxillary canines and central incisors that have an exaggerated cingulum.

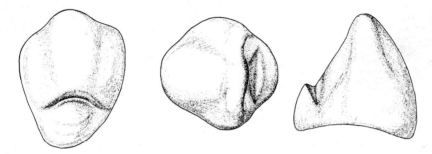

Fig. 5-17. Three views of a lingual rest seat prepared in enamel of maxillary canine. The rest seat, from lingual aspect, assumes form of a broad inverted V, maintaining natural contour sometimes seen in a maxillary canine cingulum. Inverted V notch form is self-centering for the rest and at the same time directs forces rather favorably in an apical direction. Looking at preparation from an incisal view, it will be noted that rest seat preparation is broadest at most lingual aspect of canine. As preparation approaches proximal surfaces of tooth, it is less broad than at any other areas. A proximal view demonstrates correct taper of floor of rest seat. It also should be noted that borders of rest seat are slightly rounded to avoid line angles in its preparation. Mesiodistal length of preparation should be a minimum of 2.5 to 3 mm, labiolingual width about 2 mm, and incisal-apical depth a minimum of 1.5 mm. It is a risky preparation and should not be attempted on lower anterior teeth.

Fig. 5-18. Rest seat preparation can be exaggerated for better support when it is prepared in a metallic restoration.

Fig. 5-19. A, Master cast from which a removable partial denture framework will be constructed. Properly contoured lingual rest seat was placed in a veneer crown for canine abutment. **B,** Positive vertical support for prosthesis is furnished by rest seats prepared in splinted three-quarter crowns on lateral and central incisors. These rest seats are optimally placed on incisors as near horizontal axis of rotation as possible. **C,** Lingual rest seat placed in this pin-retained inlay is cup shaped and is confined within inlay itself. **D,** Lingual rest seats on mandibular canines contained within pin onlays. Suitable rest seats could not be prepared in the enamel. Pin onlay is a more conservative and esthetically desirable restoration than is a three-quarter crown to accomplish the same end results. (Courtesy Dr. Robert Matteson, Gainesville, Fla.)

or caries is present, a veneered full crown should be used.

Incisal rests and rest seats. Incisal rests are placed at the incisal angles of anterior teeth and on prepared rest seats. Although this is the least desirable placement of rest types for reasons previously mentioned, it may be used successfully for selected patients when the abutment is sound and when a cast restoration is not otherwise indicated. Therefore incisal rests generally are placed on enamel (Fig. 5-20). Incisal rests are used predominantly as auxiliary rests or as indirect retainers.

Although the incisal rest may be used on a canine abutment in either arch, it is more applicable to the mandibular canine. This type of rest provides definite support with relatively little loss of tooth structure and little display of metal. Esthetically it is preferable to the three-quarter crown (Fig. 5-21). The same criteria apply is deciding whether to use unprotected enamel for an occlusal rest on a molar or premolar. An incisal rest is more likely to lead to some orthodontic movement of the tooth because of unfavorable leverage factors than is a lingual rest.

An incisal rest seat is prepared in the form of a rounded notch at an incisal angle or on an incisal edge, with the deepest portion of the preparation apical to the incisal edge (Fig. 5-22). The notch should be beveled both labially and lingually, and the lingual

Fig. 5-20. **A** and **B**, Incisal rest seat placed in mesial incisal edge of a lower canine. Note that contact point is not involved in preparation of rest seat to support a linguoplate (as seen in **C**). **D**, Distal incisal rest on canine furnished excellent vertical support for tooth-borne removable partial denture and is not too objectionable esthetically.

Fig. 5-21. Incisal rests are utilized on this removable partial denture and are more acceptable esthetically than three-quarter crowns in which lingual rest seats may be placed.

Fig. 5-22. Three views of an incisal rest seat preparation on a mandibular canine adjacent to a modification space. Labial view demonstrates inclination of floor of rest seat so that forces will be directed along the long axis of tooth as nearly as possible. Note that floor of rest seat has been extended slightly onto labial aspect of tooth. As seen from a proximal view, proximal edge of rest seat is rounded rather than straight. Lingual view shows that all borders of rest seat are rounded to avoid sharp line angles. It is especially important to avoid a line angle at junction of axial wall of preparation and floor of rest seat. The rest that occupies such a preparation should be able to move slightly in a lateral direction to avoid torquing the abutment tooth.

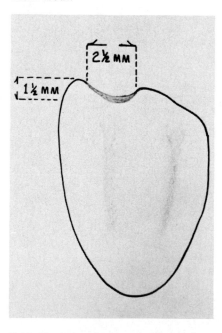

Fig. 5-23. Dimension given in illustration for an incisal rest seat preparation will provide adequate strength of framework at junction of the rest and minor connector. Rest seats of smaller dimension have proved unsatisfactory regardless of metal alloy from which framework is made.

enamel should be partly shaped to accommodate the rigid minor connector connecting the rest to the framework. An incisal rest seat should be approximately 2.5 mm wide and 1.5 mm deep so that the rest will be strong without having to exceed the natural contour of the incisal edge (Fig. 5-23).

It is, of course, essential that both the master cast and the casting be accurate if the rest is to seat properly. The incisal rest should be overcontoured slightly to allow for labial and incisal finishing to the adjoining enamel in much the same manner as a three-quarter crown or inlay margin is finished to enamel. In this way minimal display of metal is possible without jeopardizing the effectiveness of the rest.

Care in selecting the type of rest seat to be used, in preparing it, and in fabricating the framework casting does much to assure the success of any type of rest. *The topography of any rest should be such that it restores the topography of the tooth existing before the rest seat was prepared.*

SELF-ASSESSMENT AIDS

1. Define the word *rest* as a component of a removable partial denture.
2. What are the functions of a rest?
3. Rests are designated by the surface of the tooth prepared to receive the rest. Therefore rests are _____ rests, or _____ rests, or _____ rests.
4. Can you describe the form of an adequately prepared occlusal rest seat?
5. Where is the "deepest" portion of an occlusal rest seat located?
6. Can you diagram the approximate dimensions of an occlusal rest seat on a molar? A premolar?
7. Why should the angle formed by the rest and the vertical minor connector from which it originates be less than 90 degrees?
8. Under what circumstances would you elect to prepare a secondary occlusal rest seat on the same tooth?

9. Describe the form of adjacent, interproximal occlusal rest seats.

10. What advantages are gained by utilizing adjacent, interproximal occlusal rest seats rather than a single interproximal rest seat?

11. Can you describe an internal occlusal rest seat and relate the circumstances under which it may be used?

12. How do you go about fabricating an internal occlusal rest seat?

13. Rests may be placed upon sound enamel, cast restorations, or silver amalgam alloy restorations. Which of the three structures is least desirable for support of the rests? Why?

14. When preparing occlusal rest seats immediately adjacent to a proximal surface that has to be recontoured for optimal location of other components, which is accomplished first— rest seat preparation or recontouring of axial surface of abutment? Defend your answer.

15. What is the sequence of operations in preparing an occlusal rest seat in enamel? Name the cutting and polishing instruments used.

16. How is a small enamel defect encountered in preparing a rest seat handled?

17. Suppose you expose dentin in preparing an occlusal rest seat in enamel—what then?

18. Describe the form of a lingual rest seat preparation.

19. Which unrestored teeth may sometimes have such a lingual contour that an acceptable lingual rest seat may be prepared in enamel?

20. Five morphologic or anatomic factors must be evaluated in determining whether an abutment can support a lingual rest. Can you enumerate these five factors?

21. Most often, unrestored canines and incisors should not be used for supports for lingual rests. Why?

22. For what reasons should a rounded, inverted V notch form be used for a lingual rest seat?

23. Can you state the minimum dimensions for a lingual rest seat mesiodistally, labiolingually, and incisal-apically?

24. Please give the sequence of use of rotary instruments in preparing a lingual rest seat in enamel.

25. The design of a framework is such that lingual rest seats must be placed on incisor teeth, yet dentin will knowingly be exposed in preparing acceptable rest seats. What are your options for providing adequate rest seats on the incisors?

26. The adequacy of a lingual rest seat is better accomplished with a cast restoration than a preparation confined to enamel. True or false?

27. Describe the contour of an incisal rest seat preparation.

28. What are the minimum acceptable dimensions of an incisal rest seat?

29. Can you think of several indications for the use of incisal rests?

30. Which rest is the most unfavorable in relation to a possible tipping of the tooth? Which is the most favorable to avoid unfavorable leverage factors?

31. For what reasons must a rest restore the occlusal, lingual, or incisal morphology of the abutment tooth that existed prior to the rest seat preparation?

6 DIRECT RETAINERS

A removable partial denture must have *support*, derived from the abutment teeth through the use of rests and from the residual ridge through well-fitting bases. It must be *stabilized against horizontal movement* through the use of rigid components such as reciprocal clasp arms and the contact of minor connectors with vertical tooth surfaces. It must be *stabilized against rotational movement and resulting torque* through the use of rigid connectors, indirect retainers, and other stabilizing components. In addition, the removable partial denture must have sufficient *retention* to resist reasonable dislodging forces.

Retention for the removable partial denture is accomplished mechanically by placing retaining elements on the abutment teeth and by the intimate relationship of denture bases and maxillary and major connectors with the underlying tissues. The latter is similar to the retention of complete dentures and is proportionate to the accuracy of the impression registration, the accuracy of the fit of the denture bases, and the total area of contact involved.

Retention of denture bases has been described as the result of the following forces: (1) adhesion, which is the attraction of the saliva to the denture and to the tissues; (2) cohesion, which is the attraction of the molecules of the saliva for each other; (3) atmospheric pressure, which is dependent on a border seal and results in a partial vacuum beneath the denture base when a dislodging force is applied; (4) the plastic molding of the tissues around the polished surfaces of the denture; and (5) the effect of gravity on the mandibular denture. Boucher, writing on the subject of complete denture impressions, describes these forces as follows:

Adhesion and cohesion are effective when there is perfect apposition of the impression surface of the denture to the mucous membrane surfaces. These forces lose their effec-tiveness if there is any horizontal displacement of the dentures that breaks the continuity of this contact. Atmospheric pressure is effective primarily as a rescue force when extreme dislodging forces are applied to the denture. It depends on a perfect border seal to keep the pressure applied on only one side of the denture. The presence of air on the impression surface would neutralize the pressure of the air against the polished surface. Since each of these forces is directly proportional to the area covered by the dentures, the dentures should be extended to the limits of the oral cavity.

The plastic molding of the soft tissues around the polished surfaces of dentures helps to perfect the border seal. Also, it forms a mechanical lock at certain locations on the dentures, provided these surfaces are prepared for it. This lock is developed automatically and without effort by the patient if the impression is made with an understanding of the anatomic possibilities.*

Although few partial dentures are made without some mechanical retention, retention from the denture bases may contribute significantly to the overall retention of the partial denture and therefore must not be discounted as a retentive force. *Denture bases should be designed and fabricated so that they will contribute as much retention to the partial denture as possible.* However, it is questionable whether atmospheric pressure plays an important role in retention of removable partial dentures since a "border seal" cannot be obtained as can be accomplished with complete dentures. Therefore adhesion and cohesion gained by excellent apposition of the denture base and soft tissues of the basal seat do play an important retentive roll.

---

*Paraphrased from Boucher, C. O.: Complete denture impressions based upon the anatomy of the mouth, J. Am. Dent. Assoc. **31**:1174-1181, 1944.

Fig. 6-1. This intracoronal retainer consists of a key and keyway system with an extremely small tolerance. The keyway is placed totally within the metallic crown on the abutment tooth, and the key is attached to the removable partial denture framework. There is a frictional resistance to removal and placement as well as a limitation of movement of the prosthesis other than placement and removal.

Fig. 6-2. Extracoronal direct retainer (mirror view). The assembly consists of a slightly flexible retentive arm, a very limited flexing stabilizing-reciprocal arm, and a supporting element, the occlusal rest. Terminal portion of retentive arm engages a measured undercut in the abutment, and assembly remains *passive* until activated by either placement or removal of restoration or a slight rotation when a force is applied to denture. Note especially the greatly reduced taper of lingual reciprocal clasp arm to make it reasonably rigid or nonflexing.

Mechanical retention of removable partial dentures is accomplished by means of direct retainers of one type or another. A direct retainer is any unit of a removable dental prosthesis that engages an abutment tooth in such a manner as to resist *displacement* of the prosthesis away from basal seat tissues. This may be accomplished by frictional means, by engaging a depression in the abutment tooth, or by engaging a tooth undercut lying cervically to the height of contour.

There are two basic types of direct retainers. One is the *intracornal* retainer, which engages vertical walls built into the crown of the abutment tooth to create frictional resistance to removal (Fig. 6-1). The other type is the *extracoronal* retainer, which engages an external surface of the abutment tooth in an area cervical to the greatest convexity or in a depression created for that purpose. Rather than creating frictional resistance to removal, *a flexible arm is forced to deform, or a spring device is compressed, thereby generating resistance to removal.* The most common extracoronal attachment is the *retentive clasp arm* (Fig. 6-2).

The intracoronal retainer is usually spoken of as an *internal attachment,* or a *precision attachment.* The principle of the internal attachment was first formulated by Dr. Herman E. S. Chayes in 1906, and the attachment manufactured commercially carries his name. Although it may be fabricated by the dental technician as a cast dovetail fitting into a counterpart receptacle in the abutment crown, the alloys used in manufactured attachments and the precision with which they are constructed make the ready-made attachment much preferable to any of this type that can be fabricated in the dental laboratory. Much credit is due the manufacturers of precious metals used in dentistry for their continued improvements in the design of internal attachments and in the development of precise techniques for their use.

Some of the better-known internal attachments are the Ney-Chayes attachment, the Stern-Goldsmith attachment, the Brown attachment, the Baker attachment, and the Williams attachment. Descriptive literature and technique manuals are available from the manufacturers.

INTERNAL ATTACHMENTS

The internal attachment has two major advantages over the extracornal attachment: elimination of a visible retentive component and of a visible vertical support through a rest seat located more favorably in relation to the horizontal axis of the abutment tooth. For this reason the internal attachment may be preferable in selected situations. It provides some horizontal stabilization similar to that of an internal rest, but some additional stabilization extracoronally is usually desirable. It has been claimed that stimulation to the underlying tissues is greater when internal attachments are used because of intermittent vertical massage. This is probably no more than is possible with extracoronal retainers of similar construction.

Some of the disadvantages of internal attachments are that (1) they require prepared abutments and castings, (2) they require somewhat complicated clinical and laboratory procedures, (3) they eventually wear, with resulting loss of frictional resistance to denture removal, (4) they are difficult to repair and replace, (5) they are effective in proportion to their length and are therefore least effective on short teeth, and (6) they are difficult to place completely within the circumference of an abutment tooth.

Since the internal attachment must be built within the coronal limits of the tooth, a large pulp may be jeopardized by the depth of the receptacle. Because it depends on frictional resistance for retention, crown length must be sufficient to provide adequate frictional surfaces. The cost of an internal attachment prosthesis is necessarily higher than is a restoration of similar construction utilizing extracoronal retainers, even when the latter utilizes abutment castings. Limitations to the use of internal attachments are (1) size of pulp, which is usually related to age of the patient, (2) length of the clinical crown, which may prevent use on short or abraded teeth, and (3) greater cost to the patient.

Since the principle of the internal attachment does not permit horizontal movement, all horizontal, tipping, and rotational movements of the prosthesis are transmitted directly to the abutment tooth. *The internal attachment therefore should not be used in conjunction with tissue-supported distal extension denture bases unless some form of stressbreaker is used between the movable base and the rigid attachment.* Whereas stressbreakers may be used, they do have some disadvantages, which will be discussed later, and their use adds further to the cost of the partial denture. It is doubtful that the possible advantages of the stress-broken, internal-attachment denture are available to but a small percentage of the population needing a removable partial denture service.

EXTRACORONAL DIRECT RETAINERS

Although the extracoronal or clasp direct retainer is used many times more frequently than the internal attachment, it is also all too frequently misused. It is hoped that a better understanding of the principles of clasp design will lead to more intelligent use of this retainer in the future.

Clasp retention is based upon the resistance of metal to deformation. For a clasp to be retentive, it must be placed in an undercut area of the tooth, where it is forced to deform when a vertical dislodging force is applied. It is this resistance to deformation that generates retention. Such resistance is proportionate to the flexibility of the clasp arm.

It should be clearly understood that a retentive undercut exists only in relation to a given path of placement and removal, for if the path of escapement of the retentive clasp is parallel to the path of removal of the prosthesis, no retentive undercut exists.

A positive path of placement and removal is made possible by the contact of rigid parts of the denture framework with parallel tooth surfaces, which act as guiding planes. It is also made possible, to some extent, by simultaneous tooth contact on either side of the dental arch as the prosthesis is placed and removed. If some degree of parallelism does not exist during placement and removal, trauma to the teeth and supporting structures, as well as strain on the denture parts, is inevitable. This ultimately results in damage either to the teeth and their periodontal support, or to the denture itself, or both. Therefore, without guiding planes, clasp retention will either be detrimental or practically nonexistent. If clasp retention is only frictional, because of an *active* relationship of the clasp to the teeth, orthodontic movement or damage to periodontal tissues or both will result. *Instead a clasp should bear a passive relationship to the teeth except when a dislodging force is applied.*

To be retentive a tooth must have a height of contour cervical to which the surface converges. Although most any single tooth when surveyed will have a height of contour or an area of greatest convexity, areas of cervical convergence may not exist when the tooth is viewed in relation to a given path of placement. Also, certain areas of cervical convergence may not be available for the placement of retentive clasps because of their proximity to gingival tissues.

This is best illustrated by mounting a spherical object such as an egg on the adjustable table of a dental surveyor (Fig. 6-3 A). The egg now represents the cast of a dental arch or, more correctly, one tooth of a dental arch. The egg is first placed perpendicular to the base of the surveyor and surveyed to determine the height of convexity. The vertical arm of the surveyor represents the path of placement that a denture would take and, conversely, its path of removal.

With a carbon marker a circumferential line is drawn on the egg at its greatest circumference. This line, which Kennedy called the height of contour, is its greatest convexity. Cummer spoke of it as the guideline, since it is used as a guide in the placement of retentive and nonretentive clasps. To this, DeVan added the terms *suprabulge*, denoting the surfaces sloping superiorly, and *infrabulge*, denoting the surfaces sloping inferiorly. Prothero proposed that the height of convexity of a tooth be considered as the common base of two cones, the apex of one cone being somewhere above the occlusal surface and the apex of the other being somewhere below the cervical circumference of the tooth.

Any areas cervical to the height of contour may be utilized for the placement of retentive clasp arms, whereas areas occlusal to the height of contour may be utilized for the placement of nonretentive reciprocating, or stabilizing components. Obviously only flexible components may be placed gingivally to the height of contour, because if rigid elements were to be so placed, the undercut areas would be areas of interference to placement and removal rather than areas of retention.

With the original guidelines on the egg the egg is now tilted from the perpendicular to an angular relation with the base of the surveyor (Fig. 6-3, *B*). Its relation to the vertical arm of the surveyor has now been changed, just as a change in the position of a dental cast would bring about a different relationship with the surveyor. The vertical arm of the surveyor still represents the path of placement, but its relation to the egg is totally different.

Again, the carbon marker is used to delineate the greatest convexity or the height of contour. It will be seen that areas which were formerly infrabulge are now suprabulge, and vice versa. A retentive clasp arm placed below the height of contour in the original position may now be either excessively retentive or totally nonretentive, whereas a nonretentive reciprocal arm located above the height of contour in the first position now may be located in an area of undercut.

The location and degree of a tooth undercut available for retention is therefore relative to the path of placement and removal of the partial denture; at the same time, nonretentive areas on which rigid components of the clasp may be placed exist for a given path of placement only.

When the theory of clasp retention is applied to the abutment teeth in a dental arch, each tooth may be considered as an entity as far as the design of retentive and reciprocating components is concerned. This is possible because its relationship to the rest of the arch and to the design of the rest of the prosthesis has been considered previously in selecting the most suitable path of placement. Once the relation of the cast to the surveyor has been established, the height of contour on each abutment tooth becomes fixed, and the clasp design for each may be considered separately.

When the surveyor blade contacts a tooth on the cast as its greatest convexity, a triangle is formed. The apex of the triangle is at the point of contact of the surveyor blade with the tooth, and the base is the area of the cast representing the gingival tissues (Fig. 10-17). The apical angle is called the angle of cervical convergence (Fig. 6-4). This angle may be measured as described in Chapter 10, or it may be estimated by observing the triangle of light visible between the tooth and

Fig. 6-3. A, When an egg is placed with its long axis parallel to the surveying tool, the height of contour is found at its greatest circumference. Similarly, the height of contour may be identified on a single tooth when its long axis is placed parallel to the surveying tool. Rigid parts of the partial denture framework may be located in the suprabulge areas above the height of contour, whereas only the flexible portions of clasp retainers may be placed in the infrabulge areas below. Those infrabulge surfaces that will be crossed by rigid parts of a partial denture framework must be eliminated either during mouth preparations or by block-out. **B,** If the same egg is tilted in relation to the vertical arm of the surveyor, areas formerly infrabulge are now found to be suprabulge and will accommodate nonretentive denture components. At the same time, however, areas formerly suprabulge or only slightly infrabulge are found to be so severely undercut that the design and location of clasp retainers must be changed. Unfortunately, no single tooth in a partially edentulous arch may govern the relation of the cast to the surveyor and thus the path of placement of the partial denture. A compromise position must be found that, following mouth preparations, will satisfy all four factors: (1) no interference to placement, (2) effective location of retentive components, (3) most esthetic placement of all component parts, and (4) existence of guiding planes that will assure a definite path of placement and removal. (Courtesy J. M. Ney Co., Hartford, Conn.)

Fig. 6-4. Angle of cervical convergence on two teeth presenting dissimilar contours. The greater angle of cervical convergence on tooth *A* necessitates the placement of a clasp terminus, *X*, nearer the height of contour than when a lesser angle exists, as in *B*. It is apparent that uniform clasp retention depends upon the degree of tooth undercut rather than upon the distance below the height of contour at which the clasp terminus is placed.

the surveyor blade. For this reason a wide surveyor blade rather than a small cylindric tool is used so that the triangle of light may be more easily seen.

The following factors determine the amount of retention a clasp is capable of generating:

1. Size of the angle of cervical convergence
2. How far into the angle of cervical convergence the clasp terminal is placed
3. Flexibility of the clasp arm, which is the product of—
   a. Its length, measured from its point of origin to its terminal end
   b. Its relative diameter, regardless of its cross-sectional form
   c. Its cross-sectional form or shape, that is, whether it is round, half-round, or some other form
   d. The material of which the clasp is made, that is, whether it is made of of a cast gold alloy, cast chrome alloy, wrought gold alloy, or wrought chrome alloy (each alloy has its own characteristics in both cast or wrought form)

Relative uniformity of retention. The size of the angle of convergence will determine how far into that angle a given clasp arm will be placed. Disregarding, for the time being, variations in clasp flexibility, relative uniformity of retention will depend upon the location of the clasp terminal—not in relation to the height of contour but in relation to the angle of cervical convergence.

The retention on all principal abutments (of which there will be two in Class I and Class II situations and three or more in Class III situations) should be as nearly equal as possible. Whereas esthetic placement of clasp arms is desirable, it may not be possible to place all clasp arms in the same occlusocervical relationship because of variations in tooth contours. The only exceptions are when retentive surfaces may be made similar by altering tooth contours or when two cast restorations are made with similar contours.

Instead the retentive clasp arms must be located so that they lie in the same approximate degree of undercut on each abutment tooth. In Fig. 6-4 this is at point *X* on both teeth, *A* and *B*, despite the variation in the distance below the height of contour. Should both clasp arms be placed equidistantly below the height of contour, the higher location on tooth *B* would have too little retention, whereas the lower location on tooth *A* would be too retentive.

The measurement of the degree of undercut by mechanical means is therefore most important. Although experience with undercut gauges is most important, the student should graduate with a thorough comprehension of all the factors influencing clasp retention and be able to apply them intelligently.

Flexibility of clasp arm. The following factors influence the flexibility of a clasp arm.

Length of clasp arm. The longer the clasp arm, the more flexible it will be, all other factors being equal. The length of a circumferential clasp arm is *measured from the point at which a uniform taper begins.* The retentive circumferential clasp arm should

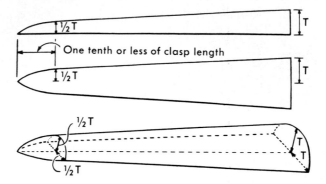

Fig. 6-5. Retentive cast clasp arm should be tapered uniformly from its point of attachment at the clasp body to its tip. The dimensions at the tip are about half those at the point of attachment. A clasp arm so tapered is approximately twice as flexible as one without any taper. *T* is clasp thickness. (Courtesy J. F. Jelenko & Co., Inc., New York, N.Y.)

be tapered uniformly from its point of origin. The length of this uniform taper is the full length of the clasp arm (Fig. 6-5).

The length of a bar clasp arm also is measured from the point at which a uniform taper begins. Generally the taper of a bar clasp arm should begin at its point of origin from a metal base or at the point at which it emerges from a resin base (Fig. 6-6). While a bar clasp arm will usually be longer than a circumferential clasp arm, its flexibility will be less because its half-round form lies in several planes, which prevents its flexibility from being proportionate to its total length. Table 1 gives an approximate depth of undercut that may be used for the cast gold retentive clasp arms of the circumferential and bar-type clasps. Based on a proportional limit of 60,000 psi and on the assumption that the clasp arm is properly tapered, the clasp arm should be able to flex repeatedly within the limits stated without hardening or rupturing because of fatigue. It has been estimated that alternate stress applications of the fatigue type are placed on a retainer arm during mastication and other force-inducing functions about 300,000 times a year.

Diameter of clasp arm. The greater the average diameter of a clasp arm, the less flexible it will be, all other factors being equal. If its taper is absolutely uniform, the average diameter will be at a point midway between its origin and its terminal end. If its taper is not uniform, a point of flexure and therefore a point of weakness will exist that will then be the determining factor in its

Fig. 6-6. Length of a cast retentive clasp arm is measured along center portion of arm until it either joins the clasp body (circumferential) or until it becomes a part of the denture base or is embedded in the base (bar-type clasp).

Table 1. *Permissible flexibilities of retentive, cast circumferential and bar-type clasp arms**

Circumferential		Bar-type	
Length (inches)	Flexibility (inches)	Length (inches)	Flexibility (inches)
to 0.3	0.01	to 0.7	0.01
0.3 to 0.6	0.02	0.7 to 0.9	0.02
0.6 to 0.8	0.03	0.9 to 1.0	0.03

*Based on the approximate dimensions of Jelenko "preformed" plastic patterns, J. F. Jelenko & Co., Inc., New York, N.Y.

Fig. 6-7. Reciprocal arm of a direct retainer assembly should be rigid. An arm tapered both lengthwise and widthwise is more flexible than an arm of the same dimensions tapered only lengthwise.

flexibility regardless of the average diameter of its entire length.

Cross-sectional form of clasp arm. Flexibility may exist in any form, but it is limited to only one direction in the case of the half-round form. The only universally flexible form is the round form, which is practically impossible to obtain by casting and polishing.

Since all cast clasps are essentially half round in form, they may flex away from the tooth, but edgewise flexing (and edgewise adjustment) is limited. For this reason cast retentive clasp arms are more acceptable in tooth-borne partial dentures in which they are called upon to flex only during placement and removal of the prosthesis. A retentive clasp arm on an abutment adjacent to a distal extension base must not only flex during placement and removal but also must be capable of flexing during functional movement of the distal extension base. It must have either universal flexibility to avoid transmission of tipping stresses to the abutment tooth or be capable of disengaging the undercut when vertical forces directed against the denture are toward the residual ridge. A round clasp form is the only circumferential clasp form that may be safely used to engage a tooth undercut on the side of an abutment tooth *away* from the distal extension base. *The location of the undercut is perhaps the most important single factor in selecting a clasp for use with distal extension partial dentures.*

Material used for clasp arm. Whereas all cast alloys used in partial denture construction possess flexibility, their flexibility is proportionate to their bulk. If this were not true, other components of the partial denture could not have the necessary rigidity. The only disadvantage of cast gold partial dentures is that their bulk must be increased to obtain needed rigidity at the expense of added weight. It cannot be denied that greater rigidity with less bulk is possible through the use of chrome alloys.

Although cast gold alloys may have greater resiliency than do cast chrome alloys, the fact remains that the structural nature of the cast clasp does not approach the flexibility and adjustability of the wrought-wire clasp. Having been formed by being drawn into a wire, the wrought-wire clasp arm has toughness exceeding that of a cast clasp arm. The tensile strength of a wrought structure is at least 25% greater than that of the cast alloy from which it was made. It may therefore be used in smaller diameters to provide greater flexibility without fatigue and ultimate fracture.

Reciprocal-stabilizing cast clasp arm. A reciprocal-stabilizing clasp arm should be rigid. Therefore it is shaped somewhat differently than is the cast retentive clasp arm, which must be flexible. Its average diameter must be greater than the average diameter of the opposing retentive arm to increase desired rigidity. Whereas a cast retentive arm is tapered in two dimensions as illustrated in Fig. 6-5, a reciprocal arm should be tapered in one dimension only, as is viewed in Fig. 6-7. To achieve such a form for the arm, freehand waxing of patterns is required.

Advantages and disadvantages of any given clasp design. In selecting a particular clasp arm for a given situation, its advantages must be weighed against its disadvantages. *The dentist should not expect the technician to make the decision as to which clasp design is to be used. The choice of clasp design must be both biologically and mechanically sound, based upon the diagnosis and treatment plan previously established.* Extracoronal direct retainers should be considered as a combination of components of a removable partial denture framework designed and located to perform the specific functions of support, stabilization and reciprocation, and retention. It matters not whether the direct retainer assembly components are physically attached directly to each other or originate from major and minor connectors of the framework (Fig. 6-8). If attention was directed to the components of the direct retainer assembly itself and to the function each component contributes to the restoration, then designing a direct retainer for a particular situation is reduced to simple rationalization.

The advantages of any particular clasp design should lie in an affirmative answer to most or all of the following questions:

1. Is it flexible enough for the purpose for which it is being used? (On an abutment adjacent to a distal extension base will tipping and torque be avoided?)
2. Does the clasp arm cover a minimum of tooth surface?
3. Will the clasp arm be as inconspicuous as possible?
4. Will tooth dimension be increased, which would relatively increase the width of the occlusal table?
5. Is the clasp design applicable to malposed or rotated abutment teeth?
6. Can it be used despite the presence of tissue undercuts?
7. Can the clasp terminal be adjusted to increase or decrease retention?
8. Will adequate stabilization be provided to resist horizontal and rotational movements?
9. Will rigidity be provided where it is needed?
10. Is the clasp arm likely to become distorted or broken? If so, can it be replaced?

The disadvantages of any given clasp design are generally the opposite of the advantages just listed. These are as follows:

1. The retentive arm is too rigid for an abutment adjacent to a distal extension base.
2. Too much tooth surface is covered, resulting in the trapping of food debris and possible caries attack.
3. There will be an objectionable display of metal, resulting in poor esthetics.
4. Tooth dimension will be increased, resulting in an increased functional load on the abutment.
5. Tooth undercuts on malposed teeth cannot be approached without encountering other disadvantages.
6. Tissue undercuts will have to be blocked out excessively, resulting in poor esthetics, annoyance to cheek and tongue, and the trapping of debris.

Fig. 6-8. Choice and definitive location of each component of a direct retainer assembly must be based on preserving the health of the periodontal attachment in spite of rotational tendencies of distal extension denture. A knowledge of the characteristics of each component of the collective assemblies for a particular arch and the rationalized rotational tendencies of the denture simplifies design of removable restorations.

7. Edgewise adjustment to increase or decrease retention is impossible.
8. Orthodontic movement of the abutment tooth is possible because of inadequate stabilization.
9. Horizontal stabilization of the partial denture is inadequate because of insufficient rigidity of stabilizing components.
10. The clasp arm may be easily distorted by careless handling.
11. If broken, the clasp arm may be difficult to replace.

With this background the various types of clasps will be considered. *The choice of a clasp is like the choice of a tool to be used in a given situation. Knowing what types are available and being familiar with their various advantages and disadvantages permits selection of a clasp design that best meets the needs of the individual situation.*

Although there are some rather complex designs for clasp arms, they may all be classified as falling into one of two categories. One is the *circumferential clasp arm*, which approaches the retentive undercut from an occlusal direction. The other is the *bar clasp arm*, which approaches the retentive undercut from a cervical direction.

A clasp assembly may be a combination of cast circumferential and bar clasp arms and wrought-wire retentive arms in one of several possible combinations as illustrated in buccal and lingual views in Fig. 6-9.

No confusion should exist between the choice of clasp arm and the purpose for which it is used. Either type of cast clasp arm may be made tapered and retentive or rigid and nonretentive, depending upon whether it is used for retention, stabilizing, or reciprocation. A clasp assembly should consist of (1) one or more minor connectors from which the clasp components originate, (2) a principal rest, (3) a retentive arm engaging a tooth undercut only at its terminus, and (4) a nonretentive arm or other component on the opposite side of the tooth for reciprocation and stabilization against horizontal movement of the prosthesis. Rigidity of this clasp arm is essential to its purpose. An auxiliary occlusal rest may be used rather than a reciprocal clasp arm if it is located to accomplish the same purpose (Fig. 6-10). The addition of a lingual apron to a cast reciprocal clasp arm

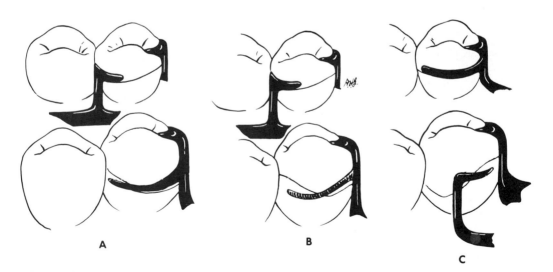

Fig. 6-9. Clasp assembly (mirror views), including a rest, may be a combination of circumferential and bar clasp arms in one of several possible combinations. These mirror views are for abutments bounding an edentulous space. **A,** Cast circumferential retentive clasp arm with a nonretentive bar clasp arm on the opposite side for stabilization and reciprocation. **B,** Tapered wrought-wire circumferential retentive clasp arm with a nonretentive bar clasp arm on the opposite side for stabilization and reciprocation. **C,** Retentive bar clasp arm with a nonretentive cast circumferential clasp arm on the opposite side for stabilization and reciprocation.

Fig. 6-11. Line drawn through illustration represents more than 180 degrees of the greatest circumference of the abutment from the occlusal rest. Unless portions of the lingual reciprocal arm and the retentive buccal arm are extended beyond the line, the clasp would not accomplish its intended purpose. If the respective arms of the retainer were not extended beyond the line, the abutment could move away from the retainer or the removable partial denture could move away from the abutment.

Fig. 6-10. Auxiliary occlusal rest (mirror view) may be used rather than a reciprocal clasp arm without violating any principle of clasp design. Its greatest disadvantages are that a second rest seat must be prepared and that an enclosed tissue space results. An auxiliary occlusal rest is also sometimes used to prevent slippage when principal occlusal rest seat cannot be inclined apically from marginal ridge. Closure of an interproximal space most often requires rests on adjacent teeth to avoid a wedging effect when a force is placed on the denture.

neither alters its primary purpose nor the need for proper location to accomplish that purpose.

Basic principles of clasp design. Any clasp assembly must satisfy the basic principle of clasp design, which is that *more than 180 degrees of the greatest circumference of the crown of the tooth must be included, passing from diverging axial surfaces to converging axial surfaces* (Fig. 6-11). This may be in the form of continuous contact when circumferential clasp arms are used, or broken contact when bar clasp arms are used. *At least three areas of tooth contact must be embracing more than one half the tooth circumference.* These are the occlusal rest area, the reten-

tive terminal area, and the reciprocal terminal area.

Other principles to be considered in the design of a clasp are as follows:

1. The occlusal rest must be designed so that movement of the clasp arms cervically is prevented.

2. Each retentive terminal should be opposed by a reciprocal arm or element capable of resisting any orthodontic pressures exerted by the retentive arm. Reciprocal and stabilizing elements must be rigidly connected bilaterally if reciprocation to the retentive elements is to be realized (Fig. 6-12).

3. Unless guiding planes will positively control the path of removal, retentive clasps should be bilaterally opposed; that is, buccal retention on one side of the arch should be opposed by buccal retention on the other, or lingual on one side opposed by lingual on the other. In Class II situations the third abutment may have either buccal or lingual retention. In Class III situations, retention may be either bilaterally or diametrically opposed.

4. The path of escapement of each retentive clasp terminal must be other than parallel to the path of removal of the prosthesis.

5. Amount of retention always should be the minimal necessary to resist reasonable dislodging forces.

6. *Clasp retainers on abutment teeth adjacent to distal extension bases should be designed so that they will avoid direct transmission of tipping and rotational forces to the*

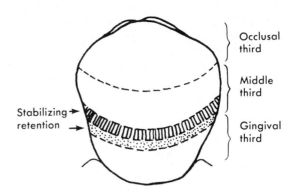

Fig. 6-12. A, Flexing action of retentive clasp arm initiates medially directed pressure on abutment teeth as its retentive tip springs over the height of contour. **B,** Reciprocation to medially directed pressure is counteracted either by lingually placed clasp arms' contacting the abutments simultaneously with buccal arms and engaging the same degree of undercut or by reciprocal elements of the framework contacting lingual guiding planes when buccal arms begin to flex.

Fig. 6-13. Simple mechanical laws demonstrate that the nearer stabilizing-reciprocal and retentive elements of direct retainer assemblies are located to the horizontal axis of rotation of the abutment, the less likely that the physiologic tolerance of the periodontal ligament will be exceeded. The horizontal axis of rotation of an abutment tooth is located somewhere in its root.

abutment. In effect, they must act as stressbreakers either by their design or by their construction. This is accomplished by proper location of the retentive terminal or by use of a more flexible clasp arm in relation to prospective rotation of the denture under varying directed forces.

7. *Ideally, reciprocal elements of the clasp assembly should be located at the junction of the gingival and middle thirds of the crowns of abutment teeth. The terminal end of the retentive arm is optimally placed in the gingival third of the crown* (Fig. 6-13). These locations will permit the abutment teeth to better resist horizontal and torquing forces than they could if the retentive and reciprocal elements were located nearer the occlusal or incisal surfaces. As a metaphor, remember that a fencepost is more easily loosened by applying horizontal forces near its top than by applying the same forces nearer ground level.

The reciprocal clasp arm has two, sometimes three, functions:

1. The reciprocal clasp arm should provide reciprocation against the action of the retentive arm. This is particularly important if the retentive arm is accidentally distorted toward the tooth, where it would become an active orthodontic force. The retentive clasp

arm should be passive until a dislodging force is applied.

During placement and removal, reciprocation is most needed as the retentive arm flexes over the height of contour. Unfortunately the reciprocal clasp arm does not usually come into contact with the tooth until the denture is fully seated and the retentive clasp arm has again become passive unless the abutment tooth has been specifically contoured. A momentary tipping force is thus applied to the abutment during each placement and removal. This may not be a damaging force, since it is transient, so long as the force does not exceed the normal elasticity of the periodontal attachments. True reciprocation during placement and removal is usually possible only through the use of crown surfaces made parallel to the path of placement. The use of a ledge on a cast restoration permits the paralleling of the surfaces to be contacted by the reciprocal arm in such a manner that true reciprocation is made possible. This will be discussed in Chapter 13.

2. The reciprocal clasp arm should be located so that the denture is stabilized against horizontal movement. This is possible only through the use of rigid clasp arms, rigid minor connectors, and a rigid major connector. Horizontal forces applied on one side of the dental arch are resisted by the stabilizing components on the opposite side. These

are not only the reciprocal clasp arms but also all rigid components contacting axial tooth surfaces. Obviously the greater the number of such components, within reason, the greater will be the distribution of horizontal stresses.

3. The reciprocal clasp arm may act to a minor degree as an indirect retainer. This is only true when it rests on a suprabulge surface of an abutment tooth lying anterior to the fulcrum line. Lifting of a distal extension base away from the tissues is thus resisted by a rigid arm, which is not easily displaced cervically. The effectiveness of such an indirect retainer is limited by its proximity to the fulcrum line, which gives it a relatively poor leverage advantage, and by the fact that slippage along tooth inclines is always possible. The latter may be prevented by the use of a ledge on a cast restoration, but enamel surfaces are not ordinarily so prepared.

Circumferential clasp arms. Although a thorough knowledge of the principles of clasp design should lead to a logical application of those principles, it is better that some of the more common clasp designs be considered individually. The circumferential clasp will be considered first as an all-cast clasp.

The circumferential clasp is usually the most logical clasp to use with all tooth-supported partial dentures because of its retentive and stabilizing ability. Only when the retentive undercut may be approached better with a bar clasp arm or when esthetics will be enhanced should the latter be used (Fig. 6-14). The circumferential clasp arm does have the following disadvantages:

1. More tooth surface is covered than with a bar clasp arm because of its occlusal direction of approach.

2. On some tooth surfaces, particularly the buccal surface of mandibular teeth and the lingual surfaces of maxillary teeth, its occlusal approach may increase the width of the occlusal surface of the tooth.

3. In the mandibular arch more metal may be displayed than with a bar clasp arm.

4. As with all cast clasps, its half-round form prevents edgewise adjustment to increase or decrease retention. Adjustments in the retention afforded by a clasp arm should be made by moving a clasp terminal cervically into the angle of cervical convergence or occlusally into a lesser area of undercut. Tightening a clasp against the tooth or loosen-

Fig. 6-14. Example of the two types of cast clasps in use. Molar abutment is engaged by a circumferential clasp originating above (or occlusal to) the height of contour, whereas premolar abutment is engaged by a bar clasp originating from the base below (or gingival to) the height of contour. However, only the terminal tip of this clasp is placed in a measured undercut.

ing it away from the tooth increases or decreases frictional resistance and does not affect the retentive potential of the clasp. *True adjustment is, therefore, impossible with most cast clasps.*

Despite its disadvantages the cast circumferential clasp arm may be used effectively, and many of these disadvantages may be minimized by proper design. Adequate mouth preparation will permit its point of origin to be placed far enough below the occlusal surface to avoid poor esthetics and increased tooth dimension (Fig. 6-15). Although some of the other disadvantages listed imply that the bar-type clasp may be preferable, the circumferential type clasp is actually superior to a bar clasp arm that is improperly used or poorly designed. Experience has shown that the possible advantages of the bar clasp arm are too often negated by faulty application and design, whereas the circumferential clasp arm is less easily misused.

The basic form of the circumferential type clasp is a buccal and lingual arm originating from a common body (Fig. 6-16). *This clasp is used improperly when two retentive clasp arms originate from the body and occlusal rest areas and approach bilateral retentive areas on the side of the tooth away from the point of origin. The correct form of this clasp has only one retentive clasp arm, opposed by*

Fig. 6-15. Cast circumferential retentive clasp arms properly designed. They originate on or occlusally to the height of contour, which they then cross in their terminal third, and engage retentive undercuts progressively as their taper decreases and their flexibility increases.

Fig. 6-16. Cast circumferential retentive clasp arm.

A   B

Fig. 6-17. Ring clasp(s) encircling nearly all the tooth from its point of origin. **A,** Clasp originates on mesiobuccal surface and encircles the tooth to engage a mesiolingual undercut. **B,** Clasp originates on mesiolingual surface and encircles the tooth to engage a mesiobuccal undercut. In either case a supporting strut is used on the nonretentive side. (Drawn both as a direct view of the near side of the tooth and as a mirror view of the opposite side.)

a nonretentive reciprocal arm on the opposite side. A common error is to use this clasp improperly by making both clasp terminals retentive. This is not only unnecessary but also disregards the need for reciprocation and bilateral stabilization.

The circumferential type clasp may be used in several other forms. One is the *ring-type clasp,* which encircles nearly all of a tooth from its point of origin (Fig. 6-17). It is used when a proximal undercut cannot be approached by other means. For example, when a mesiolingual undercut on a lower molar abutment cannot be approached directly because of its proximity to the occlusal rest area, yet cannot be approached with a bar clasp arm because of lingual inclination of the tooth, the ring clasp encircling the tooth allows the undercut to be approached from the distal aspect of the tooth.

The clasp should never be used as an unsupported ring (Fig. 6-18) because if it is free to open and close as a ring, it cannot provide either reciprocation or bracing. Instead the ring-type clasp should always be used with a supporting strut on the nonretentive side, with or without an auxiliary occlusal rest on the opposite marginal ridge. The advantage of an auxiliary rest is that further movement of a mesially inclined tooth is prevented by the presence of a distal rest. In any event the supporting strut should be regarded as being

a minor connector from which the flexible retentive arm originates. Reciprocation then comes from the rigid portion of the clasp lying between the supporting strut and the principal occlusal rest. (See Figs. 6-19 and 6-20.)

The ring-type clasp should be used on protected abutments whenever possible because it covers such a large area of tooth surface. Esthetics usually need not be considered on such a posteriorly located tooth.

A ring-type clasp may be used in reverse on an abutment located anterior to a tooth-bounded edentulous space (Fig. 6-21). Although potentially an effective clasp, this clasp covers an excessive amount of tooth surface and is esthetically objectionable. The only justification for its use is when a distobuccal or distolingual undercut cannot be ap-

Fig. 6-18. Improperly designed clasp lacking necessary support. Such a clasp lacks any reciprocating or stabilizing action, since the entire circumference of the clasp is free to open and close. Instead, a supporting strut should always be added on the nonretentive side of the abutment tooth, which then becomes, in effect, a minor connector from which a tapered and flexible retentive clasp arm originates.

Fig. 6-19. Buccal strut supporting a mesially originating ring clasp. The flexible retentive arm begins at the distal occlusal rest and engages a mesiolingual undercut. Despite its resemblance to a bar-type clasp, this is a circumferential clasp by reason of its point of origin, the strut being actually an auxiliary minor connector.

Fig. 6-20. Ring clasp engaging a mesiobuccal undercut on a mesially inclined lower right molar requires a supporting bar on lingual surface to limit flexure to only the retentive portion of the clasp.

Fig. 6-21. Ring-type clasp may be used in reverse on an abutment located anterior to a tooth-bound edentulous space.

proached directly from the occlusal rest area, yet tissue undercuts prevent its approach from a gingival direction with a bar clasp arm.

The *back-action clasp* is a modification of the ring clasp, with all of its disadvantages and no apparent advantages (Fig. 6-22). *It is difficult to ever justify its use.* The undercut can usually be approached just as well using a conventional circumferential clasp, with less tooth coverage and less display of metal. With the circumferential clasp the proximal tooth surface can be used properly as a guiding plane, as it should be, and the occlusal rest can have the rigid support it requires. An occlusal rest always should be attached to some rigid minor connector and should never be supported by a clasp arm alone. If the occlusal rest is part of a flexible assembly, it cannot function adequately as an occlusal rest. *Unfortunately the back-action clasp is still being used, despite the fact that it is biologically and mechanically unsound.*

In the construction of an unmodified Class II or Class III partial denture there are no edentulous spaces on the opposite side of the arch to aid in clasping. Mechanically this is a disadvantage. However, when the teeth are sound and retentive areas are available or when multiple restorations are justified, clasping is accomplished by means of an *embrasure clasp* (Figs. 6-23 and 6-24).

Fig. 6-22. Back-action circumferential clasp used on a premolar abutment anterior to an edentulous space. It is difficult to justify its use.

Sufficient space must be provided between the abutment teeth in their occlusal third to make room for the common body of the embrasure clasp (Fig. 6-25), yet the contact area should not be eliminated entirely. Since vulnerable areas of the teeth are involved, abutment protection with inlays or crowns is indicated in almost every instance. The decision to use unprotected abutments must be made at the time of oral examination and should be based on the age of the patient, caries index, and oral hygiene as well as on whether existing tooth contours are favorable. Preparation

Fig. 6-23. Embrasure clasp is used where no edentulous space exists. Although in this drawing both retentive clasp arms are located on the buccal surface and the nonretentive arms on the lingual surface, retention and reciprocation can be reversed on both teeth or on either tooth, depending on the respective contours of the teeth. However, if the second molar is sound and suitable stabilizing and retentive areas can be found, a circumferential clasp may be used originating on the distal surface of the abutment.

Fig. 6-24. Multiple clasping in a surgically mutilated mouth. On the right are an embrasure clasp, a bar clasp arm, and a conventional circumferential clasp engaging lingual undercuts on three abutment teeth. On the left is a well-designed ring clasp engaging a lingual undercut, with supporting strut on the buccal surface and auxiliary occlusal rest to prevent mesial tipping. Note rigid design of major connector.

Fig. 6-25. Embrasure and hairpin circumferential retentive clasp arms. The terminus of each engages a suitable retentive undercut. Use of hairpin-type clasp on second molar is made necessary by the fact that the only available undercut lies directly below point of origin of clasp arm.

Fig. 6-26. A, Example of the use of an embrasure clasp for a Class II partially edentulous arch. Embrasure clasp on two left molar abutments was utilized in the absence of a posterior modification space. **B,** Occlusal and proximal surfaces of adjacent molar and premolar prepared for an embrasure clasp. Note that rest seat preparations are extended both bucally and lingually to accommodate retentive and reciprocal clasp arms. An adequate preparation confined to enamel can rarely be accomplished for such a clasp, especially when the teeth are opposed by natural teeth.

of adjacent, contacting, uncrowned abutments to receive any type of embrasure clasp of adequate interproximal bulk is difficult, especially when apposed by natural teeth.

The embrasure clasp always should be used with double occlusal rests, even when definite proximal shoulders can be established (Fig. 6-26). This is to avoid interproximal wedging by the prothesis, which could cause separation of the abutment teeth and result in food impaction and clasp displacement. In addition to providing support, occlusal rests also serve to shunt food away from contact areas. For this reason occlusal rests should always be used whenever food impaction is possible.

Embrasure clasps should have two retentive clasp arms and two reciprocal clasp arms, either bilaterally or diagonally opposed. An auxiliary occlusal rest or a bar clasp arm can be substituted for a circumferential reciprocal arm as long as definite reciprocation and stabilization result. A lingually placed retentive bar clasp arm may be substituted if a rigid circumferential clasp arm is placed on the buccal surface for reciprocation, provided lingual retention is utilized on the opposite side of the arch.

Other modifications of the cast circumferential clasp are the multiple clasp, the half-and-half clasp, and the reverse action clasp. The *multiple clasp* is simply two opposing circumferential clasps joined at the

Fig. 6-27. Multiple clasp is actually two opposing circumferential clasps joined at the terminal end of the two reciprocal arms (mirror view).

terminal end of the two reciprocal arms (Fig. 6-27). It is used when additional retention is needed, usually on tooth-borne partial dentures. It may be used for multiple clasping in instances in which the partial denture replaces an entire half of the dental arch. It may be used rather than an embrasure clasp when the only available retentive areas are adjacent to each other. Its disadvantage is that two embrasure approaches are necessary rather than a single common embrasure for both clasps.

The *half-and-half clasp* consists of a circumferential retentive arm arising from one direction and a reciprocal arm arising from

Fig. 6-28. Half-and-half clasp consists of one circumferential retentive arm arising from the distal and a second circumferential arm arising from the mesial on the opposite side, with or without a secondary occlusal rest. Broken line illustrates a nonretentive reciprocal clasp arm used without a secondary occlusal rest (mirror view).

Fig. 6-29. Reverse-action or hairpin clasp arm may be used on abutments of a tooth-borne denture when a proximal undercut lies below point of origin of clasp (mirror view). It may be esthetically objectionable and covers considerable tooth surface and should be used only when a bar-type retentive arm is contraindicated because of a tissue undercut cervical to gingival margin.

another (Fig. 6-28). Since the second arm must arise from a second minor connector, this arm is actually a bar clasp used with or without an auxiliary occlusal rest. Reciprocation arising from a second minor connector can usually be accomplished with a short bar or with an auxiliary occlusal rest, thereby avoiding so much tooth coverage. Thus it is apparent that there is little justification for the use of the half-and-half clasp in bi-

lateral dentures. Its design was originally intended to provide dual retention, a principle that should be applied only to unilateral denture design.

The *reverse action* or *hairpin clasp arm* is designed to permit engaging a proximal undercut from an occlusal approach (Fig. 6-29). Other methods of accomplishing the same result are with a ring clasp originating on the opposite side of the tooth or with a bar clasp arm originating from a gingival direction. However, when a proximal undercut must be used on a posterior abutment and when tissue undercuts or high tissue attachments prevent the use of a bar clasp arm, the reverse action clasp may be used successfully. Although the ring clasp may be preferable, lingual undercuts may prevent the placement of a supporting strut without tongue interference. In this limited situation the hairpin clasp arm serves adequately, despite its several disadvantages. The clasp covers considerable tooth surface and may trap debris; its occlusal origin may increase the functional load on the tooth, and its flexibility is limited. Esthetics usually need not be considered when the clasp is used on a posterior abutment, but the hairpin clasp arm does have the additional disadvantage of displaying too much metal for use on an anterior abutment.

Properly designed, the reverse action clasp should make a hairpin turn to engage an undercut below the point of origin (Fig. 6-29). The upper arm of this clasp should be considered a minor connector giving rise to the tapered lower arm. Therefore only the lower arm should be flexible; with the retentive portion beginning beyond the turn, only the lower arm should flex over the height of contour to engage a retentive undercut. The clasp should be designed and fabricated with this in mind.

These are the various types of cast circumferential clasps. As mentioned previously, they may be used in combination with bar clasp arms as long as differentiation is made by their location and bulk between retention and reciprocation. Circumferential and bar clasp arms may be made either flexible (retentive) or rigid (reciprocal) in any combination as long as each retentive clasp arm is opposed by a rigid reciprocal arm.

The use of many of the less desirable clasp forms can be avoided by changing the crown forms of the abutments with full restorations. In fabricating abutment coverage, tooth contours should be established that will permit the use of the most desirable clasp forms rather than reproduce a form that makes necessary the use of less desirable clasp designs.

Bar clasp arms. The berm *bar clasp arm* is generally preferred over the less descriptive term *Roach clasp arm.* Reduced to its simplest terms, the bar clasp arm arises from the denture framework or a metal base and approaches the retentive undercut from a gingival direction (Fig. 6-14).

The bar clasp arm has been classified by the shape of the retentive terminal. Thus it has been identified as a T, modified T, I, Y, or almost any letter clasp arm. All have the same characteristics in common: they originate from the framework or base and approach the undercut from a gingival direction. *The form the terminal takes is of little significance as long as it is mechanically and functionally effective, covers as little tooth surface as possible, and displays as little metal as possible.*

The T and Y clasp arms are the most frequently misused. It is unlikely that the full area of a T or Y terminal is ever necessary for adequate clasp retention. Whereas the larger area of contact would provide greater frictional resistance, this is not true clasp retention, and only that portion engaging an undercut area should be considered retentive. Only one terminal of such a clasp arm is placed in an undercut area. The remainder of the clasp arm may be superfluous unless it is needed as part of the clasp assembly to encircle the abutment tooth more than 180 degrees of its greatest circumference, passing from diverging axial surfaces to converging axial surfaces. If the bar clasp arm is made to be flexible for retentive purposes, any suprabulge portion of the clasp will provide only limited stabilization, since it is also part of the flexible arm. Therefore in many instances the suprabulge portion of a T or Y clasp arm may be dispensed with, and the clasp terminal placed in an undercut. The terminal of the bar clasp should be designed to be biologically and mechanically sound rather than to conform to any alphabetical connotation.

With just one exception the bar clasp arm should be used only with tooth-borne partial dentures or tooth-borne modification areas. This exception is when an undercut that logically can be approached with a bar clasp arm lies on the side of an abutment tooth adjacent to a distal extension base (Figs. 6-30 to 6-34). If a tissue undercut prevents such use of a bar clasp arm, a mesially originating ring clasp, a cast, or a wrought-wire reverse action clasp may be

Fig. 6-30. Bar clasp arm properly used on a terminal abutment. A mesial extension or T is neither advantageous nor desirable in this situation, since abutment tooth was encompassed more than 180 degrees.

Fig. 6-31. Bar clasp arm on a distal abutment must be made light enough to be flexible and may be used only when it can engage a proximal undercut adjacent to extension base. Mesial T portion of clasp arm had to be placed to encompass the abutment by more than 180 degrees. It is placed on the height of contour. Note finishing line where clasp and denture base will join.

Fig. 6-32. Bar clasp arm on a maxillary terminal abutment. Note uniform taper from point where it will emerge from a resin base and that it engages tooth undercut on *side adjacent* to distal extension base. A butt-type joint for a finishing line between direct retainer and acrylic resin base is provided.

Fig. 6-33. Bar clasp arm on a lower molar abutment engaging a mesiobuccal undercut. Note proper utilization of parallel proximal guiding planes.

Fig. 6-34. Bar clasps used for both retention and reciprocation. Bar-type retainer on right second premolar engages a distobuccal undercut. Bar-type configuration of the lingual of the molar is utilized for reciprocation and stabilization and does not engage an undercut.

Fig. 6-35. Bar retainer is used on anterior abutment of modification space, and its terminus engages a distobuccal undercut. Denture will rotate around terminal abutments when a force is directed toward basal seat on left. Such rotation will impart a force on right premolar directed superiorly and anteriorly. However, this direction of force is resisted in great part by the mesial contact with canine. A direct retainer on right premolar engaging a mesiobuccal undercut would tend to force tooth superiorly and posteriorly.

used. Preparation of adjacent abutments (natural teeth) to receive any type of interproximal direct retainer, traversing from lingual to buccal surfaces, is most difficult to adequately accomplish. Inevitably the relative size of the "occlusal table" is increased, contributing to undesirable and additional functional loading.

A bar clasp arm should not be used on a terminal abutment if the undercut lies on the side of the tooth away from the extension base. The bar clasp arm is not a particularly flexible clasp arm because of the effect its half-round form and its several planes of origin have. Although the cast circumferential clasp arm can be made more flexible than can the bar clasp arm, the combination clasp is much preferred for use on terminal abutments when torque and tipping are possible because of engaging an undercut away from the distal extension base. Situations often exist in which a bar clasp arm may be used to advantage without jeopardizing a terminal abutment. A bar clasp arm swinging distally into the undercut is a logical choice, since movement of the abutment as the distal extension base moves tissueward is prevented by the distal location of the clasp terminal.

The specific indications for using a bar clasp arm are (1) when a small degree of undercut (0.25 mm [0.01 in]) exists in the cervical third of the abutment tooth, which

may be approached from a gingival direction, and (2) with a single exception, on abutment teeth when they support tooth-borne partial dentures or tooth-borne modification areas (Fig. 6-35). Thus use of the bar clasp arm is contraindicated when a deep cervical undercut exists or when a severe tissue undercut exists, either of which must be bridged by excessive blockout. When severe tooth and tissue undercuts exist, which must be blocked out, a bar clasp arm usually is an annoyance to tongue and cheek and also traps food debris.

Combination clasp. The combination clasp consists of a wrought-wire retentive clasp arm and a cast reciprocal clasp arm (Fig. 6-36). Although the latter may be in the form of a bar clasp arm, it is usually a circumferential arm. The retentive arm is almost always circumferential, but it also may be used in the manner of a bar, originating gingivally from the denture base.

The advantages of the combination clasp lie in the *flexibility*, the *adjustability*, and the *appearance* of the wrought-wire retentive arm. It is used when maximum flexibility is desirable, such as on an abutment tooth adjacent to a distal extension base

Fig. 6-36. A, Combination clasp consists of a cast reciprocal arm and a tapered, round wrought-wire retentive clasp arm. The latter is either cast to, or soldered to, the cast framework. This design is recommended for the anterior abutment of a posterior modification space in the Class II partially edentulous arch, where only a mesiobuccal undercut exists, to minimize the effects of a first-class lever system. **B,** In addition to the advantages of flexibility, adjustability, and appearance, the wrought-wire retentive arm makes only a line contact with the abutment tooth, rather than the broader contact of the cast clasp.

or on a particularly weak abutment when a bar-type direct retainer is contraindicated. It may be used for its adjustability when precise retentive requirements are unpredictable and later adjustment to increase or decrease retention may be necessary. A third justification for its use is its esthetic advantage over cast clasps. Being wrought in structure, it may be used in smaller diameters than may a cast clasp, with less danger of fracture. Since it is round, light is refracted is such a manner that the display of metal is less noticeable than with the broader surfaces of a cast clasp.

The most common use of the combination clasp is on an abutment tooth adjacent to a distal extension base where only a mesiogingival undercut exists in the abutment or where a gross tissue undercut contraindicates a bar-type retainer. When a distal undercut exists that may be approached with a properly designed bar clasp arm or with a ring clasp (despite its several disadvantages), a cast clasp can be located so that it will not cause abutment tipping as the distal extension base moves tissueward. *When the undercut is on the side of the abutment away from the extension base, the tapered wrought-wire retentive arm offers greater flexibility than does the cast clasp arm and therefore better dissipates functional*

stresses. For this reason the combination clasp is preferred (Fig. 6-37).

The combination clasp has two disadvantages: (1) the extra steps in fabrication, particularly when high-fusing chrome alloys are used, and (2) the fact that it may be distorted by careless handling on the part of the patient. The disadvantages of the wrought-wire clasp are offset by its several advantages, which are (1) its flexibility, (2) its adjustability, (3) its esthetic advantage over other retentive circumferential clasp arms, (4) the fact that a minimum of tooth surface is covered because of its line contact with the tooth rather than having the surface contact of a cast clasp arm, and (5) the fact that fatigue failures in service are less likely to occur with the tapered wrought-wire retentive arm than with the cast, half-round retentive arm.

The disadvantages listed previously should not prevent its use regardless of the type of alloy being used for the cast framework. Technical problems are minimized by selecting the best wrought wire for this purpose and then either casting to it or soldering it to the cast framework. Selection of wrought wire, attachment of it to the framework, and subsequent laboratory procedures to maintain its optimal physical properties are presented in Chapter 11.

Fig. 6-37. Five types of extracoronal direct retainer assemblies that may be used on an abutment adjacent to a distal extension base to avoid or minimize the effects of a cantilever design. Arrows indicate general direction of movement of retentive tips of retainer arms when denture base rotates toward and away from edentulous ridge. **A,** Distobuccal undercut engaged by a one-half T-type bar clasp. Portion of clasp arm on and above height of contour will afford some bracing against horizontal rotation of denture base. **B,** An I bar placed in an undercut at middle (anteroposteriorly) of buccal surface. This retainer contacts tooth only at its tip. Note that guiding plane on distal of abutment is contacted by metal of denture framework and that a mesial rest is utilized. **C,** Interproximal ring-type clasp engaging a distobuccal undercut. A bar-type retainer cannot be used because of tissue undercuts inferior to buccal surface of abutment. **D,** Round, uniformly tapered 18-gauge wrought-wire circumferential retainer arm engaging a mesiobuccal undercut. A wrought-wire arm, instead of a cast arm, must be used in this situation because of the ability of the wrought wire to flex omnidirectionally. A cast half-round retainer arm would not flex edgewise, resulting in excessive stress on tooth when rotation of denture base occurs. **E,** Hairpin-type clasp may be used when undercut lies cervical to origin of retainer arm. Both hairpin and interproximal ring types of clasps may be used to engage a distobuccal undercut on terminal abutment of a distal extension denture. However, a distobuccal undercut on terminal abutment should be engaged by a bar-type clasp in the absence of a gross buccal tissue undercut cervical to terminal abutment. Hairpin and interproximal ring clasps are the least desirable of clasping situations illustrated here. **F,** Lingual view shows use of double occlusal rests, connected to lingual bar by a minor connector in the illustrated designs. This design eliminates the need for a lingual clasp arm, places fulcrum line anteriorly to better utilize residual ridge for support, and provides stabilization against horizontal rotation of denture base.

The patient may be taught to avoid distortion of the wrought wire by explaining that the fingernail should always be applied to its point of origin, where it is held rigid by the casting, rather than to the flexible terminal end. Frequently, lingual retention may be used rather than buccal retention, especially on a mandibular abutment, so that the wrought-wire arm is never touched by the patient during removal of the denture. Instead removal may be accomplished by lifting against the cast reciprocal arm located on the buccal side of the tooth. However, this negates the esthetic advantage of the wrought-wire clasp arm, and esthetics may be given preference when the choice must be made between buccal and lingual retention. Frequently, however, retention must be used where it is found and the clasp designed accordingly.

Lingual retention in conjunction with internal rests. The internal rest is covered in Chapter 5. It is emphasized that the internal rest is not utilized as a retainer but

Fig. 6-38. Infrabulge clasp designed by Dr. M. M. DeVan. In **A** the clasp arm arises from border of a metal base and is separated from it with a saw cut or by having been cast against a separating shim, which is later removed. A wrought-wire retentive arm may be soldered to the metal base to serve the same purpose. In **B** the clasp arm is attached to border of a resin base. This is usually a wrought-wire clasp arm partially embedded in resin base at the border.

that its near-vertical walls provide for reciprocation against a lingually placed retentive clasp arm. For this reason visible clasp arms may be eliminated, thus meeting one of the principal objections to the extracoronal retainer.

Such a retentive clasp arm, terminating in an existing or prepared infrabulge area on the abutment tooth, may be of any acceptable design. It is usually a circumferential arm arising from the body of the denture framework at the rest area. It should be wrought, for the advantages of adjustability and flexibility make the wrought clasp arm preferable. It may be cast-to with gold or low fusing chrome-cobalt alloy or be assembled by being soldered to one of the higher fusing chrome-cobalt alloys. In any event, future adjustment or repair is facilitated.

The use of lingual extracoronal retention avoids much of the cost of the internal attachment yet disposes of a visible clasp arm when esthetics must be considered. Frequently its use with a tooth-supported partial denture is employed only on the anterior abutments, and the posterior abutments, when esthetics is not a consideration, are clapsed in the conventional manner. (See Figs. 5-10 to 5-12.)

Other types of clasps. Several other types of clasps will be considered briefly. The *infrabulge clasp* is a bar clasp arm arising from the border of the base, either as an extension of a cast base or attached to the border of a resin base (Fig. 6-38). It is made more flexible than the usual bar clasp arm in that the portion of the cast base that gives rise to the clasp arm is separated from the clasp arm itself, either by a saw cut or by being casted against a separating shim of matrix metal, which is later removed with acid. It may be made more flexible through the use of wrought wire, which either is attached to a metal base by soldering or is embedded in the border of a resin base.

Some of the advantages attributed to the infrabulge clasp are (1) its interproximal location, which may be used to esthetic advantage, (2) increased retention without tipping action on the abutment, and (3) less chance of accidental distortion due to its proximity to the denture border. The wearer should be meticulous in his care of a denture so made, not only for reasons of oral hygiene but also to prevent cariogenic debris being held against tooth surfaces.

Oddo developed the *"movable-arm" clasp* (Fig. 6-39). Support in the form of occlusal rests and stabilization in the form of other elements are used in conjunction with the movable-arm clasp.

The retentive portions of the clasp are placed in undercut regions of the abutment tooth after the denture is seated in the mouth. This of course will eliminate the spring tension exhibited by conventional extracoronal direct retainers when the partial denture is seated and removed.

Advantages of the movable-arm partial

Fig. 6-39. A, Components for fabricating the movable-arm clasp are available in kit form. Metal spring-lock box (left) and rigid plastic burnout pattern used to fabricate the cast retentive arm. **B,** Cast retentive arm of direct retainer assembled in spring-lock box (open position). **C,** Assembled unit is located in a waxed denture base prior to processing in acrylic resin (right figure). Movable-arm clasp assembly in acrylic resin base (left figure). Projecting portions of spring-lock box are finished flush with resin base. Spring tension on movable-arm can be varied by adjusting upper and lower edges of spring-lock box. **D,** Interproximal movable-arm clasp in closed position. (**A** to **C** redrawn from Oddo, Vincent, J., Jr.: J. Am. Dent. Assoc. **74:**1008-1015, April, 1967; **D,** courtesy Dr. Vincent J. Oddo, Jr.)

denture, according to Dr. Oddo, include the following:

1. Each clasp is treated separately, and as a result a common path of placement of a number of clasps on one partial denture is no longer a concern.
2. Clasp tension, loosening, flexibility, and breakage are not considered, since passivity eliminates stress and flexibility.
3. Since the retentive arm can be placed anywhere in the undercut region, esthetics is improved.

Continued clinical evaluation of the movable-arm denture is most worthy. However, the occurrence of inherent problems with movable portions of partial dentures in construction, cost, service, adjustment, and occasional replacement must also be weighed as well as their advantages.

The choice of clasp designs should be based upon biologic as well as mechanical principles. The dentist responsible for the treatment being rendered the patient must be able to justify the clasp design used for each abutment tooth in keeping with these principles.

Hart-Dunn attachment for unilateral distal extension partial dentures.* Objections to the use of embrasure clasp retainers on the nonedentulous side of a Class II partially edentulous arch can be met with the use of the Hart-Dunn attachment partial denture. Retention is by an embrasure hook consisting of 18- or 19-gauge round wrought wires placed just beneath the contact areas in the mesial and distal areas of the selected abutment tooth, slightly curved to allow easy placement from the lingual direction and protection of the interdental papillae. Stabilization is provided by occlusal rests mesially and distally, which also serve to prevent the wires from settling into the interdental papillae (Fig. 6-40).

Mann has emphasized that because the Hart-Dunn attachment is placed in a horizontal direction just prior to seating the

---

*Dunn, A. L.: A safe temporary partial denture J. Am. Dent. Assoc. **23:**96-99, 1936.

Fig. 6-40. Hart-Dunn attachment for distal extension partial dentures. **A,** Mandibular Class II distal extension partial denture retained by circumferential clasping on terminal abutment on edentulous side and embrasure wires on either side of left second premolar. **B,** Partial denture off of cast, showing occlusal rests and embrasure wires. **C,** Maxillary Clasp II partial denture of similar design with split palatal bar stressbreaker leading from clasp retainer on edentulous side abutment. The soundness of using a cast circumferential direct retainer on terminal abutment of edentulous side in these illustrations is questioned.

clasp on the opposite or denture base side, conventional surveying of the abutment teeth cannot be used. This is to say that guiding planes to placement and removal are not used. Instead, a divider is used for surveying the cast. Mann is quoted directly, as follows:

One point of the divider is placed on the center of rotation for the attachment (at a point midway between the embrasure hook and the occlusal rests), and the other end of the divider is swept over the buccal and lingual surfaces of the abutment tooth on the opposite side and over the lingual denture base area on the study [diagnostic] cast. Either a precision [internal] attachment or a circumferential clasp can be used on the denture base side to lock the partial denture in position. However, *these retainers must be on the arc scribed by the divider* in order that the attachment can first be seated horizontally, then the clasp or attachment on the denture base side is seated occlusogingivally. If the abutment on the denture base side is inclined toward the buccal, it presents an undercut problem. This can be solved best by constructing a cast crown to eliminate the undercut.*

Either a nonlocking internal attachment or a clasp ideal for a terminal abutment on the denture base side may be used. On the opposite side the hook may be fitted into the pontic casting of a fixed partial denture rather than embrasure hooks. A prefabricated hook suggested and designed by Dr. George M. Hollenback for this puspose is commercially available.†

OTHER TYPES OF RETAINERS

Numerous other types of retainers for partial dentures have been devised that cannot be classified as being primarily of the intracoronal or extracoronal type. Neither can they be classified as relying primarily on frictional resistance or placement of an element in an undercut to prevent displacement of the denture. However, all these utilize some type of locking device, located either intracoronally or extracoronally, for providing retention without visible clasp retention. Although the motiva-

tion behind the development of other types of retainers has usually been a desire to eliminate visible clasp retainers, the desire to minimize torque and tipping stresses on the abutment teeth has also been given consideration.

All of the few retainers that will be discussed herein have merit, and much credit is due those who have developed specific devices and techniques for the retaining of partial dentures. Unfortunately not all can be included without devoting considerable space to the history and development of partial denture retaining devices. Also the use of patented retaining devices and other techniques falls in the same limited category as the internal attachment prosthesis and is, for economic and technical reasons, available to only a small percentage of those patients needing partial denture service.

Neurohr spring-lock attachment. One of the earlier attempts at eliminating partial denture clasps and at the same time providing adequate extracoronal retention was the spring wire lock system of attachment devised by Dr. F. G. Neurohr and patented in 1930 (Fig. 6-41). The Neurohr method employs tapered vertical rests retained within the contours of the abutment tooth. A single buccal clasp arm, with a ball terminus, engages an undercut in the abutment casting and retains the partial denture in place. Occlusal stress is transmitted to the abutment tooth in a near vertical direction.

• • •

Dr. Franklin Smith makes use of the Neurohr-Williams shoe in a manner similar to the Nuerohr spring-lock attachment (Fig. 6-42). A single, short retentive clasp arm of 20-gauge wrought wire engages a small distobuccal, horizontal groove in the abutment casting. The lateral walls of the rest shoe are parallel and as such offer some resistance to horizontal rotational tendencies of the denture. Additionally, this attachment permits some vertical rotation of the denture bases toward the residual ridges. It will also resist rotary displacement of the denture bases away from the residual ridges.

Smith lists the following indications, advantages, contraindications, and disadvantages for his use of the Neurohr-Williams

---

* From Mann, A. W.: The lower distal extension partial denture using the Hart-Dunn Attachment, J. Prosthet. Dent. 8:282-288, 1958.
†Williams hook attachment, Williams Gold Refining Co., Buffalo, N.Y.

Fig. 6-41. Neurohr spring-lock attachment. **A,** Tapered mandrel used in surveyor to form vertical rest. **B,** Spring wire lock soldered to denture base, engaging a depression in abutment tooth casting.

Fig. 6-42. A, Premolar abutment crown containing preformed rest seat. Groove one half the depth of a No. 557 bur is prepared at height of gingival seat of female portion. **B,** Retentive arm is fabricated from 20-gauge wrought wire. **C,** An assembled unit (schematic). Retentive arm is passive until a dislodging force is applied to denture. (**B** courtesy Dr. Franklin Smith.)

rest shoe. The indications and advantages claimed are as follows:

1. Stress-breaking action in respect to distal rotation
2. Lowered leverage point of applied force
3. Multiple options of retentive area placement
4. Internal reciprocal action and indirect retention
5. Esthetics
6. Stability, simplicity (in form)
7. Amenability to tilted teeth where "draw" is a problem with conventional approaches
8. Amenability to anterior abutments

The contraindications and disadvantages are as follows:

1. Anticipation of possible tooth (abutment migration in an anterior direction
2. Preclusion where poor retentive qualities of an abutment casting are antici-

pated (for example, short or tapered crowns)

3. Any problem of inadequate crown length to retain the casting or house the intracoronal receptable (for example, short crown, deep impinging vertical overlap, large pulps)
4. Time, cost, and complexity of total procedure

Dowel rest attachment. Dr. Morris J. Thompson and others have developed what is called the *dowel rest attachment* (Figs. 6-43 to 6-46). A boxlike rest seat is machined in the abutment casting for support of the partial denture, and a dimple is provided on the lingual surface of the abutment casting for retention. This dimple is engaged by a boss on a lingual arm on the denture framework, thereby affording retention without the use of a visible clasp arm. The lingual arm is an extension of the major connector,

Fig. 6-43. Bilateral dowel rest attachments used on a Class I (bilateral distal extension) cast gold partial denture skeleton. *A*, Stabilizing bar; *B*, lug rest, which fits into notch *F* of the abutment; *C*, slit made with a gold saw to provide spring for stabilizing bar; *D*, boss, which fits into round recess *H* of the abutment; *E*, dowel which fits into well *G* of the abutment; *F*, notch into which lug rest fits; *G*, well into which dowel fits; *H*, round recess into which the boss fits. (From Thompson, M. J.: Solution for specific problems in replacing missing teeth with partial dentures, Illinois State Dental Society's Seminar Manual, 1957.)

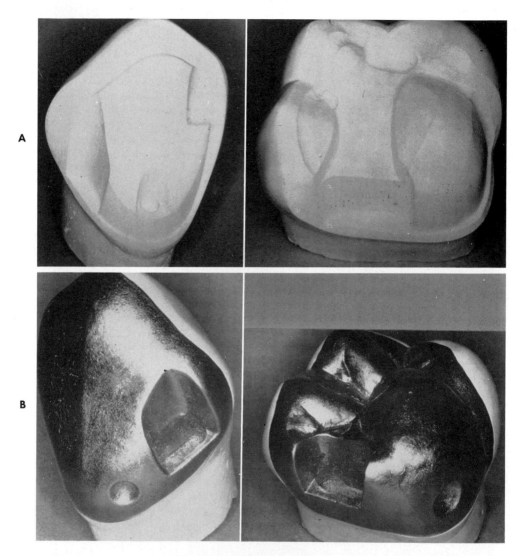

Fig. 6-44. A, Preparations for canine and molar abutment teeth upon which dowel rest attachments will be constructed. **B,** Dowel rest attachments constructed on canine and molar abutment teeth. Note tapered nonlocking rest seat and dimple recessed in lingual surface, which will be engaged by a corresponding boss on retentive arm of denture framework. (From Harris, F. N.: J. Prosthet. Dent. **5:**43-48, 1955.)

Fig. 6-45. Maxillary partial denture framework with nonlocking rest and lingual retentive arm originating from palatal major connector but separated from it with a fine saw cut. Note the boss on spring arm, which engages a corresponding dimple in abutment restoration. (From Harris, F. N.: J. Prosthet. Dent. **5**:43-48, 1955.)

separated from it by a saw cut in the completed casting.

This attachment is most applicable to maxillary partial dentures, where the saw cut may be made in the palatal major connector. A stainless steel shim may be used rather than a saw cut to provide the necessary separation, which is then removed from the casting with acid. Flexibility of the retentive arm will be in proportion to its length as determined by the distance the separation is carried into the major connector.

The advantages that are given for this attachment are (1) no contact of the prosthesis with tooth structure, (2) stress-breaking effect, due to the flexibility of the lingual arm engaging the dimple on the abutment casting, (3) hygienic contours, and (4) no visible clasp arms. One of the most obvious disadvantages of this type of attachment is the lack of other than minimal stabilization against horizontal movement of the partial denture. Abutment torque is avoided by making the rest seat free of any locking effect; but by so doing, since the only external arm is a flexible one, stabilization against horizontal movement may be minimal. Thus, as with many stressbreaker designs, the edentulous ridge is called upon to resist horizontal movement of the prosthesis when only slightly aided by two opposing parallel walls and not by any rigid components located on the abutment teeth. The addition of anteriorly placed indirect retainers, one on each lingual side of the arch,

seemingly would add much to the dowel rest denture.

A dowel rest attachment may be used in conjunction with a fixed partial denture (Fig. 6-47). It would not be a complicated procedure, provided the fixed restoration was fabricated in conjunction with the removable restoration. However, it is doubted that adequate preparation of the rest seat could be accomplished intraorally on an existing pontic. The attachment may also be utilized in the pontic involving only the lingual and lingual occlusal of the pontic.

Internal attachments of the locking or dovetail type unquestionably have many advantages over the clasp-type denture for tooth-borne situations. It is, however, questionable whether the locking type of internal attachments for distal extension removable partial dentures are indicated, with or without stressbreakers and with or without splinted abutments, because of inherent excessive leverages most often associated with these attachments.

The nonlocking type of internal attachments, when used in conjunction with sound prosthodontic principles, can be advantageously used in many instances in Class I and II partially edentulous situations. However, unless the cross-arch axis of rotation is common to the bilaterally placed attachments, torque on the abutments may be experienced (Fig. 6-48). Excellent textbooks devoted to the use of manufactured intracoronal and extracoronal retainer systems are available.

Fig. 6-46. A, Dowel rest preparation (schematic) in a lower premolar full crown (buccal view). **B,** Proximal view (schematic) of dowel rest preparation and lingual dimple in a lower left premolar full crown. **C,** Lingual view (schematic) of dowel rest attachment. Spring arm terminating in a boss that engages a dimple in abutment crown is separated from major connector by a saw cut, or a split lingual bar is cast around a metal shim, which is later eliminated with acid. **D,** Removable partial denture framework incorporating the construction specifications illustrated in **A, B,** and **C.** (**A** to **C** courtesy Dr. R. C. Van Dam; **D** courtesy Dr. L. E. Knowles.)

Fig. 6-47. A, Dowel rest preparation in pontic of a fixed partial denture. Preparation provides for a "snubber" arm on buccal surface of pontic to facilitate removal of denture by patient. **B,** Denture is in its resting position. Note that occlusal surface of pontic has been restored by the framework. (Courtesy Dr. L. E. Knowles.)

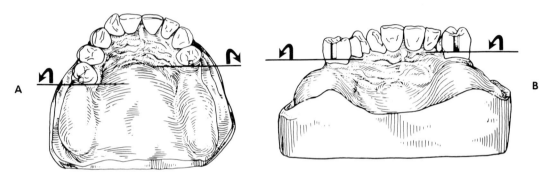

Fig. 6-48. A, Axes of rotation, although parallel, are not common since one axis is located anterior to the other axis. **B,** When one nonlocking internal attachment is elevated farther from the residual ridge than its cross-arch counterpart, the axes of rotation do not fall on a common line; thus some torquing of abutments should be anticipated. However, in many instances the effect produced by this situation will not exceed the physiologic tolerance of the supporting structures of the abutments—all other torquing factors being equal.

For this reason, this text concerns itself primarily with the extracoronal type of direct retainer assemblies (clasps).

SELF-ASSESSMENT AIDS

1. The framework of a removable partial denture must furnish *support, stabilization against horizontal (off vertical) movement, and mechanical retention.* How is mechanical retention accomplished?
2. What factor other than mechanical retention contributes to resistance of the denture to dislodging forces?
3. What is the function of a direct retainer (clasp)?
4. There are basically two types of direct retainers. Can you picture and name them?
5. Describe the principles by which the extracoronal direct retainer and the intracoronal retainer provide retention for the removable partial denture.
6. What is meant by the "height of contour" of an abutment tooth?
7. Draw a diagram of an abutment tooth and illustrate the angle of cervical convergence.
8. A direct retainer is an assembly of three components that perform individual function: (1) support, by a rest, (2) stabilization-reciprocation, by a clasp arm or other component, and (3) a retentive element. Do these elements necessarily have to arise from a common source?
9. Flexibility is permitted for only one component of a clasp assembly. Which one?
10. The amount of retention that a direct retainer is capable of generating depends on three factors. Can you visualize what these factors are?
11. The retentive arm of a direct retainer must be flexible to engage an undercut in its terminal portion. Flexibility of the arm is a product of four physical and composition factors.

Do you know what these important factors are?

12. Retention on all principal abutments should be as nearly equal as possible. To obtain this, which is the more important factor—the relation of the tip of the retentive arm to the height of contour or its depth in the angle of cervical convergence?

13. Can you describe the proportionate tapers of a cast, half-round retentive arm?

14. Can you describe the taper of a cast, half-round reciprocal-stabilizing arm of a direct retainer assembly? For what reason must there be a difference in form between a retentive arm and a reciprocal or stabilizing arm?

15. Name the two basic types of retentive clasp arms.

16. If a circumferential clasp arm approaches the retentive undercut from an occlusal direction, from which direction does a bar clasp arm approach the undercut?

17. A clasp assembly may be a combination of cast circumferential and bar clasp arms and wrought-wire retentive arms in one of several combinations. True or false?

18. A bar clasp arm is tapered in exactly the same way that a cast, half-round circumferential retentive clasp arm is tapered, differing only in configuration. Which arm is the more flexible if the two different arms are the same length? Why?

19. Permissible flexibilities of retentive cast circumferential and bar-type clasp arms based on length have been given in Table I in this chapter. Can a 0.7-inch bar-type arm be safely placed in the same depth of undercut that a 0.7-inch circumferential arm can?

20. Cast clasp arms are essentially half-round in form, permitting flexing in only one direction. Which direction is this?

21. Wrought wire, 18-gauge round, is often used as a circumferential clasp arm. Its round form will permit flexing in what directions?

22. We speak of a reciprocal clasp arm. Can you explain what is meant by reciprocation and describe the condition that must be met for true reciprocation to occur?

23. A basic principle of direct retainer (clasp) design is that the retentive and reciprocal arms must encompass more than 180 degrees of the greatest circumference of the tooth, passing from diverging to converging axial surfaces. What would probably happen if a clasp designed otherwise was used?

24. Simple mechanical laws (of levers) demonstrate that the closer a direct retainer assembly is located to the tipping axis of the tooth, the less likely that the periodontal ligament will be taxed from rotation tendencies of the denture. Can you draw the coronal portion of an abutment, divide the enamel crown into thirds, and locate retentive, reciprocal, and stabilizing components optimally?

25. Clasp retainers on abutment teeth adjacent to distal extension bases should be designed so that they will avoid direct transmission of tipping and rotational forces to the abutment. Is this statement true or false?

26. The location of a usable undercut is perhaps the most important single factor in selecting a clasp for use with distal extension partial dentures. True or false?

27. There are many types and configurations of clasps. This can be most confusing, especially to the student dentist. However, if you will simply remember the three components necessary for a clasp assembly and their functions, locate the components to assure proper function, know that a distal extension denture will rotate under forces, and design accordingly, always thinking kindness to the periodontium, your difficulties in choosing the correct retainer will be minimized.

28. Under what circumstances may circumferential embrasure clasps be used? What are some real disadvantages of this type of retainer, including preparation of abutment teeth?

29. Give the indications for using a cast circumferential direct retainer.

30. What observations would lead you to select a bar-type clasp?

31. What is a combination clasp and what are the indications for its use?

32. State three advantages of the combination clasp.

33. Selection of wrought wire, attachment of it to the framework, and quality control in its use are discussed at the end of Chapter 11, You should have a thorough knowledge of the information presented there. It will assist you in decision making and maintaining quality control.

34. Nonlocking internal attachments we have used were discussed at the end of this chapter. Several good texts are available on manufactured intracoronal and extracoronal attachments. Self-assessment aids on internal attachments are not included in this text.

7 INDIRECT RETAINERS

Movement of the base of an entirely tooth-borne partial denture *toward* the edentulous ridge is prevented primarily by rests placed on the abutment teeth located at each end of each edentulous space. Presuming that the denture framework is rigid and the rests are properly placed, occlusal forces are transmitted directly to the abutment teeth through the rests placed on those teeth. Movement of the base *away* from the edentulous ridge is prevented by the activation of the otherwise passive direct retainers on the same abutment teeth. Horizontal movement of the partial denture and longitudinal rotational movement of the denture base are prevented by stabilizing components on the same abutment teeth, plus any auxiliary abutments contacted for stabilization. Rotation of the tooth-borne partial denture is therefore relatively nonexistent.

In contrast, all Class I and Class II partial dentures having one or more distal extension bases are not totally tooth supported; neither are they completely retained by bounding abutments. Any Class III or Class IV partial denture that does not have adequate abutment support falls into the same category. These latter may derive some support from the edentulous ridge and therefore may have a composite support from both teeth and ridge tissues.

Movement of a distal extension base *toward* the ridge tissues will be proportionate to the quality of those tissues, the accuracy of the denture base, and the total functional load applied. Movement of a distal extension base *away* from the ridge tissues will occur either as a rotational movement about an axis or as displacement of the entire denture. The forces that tend to displace any denture are also the forces that cause rotation of a distal extension partial denture.

Denture rotation about an axis. Presuming that direct retainers are functioning to prevent total displacement, rotational movement will occur about some axis as the distal extension base or bases either move toward or away from the underlying tissues. This axis is an imaginary line passing through teeth and *direct retainers*, around which line the denture rotates slightly when subjected to various forces directed toward residual ridges. It is called the *fulcrum line*. More than one fulcrum line may be present for the same removable partial denture (Fig. 7-1).

When the base(s) of an extension denture move away from the basal seat, an axis of rotation will pass through the most anteriorly located supporting elements of the denture framework, assuming that these anteriorly located elements are in their planned positions. In the absence of indirect retainers or components that function as indirect retainers, the axis of rotation will pass through the most posterior and bilaterally located tips of retainer arms engaging an undercut.

For the sake of clarity in discussing the location and functions of indirect retainers, the term fulcrum line should be considered the axis about which the denture will rotate when the bases move toward the residual ridge.

The fulcrum line is identified on a Class I partial denture as passing through the rigid components of the direct retainer assemblies occlusal to the height of contour on the most posterior abutment on either side of the arch (Fig. 7-2, A and B). On a Class II partial denture the fulcrum line is always diagonal, passing through the abutment on the distal extension side and the most distal abutment on the other side (Fig. 7-2, C). If a modification area is present on that side, the additional abutment lying between the two principal abutments may be used for support of the indirect retainer if it is far enough removed from the fulcrum line (Fig. 7-2, D).

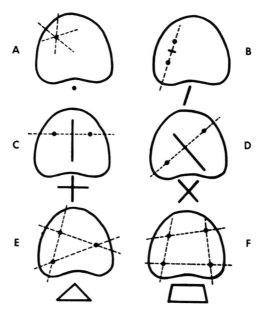

Fig. 7-1. **A,** Broken lines represent imaginary fulcrum lines passing through vertical support areas of a direct retainer. The dot represents a single-clasp restoration. Any number of fulcrum lines could pass through the one supporting point. Such a restoration could not have stability by means of cross-arch leverage. **B,** A two-clasp unilateral partial denture situation is represented by a straight line, the fulcrum line passing through the support areas and in line with the partial denture. This design derives its stability against tipping from only the short leverages supplied by the clasp arms with no cross-arch assistance. **C,** The imaginary + represents the two-clasp, diametrically opposed, distal extension partial denture situation. The fulcrum line forms the cross bar, and the unseating leverage (afforded by the extension bases), combined with the controlling leverage (the indirect retainer anterior to the fulcrum line), completes the upright. A partial denture designed to counteract unseating leverages in accordance with this imaginary figure would be stable. **D,** The imaginary x with two diagonally opposed clasps providing the guide for the fulcrum line. The leverage below this line from the single base extension, added to the length of the indirect leverage anterior to the line, completes the geometric figure that represents a stable denture design. **E,** The triangular design results from the use of three clasps, with the abutments being selected as far apart as feasible to include the largest area within the triangle and to provide the longest controlling leverages against tipping strains. Usually this is a stable design. **F,** The quadrangular figure is representative of a four-clasp restoration. Its area is large enough to circumscribe most unseating stresses so that they would fall within the quadrangle and tend to seat the restoration instead of dislodging it. (Paraphrased from Steffel, V. L.: J. Prosthet. Dent. **12:** 524-535, 1962.)

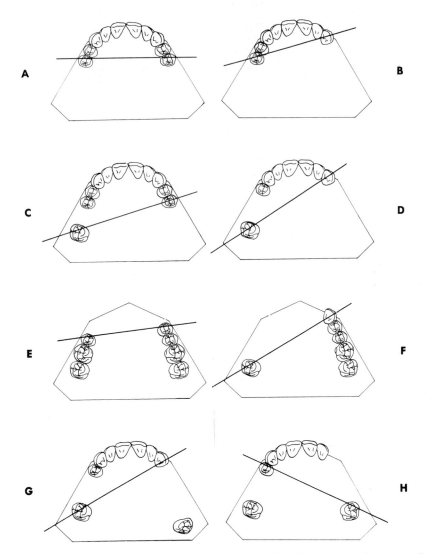

Fig. 7-2. Fulcrum line found in various types of partially edentulous arches around which the denture will probably rotate when the bases are subjected to forces directed toward the residual ridge. **A** and **B,** In a Class I arch the fulcrum line passes through the most posterior abutments, provided some rigid component of the framework is occlusal to the abutments' heights of contour. **C,** In a Class II arch the fulcrum line is diagonal, passing through the abutment on the distal extension side and the most posterior abutment on the opposite side. **D,** If an abutment tooth anterior to a modification space lies far enough removed from the fulcrum line, it may be used effectively for the support of an indirect retainer. **E** and **F,** In a Class IV arch the fulcrum line passes through the two abutments adjacent to the single edentulous space. **G,** In a Class III arch with a posterior tooth on one side, which possibly will eventually be lost, the fulcrum line is considered the same as though the posterior tooth were not present. Thus its loss at some future date will not necessitate altering the design of the partial denture. **H,** In a Class III arch with nonsupporting anterior teeth the adjacent edentulous area is considered to be a tissue-supported end, with a diagonal fulcrum line passing through the two principal abutments as in a Class II arch.

Fig. 7-3. Planning location for indirect retainers for a Class I partial denture. The greatest distance from axis of rotation (fulcrum line) would fall on incisor teeth, which are ill-suited to provide adequate support without tooth movement or slippage of retainer or both. Dual occlusal rests on prepared rest seats at mesial marginal ridge of first premolars provide effective indirect retention with optimal tooth support.

Fig. 7-4. Example of indirect retention used in conjunction with palatal plate–type major connector. Indirect retainers are located on first premolars. A secondary function of auxiliary occlusal rest assemblies is to prevent settling of anterior portion of major connector and to provide stabilization against horizontal rotation.

In a Class IV partial denture the fulcrum line passes through the two abutments adjacent to the single edentulous space (Fig. 7-2, *E* and *F*). In a tooth- and tissue-supported Class III partial denture the fulcrum line is determined by considering the weaker abutment as nonexistent and that end of the base as being a distal extension (Fig. 7-2, *G* and *H*).

Movement of the denture base away from the tissues and about the fulcrum line is prevented by units of the partial denture framework that are located on definite rest seats on the opposite side of the fulcrum line from the distal extension base and the activation of the retentive element of the direct retainer assembly. These anteriorly located components should be placed as far as possible from the distal extension base affording the best possible leverage advantage against lifting of the distal extension base. Such units are called *indirect retainers.*

As indirect retainer consists of one or more rests and their supporting minor connectors (Figs. 7-3 and 7-4). Although it is customary to identify the entire assembly as the indirect retainer, it should be remembered it is the rest that is actually the indirect retainer, united to the major connector by a minor connector. This is to avoid

interpreting any contact with tooth inclines as being part of the indirect retainer. *An indirect retainer should be placed as far from the distal extension base as possible in a prepared rest seat on a tooth capable of supporting its function.*

Whereas the most effective location of an indirect retainer is frequently in the vicinity of an incisor tooth, that tooth may not be strong enough to support an indirect retainer and may have steep inclines that cannot be favorably altered to support a rest. In such case the nearest canine tooth or the mesial occlusal surface of the first premolar may be the best location, despite the fact that it is not as far removed from the fulcrum line. Whenever possible, two indirect retainers closer to the fulcrum line are then used to compensate for the compromise in distance.

Factors influencing effectiveness of indirect retainers. The factors influencing the effectiveness of an indirect retainer are as follows:

1. Effectiveness of the direct retainers. Unless the principal occlusal rests are reasonably held in their seats by the retentive arms of the direct retainers, rotation about an axis will not occur, but total displacement will occur. Therefore an indirect re-

tainer cannot activate the direct retainer to prevent lifting of the distal extension base away from the tissues.

2. Distance from the fulcrum line. Three areas must be considered:

    a. Length of the distal extension base

    b. Location of the fulcrum line

    c. How far beyond the fulcrum line the indirect retainer is placed

3. Rigidity of the connectors supporting the indirect retainer. All connectors must be rigid if the indirect retainer is to function as intended.

4. Effectiveness of the supporting tooth surface. The indirect retainer must be placed on a definite rest seat on which slippage or tooth movement will not occur. Tooth inclines and weak teeth should never be used for the support of indirect retainers.

Auxiliary functions of indirect retainers. In addition to effectively activating the direct retainer to prevent movement of a distal extension base away from the tissues, an indirect retainer may serve the following auxiliary functions:

1. It tends to reduce anteroposterior tilting leverages on the principal abutments. This is particularly important when an isolated tooth is being used as an abutment, a situation that should be avoided whenever possible. Ordinarily, proximal contact with the adjacent tooth prevents such tilting of an abutment as the base lifts away from the tissues.

2. Contact of its minor connector with axial tooth surfaces aids in stabilization against horizontal movement of the denture. Such tooth surfaces, when made parallel to the path of placement, may also act as auxiliary guiding planes.

3. Anterior teeth supporting indirect retainers are splinted against lingual movement.

4. It may act as an auxiliary rest to support a portion of the major connector. For example, a lingual bar may be supported against settling into the tissues by the indirect retainer acting as an auxiliary rest. One must be able to differentiate between an auxiliary rest placed for support for a major connector, one placed for indirect retention, and one serving a dual purpose. Some auxiliary rests are added solely to provide rest support to a segment of the denture and should not be confused with indirect retention.

Forms of indirect retainers. The indirect retainer may take any one of several forms. All are effective in proportion to their *support* and the *distance from the fulcrum line.*

Auxiliary occlusal rest. The most frequently used indirect retainer is an auxiliary occlusal rest located on an occlusal surface as far away from the distal extension base as possible. In a mandibular Class I arch this is usually on the mesial marginal ridge of the first premolar on each side (Fig. 7-3). The longest perpendicular to the fulcrum line would be in the vicinity of the central incisors, which are too weak and have lingual surfaces that are too perpendicular to support a rest. Bilateral rests on the first premolars are quite effective, even though located closer to the axis of rotation.

The same principle applies to any maxillary Class I partial denture when indirect retainers are used. Bilateral rests on the mesial marginal ridge of the first premolars are almost always used in preference to rests on incisor teeth (Fig. 7-4). Not only are they effective without jeopardizing the weaker single-rooted teeth, but also interference to the tongue is far less when the minor connector can be placed in the embrasure between canine and premolar rather than anterior to the canine teeth.

Indirect retainers for Class II partial dentures are usually placed on the marginal ridge of the first premolar tooth on the opposite side of the arch from the distal extension base (Fig. 7-5). Bilateral rests are seldom indicated except when an auxiliary occlusal rest is needed for support of the major connector or when the prognosis of the distal abutment is poor and provision must be made for later conversion to a Class I partial denture should that tooth be lost.

Canine extensions from occlusal rests. Occasionally a finger extension from a premolar rest is placed on the prepared lingual slope of the adjacent canine tooth (Fig. 7-6). Such an extension is used to effect indirect retention by increasing the distance of a resisting element from the fulcrum line. This is particularly applicable when a first premolar must serve as a primary abutment. The distance anterior to the fulcrum line is only the distance between the mesial occlusal rest and the anterior terminal of the finger extension. In this instance, although the ex-

Fig. 7-5. Lower Class II design utilizing embrasure clasping on nonedentulous side. Indirect retainer on distal marginal ridge of rotated first premolar is favorably located in relation to fulcrum line. Note use of wrought-wire retentive clasp arm on buccal surface of left first premolar. Bar-type retainer could not be used because of presence of a gross tissue undercut (buccal) below first premolar and absence of a usable undercut on its distobuccal surface.

Fig. 7-6. Mandibular Class I design utilizing canine extensions from occlusal rests as indirect retainers. Canine extensions must be placed in prepared rest seats so that resistance will be directed as nearly as possible along long axes of canine abutments.

tension rests on a prepared surface, it is used in conjunction with a terminal rest on the mesial marginal ridge of the premolar tooth. Tipping leverage on the canine tooth is predominantly avoided. *Even when not used as indirect retainers, canine extensions, continuous bar retainers, and linguoplates should never be used without terminal rests because of the resultant forces effective when they are placed on inclined planes alone.*

Canine rests. When the mesial marginal ridge of the first premolar is too close to the fulcrum line or when the teeth are lapped so that the fulcrum line is not accessible, a rest on the adjacent canine tooth may be used. Such a rest may be made more effective by placing the minor connector in the embrasure anterior to the canine, either curving back onto a prepared lingual rest seat or extending to a mesioincisal rest. The same types of canine rests as those previously outlined may be used, which are the lingual or incisal rests. (See Chapter 5.)

Continuous bar retainers and linguoplates. Technically, continous bar retainers and linguoplates are not indirect retainers, since they rest on unprepared lingual inclines of anterior teeth. The indirect retainers are actually the terminal rests at

either end, in the form of auxiliary occlusal rests or canine rests.

In Class I and Class II partial dentures a continuous bar retainer or linguoplate may extend the effectiveness of the indirect retainer if used with a terminal rest at each end. In tooth-borne partial dentures they are placed for other reasons but always with terminal rests. (See Chapter 4.)

In Class I and Class II partial dentures especially, a continuous bar retainer or the superior border of the linguoplate should never be placed above the middle third of the teeth so that orthodontic movement during the rotation of a distal extension denture is avoided. This is not so important when the six anterior teeth are in nearly a straight line, but when the arch is narrow and tapering, a continuous bar retainer or linguoplate on anterior teeth extends well beyond the terminal rests, and orthodontic movement of those teeth is more likely. Whereas these are intended primarily to stabilize weak anterior teeth, they may have the opposite effect if not used with discretion.

Modification areas. Occasionally the occlusal rest on a secondary abutment in a Class II partial denture may be used also as an indirect retainer. This will depend on how far from the fulcrum line the secondary abutment is located.

The primary abutments in a Class II,

Fig. 7-7. Class II, modification 1, removable partial denture framework. The fulcrum line, when denture base is displaced toward residual ridge, runs from left second premolar to right second molar. When forces tend to displace denture away from its basal seat, supportive element of direct retainer assembly on right first premolar "acts" as an indirect retainer.

Fig. 7-8. Class II maxillary removable partial denture framework design. The fulcrum line runs from patient's right canine to left second molar. Forces that tend to unseat denture from its basal seat will be resisted by activation of retentive elements on canine and molar, utilizing supportive elements on first premolar as terminus of a resistance arm.

modification 1, partial denture are the abutment adjacent to the distal extension base and the most distal abutment on the tooth-borne side. The fulcrum line is a diagnoal axis between the two terminal abutments (Fig. 7-7.)

The anterior abutment on the tooth-borne side is a secondary abutment, serving to support and retain one end of the tooth-borne segment, as well as adding horizontal stabilization to the denture. If the modification space were not present, as in an unmodified Class II arch, auxiliary occlusal rests and stabilizing components would still be essential to the design of the denture (Fig. 7-8). But the presence of a modification space conveniently provides an abutment tooth for retention, stabilization, and support.

If the occlusal rest on the secondary abutment lies far enough from the fulcrum line, it may serve adequately as an indirect retainer. Its dual function then is tooth support for one end of the modification area and support for an indirect retainer. The most typical example is a distal occlusal rest on a first premolar, when second premolar and first molar are missing and the second molar serves as one of the primary abutments. The longest perpendicular to the fulcrum line falls in the vicinity of the first pre-

molar, making the location of the indirect retainer nearly ideal.

On the other hand, if only one tooth, such as a first molar, is missing on the modification side, the occlusal rest on the second premolar abutment is too close to the fulcrum line to be effective. In such case an auxiliary occlusal rest on the mesial marginal ridge of the first premolar is needed, both for indirect retention and for support for an otherwise unsupported major connector.

Support for a modification area extending anteriorly to a canine abutment is obtained by any one of the accepted canine rest forms, as previously outlined. In this situation the canine tooth provides nearly ideal indirect retention, and support for the major connector as well.

Rugae support. Some authorities consider coverage of the rugae area of the maxillary arch as a means of indirect retention, since the rugae area is firm and usually well situated to provide indirect retention for a Class I denture. While it is true that broad coverage over the rugae area can conceivably provide some support, the facts remain that tissue support is less effective than positive tooth support and that rugae coverage is undesirable if it can be avoided.

The use of rugae support for indirect retention is usually part of a palatal horseshoe design. Since posterior retention is usually inadequate in this situation, the requirements for indirect retention are probably greater than can be satisfied by tissue support alone.

Direct-indirect retention. In the mandibular arch, retention from the distal extension base alone is usually inadequate to prevent lifting of the base away from the tissues. In the maxillary arch, where only anterior teeth remain, full palatal coverage is usually necessary. In fact, with any Class I partial denture extending distally from the first premolar teeth, except when a maxillary torus prevents its use, palatal coverage may be used to advantage. While full coverage may be in the form of a resin base, the added retention and lesser bulk of the cast metal palate makes the latter preferable. (See Chapter 4.) However, in the absence of full palatal coverage an indirect retainer should be used with other designs of major palatal connectors for the Class I removable partial denture.

SELF-ASSESSMENT AIDS

1. What elements prevent movement of the base(s) of a tooth-borne denture toward the basal seats?
2. Support of a distal extension removable partial denture is shared by abutment teeth and residual ridges. The quality of support furnished by the residual ridges is proportionate to at least three factors. Can you name them?
3. Movement of a distal extension base away from basal seats will occur as a rotational movement or _____?
4. What is the difference between fulcrum line and axis of rotation?
5. Can you identify the fulcrum line on a Class I arch? Class II, modification 1? Class IV?
6. Define the term *indirect retainer*.
7. What components of a removable partial denture framework usually make an indirect retainer?
8. From the standpoint of leverage advantage, where should an indirect retainer be located?
9. An indirect retainer performs one major function and four auxiliary functions. Can you state these five functions?
10. The effectiveness of an indirect retainer is influenced by four factors. What are they?
11. What are the probable sequelae of trying to use a continuous bar retainer or linguoplate to serve the purpose of an indirect retainer?
12. In a Class II, modification 1 arch, especially if the modification is a long edentulous space, what component may act as an indirect retainer?
13. Discuss the inadequacy of utilizing coverage of rugae to act as support for indirect retention.
14. Each design of the extension type removable partial denture should include an indirect retainer or some component that will act as an indirect retainer. True or false?
15. Bilaterally placed indirect retainers contribute to stability of the Class I restoration to a greater extent that does a single indirect retainer. True or false?

8 DENTURE BASES AND STRESSBREAKERS (STRESS EQUALIZERS)

DENTURE BASES

The denture base supports the supplied teeth and effects the transfer of occlusal stresses to the supporting oral structures (Fig. 8-1).

Although its primary purpose is related to masticatory function, the denture base also may add to the cosmetic effect of the replacement, particularly when modern techniques for tinting and the reproducing of natural looking contours are used. Most of the modern techniques for creating naturalness in complete denture bases are applicable equally well to partial denture bases.

Still another function of the denture base is the stimulation, by massage, of the underlying tissues of the residual ridge. Some vertical movement occurs with any denture base, even those supported entirely by abutment teeth, because of the physiologic movement of those teeth under function. It is clearly evident that oral tissues placed under functional stress within their physiologic tolerance maintain their form and tone better than do similar tissues suffering from disuse. The term *disuse atrophy* is applicable to both periodontal tissues and the tissues of a residual ridge.

Functions of tooth-supported partial denture base. Denture bases differ in functional purpose and may differ in the material of which they are made. In a tooth-borne prosthesis the denture base is primarily a span between two abutments supporting artificial occlusal surfaces. Thus occlusal forces are transferred directly to the abutment teeth through rests. Also, the denture base and the supplied teeth serve to prevent horizontal migration of the teeth in the partially

edentulous arch and vertical migration of teeth in the opposing arch.

When only posterior teeth are being replaced, esthetics is usually a secondary consideration. On the other hand, when anterior teeth are replaced, esthetics may be of primary importance. Except for esthetic considerations, the tooth-borne partial denture base is essentially a framework supporting occlusal surfaces. Theoretically, occlusal surfaces alone would accomplish masticatory efficiency and maintain the relative position of the natural teeth. However, they would lack desirable esthetics, create undesirable food traps, and deprive the tissues of the stimulation by massage that they would receive from an accurate denture base. The reasons, then, for providing more than only the necessary support for occlusal surfaces in a tooth-borne denture are (1) esthetics, (2) cleanliness, and (3) stimulation of underlying tissues.

Functions of distal extension partial denture base. In a distal extension partial denture the denture bases other than those in tooth-supported modifications must contribute to the support of the denture. Close to the terminal abutment only a framework supporting occlusal surfaces is necessary. However, farther from the abutment the support from the underlying ridge tissues becomes increasingly important. Maximum support from the residual ridge may be obtained only by using broad, accurate denture bases, which spread the occlusal load equitably over the entire area that is available for such support. The space that is available for a denture base is controlled by the structures surrounding the space and their movement during function. Maximum sup-

Fig. 8-1. A, Maxillary bilateral distal extension removable partial denture with acrylic resin denture bases. Bases are extended bucally within physiologic tolerance of border structures, and they cover tuberosities being extended into pterygomaxillary notches. B, Mandibular bilateral distal extension removable partial denture with acrylic resin denture bases. As in A, bases are fully extended. Lingual flanges are extended into retromylohyoid fossae. The impression procedure utilized established the buccal shelves as primary stress-bearing areas of basal seats.

Fig. 8-2. Mandibular Class II, modification 1, design wax pattern developed on an investment cast. Adequate provision is made for attaching major connector to resin base on edentulous side by way of a ladderlike minor connector and a butt-type joint. A cast base will be used for modification space. Note finishing lines on cast base pattern and "nail–head" minor connectors for retention of acrylic resin supporting prosthetically supplied teeth.

In addition to their difference in functional purposes, denture bases vary in material of construction. This is related to their function because of the need for future rebasing in one instance and usually not in another.

Since the tooth-supported base has an abutment tooth at each end upon which a rest has been placed, future relining or rebasing may not be necessary to reestablish support. Relining is necessary only when tissue changes have occurred beneath the tooth-borne base to the point that poor esthetics and the accumulation of debris result. For these reasons alone, tooth-borne bases that are made soon after extractions should be constructed of a material that permits later relining. Such materials are the denture resins, the most common of which are copolymer and methyl methacrylate resins.

Resin bases are attached to the partial denture framework by means of a retentive framework designed so that a space exists between it and the underlying tissues of the residual ridge (Fig. 8-2). A blockout of at least 20-gauge thickness over the master cast is used to create a raised platform on the investment cast on which the pattern for the retentive frame is formed. Thus, after casting, the portion of the retentive framework to which the resin base will be attached will stand away from the tissue

port for the denture base therefore can be accomplished only by utilizing·a knowledge of the limiting anatomic structures, knowledge of the histologic nature of the basal seat areas, accuracy of the impression, and accuracy of the denture base. A principle as old as the snowshoe is that broad coverage furnishes the best support with the least load per unit area. Therefore support should be the primary consideration in selecting, designing, and fabricating a distal extension partial denture base. Of secondary importance, but to be considered nevertheless, are esthetics, stimulation of the underlying tissues, and oral cleanliness. Methods we have used to accomplish maximum support of the restoration through its base(s) are presented in Chapter 14.

Fig. 8-3. Replaced lateral incisor and canine are abutted to residual ridge for better esthetics. Occasionally first premolar is treated similarly, depending on how visible this tooth is. Retentive framework for resin base must be designed so that interference with proper placement and arrangement of artificial teeth will not be encountered.

surface sufficiently to permit a flow of resin base material beneath the surface.

The retentive framework should be embedded in the base material with sufficient thickness of resin to allow for relieving if this becomes necessary during denture adjustment over tender areas or during relining procedures. Thickness is also necessary to avoid weakness and subsequent fracture of the resin base material surrounding the metal framework.

The use of plastic mesh patterns in forming the retentive framework is generally less satisfactory than is a more open framework. Less weakening of the resin by the embedded framework results from the use of the more open form. Pieces of 12- or 14-gauge half-round wax and 18-gauge round wax are therefore used to form a ladderlike framework rather than the finer latticework of the mesh pattern. The precise design of the retentive framework, other than that it should be located both bucally and lingually, is not so important as its effective rigidity and strength when embedded in the resin base—free of interference to future adjustment and to arrangement of artificial teeth and open enough to avoid weakening any portion of the attached resin (Fig. 8-3). Designing the retentive framework for a denture base by having elements both buccal and lingual to the residual ridge not only will strengthen the resin base but also will minimize distortion of the base created by the release of inherent strains in the acrylic resin base during use or storage of the restoration (Fig. 8-4).

Fig. 8-4. Note that minor connectors by which acrylic resin denture bases will be attached to framework are open, ladderlike configurations extending on both buccal and lingual surfaces. This not only provides excellent attachment of acrylic resin bases but also minimizes warping of bases due to release of inherent strains in compression-molded acrylic resin.

Ideal denture base. The requirements for an ideal denture base are as follows:

1. Accuracy of adaptation to the tissues, with low volume change
2. Dense, nonirritating surface that is capable of receiving and maintaining a good finish
3. Thermal conductivity
4. Low specific gravity; lightness in the mouth
5. Sufficient strength; resistance to fracture or distortion
6. Self-cleansing factor, or easily kept clean
7. Esthetic acceptability
8. Potential for future relining
9. Low initial cost

Obviously such an ideal denture base material does not exist; nor is it likely to be developed in the near future. However, any denture base—whether of resin or metal and regardless of the method of fabrication—should come as close to this ideal as possible.

Advantages of metal bases. Except for those edentulous ridges with recent extractions, metal is preferred to resin for tooth-supported bases because of the several advantages of the metal base. Its principal disadvantage is that it can be relined only with difficulty, if at all. Nevertheless the stimulation that it gives to the underlying tissues is so beneficial that it probably prevents some alveolar atrophy that would otherwise occur under a resin base and thereby prolongs the health of the tissues that it contacts. Some of the advantages of a metal base are as follows:

1. *Thermal conductivity.* Temperature changes are transmitted through the metal base to the underlying tissues, thereby helping to maintain the health of those tissues. Freedom of interchange of temperature between the tissues covered and the surrounding external influences (temperature of liquid and solid foods and inspired air) contributes much to the patient's acceptance of a denture and may help avoid the feeling of the presence of a foreign body. Denture resins, on the other hand, all have insulating properties that prevent interchange of temperature between the inside and the outside of the denture base.

2. *Accuracy and permanence of form.* Cast metal bases, whether of gold or chrome alloys, not only may be cast more accurately than denture resins but also maintain their accuracy of form without change in the mouth. Internal strains that may be released later to cause distortion are not present. Although some resins and some processing techniques are superior to others in accuracy and permanence of form, modern cast alloys are generally superior in this respect. Evidence of this fact is that an additional posterior palatal seal may be eliminated entirely when a cast palate is used for a complete denture, as compared with the need for a definite attempt in this regard when the palate is made of resin. Distortion of a resin base is manifest in the maxillary denture by a distortion away from the palate in the midline and toward the tuberosities on the buccal flanges. The greater the curvature of the tissues, the greater is this distortion. Similar distortions occur in a mandibular denture but are less easily detected. Accurate metal castings are not subject to distortion by the release of internal strains as are most denture resins.

Because of its accuracy, the metal base provides an intimacy of contact that contributes considerably to the retention of a denture prosthesis. Sometimes called *interfacial surface tension*, direct retention from a cast denture base is significant in proportion to the area involved. This has been previously mentioned as an important factor in both direct and direct-indirect retention of maxillary restorations. Such intimacy of contact is not possible with resin bases.

Permanence of form of the cast base is also assured because of its resistance to abrasion from denture cleaning agents. Cleanliness of the denture base should be stressed; however, constant brushing of the tissue side of a resin denture base, if effective, inevitably causes some loss of accuracy by abrasion. Intimacy of contact, which was never as great with a resin base as with a metal base, is therefore jeopardized further by cleaning habits. The metal bases, particularly the harder chrome alloys, withstand repeated cleaning without significant changes in surface accuracy.

3. *Cleanliness.* Cleanliness is listed apart from resistance to abrasion because the inherent cleanliness of the cast base contributes to the health of the tissues regardless of the patient's cleaning habits. Resin bases tend to accumulate mucinous deposits containing food particles, as well as calcareous deposits. Unfavorable tissue reaction to de-

composing food particles and bacterial enzymes and to mechanical irritation from calculus results if the denture is not kept mechanically clean. Whereas calculus, which must be removed periodically, does precipitate on a cast metal base, other deposits do not accumulate as they do on a resin base. For this reason a metal base is naturally cleaner than is a resin base.

4. *Weight and bulk.* Metal alloy may be cast much thinner than resin and still have adequate strength and rigidity. Still less weight and bulk are possible when the denture bases are made of chrome alloys. Cast gold must be given slightly more bulk to provide the same amount of rigidity but may still be made with less thickness than resin materials.

There are times, however, when both weight and thickness may be used to advantage in denture bases. In the mandibular arch, weight of the denture may be an asset in regard to retention, and for this reason a cast gold base may be preferred. On the other hand, extreme loss of residual alveolar bone may make it necessary to add fullness to the denture base to restore normal facial contours and to fill out the buccal vestibule with a denture contour that will prevent food from being lost in the cheek and from working beneath the denture. In such situations a resin base may be preferred to the thinner metal base.

In the maxillary arch a resin base may be preferred to the thinner metal base to provide fullness when needed, such as in buccal flanges or to fill a maxillary buccal vestibule. Resin may also be preferred over the thinner metal base for esthetic reasons. In these several instances the thinness of the metal base may be of no advantage, but in areas where the tongue and cheek needed maximum room, thinness may be desirable.

Denture base contours for functional tongue and cheek contact can best be accomplished with resin. Whereas metal bases are usually made thin to minimize bulk and weight, resin bases may be contoured to provide ideal polished surfaces that contribute to the retention of the denture, restore facial contours, and avoid the accumulation of food at denture borders. Lingual surfaces usually are made concave except in the distal palatal area. Buccal surfaces are made convex at gingival margins, over root prominences,

Fig. 8-5. Partial metal bases used with a full palatal plate and "pressed-on" anterior teeth. Attachment of artificial posterior teeth with resin is accomplished by diagonal spurs and lingual undercut finishing line. The visible buccal flange will be of resin, yet without sacrificing most of the advantages of a metal base. Support anteriorly is by a mesioincisal rest on a canine and by lingual rests on all remaining anterior teeth.

and at the border to fill the area recorded in the impression. Between the border and the gingival contours the base is made concave to aid in retention and to facilitate the food bolus's being returned to the occlusal table during mastication. Such contours prevent food from being lost in the cheek and from working under the denture. This cannot usually be accomplished with metal bases.

However, the advantages of a metal base need not necessarily be sacrificed for the sake of esthetics or desirable denture contours when the use of such a base is otherwise indicated. Denture bases may be designed to provide almost total metallic coverage, yet with resin borders to avoid a display of metal and to add buccal fullness when needed (Fig. 8-5). The advantages of thermal conductivity are not necessarily lost by covering a portion of the metal base so long as other parts of the denture are exposed to effect temperature changes through conduction.

Attaching artificial teeth to metal bases. Artificial teeth may be added to denture bases by several means. Some of these are as follows:

1. *Porcelain or resin artificial teeth attached to a metal base with resin.* Retention of the resin to the metal base may be accomplished by nailhead retention, retention loops, or diagonal spurs placed at random.

Nailheads should be placed so that they will not interfere with the placement of the teeth on the metal base (Fig. 8-5).

Any junction of resin with metal should be at an undercut finishing line or associated with some retentive undercut. Since only a mechanical attachment exists between metal and resin, every attempt should be made to avoid separation and seepage, which results in discoloration and uncleanliness. Denture odors are frequently caused by accretions at the junction of resin with metal when only mechanical union exists. Separation occurring between resin and metal leads eventually to some loosening of the resin base.

2. *Porcelain or resin tube teeth and facings cemented directly to metal bases* (Fig. 8-6). Some disadvantages of this type of attachment are the difficulties in obtaining satisfactory occlusion, lack of adequate contours for functional tongue and cheek contact, and unesthetic display of metal at gingival margins. The latter is avoided when the tooth is butted directly to the ridge, but then the retention for the tooth frequently becomes inadequate.

A modification of this method is the attachment of ready-made resin teeth to the metal base with acrylic resin of the same shade. This is called *pressing on* a resin tooth and is not the same as using resin for cementation. It is particularly applicable to anterior replacements, since it is desirable to know in advance of making the casting that the shade and contours of the selected tooth will be acceptable (Fig. 8-5). After a labial index of the position of the teeth has been made, the lingual portion of the tooth then is cut away to make room for retention on the casting. Subsequently the tooth is attached to the denture with acrylic resin of the same shade. Since this is done under pressure, the acrylic resin attachment is comparable to the manufactured tooth in hardness and strength.

Tube or side-groove teeth must be selected in advance of waxing the denture framework. Yet, for best occlusal relationships, jaw relation records always should be made with the denture casting in the mouth. This problem may be solved by selecting tube teeth for width but with occlusal surfaces slightly higher than will be necessary. The teeth are ground to fit the ridge with sufficient clearance beneath for a thin metal base and beveled to accommodate a boxing of

Fig. 8-6. Class III, modification 2, partial denture with palatal major connector supporting tubed teeth posteriorly and Steele's facings anteriorly. The design is actually an anatomic replica palatal major connector extended anteriorly to support anterior replacements. The entire major connector is as thin as mechanically feasible and of uniform thickness, made possible by using an anatomic replica pattern. Esthetics dictated the spacing between incisor teeth, which could not easily have been accomplished with a fixed partial denture. Note also the clearance lingual to premolar abutments. **A,** Wax and plastic pattern for this casting, with a plaster index for positioning anterior Steele's facings. Backings are plastic waxed to anatomic replica palatal pattern. **B,** Completed casting.

metal. If a plastic tube tooth is used, the diatoric hole should be made slightly larger than provided. The casting is completed and tried in, occlusal relationships are recorded, and then the teeth are ground to harmonious occlusion with the opposing dentition. As will be discussed in Chapter 16, artificial posterior teeth on partial dentures should hardly ever be used unaltered but rather should be considered material from which occlusal forms may be created to function harmoniously with the remaining natural occlusion.

Fig. 8-7. Direct attachment of resin teeth to metal bases. These are waxed to fit the space and opposing occlusion and processed to retention previously provided on metal framework. Occlusal surfaces of acyrlic resin posterior teeth should be duplicated in cast inlay gold.

Fig. 8-8. Occlusal surfaces cast with inlay-type gold and attached to prosthetically supplied teeth.

3. *Resin teeth processed directly to metal bases.* Modern cross-linked copolymers enable the dentist or technician to process acrylic resin teeth that have satisfactory hardness and abrasion resistance for many situations. Thus occlusion may be created without resorting to the modification of ready-made artificial teeth (Fig. 8-7). Recesses in the denture pattern are either carved by hand or created around manufactured teeth that are used only to form the recess in the pattern. Occlusal relations may be established either in the mouth on the denture framework or by the use of an articulator, and then the teeth are carved and processed in acrylic resin of the proper shade to fit the opposing occlusal record. Better attachment to the metal base than by cementation is thus possible. In addition, unusually long, short, wide, or narrow teeth may be created when necessary to fill spaces not easily filled by the limited selection of commercially available teeth.

Occlusion on resin teeth may be reestablished to compensate for wear or settling by reprocessing new acrylic occlusal surfaces at a later date when this becomes necessary. Distinction always should be made between the need for relining to reestablish occlusion (on a distal extension partial denture) or the need for rebuilding occlusal surfaces on an otherwise satisfactory base (on either a tooth-supported or a tooth-and-tissue supported partial denture).

Reestablishment of occlusion also may be accomplished by placing gold inlays on existing resin teeth. Although this may be done also on porcelain teeth, it is difficult to cut inlay recesses in porcelain teeth unless air abrasive methods are used. Therefore, if later additions to occlusal surfaces are anticipated, plastic teeth should be used, thereby facilitating the addition of new resin or cast gold surfaces (Fig. 8-8). A simple technique to fabricate cast gold occlusal surfaces and attach them to resin teeth is illustrated in Chapter 17.

4. *Metal teeth.* Occasionally a second molar tooth may be replaced as part of the partial denture casting. This is usually done when space is too limited for the attachment of an artificial tooth and yet the addition of a second molar is desirable to prevent migration of an opposing second molar. Since the occlusal surface must be waxed prior to casting, perfect occlusion is not possible. Since metal, particularly a chrome alloy, is abrasion resistant, the area of occlusal contact should be held to a minimum to avoid damage to the periodontium of the opposing tooth and the associated discomfort to the patient. Whereas occlusal adjustment on gold occlusal surfaces is readily accomplished, metal teeth made of chrome alloys are difficult to adjust and are objectionably hard for use as occlusal surfaces. Therefore they should be used only to fill a space and to prevent tooth migration and no more.

Need for relining. The distal extension base differs from the tooth-borne base in several respects, one of which is that it must be made of a material that can be relined or rebased when it becomes necessary to reestablish tissue support for the distal extension base. Therefore resin denture base materials that can be relined are generally used.

Although satisfactory techniques for making distal extension partial denture bases of cast metal are available (Chapter 15), the fact that metal bases are difficult if not impossible to reline limits their use to stable ridges that will change little over a long period of time.

Changes in ridge form over a period of time may not be visible. Manifestations of change may be seen, however. One of these is a *loss of occlusion* between the distal extension denture base and the opposing dentition, increasing as the distance from the abutment increases. This is proved by having the patient close on strips of 28-gauge green casting wax, or any similar wax, tapping in *centric occlusion* only. Indentations in a wax strip of known thickness are quantitative, whereas marks made with articulating ribbon are only qualitative. In other words, indentations in the wax may be interpreted as being light, medium, or heavy, whereas it is difficult if not impossible to interpret a mark made with articulating ribbon as being light or heavy. In fact, the heaviest occlusal contact may perforate paper articulating ribbon and make a lesser mark than areas of lighter contact. Therefore the use of any articulating ribbon is of limited value in checking occlusion intraorally. In making occlusal adjustments, articulating ribbon should be used only to indicate *where* to relieve after the *need for relief* has been established by using wax strips of known thickness. For this purpose, 28-gauge green or blue casting wax is generally used, although the thinner 30-gauge or the thicker 26-gauge wax may also be used for better evaluation of the clearance between areas not in contact.

Loss of support for a distal extension base will result in a loss of occlusal contact between the prosthetically supplied teeth and the opposing dentition and a return to heavy occlusal contact between the remaining natural teeth. Usually this is an indication that relining is needed to reestablish the original occlusion by reestablishing supporting contact with the residual ridge. It must be remembered, however, that occlusion on a distal extension base is sometimes maintained at the expense of migration of the opposing natural teeth. In such case, checking the occlusion alone will not show that settling of the extension base has occurred because changes in the supporting ridge may have also taken place.

A second manifestation of change also must be observable to justify relining. This second manifestation of change in the supporting ridge is evidence of rotation about the fulcrum line with the indirect retainers lifting from their seats as the distal extension base is pressed against the ridge tissues. Originally, if the distal extension base was made to fit the supporting form of the residual ridge (Chapter 15), rotation about the fulcrum line is not visible. At the time the denture is initially placed, no teeter-totter should exist when alternating finger pressure is applied to the indirect retainer and the distal end of a distal extension base or bases. After changes in the ridge form, which causes some loss of support, rotation occurs about the fulcrum line when alternating finger pressure is applied. This is evidence of changes in the supporting ridge that must be compensated for by relining or rebasing.

If occlusal contact has been lost and rotation about the fulcrum line is evident, then relining is indicated. On the other hand, if occlusal contact has been lost without any evidence of denture rotation, and if stability of the denture base is otherwise satisfactory, then reestablishing the occlusion is the remedy rather than relining. For the latter the original denture base may be used in much the same manner as the original trial base was used to record occlusal relation. Teeth may then be reoccluded to an opposing cast or to an occlusal template, using new teeth or cast gold occlusal surfaces. In any event new occlusion may be established on the existing bases. Relining in this instance would be the wrong solution to the problem.

More often, however, loss of occlusion is accompanied by settling of the denture base to the extent that rotation about the fulcrum line is manifest. Since relining is the only remedy short of making completely new bases, use of a resin base originally facilitates later relining. For this reason resin bases are generally preferred for distal extension partial dentures.

The question remains as to when, if ever, metal bases with their several advantages may be used for distal extension partial dentures. It is debatable as to what type of ridge will be the most likely to remain stable under functional loading without apparent change. Certainly the age and general health of the patient will influence the ability of a residual ridge to support function. Minimal and harmonious occlusion and the accuracy with which the base fits the underlying tissues will influence the amount of trauma that will occur under function. Undoubtedly the absence of trauma plays a big part in the ability of the ridge to maintain its original form.

The best risk for the use of metal distal extension bases is a ridge that has supported a previous partial denture without having become narrowed or flat or consisting primarily of easily displaceable tissues. When such changes have occurred under a previous denture, further change may be anticipated because of the possibility that the oral tissues in question are not capable of supporting a denture base without retrogressive change. Despite every advantage in their favor, apparently there are some individuals whose ridges respond unfavorably to being called on to support any denture base.

In other instances, such as when a new partial denture is to be made because of the loss of additional teeth, the ridges may still be firm and healthy. Since the ridges have previously supported a denture base and have sustained occlusion, bony trabeculae will have become arranged to best support vertical and horizontal loading, cortical bone may have been formed, and tissues will have become favorable for continued support of a denture base.

Admittedly there are relatively few instances in which the need for future relining of a distal extension base need not be considered and metal bases may be used. There are, however, many instances that may be considered borderline. In these, metal bases may be used with full understanding on the part of the patient that a new or rebuilt denture may become necessary in the future if unforeseen tissue changes occur. A technique is given in Chapter 15 that permits replacing metal distal extension bases without having to remake the entire denture. This method should be seriously considered any time a distal extension partial denture is to be made with a metal base or bases.

For reasons previously outlined the possibility that tissues will remain healthier beneath a metal base than they will beneath a resin base may justify wider use of metal bases for distal extension partial dentures. Through careful treatment planning, better patient education of the problems involved in making a distal extension denture, and greater care in the fabrication of the denture bases, metal may be used to advantage in some situations in which resin bases are ordinarily used.

STRESSBREAKERS (STRESS EQUALIZERS)

The previous chapters on component parts of a partial denture have presumed absolute rigidity of all parts of the partial denture framework except the retentive arm of the direct retainer assembly. All vertical and horizontal forces applied to the supplied teeth are thus distributed throughout the supporting portions of the dental arch. Broad distribution of force is accomplished through the rigidity of the major and minor connectors. The effect of the stabilizing components is also made possible by the rigidity of the connectors.

In a distal extension restoration, strain on the abutment teeth is minimized through the use of functional basing, broad converage, harmonious occlusion, and correct choice of direct retainers. Retentive clasp arms may be cast only if they engage undercuts on the abutment teeth in such a manner that tissue-ward movement of the extension base transmits only minimal leverage to the abutment. Otherwise, tapered wrought-wire retentive clasp arms should be used because of their greater flexibility. Because of its flexibility, the tapered, round wrought-wire clasp arm may be said to act somewhat as a stressbreaker between the denture base and the abutment tooth.

A concept of stress breaking exists, however, that insists on separating the action of the retaining elements from the movement of the distal extension base. Thus, when the term stressbreaker is used, it is generally applied to a device that allows some movement between the denture base or its supporting framework and the direct retainers, whether they are intracoronal or extracoronal in design.

A stressbreaker is also sometimes referred to as a *stress equalizer*. The term *articulated prosthesis* is also frequently applied to a broken-stress partial denture.

Almost forty years ago Kennedy wrote as follows:

Since the advent of the cast clasp and the removable bridge, a great number of men have advocated the use of "stress breakers" between their saddles and the clasps. These have been shown to be absolutely essential by dentists who have used cast clasps for partial dentures. They found that in a short time the teeth to which such clasps were attached loosened, and that this was due mainly to the rigidity of the clasp.

A well-designed round wire clasp is, in itself, a stress breaker, and allows sufficient saddle movement to prevent excessive strain upon the abutment teeth. . . .

In my hands, stress breakers used on partial dentures have permitted so much movement of the saddles, that they produce excessive soreness, and, after many trials, especially after patients have worn them for some time, I found that a greater number of abutment teeth were loosened than where we used the double bar, . . . the "continuous clasp" [what is now known as the secondary lingual bar or Kennedy bar]. It is only where we have too few teeth in the mouth that it is necessary to use some form of specially designed stress breaker between the clasps and saddles.

. . . Clasps should not be made so rigid that they hold the denture in place. We must depend on the inherent stability of the saddles to prevent strain on the teeth. . . . If there are only one or two teeth present, we would not expect these teeth to do the work of fourteen, without excessive strain being placed upon them, and it is in such conditions that some form of stress breaker becomes useful.*

Several partial denture textbooks have little to say about stressbreakers, as though to avoid a controversial subject. That the subject is controversial is evidenced by the rigid adherence to their use by some with apparent success, whereas properly designed rigid restorations are routinely used by others without harm to abutments. *It is only the improperly designed or ineffectively fabricated rigid restoration that has proved to be harmful to abutment teeth.* There is little question that some form of mechanical stressbreaker is preferable to a poorly designed and ineffectively fabricated rigid restoration!

It is interesting and significant to note that the development and promotion of stressbreaker designs in this country has been largely through the efforts of the commercial

*From Kennedy, E.: Partial denture construction, Brooklyn, 1942, Denture Items of Interest Publishing Co., Inc.

dental laboratory. In most instances this has been due to the failure of the dentist to furnish the laboratory with a master cast that provides for adequate denture base support. If the dentist is not inclined to employ carefully contoured abutment retainers that permit the use of proper clasp designs and is not willing to take the steps necessary to provide maximum support for tissue-supported denture bases, then he probably should utilize one of the stressbreaker designs offered by the commercial dental laboratory if he insists on including removable partial prosthodontics in his practice.

Types of stressbreakers. Stressbreakers may be divided into two groups. In the first are those having a movable joint between the direct retainer and the denture base (Figs. 8-9 and 8-10). In this group fall the hinges, sleeves and cylinders, and ball-and-socket devices (some of which are spring loaded). Being placed between the direct retainer and the denture base, they may permit both vertical movement and hinge action of the distal extension base. This serves to prevent some direct transmission of tipping forces to the abutment teeth as the base moves tissueward under function.

Examples of this group are the various hinges, the Swiss-made Dalbo attachment, the Crismani attachment, the C & M 637 attachment, and the ASC 52 attachment. Most of these attachments are prefabricated, but the laboratory may utilize dual-casting techniques for fabricating the attachment. Because of the rapid wear likely to occur with gold, such attachments are usually made of a harder alloy and therefore are usually machine made.

The articulated partial denture designs comprise the second group and include those designs having a flexible connection between the direct retainer and the denture base. These include the use of wrought-wire connectors, divided major connectors, and other flexible devices for permitting movement of the distal extension base (Figs. 8-11 and 8-12). Included also in this group are those utilizing a movable joint between two major connectors. These are generally fabricated by the laboratory with a dual-casting technique. The earliest of such connectors were double lingual bars of wrought metal, one supporting the clasps and other components and the other supporting and connecting the distal

Fig. 8-9. D-E hinge-type stressbreaker utilizing a vertical stop to limit movement of denture base away from tissues. The trunnion design of the stressbreaker also prevents lateral movement. (Courtesy Austenal, Inc., Chicago, Ill.)

Fig. 8-10. Kennedy Class II, modification 1, partial denture utilizing a hinge stressbreaker of Baca design. Hinge and vertical movements are permitted by the fact that the action is protected by a metal sleeve (Courtesy Ticonium Division of CMP Industries, Inc., Albany, N.Y.)

Fig. 8-11. Stressbreaking effect of a split bar major connector. Vertical and diagonal forces (arrow) applied to tissue-supported base must pass anteriorly along lower bar and then back along the more rigid upper bar to reach abutment tooth. Thus tipping forces that would otherwise be transmitted directly to abutment tooth are supposedly dissipated by the flexibility of lower bar and distance traveled.

Fig. 8-12. Early type of stress equalizer. The direct retainers (clasps) are connected by a 16-gauge, round, wrought wire. An inferiorly placed cast major connector joins the denture bases. Heavy wrought wire and cast major connector are joined with solder at midline only. A need for indirect retention still exists even though a stress equalizer is utilized.

extension bases. The two bars were usually but not always united at the midline by binding with fine wire and soldering.

The double bar principle is still used in the form of split major connectors. Instead of using wrought metal, a single cast connector is made flexible by separating a portion of its length. This may be done by making a saw cut part way through a gold casting with a jeweler's saw or by casting to a thin shim; this is then removed, leaving a separation.

Although mica and other materials have been used for this purpose, stainless steel is generally used (0.02 band material), which is then removed by acid. The nature of chrome-cobalt alloys permits making one casting first and then waxing and casting the second part to the first without union. This facilitates making split bars and movable joints with fine precision and nearly imperceptible junction lines. In any event, the resulting flexibility of the major connector acts to prevent some direct transmission of forces to the abutment tooth.

A design utilizing a dual-casting technique is the Ticonium hidden-lock design (Fig. 8-13). This is a two-piece casting. The top half, which is the major connector supporting the direct retainers and other rigid components, is cast first, and the bottom half, which is the connector between the denture bases, is cast to the major connector. The latter is completely independent of the first except that it is locked in by a circle-type retention, prepared in the wax pattern.

The hidden-lock is created by mechanical means, and the split between the two connectors is made possible by the thin oxide shell that forms during the making of the two sections. What appears to be a conventional lingual bar or linguoplate actually is two bars connected by a movable joint at the midline.

Still other devices permit disassembly of the denture by the patient for cleaning. All mechanical devices that are free to move in

Fig. 8-13. Ticonium hidden-lock partial denture. **A,** Lower half of framework, consisting of lower half of lingual bar and denture base retainer, is cast first with a bi-bevel circle formed in wax pattern by waxing around a lightly oiled mandrel, which is removed to provide a perfect circle within wax. This half is cast as illustrated. **B,** On a second investment cast, original bar is replaced and remainder of framework is waxed to it. This portion consists of the clasps, the indirect retainers, and the remainder of the bar. The hidden-lock and split bar are made possible because of the thin oxide shell that forms during the second casting, leaving an almost imperceptible junction line between the two sections. Hinge movement occurs at circle in the midline. (Courtesy Ticonium Co., Albany, N.Y.)

the mouth collect debris and become unclean; therefore disassembly is a desirable feature whether done daily by the patient or periodically by the dentist (some hinged devices have small screws that may be removed for cleaning or adjusting the action of the device).

In addition to the trapping of debris, some split connectors used as stressbreakers have been known to pinch the underlying soft tissues or the tongue as they open and close under function. Furthermore, such flexible connectors, especially those made of cast alloys, become fatigued through repeated flexing, resulting in permanent distortion of the denture framework and possible ultimate failure through fracture.

Regardless of their design, most all stressbreakers effectively dissipate vertical stresses, which is the purpose for which they are used. At the same time their flexibility or mechanical movement may eliminate the horizontal stability at the distal extension base that is inherent in a rigid partial denture design. The effectiveness of minor connectors, stabilizing components, occlusal rests, and indirect retainers is either lost or dissipated by the action of the stressbreakers. *As a result, consideration of the abutments is at the expense of the tissues of the residual ridge.* This is evidenced by the fact that the stress-broken denture will often require relief on the tissue side of the buccal flange.

Since horizontal stresses cannot be resisted by rigid stabilizing components elsewhere in the arch, the residual ridge is forced to bear those horizontal forces alone. This and the added cost are the most obvious disadvantages to the use of stressbreakers in distal extension partial denture designs.

Advantages of stressbreakers. Some of the claimed advantages of stressbreakers by those who use them may be listed as follows:

1. Since the horizontal forces acting on the abutment teeth are minimized, the alveolar support of these teeth is preserved.

2. By careful choice of the type of flexible connector, it is possible to obtain a balance of stress between the abutment teeth and the residual ridge.

3. Intermittent pressure of the denture bases massages the mucosa, thus providing physiologic stimulation, which prevents bone resorption and eliminates the need for relining.

4. If relining is needed but not done, the abutment teeth are not damaged as quickly.

5. Splinting of weak teeth by the denture is made possible despite the movement of a distal extension base.

Disadvantages of stressbreakers. Some of the disadvantages of the stress-breaking principle are as follows:

1. The broken-stress denture is usually more difficult to construct and therefore more costly.

2. Vertical and horizontal forces are concentrated on the residual ridge, resulting in increased ridge resorption. Many stressbreaker designs are not well stabilized against horizontal forces. Proponents of broken-stress dentures claim that this is avoided by the intermittent massage, which stimulates and promotes better health of the residual ridge.

3. If relining is not done when needed, excessive resorption of the residual ridge may result. This is offset to some extent by the fact that such a denture base is no longer in occlusion and that therefore resorption may not be progressive.

4. The effectiveness of indirect retainers is reduced or eliminated altogether.

5. The more complicated the prosthesis, the less it may be tolerated by the patient. Spaces between components are sometimes opened up in function, thus trapping food and, occasionally, the tissues of the mouth.

6. Flexible connectors may be bent and distorted by careless handling. Even a slightly distorted connector may bring more stress to bear on the abutment rather than less.

7. Repair and maintenance of any stressbreaker is difficult, costly, and frequently required.

Advantages of a rigid design. Some of the advantages of the rigid partial denture design may be listed as follows:

1. Mechanically the framework is easier and less costly to make.

2. Equitable distribution of stress between abutments and the residual ridge(s) is possible with a rigid design.

3. The need for relining the rigid prosthesis is less frequent, since the residual ridge does not have to carry the functional load unaided.

4. Indirect retainers and other rigid components may act to prevent rotational movement of the denture and will provide horizontal stabilization that is not possible when stressbreakers are used.

5. By reducing the number of flexible or movable parts, there is less danger of distortion by careless handling on the part of the patient.

6. Moving parts being absent, the prosthesis is more easily kept clean.

Disadvantages of a rigid design. Some of the possible disadvantages of the rigid denture design are as follows:

1. Objectionable torque will be applied to the abutment teeth if abutment retainers are not passive and correctly designed.

2. Rigid continuous clasping may be hazardous when stressbreakers are not used.

3. Locking-type (dovetail) intracoronal retainers may not be used at all without stressbreakers on distal extension dentures because they are locked within the abutment, and tipping forces would be transmitted directly to the abutment tooth. Even when used in conjunction with multiple splinting of abutments, coupled with a minimum of occlusion on the distal extension denture base, locking-type retainers are still risky.

4. The use of tapered wrought-wire retentive clasp arms as stressbreakers may present some technical difficulties, particularly when high-fusing chrome alloys are used. Wrought wire may be crystalized by improper application of heat during casting or soldering operations, resulting in early fracture. Use of the type II wire will minimize problems associated with the application of heat. It also may be distorted by careless handling, leading to excessive or insufficient retention, or ultimate fracture due to repeated adjustment.

5. If relining is not done when needed, the abutment tooth may be loosened and suffer permanent periodontal damage because of the repeated application of torque and tipping stresses.

The student is referred to three textbooks that describe in detail the use of stressbreakers and articulated partial denture designs: (1) *Precision Attachments in Dentistry*, ed. 3, by H. W. Preiskel, (2) *Precision Work for Partial Dentures* by Alfred A. Steiger and Raoul H. Boitel of Zurich, and (3) *Protesis Parcial Removible* by Adalberto D. Rebossio of Buenos Aires. The latter is available in Spanish only.

SELF-ASSESSMENT AIDS

1. What is a denture base?
2. What is meant by the term *basal seat?*
3. Is the primary purpose of a denture base related to masticatory function?
4. To what extent may the denture base contribute to the factor of appearance?
5. Are the functions of tooth-supported and extension type bases somewhat different?
6. What are the functions of a tooth-supported partial denture base?
7. Describe the functions of a distal extension denture base.

8. The space available for a denture base is controlled by the structures surrounding the space and their movements during function. True or false?

9. We hear of the term *snowshoe effect* in designing denture bases. What does this mean to you?

10. By what means is an acrylic resin base attached to a framework?

11. A ladderlike minor connector is employed to attach an acrylic resin base to frameworks. Should this minor connector be rigid or flexible?

12. Is it important that a minor connector for an extension type acrylic resin base be located on both the buccal and lingual sides of the residual ridge? Can you defend your answer?

13. Is an open ladder type of design for connecting an acrylic resin base to a major connector preferred to a close "meshwork" design? Why?

14. Can you give a rule of thumb for the distal extent of a minor connector attaching the resin base to the major connector?

15. Quite obviously the minor connector for resin bases must be embedded totally in the resin base. What thickness of acrylic resin is necessary between the residual ridge and minor connector to allow adjustment of the base if it should become necessary?

16. Nine requirements for an ideal denture base are given in this chapter. Can you think of six of them?

17. Metal bases have distinct advantages over resin bases, such as thermal conductivity and accuracy and permanence of form. Do they have any other advantages?

18. What are the indications and contraindications for metal bases?

19. Denture base contours for functional cheek and tongue contact can best be accomplished with (resin) (metal)?

20. Relining of extension bases becomes necessary to reestablish support of the base. Could this be a factor in selecting the material for a denture base?

21. How can it be determined when a denture base requires relining?

22. What is meant by the word stressbreaker in removable partial prosthodontics?

23. By what means can the action of the retaining elements be separated from movements of the extension base?

24. Stressbreakers may be divided into two broad groups. Can you give a couple of examples of each group?

25. What is meant by a dual-casting technique and how is it accomplished?

26. Most designs of stressbreakers will rather effectively dissipate vertical forces to terminal abutments. However, this occurs at the expense of what supporting entity?

27. Contrast stressbreaker and rigid designs by giving advantages and disadvantages of each.

9 PRINCIPLES OF REMOVABLE PARTIAL DENTURE DESIGN

BIOMECHANICAL CONSIDERATIONS

As Maxwell stated, "Common observations clearly indicates that the ability of living things to tolerate force is largely dependent upon the magnitude or intensity of the force." The supporting structures for removable partial dentures (abutment teeth and residual ridges) are "living things" and are subjected to forces. In consideration of maintaining the health of these structures, the dentist must also consider direction, duration, and frequency of force application as well as magnitude of the force.

In the final analysis it is bone that provides the support for a removable restoration, that is, alveolar bone by way of the periodontal ligament and bone of the residual ridge through its soft tissue covering. If potentially destructive forces can be minimized, then the physiologic tolerances of the supporting structures need not be tested. To a great extent the forces accruing through a removable restoration can be widely distributed, directed, and minimized by the selection, the design, and the location of components of the removable partial denture and by developing a harmonious occlusion.

Unquestionably the design of removable partial dentures requires a consideration of mechanics as well as biologic considerations. It is not required that a dentist be a mechanical genius to apply certain fundamental principles to minimize or distribute potentially destructive forces by a rational design of a restoration. Imbued in most dentists, just through the maturing process, is an appreciation—perhaps unrecognized—for the application of mechanical laws. For example, the lid of a paint can is more easily pried off with a screwdriver than it is with a half dollar! The longer the handle, the less effort (force) it takes. We are then applying

the mechanics of levers. By the same token a lever system built into a distal extension removable restoration can magnify, so to speak, the applied force to the terminal abutments, which is most undesirable.

Tylman correctly stated, "Great caution and reserve are essential whenever an attempt is made to interpret biological phenomena entirely by mathematical computation." However, an understanding of certain things mechanical and of simple machines should enhance our rationalization of the design of removable partial dentures to accomplish an objective of preservation of oral structures. A removable partial denture can be, and often is, unknowingly designed as a destructive machine.

Machines may be classified into two general categories: simple and complex. Complex machines are combinations of many simple machines. There are six simple machines: lever, wedge, screw, wheel and axle, pulley, and inclined plane (Fig. 9-1). Of the simple machines the lever and the inclined plane most deserve our consideration in designing removable partial dentures—a consideration based on *avoiding* lever and inclined plane designs to the greatest extent possible.

In its simplest form a lever is a rigid bar supported somewhere along its length. It may rest on the support or may be supported from above. The support point of the lever is called the fulcrum, and the lever can move around the fulcrum (Fig. 9-2). There are three types of levers: first, second, and third class (Fig. 9-3). The potential of a lever system to relatively magnify a force is illustrated in Fig. 9-4.

An extension-type removable partial denture will rotate when a force is placed on the denture base. It will rotate in relation to the three cranial planes because of differences in

Fig. 9-1. Scientists today recognize six simple machines: lever, wedge, screw, wheel and axle, pulley, and inclined plane (*F* = fulcrum).

Fig. 9-2. A lever is simply a rigid bar supported somewhere between its two ends. It can be used to move objects by the application of a force (weight) much less than the weight of the object being moved.

Fig. 9-3. There are three classes of levers. The classification is based on the location of a fulcrum, *F*; a resistance, ⟨*R*⟩, and the direction of an effort (force), *E*. Examples of each class are illustrated on the right.

Fig. 9-4. The length of the lever from the fulcrum, *F*, to the resistance, ⟨*R*⟩, is called the resistance arm. That portion of the lever from the fulcrum to the point of application of a force, *E*, is called the effort arm. Whenever the effort arm is longer than the resistance arm, the mechanical advantage is in favor of the effort arm, proportional to the difference in length of the two arms. In other words, when the effort arm is twice the length of the resistance arm, a 25-pound weight on the effort arm will balance a 50-pound weight at the end of the resistance arm.

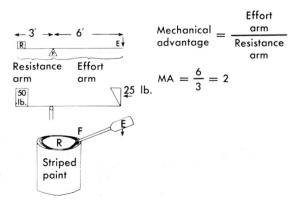

$$\text{Mechanical advantage} = \frac{\text{Effort arm}}{\text{Resistance arm}}$$

$$MA = \frac{6}{3} = 2$$

the support characteristics of the abutment teeth and the soft tissues covering the residual ridge (Fig. 9-5). Even though the gross movement may be small, there still exists the potential for detrimental, lever-like imposed forces to accrue to abutment teeth, depending on design of the prosthesis, especially when servicing of the prosthesis is neglected over a long period of time.

A cantilever is a beam supported only at one end and can "act" as a first-class lever (Fig. 9-6). A cantilever design should be avoided (Fig. 9-7). Examples of other lever-like designs as well as suggestions for alternative designs to avoid or to minimize their destructive potential are illustrated in Figs. 9-8 and 9-9.

A tooth is apparently better able to tolerate vertically directed forces than off-

vertical or near horizontal forces. This characteristic is observed clinically and was substantiated many years ago by the work of Dr. Box and Mr. Synge of Toronto, Canada. It seems rational that more periodontal fibers are activated to resist the application of vertical forces to teeth than are activated to resist the application of off-vertical forces (Fig. 9-10).

Again, a distal extension removable partial denture rotates when forces are applied. Since it can be assumed that this rotation must create predominantly off-vertical forces, location of stabilizing and retentive components in relation to the horizontal axis of rotation of the abutment becomes extremely important. In other words an abutment tooth will better tolerate off-vertical forces if these forces accrue as near as

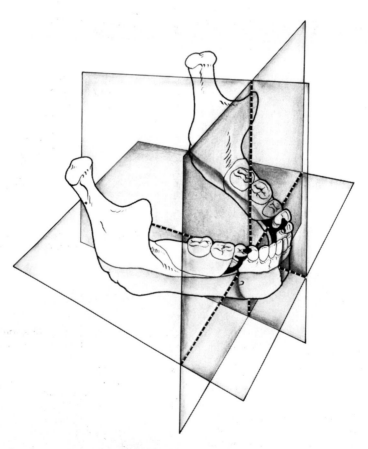

Fig. 9-5. A distal extension removable partial denture will rotate when a force is directed on the denture base. The differences in the displaceability of the periodontal ligament and the soft tissues covering the residual ridge permit this rotation. It would seem that rotation of the denture is in a combination of directions rather than unidirectional. In other words, the distal extension denture can pitch, roll, and yaw.

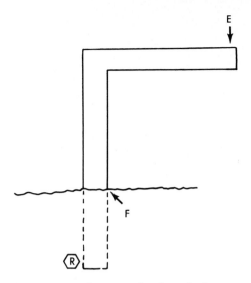

Fig. 9-6. A cantilever can be described as a rigid beam supported at one end. When a force is directed against the unsupported end of the beam, a cantilever can act as a first-class lever. The mechanical advantage in this illustration is in favor of the effort arm, so to speak.

Fig. 9-7. A design often seen for a distal extension removable partial denture. A cast circumferential direct retainer engages a mesiobuccal undercut and is supported by a distocclusal rest. The only difference in this design and a locking-type internal attachment on the distal of the premolar is in the firmness of the attachment to the abutment. *This is a cantilever design,* and it will impart a detrimental first-class lever force to the abutment.

Fig. 9-8. The potential for a first-class lever action exists in this Class II, modification 1, removable partial denture framework. If a cast circumferential direct retainer utilizing a mesiobuccal undercut on the right first premolar were used, a force placed on the denture base would impart an upward and posteriorly moving force on the premolar, probably resulting in a loss of contact between the premolar and canine, with its soon-following sequelae. As designed with the bar-type retainer, the force during rotation of the denture would be more anteriorly directed, thus maintaining contact. The other alternatives to the first premolar design of a direct retainer would be a tapered wrought-wire retentive arm that utilizes a mesiobuccal undercut or just has a buccal stabilizing arm above the height of contour or uses an I-bar retentive arm on the buccal surface.

Fig. 9-9. Upper illustration utilizes a bar-type retainer, a minor connector contacting a guiding plane on distal surface of a premolar, and a mesiocclusal rest, thus eliminating a cantilever or first-class lever force when denture rotates toward residual ridge. An I-bar-type retentive arm could also be used. Lower figure utilizes a tapered wrought-wire retentive arm, a minor connector contacting a guiding plane on distal surface of a premolar, and a mesiocclusal rest. This design is applicable when a distobuccal undercut (anteriorly tilted terminal abutments) cannot be found or created or when a tissue undercut contraindicates placing a bar-type retentive arm. It is a compromise; however, this design would probably be much more kind to the periodontal ligament than would the use of a cast, half-round retentive arm.

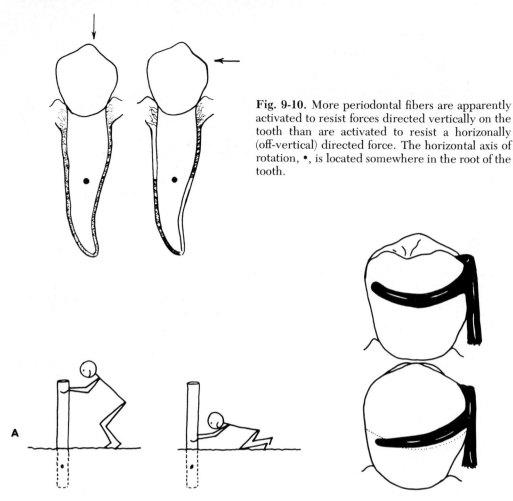

Fig. 9-10. More periodontal fibers are apparently activated to resist forces directed vertically on the tooth than are activated to resist a horizonally (off-vertical) directed force. The horizontal axis of rotation, •, is located somewhere in the root of the tooth.

A

B

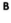

Fig. 9-11. A, Fencepost is more readily removed by an application of force near its top than by applying the same force nearer ground level. **B,** The retentive and reciprocal components (mirror view) of this direct retainer assembly are located much nearer the occlusal surface than they should be. This is similar to left-hand figure in **A.**

Fig. 9-12. Abutment has been contoured to allow a rather favorable location of retentive and reciprocal-stabilizing components (mirror view). This is similar to the right-hand figure in Fig. 9-11, *A.*

possible to the horizontal axis of rotation of the abutment (Fig. 9-11). The axial surface contours of abutment teeth must usually be altered to locate components of direct retainer assemblies more favorably in relation to the abutment's horizontal axis (Fig. 9-12).

OTHER FACTORS INFLUENCING THE DESIGN OF REMOVABLE PARTIAL DENTURES

As a direct result of examination and diagnosis the design of the removable partial denture must originate on the diagnostic cast so that all mouth preparations may be planned and performed with a specific design in mind. This will be influenced by many factors, some of which follow:

1. Which arch is to be restored and if both, their relationship to one another.

2. Type of major connector indicated, based on existing and correctable situations.

3. Whether the denture will be entirely tooth borne. If one or more distal extension bases are involved, the following must be considered:

    a. Need for indirect retention

    b. Clasp designs that will best minimize the forces applied to the abutment teeth during function

    c. Need for later rebasing, which will influence the type of base material used

    d. Secondary impression method to be used

4. Materials to be used, both for the framework and for the bases.

5. Type of replacement teeth to be used. This may be influenced by the opposing dentition.

6. Need for abutment restorations, which may influence the type of clasp arms to be used and their specific design.

7. Patient's past experience with a removable partial denture and the reasons for making a new denture. If, for example, a lingual bar has been objectionable, was it because of design, fit, or the patient's inability to accept it? Frequently an appraisal of these factors alone justifies the use of a contoured linguoplate rather than a lingual bar. If an anterior palatal bar has proved objectionable, was it due to bulk, location, or flexibility, or to tissue irritation? A design using a thin palatal major connector located more posteriorly may be preferable to an anterior bar or palatal horseshoe design located anteriorly.

8. Periodontal condition of the remaining teeth, the amount of abutment support remaining, and the need for splinting. This may be accomplished either by means of fixed restorations or by the design of the denture framework.

9. Method to be used for replacing single teeth or missing anterior teeth. The decision

Fig. 9-13. A, Diagnostic cast of partially edentulous maxillary arch. Ideally, missing lateral incisors should be restored with fixed partial dentures. By so doing, not only will design of removable partial denture be simplified but canines will be spared some leverages created by rotation of denture in use. Prognosis for canines and central incisors will be greatly enhanced. **B,** The lone standing premolar in this mandibular arch should be splinted to right central and right lateral incisors, with a fixed partial denture replacing missing canine. If it is utilized as a lone standing abutment for a removable restoration, first class lever or cantilever forces cannot be avoided regardless of design.

to use fixed restorations for these spaces rather than replacing them with the removable partial denture must be made at the time of treatment planning (Fig. 9-13). Such a decision will necessarily influence the design of the denture framework.

DIFFERENTIATION BETWEEN TWO MAIN TYPES

It is clear that two distinctly different types of removable partial dentures exist. Certain points of difference are present between the Class I and Class II types of partial dentures on the one hand and the Class III type of partial denture on the other. The first consideration is the *manner in which each is supported.* The Class I type and the distal extension side of the Class II type derive their support to a great extent from the tissues underlying the base and only to a limited degree from the abutment teeth (Fig. 9-14), whereas the Class III type derives all its support from the abutment teeth at each end of the edentulous space (Fig. 9-15).

Second, for reasons directly related to the manner of support, the *method of impression registration* required for each type will vary.

Third, the *need for some kind of indirect retention* exists in the distal extension type of partial denture, whereas in the tooth-borne, Class III type there is no extension base that can lift away from the supporting tissues because of the action of sticky foods and movements of the tissues of the mouth against borders of the denture. This is because each end of each denture base is secured by a direct retainer on an abutment tooth unless anterior teeth are replaced by the denture. Therefore the tooth-borne partial denture does not rotate about a fulcrum as does the distal extension partial denture.

Fourth, the manner in which the distal extension type of partial denture is supported often necessitates the *use of a base material that can be relined* to compensate for tissue changes. Acrylic resin is generally used as a base material for distal extension bases. The Class III partial denture, on the other hand, being entirely tooth supported, does not require rebasing except when it is advisable to eliminate an unhygienic, unesthetic, or uncomfortable condition resulting from loss of tissue contact. Metal bases therefore are more frequently used in tooth-borne restorations, since rebasing is not as likely to be necessary with them.

Differences in support. The distal extension partial denture derives its major support from the residual ridge with its fibrous connective tissue covering. Some areas of this residual ridge are firm, with limited displaceability, whereas other areas are displaceable, depending on the thickness and structural character of the tissues overlying the residual alveolar bone. The movement of the base under function determines the occlusal efficiency of the partial denture and also the degree to which the abutment teeth are subjected to torque and tipping stresses.

Fig. 9-14. Kennedy Class I partially edentulous arch. The major support for denture bases must come from residual ridges, tooth support from occlusal rests being effective only at anterior portion of each base.

Fig. 9-15. Kennedy Class III, modification 1, partially edentulous arch, which provides total tooth support for prosthesis. A removable partial denture made for this arch is totally supported by rests on properly prepared occlusal rest seats on the four abutment teeth.

Impression registration. An impression registration for the construction of a partial denture must fulfill the following two requirements:

1. The anatomic form and the relationship of the remaining teeth in the dental arch, as well as the surrounding soft tissues, must be recorded accurately so that the denture will not exert pressure on those structures beyond their physiologic limits and so that its retentive and stabilizing components may be properly placed. Some impression material that can be removed from undercut areas without permanent distortion must be used to fulfill this requirement. The elastic impression materials such as reversible hydrocolloid agar or irreversible hydrocolloid alginate, mercaptan rubber base (Thiokol), and silicone impression materials are therefore used for this purpose.

2. The supporting form of the soft tissues underlying the distal extension base of the partial denture should be recorded so that firm areas are used as primary stress-bearing areas and readily displaceable tissues are not overloaded. Only in this way can maximum support of the partial denture base be obtained. An impression material capable of displacing tissue sufficiently to register the supporting form of the ridge will fulfill this second requirement. One of the fluid mouth-temperature waxes or any of the readily flowing materials (rubber base, zinc oxide–eugenol impression paste, or silicone impression material [provided an individual, corrected tray is used]) may be employed for registering the supporting form.

No single impression material can satisfactorily fulfill both of the previously mentioned requirements. The compromise by recording just the anatomic form of both teeth and supporting tissues can result only in inadequate support for the distal extension base of the partial denture.

Differences in clasp design. A fifth point of difference between the two main types of partial dentures lies in their *requirements for direct retention.*

Direct retainers may be classified as being either intracoronal or extracoronal. The clasp-type partial denture, utilizing the extracoronal direct retainer, is probably used a hundred times more frequently than is the intracoronal, or internal attachment, partial denture. This is not necessarily an indication of increasing preference for the clasp denture, nor is it a reflection on the excellence of the internal attachment denture. The fact remains, however, that although the internal attachment was devised more than forty-five years ago, for economic and other reasons the clasp denture is the more widely used. *The clasp-type denture permits the rendering of a physiologically sound partial denture service to the greatest number of patients in keeping with the ability of the majority of patients to pay for such service.*

The tooth-borne partial denture, being totally supported by abutment teeth, is retained and stabilized by a clasp at each end of each endentulous space. The only requirement of such clasps is that they flex sufficiently during placement and removal of the denture to pass over the height of contour of the teeth in approaching or escaping from an undercut area. *While in its terminal position on the tooth, a retentive clasp should be passive and should not be called on to flex except when engaging the undercut area of the tooth for resisting a vertical dislodging force.*

Cast retentive arms are generally used for this purpose. These may be either of the circumferential type, arising from the body of the clasp and approaching the undercut from an occlusal direction, or of the bar type, arising from the base of the denture and approaching the undercut area from a gingival direction. A modification of the latter type is the infrabulge clasp. Each of these two types of cast clasps has its advantages and disadvantages.

The direct retainer adjacent to a distal extension base must perform still another function in addition to that of resisting vertical displacement. Because of the lack of tooth support distally, the denture base will move tissueward under function *proportionate to the quality of the supporting tissues, the accuracy of the impression registration, the accuracy of the denture base, and the total occlusal load applied.* Because of this tissueward movement, those elements of the circumferential clasp that lie in a mesial undercut area must be able to flex sufficiently to dissipate stresses, which otherwise would be transmitted directly to the abutment tooth as leverage. On the other hand, a bar-type retainer placed to take advantage of a distal undercut moves farther into the undercut and does not overly stress the abutment tooth.

The cast circumferential clasp cannot effectively act to dissipate this stress for two reasons. First, the material itself can have only a limited flexibility, or else other parts of the casting (which must be rigid, such as lingual and palatal bars) would also tend to be flexible. The material employed being the same, the only variable factors are the bulk and diameter used in each component part. Second, and probably more important, the cast circumferential clasp is of necessity made half-round in shape. Since edgewise flexing is negligible, the clasp can flex in only one direction and therefore cannot effectively dissipate, by flexing, the torque stresses placed upon it. For this reason some torque is inevitably transmitted to the abutment tooth and is magnified by the length of the lever arm.

Immediately there come to mind the stressbreakers, which are often incorporated into the partial denture design for this reason. Some dentists strongly believe that a stressbreaker is the best means of preventing leverage from being transmitted to the abutment teeth. Others believe just as strongly that a wrought-wire or bar-type retentive arm more effectively accomplishes this purpose with greater simplicity and ease of application. It cannot be denied that a retentive clasp arm made of wrought wire can flex more readily in all directions than can the cast half-round clasp arm and thereby more effectively dissipate those stresses that would otherwise be transmitted to the abutment tooth. The advantages and disadvantages of stressbreakers have been considered in detail in Chapter 8.

Only the retentive arm of the circumferential clasp, however, should be made of wrought metal. Reciprocation and stabilization against lateral movement must be obtained through the use of rigid cast elements that make up the remainder of the clasp. This is called a combination clasp, being a combination of both cast and wrought materials incorporated into one direct retainer. It is frequently used on the terminal abutment for the distal extension partial denture and is indicated where a mesiobuccal but no distobuccal undercut exists or can be made, or where a gross tissue undercut, cervical and buccal to the abutment tooth, exists. It must always be remembered that the factor of length contributes to the flexibility of clasp arms. *A short wrought-wire arm can be a destructive element because of its reduced ability to flex compared with a longer wrought-wire arm.* However, in addition to its greater flexibility compared to the cast circumferential clasp, the combination clasp has further advantages of adjustability, minimal tooth contact, and better esthetics, which justifies its occasional use in tooth-borne designs also.

ESSENTIALS OF PARTIAL DENTURE DESIGN

The design of the partial denture framework should be carefully planned and outlined on an accurate diagnostic cast. After the making of necessary mouth changes to provide for rests, optimal location of framework components, and guiding planes, the master cast is made and carefully surveyed to determine the location of undercut areas that are either to be blocked out or utilized for retention. The design should provide for occlusal rests and rigid reciprocal arms on all abutment teeth to assure vertical and horizontal stability of the partial denture.

The design must include provision for adequate indirect retention that will function to counteract any lifting of the distal extension base away from the tissues. The indirect retainers should be placed in relation to a line drawn through the two principal abutments, which is the axis of rotation, or the *fulcrum line.* The indirect retainer may be in the form of an auxiliary occlusal rest, a continuous bar retainer in combination with terminal rests, a linguoplate with terminal rests, or an incisal rest on an anterior tooth. The indirect retainer should be placed as far as possible from this fulcrum line and should not terminate on a tooth incline, such as the lingual surface of an anterior tooth.

Some retentive elements for the attachment of the resin bases must be provided for to complete the partial denture framework.

Class III removable partial denture (Figs. 9-16 to 9-21). The Kennedy Class III removable partial denture, being entirely tooth supported, may be made entirely to fit the anatomic form of the teeth and surrounding structures. It does not require an impression of the functional form of the ridge tissues nor does it require indirect retention. Cast clasps of either the circumferential or the bar type may be used, or the combination clasp may be used if preferred. Unless a need for later

Fig. 9-16. Removable partial denture in a maxillary Class III arch. The design consists of anterior and posterior palatal bar major connectors, resin-supported artificial teeth, and bar clasp arms throughout. (From McCracken, W. L.: J. Prosthet. Dent. 8:71-84, 1958.)

Fig. 9-17. Removable partial denture framework in a maxillary Class III arch. The design consists of a single palatal major connector, bar and circumferential clasp arms, and means to attach resin-supported artificial teeth.

Fig. 9-18. Removable partial denture in a mandibular Class III arch. The design consists of a lingual bar major connector, metal bases and tube teeth, and bar clasp arms. Note the mesially inclined left third molar with onlay-type reciprocal clasp arm. (From McCracken, W. L.: J. Prosthet. Dent. 8:71-84, 1958.)

rebasing is anticipated, as in the case of recently extracted teeth, the denture base may be made of metal, which has several advantages.

The Class III partial denture can frequently be utilized as a valuable aid to periodontal treatment because of its stabilizing influence on the remaining teeth (Fig. 9-20).

Class I, bilateral, distal extension partial dentures. The Class I, bilateral, distal extension partial denture is as completely unlike

the Class III type as any two dental restorations could be. Since it derives its principal support from the tissues underlying its base, a Class I partial denture made to anatomic ridge form cannot have uniform and adequate support. Yet, unfortunately, many Class I mandibular partial dentures are being made from a single hydrocolloid impression. In such situations both the abutment teeth and the residual ridges suffer because the occlusal load placed upon the remaining teeth

Fig. 9-19. A, Carefully designed tooth-borne denture framework outlined on master cast, in this particular instance to support anterior teeth in the mouth of a musician being traumatized by constant trumpet playing. Note positive lingual rest seats on canines. **B,** Cast framework as returned from laboratory, following precisely design prescribed by dentist.

Fig. 9-20. Maxillary Class III partial denture framework designed for maximum periodontal support. Posterior occlusal rest and clasp arm on nonedentulous side are added for stabilization and to prevent settling of major connector at that point. A partial metal base is used to avoid any display of base metal anteriorly.

Fig. 9-21. Maxillary Class III, modification 1, partial denture designed as a periodontal splint. Full crowns on patient's right premolar and molar are splinted together with continuous lingual ledges. Patient's left premolar is a full crown with lingual ledge. Left molar abutment is unrestored but altered somewhat by recontouring. All gold guiding plane surfaces, lingual and proximal, were machined parallel to path of placement. Unilateral fixed partial dentures would not provide the bilateral stabilization needed for this patient.

is inevitably made greater by the lack of adequate posterior support.

Many dentists, recognizing the need for some type of impression registration that will record the supporting form of the residual ridge, attempt to record this form with a metallic oxide, rubber base, or silicone impression material. Such materials actually only record the anatomic form of the ridge, except when special design of the impression trays permits placement of tissues overlying primary stress-bearing areas. Others prefer to place a base that was made to fit the anatomic form of the ridge under some pressure at the time that it is related to the remaining teeth, thus obtaining functional support. Any impression record will be influenced by the consistency of the impression material and the amount of hydraulic pressure exerted by its confinement within the impression tray. Still others, believing that a properly compounded mouth-temperature wax will displace only those tissues that are incapable of providing support to the denture base, use a wax secondary impression to record the supporting, or functional, form of the edentulous ridge.

Class II partial dentures (Figs. 9-22, and 9-23). The Kennedy Class II partial denture actually may be a combination of both tissue-borne and tooth-borne restorations. The distal extension base must have adequate tissue support, whereas tooth-borne bases elsewhere in the arch may be made to fit the anatomic form of the underlying ridge. Indirect retention must be provided for, but occasionally the anterior abutment on the tooth-borne side will serve to satisfy this requirement. If additional indirect retention is needed, provisions must be made for it.

Cast clasps are generally used on the tooth-borne side, whereas some clasp design must be used on the abutment tooth adjacent to the distal extension, which will prevent the application of torque to that tooth. The use of a cast circumferential clasp engaging a mesiobuccal undercut on the anterior abutment of the tooth-borne modification space is questioned as being sound. A class II, modification 1 (posterior space), situation results in a Class I leverlike design of the denture. It seems rational in this instance to use a bar-type retainer engaging a distobuccal undercut (Fig. 9-24). Should the bar type retainer be contraindicated because of a gross tissue undercut or the existence of only

Fig. 9-22. Mandibular Class II, modification 1, partial denture framework for a resin distal extension base and a cast base on tooth-borne modification space. Bar-type retainers engage distobuccal undercuts on premolar abutments.

Fig. 9-23. Mandibular Class II partial denture with metal distal extension base. Acrylic resin attachment of prosthetically supplied teeth to metal base is with suitable mechanical retention (nailheads, loops, or spurs, plus an undercut finishing line). Embrasure clasps are used on nonedentulous side, with an indirect retainer located favorably in relation to fulcrum line. Because of a tissue undercut cervical to buccal surface of right second premolar and the lack of a distobuccal undercut, a wrought-wire (tapered) retainer arm was used.

a mesiobuccal undercut on the anterior abutment, then a combination direct retainer should be used having the retentive arm made of tapered wrought wire. *A thorough understanding of the advantages and disadvantages of various clasp designs is necessary in determining the type of direct retainer that is to be used for each abutment tooth.*

The steps in the completion of the Class II

Fig. 9-24. Mandibular Class II, modification 1, partially edentulous arch. Note that bar-type retentive arms are utilized on both premolar abutments, engaging distobuccal undercuts at their terminal ends. Leverlike forces will not be as readily imparted to right premolar, contrasted with a cast circumferential direct retainer engaging a mesiobuccal undercut.

partial denture follow closely those of the Class I partial denture, except that the distal extension base is usually made of a resin material, whereas the base for any tooth-borne areas is frequently made of metal. This is permissible because the residual ridge beneath tooth-borne bases is not called on to provide support for the denture, and later rebasing is not as likely to be necessary.

COMPONENTS OF PARTIAL DENTURE

All partial dentures have two things in common: (1) they must be supported by oral tissues and (2) they must be retained against reasonable dislodging forces.

In the Class III partial denture three components are necessary: the connectors, the retainers, and the stabilizing components.

The partial denture that does not have the advantage of tooth support at each end of each edentulous space still must have support, but in this instance the support comes from both the teeth and the underlying ridge tissues rather than from the teeth alone. This is a composite support, and the prosthesis must be fabricated so that the resilient support provided by the edentulous ridge is coordinated with the more stable support offered by the abutment teeth. The three essentials—connectors, retainers, and stabilizing components—must be even more carefully designed and executed because of the movement of tissue-supported denture base areas. In addition, provision must be made for three other essentials, as follows:

1. The best possible support must be obtained from the resilient ridge tissues. This is accomplished by the impression technique more than by the partial denture design, although the amount of area covered by the partial denture is a contributing factor in such support.

2. The method of direct retention must take into account the inevitable tissueward movement of the distal extension base (s) under the stresses of mastication and occlusion. Either some kind of stressbreaker must be used or direct retainers must be designed so that some flexing or stressbreaking under occlusal loading will occur to prevent the direct transmission of this loading instead of leverage to the abutment teeth.

3. The partial denture having one or more distal extension denture bases must be designed so that movement of the unsupported and unretained end away from the tissues will be prevented or minimized. This is often referred to as indirect retention and is best described in relation to an axis of rotation through the rest areas of the principal abutments. However, retention from the partial denture base itself frequently can be made to prevent this movement of the denture base away from the tissues and, in such instances, may be discussed as direct-indirect retention.

The support of the partial denture by the abutment teeth is dependent on the alveolar support of those teeth, the rigidity of the partial denture framework, and the design of the occlusal rests. Through clinical and roentgenographic interpretation the dentist may evaluate the abutment teeth and decide whether they will provide adequate support. In some instances the splinting of two or more teeth is advisable, either by fixed partial dentures or by soldering two or more individual restorations together. In other instances a tooth may be deemed too weak to be used as an abutment, and extraction is indicated in favor of obtaining better support from an adjacent tooth.

Having decided on the abutments, the dentist is responsible for the preparation of the abutment teeth, for the design of cast restorations, and for the form of the occlusal rest seats. These may be prepared either in sound tooth enamel or in the cast restorations. The technician cannot be blamed for inadequate occlusal rest support. On the other hand, the technician is solely to blame if he extends the casting beyond or fails to include the total prepared area. If a definite occlusal rest seat is faithfully recorded in the master cast and delineated in the penciled design, no excuse can be made for poor occlusal rest form on the partial denture if the dentist has sufficiently reduced the marginal ridge area of the rest seat to avoid interference from opposing teeth.

Major connectors. A major connector should be properly located in relation to gingival and moving tissues and should be designed to be rigid. Rigidity in a major connector is necessary to provide proper distribution of forces to and from the supporting components.

A lingual bar connector should be tapered superiorly with a half-pear shape in cross section and should be relieved sufficiently but not excessively over the underlying tissues when such relief is indicated. The addition of a continuous bar retainer or a lingual apron does not alter the basic design of the lingual bar. These are added solely for support, stabilization, rigidity, and protection of the anterior teeth and specifically are neither connectors nor indirect retainers. The finished inferior border of either a lingual bar or a linguoplate should be gently rounded to avoid irritation to subadjacent tissues when the restoration moves even slightly in function.

The use of a linguoplate is indicated when the lower anterior teeth are weakened by periodontal disease. It is also indicated in Class I partially edentulous arches wherein the need for additional resistance to horizontal rotation of the denture is occasioned by excessively resorbed residual ridges. Still another indication is in those situations in which the floor of the mouth so closely approximates the lingual gingiva of anterior teeth that an adequately inflexible lingual bar cannot be positioned without impinging the gingival tissues.

Experience with the linguoplate has shown that with good oral hygiene the underlying tissues remain healthy and there are no harmful effects to the tissues from the metallic coverage per se. However, adequate relief must be provided whenever a metal component crosses the gingival margins and the adjacent gingivae. Excessive relief should be avoided because tissues tend to fill a void, resulting in the overgrowth of abnormal tissue. The amount of relief used, therefore, should be only the minimum necessary to avoid gingival impingement.

It does not seem that there are any advantages to be found in the use of the continuous bar retainer versus the linguoplate. In rare instances, when a linguoplate would show through multiple interproximal embrasures, the continuous bar retainer may be preferred for esthetic reasons only. In other instances, when a single diastema exists, a linguoplate may be cut out in this area to avoid display of metal, without sacrificing its use when otherwise indicated.

Rigidity of a palatal major connector is just as important and its location and design just as critical as is rigidity of a lingual bar. A horseshoe-shaped palatal connector is rarely justified except to avoid an inoperable palatal torus that extends to the junction of the hard and soft palates. Neither can the routine use of a narrow, single palatal bar be justified. The anterior and posterior palatal bar is mechanically and biologically sound if it is located so that it does not impinge on tissues. The broad, anatomic palatal major connector is frequently preferred because of its rigidity, better acceptance by the patient, and greater stability without tissue damage. In addition, this type of connector may provide direct-indirect retention that may sometimes, but rarely, eliminate the need for separate indirect retainers.

Direct retainers for tooth-borne partial dentures. Retainers for tooth-borne partial dentures have only two functions, and these are to retain the prosthesis against reasonable dislodging forces without damage to the abutment teeth and to aid in resisting any tendency of the denture to be displaced in a horizontal plane. There can be no movement of the prosthesis tissueward because each terminus is supported by a rest. There can be no movement away from the tissues, and therefore no rotation about a fulcrum, because each terminus is secured by a direct retainer.

Any type of direct retainer is acceptable as long as the abutment tooth is not jeopardized by its presence. Intracoronal (frictional) retainers are ideal for tooth-borne restorations and offer esthetic advantages not possible with extracoronal (clasp) retainers. Nevertheless the circumferential and bar-type clasp retainers are mechanically effective and are more economically constructed than are intracoronal retainers. Therefore they are more universally used.

Vulnerable areas on the abutment teeth must be protected by restorations with either type of retainer. The clasp retainer must not impinge on gingival tissues. The clasp must not exert excessive torque on the abutment tooth during placement and removal. It must be located the least distance into the tooth undercut for adequate retention, and it must be designed with a minimum of bulk and tooth contact.

The bar clasp arm should be used only when the area for retention lies close to the gingival margin of the tooth and little tissue blockout is necessary. If the clasp must be placed high occlusally or if an objectional space would exist beneath the bar clasp arm because of blockout of tissue undercuts, the bar clasp arm should not be used.

Direct retainers for distal extension partial dentures. Retainers for distal extension partial dentures, while retaining the prosthesis, must also be able to flex or disengage when the denture base moves tissueward under function. Thus the retainer may act as a stressbreaker. Mechanical stress-breakers accomplish the same thing, but they do so at the expense of horizontal stabilization. When some kind of mechanical stressbreaker is used, the denture flange must be able to act to prevent horizontal movement. Clasp designs that allow for flexing of the retentive clasp arm may accomplish the same purpose as that of mechanical stressbreakers, without sacrificing horizontal stabilization and generally with less complicated techniques.

In evaluating the ability of a clasp arm to act as a stressbreaker, one must realize that flexing in one plane is not enough. Rather the clasp arm must be freely flexible in any direction, as dictated by the stresses applied. Bulky, half-round clasp arms cannot do this and neither can a bar clasp engaging an undercut on the side of the tooth away from the denture base. Round, tapered clasp forms offer advantages of greater and more universal flexibility, less tooth contact, and better es-

thetics. *Either the combination circumferential clasp with its tapered wrought-wire retentive arm or the carefully located and properly designed bar clasp should be used on all abutment teeth adjacent to extension denture bases.*

Stabilizing components. Stabilizing components of the partial denture framework are those rigid components that assist in stabilizing the denture against horizontal movement. The purpose of all stabilizing components should be to distribute stresses equally to all supporting teeth without overworking any one tooth.

All minor connectors that contact vertical tooth surfaces (and all reciprocal clasp arms) act as stabilizing components. It is necessary that minor connectors have sufficient bulk to be rigid and yet that they present as little bulk to the tongue as possible. This means that they should be confined to interdental embrasures whenever possible. When minor connectors are located on vertical tooth surfaces, it is best that these surfaces be parallel to the path of placement. When cast restorations are used, these surfaces of the wax patterns should be made parallel on the surveyor prior to casting.

Reciprocal clasp arms also must be rigid, and they must be placed occlusally to the height of contour of the abutment teeth where they will be nonretentive. By their rigidity these clasp arms reciprocate the opposing retentive clasp, and they also prevent horizontal movement of the prosthesis under functional stresses. For a reciprocal clasp arm to be placed favorably, some reduction of the tooth surfaces involved is frequently necessary to increase the suprabulge area.

When crown restorations are used, a lingual reciprocal clasp arm may be inset into the tooth contour by providing a ledge on the crown upon which the clasp arm may rest. This permits the use of a wider clasp arm and restores a more nearly normal tooth contour, at the same time maintaining its strength and rigidity.

Guiding planes. The term *guiding planes* is defined as two or more parallel, vertical surfaces of abutment teeth, so shaped as to direct a prosthesis during placement and removal. After the most favorable path of placement has been ascertained, axial surfaces of abutment teeth are found or are prepared parallel to the path of placement and therefore become parallel to each other. Guiding planes may be contacted by various components of the restoration—the body of an extracoronal direct retainer, the stabilizing arm of a direct retainer, the minor connector portion of an indirect retainer—or by a minor connector specifically designed to contact the guiding plane surface.

The functions of guiding plane surfaces are (1) to provide for one path of placement and removal of the restoration; (2) to ensure the planned and intended action of reciprocal stabilizing, and retentive components; (3) to eliminate detrimental strain to abutment teeth and framework components in placing and removing the restoration, (4) to eliminate gross food traps between abutment teeth and denture bases, (5) to provide retentive characteristics against dislodgement of the restoration when the disloding force is directed other than parallel to the path of removal, and (6) to provide stabilizing characteristics against horizontal rotation of the denture.

Guiding plane surfaces should be found or created so that they are as nearly parallel to the long axes of abutment teeth as possible. Establishing guiding planes on several abutment teeth (preferably more than two teeth), located at widely separated positions in the dental arch, provides for a more effective use of these surfaces. The effectiveness of guiding plane surfaces is also enhanced if these surfaces lie in more than one common axial surface of the abutment teeth (Fig. 9-25).

As a rule of thumb, proximal guiding plane surfaces should be about two thirds as wide as the distance between the tips of adjacent buccal and lingual cusps and should extend vertically about two thirds the length of the "enamel crown" portion of the tooth from the marginal ridge cervically. In preparing guiding plane surfaces, care must be exercised to avoid creating buccal or lingual line angles (Fig. 9-26). Assuming that the stabilizing or retentive arm of a direct retainer may originate in the guiding plane region, a line angle preparation would weaken either or both components of the clasp assembly. Another precaution that should be observed is to avoid preparing guiding plane surfaces on *both* proximal surfaces of a lone-standing terminal abutment supporting a distal extension denture base. A terminal abutment so prepared would be subjected to a "monkey

Fig. 9-25. Prospective guiding plane surfaces are indicated by wires placed on abutment teeth. All these surfaces, when utilized, can be made vertically parallel to path of placement. However, by including guiding plane surfaces, which are divergent cross-arch, resistance to horizontal rotation of denture is enhanced.

Fig. 9-26. A, Guiding plane surface should be like an area on a cylindric object. It should be a continuous surface unbounded by even "rounded" line angles. **B,** Minor connector contacting a guiding plane surface has the same curvature as does that surface. From the occlusal view it tapers buccally from a thicker lingual portion, thus permitting a closer contact of abutment tooth and prosthetically supplied tooth. Viewed from the buccal, minor connector contacts "enamel" crown of tooth on its proximal surface only about two thirds its length.

wrench" leverage effect, which could only result in exceeding the physiologic tolerance of the supporting tissues of the abutment.

Ridge support. Support for the tooth-borne denture or the tooth-borne modification space comes entirely from the abutment teeth by means of rests. Support for the distal extension denture base comes primarily from the soft tissues overlying the residual alveolar bone. In the latter, rest support is effective only at the abutment end of the denture base.

The effectiveness of tissue support is dependent on four things: (1) the quality of the residual ridge, (2) the total occlusal load applied, (3) the accuracy of the denture bases, and (4) the accuracy and type of impression registration.

The quality of the ridge cannot be influenced, except to modify it or improve it by surgical intervention. Such modification is frequently advisable but is less frequently done.

The total occlusal load applied to the residual ridge may be influenced by reducing the occlusal area. This is done by the use of fewer, narrower, and more effectively shaped artificial teeth.

The accuracy of the denture base is influenced by our choice of materials and by the exactness of the processing techniques. Inaccurate and warped denture bases influence adversely the support of the partial denture. Materials and techniques that will assure the greatest dimensional stability should be selected.

The accuracy of the impression technique is entirely in the hands of the dentist. Maximum tissue coverage for support and the use of primary stress-bearing areas should be the primary objectives in any partial denture impression technique. The manner in which this is accomplished should be based on a biologic comprehension of what happens beneath a distal extension denture base when an occlusal load is applied.

The distal extension partial denture is unique in that its support is derived both from abutment teeth, which are comparatively unyielding, and from soft tissues, which may be comparatively yielding under occlusal forces. Resilient tissues, being unable to provide support for the denture base comparable to that offered by the abutment teeth, are displaced by the occlusal load. Only the projections of the underlying resid-

ual bone remain to be traumatized by occlusal forces. This problem of support is further complicated by the fact that the patient has natural teeth remaining on which he may exert far greater force than he would were he completely edentulous. This fact is clearly evident from the damage often occurring to an edentulous ridge when it is opposed by a few remaining anterior teeth in the other arch and especially when the opposing occlusion of anterior teeth has been arranged so that contact exists in both centric and eccentric positions.

Ridge tissues recorded in their resting or nonfunctioning form are incapable of providing the composite support needed for a denture that derives its support from both hard and soft tissue. It is necessary that three factors be taken into consideration in the acceptance of an impression technique for distal extension partial dentures: (1) the material should record the tissues covering the primary stress-bearing areas in their supporting form, (2) tissues within the basal seat area other than primary stress-bearing areas must be recorded in their anatomic form, and (3) the total area covered by the impression should be as great as possible, to distribute the load over as large an area as can be tolerated by the border tissues. This is an application of the principle of the snowshoe.

Anyone who has had the opportunity of comparing two master casts for the same partially edentulous arch—one cast having the distal extension area recorded in its anatomic, or resting, form and the other cast having the distal extension area recorded in its functional form—has been impressed by the differences in the two. A denture base processed to the functional form is generally less irregular, and it has greater area coverage than does a denture base processed to the anatomic, or resting, form. Moreover, and of far greater significance, a denture base made to anatomic form exhibits less stability under rotating forces than does a denture base processed to functional form and thus fails to maintain its occlusal relation with the opposing teeth. By having the patient close onto strips of soft wax, it is evident that occlusion is maintained at a point of equilibrium over a longer period of time when the denture base has been made to the functional form. In contrast, evidence exists that there has been a rapid settling of the denture base when it has been made to the anatomic form, with an early return of the occlusion to natural tooth contact only. Such a denture not only fails to distribute the occlusal load equitably but it also allows rotational movement, which is damaging to the abutment teeth and their investing structures.

Indirect retainers. An indirect retainer must be placed as far anteriorly from the fulcrum line as adequate tooth support permits if it is to function with the direct retainer to restrict movement of a distal extension base away from the basal seat tissues. It must be placed on a rest seat prepared in an abutment tooth that is capable of withstanding the forces placed on it. An indirect retainer cannot function effectively on an inclined tooth surface, nor can a single weak incisor tooth be used for this purpose. Either a canine or premolar tooth should be used for the support of an indirect retainer, and the rest seat must be prepared with as much care as is given any other rest seat. An incisal rest or a lingual rest may be used on an anterior tooth, provided a definite seat can be obtained either in sound enamel or on a cast restoration.

A second purpose that indirect retainers serve in partial denture design is that of support for major connectors. A long lingual bar or an anterior palatal major connector is thereby prevented from settling into the tissues. Even in the absence of a need for indirect retention, provision for such auxiliary support is sometimes indicated.

Contrary to common usage, a continuous bar retainer or a linguoplate does not in itself act as an indirect retainer. Since these are located on inclined tooth surfaces, they serve more as *an orthodontic appliance* than as support for the partial denture. When a linguoplate or a continuous bar retainer is used, terminal rests should always be provided at either end to stabilize the denture and to prevent orthodontic movement of the teeth contacted to the greatest extent possible. Such terminal rests may function also as the indirect retainers, but these would function equally well in that capacity without the continuous bar retainer or linguoplate.

OTHER CONSIDERATIONS INFLUENCING DESIGN

Every effort should be made by the dentist to gain the greatest support possible for removable restorations by utilizing abutments bounding edentulous spaces. Not only

will the residual ridges be relieved of some support contribution, but design of the framework may be greatly simplified. To this end, use of splint bars, internal clip attachments, and overlay abutments should be considered.

Use of a splint bar for denture support. In Chapter 13 under Missing Anterior Teeth, mention is made of the fact that missing anterior teeth are best replaced with a fixed partial denture that also replaces posterior teeth elsewhere in the arch. The following is quoted from that chapter: "From a biomechanical standpoint, . . . a removable partial denture should replace only the missing posterior teeth, *after* the remainder of the arch has been made intact by means of fixed restorations."

Occasionally a situation is found in which, economics aside, it is necessary that several missing anterior teeth be replaced with the removable partial denture rather than by fixed restorations. This may be due to the length of the edentulous span, to the loss of sufficient residual ridge by resorption, accident, or surgery, or to a situation in which the amount of vertical space prevents the use of a fixed partial denture or in which esthetic requirements can better be met through the use of teeth added to the denture framework. In such instances it is necessary that the best possible support for the replaced anterior teeth be provided. Ordinarily this is done through the placement of occlusal or lingual rests or both on the adjacent natural teeth, but when the edentulous span is too large to assure adequate support from the adjacent teeth, another method must be used. This is included here only because it influences the design of the major connector that must then be used.

An anterior splint bar may be attached to the adjacent abutment teeth in such a manner that a fixed splint results, but with a smooth, contoured bar resting lightly on the gingival tissues to support the removable partial denture (Fig. 9-27, A). As with any fixed partial denture, the type of abutment retainers and the decision to use multiple abutments will depend on the length of the span and the stability of the teeth being used as abutments. Regardless of the type of abutment retainers used, the connecting bar must be cast separately and of a rigid alloy, or a commercially available bar may be used and attached to the abutments by soldering.

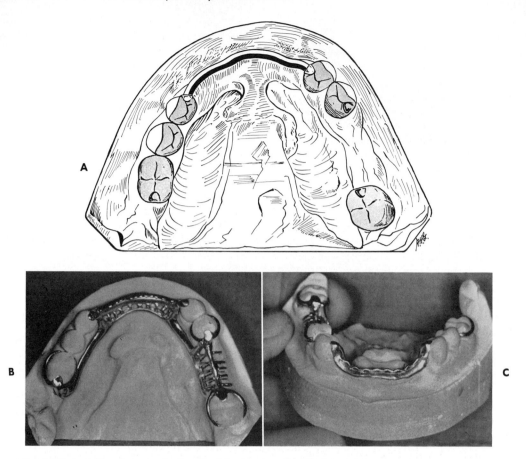

Fig. 9-27. A, Splint bar attached to double abutments on either side of arch. Although this may be made of a hard gold alloy, its rigidity is better assured by making the bar of a chromium-cobalt alloy that fits into recesses prepared in abutment pieces, attaching it by electric soldering. **B** and **C,** Denture framework designed to fit and be supported by splint bar.

Rather than rely on soldered junctions alone, it is best that recesses be formed in the abutment pieces and that the connecting bar, which rests lightly on the tissues, be cast or made to fit into these recesses; they are then attached by soldering.

Because of the greater rigidity of the chromium-cobalt alloys, the splint bar is preferably cast in one of these materials and then attached to the gold abutment pieces by electric soldering. The complete assembly (abutment pieces and connecting bar) is then cemented permanently to the abutment teeth, the same as a fixed partial denture. The impression for the partial denture than is made and a master cast obtained that accurately reproduces the contours of the tissue bar. The denture framework is then made to fit this

bar by extending the major connector to cover and rest upon the splint bar. Either retention for the attachment of a resin base or any other acceptable means of attaching the replaced anterior teeth is incorporated into the denture design (Fig. 9-27, *B* and *C*.) In those situations wherein the removable restoration will be practically tooth supported, the splint bar may be curved to follow the crest of the residual ridge, as seen in Fig. 9-27, *A.* However, in a distal extension situation, because of the vertical rotation of the denture, caution must be exercised to so form the splint bar that excessive torque will not accrue to its supporting abutments (Fig. 9-28).

The resulting partial denture will have the esthetic and other advantages of removable

Fig. 9-28. A, Insofar as possible, "incisal" portion of splint bar should be flat when viewed frontally. Provision must be made in the construction and location of bar so that dental floss may be threaded underneath bar to allow proper cleaning by patient. **B,** As viewed from above, bar is in a straight line between the abutments. This is especially critical for distal extension dentures to avoid excess torque on abutments as denture rotates in function. **C,** Sagittal section through bar demonstrates rounded form of bar making a point contact with residual ridge. The whole "tissue" surface of bar is easily accessible for cleaning with dental floss. Pear-shaped bar (in cross section) will permit rotation of removable partial denture without appreciable resistance or torque.

Fig. 9-29. A, Lower canines splinted together with a splint bar. The longevity of these teeth is greatly enhanced by splinting. Tissue surfaces are minimally contacted by rounded form of lower portion of bar. Anterior and posterior slopes of splint bar must be compatible with path of placement of denture. **B,** Floss is used by patient to clean inferior portion of splint bar.

anterior replacements but will have positive support from the underlying splint bar (Fig. 9-29).

Internal clip attachment. The internal clip (or grip) attachment differs from the splint bar in that the internal clip attachment provides both support and retention at the connecting bar (Fig. 9-30).

The connecting bar is made of 11-gauge platinum alloy wire, and the female grip is made of 27-gauge plate metal. Rather than resting on the tissues of the residual ridge as does the splint bar, the wire bar is located slightly above the tissues. Retention is provided by the plate metal grip, which is contoured to fit the bar and is partially embedded by means of retention spurs or loops into the overlying resin denture base.

The internal clip attachment thus provides both support and retention for the anterior modification area and may serve to eliminate both occlusal rests and retentive clasps on the adjacent abutment teeth.

Overlay abutment as support for a denture base. Every consideration should be directed to preventing the need for a distal ex-

Fig. 9-30. **A,** Canines have been endodontically treated and are splinted together with a round, straight connecting bar, slightly elevated from residual ridge. Retaining left molar as an abutment will immeasurably contribute to stability of removable partial denture. **B,** Tissue surface of completed mandibular restoration containing internal clip attachment. **C,** Complete denture and removable partial denture have been initially placed for patient. (Courtesy Dr. Bernard Wilkie, Charlotte, N.C.)

Fig. 9-31. **A,** Master cast has been prepared for duplicating in a refractory investment to develop wax pattern for removable partial denture framework, supported by an overlay abutment second molar. Molar could not be restored by conventional means. It was endodontically treated, and crown was reduced to a slightly elevated dome shape. Pulp chamber was filled with a silver amalgam alloy. **B,** Wax pattern has been developed on investment cast and provision has been made to attach a properly extended acrylic resin denture base. A bilateral distal extension denture has been avoided by planning an overlay prosthesis.

tension removable partial denture. In many instances it is possible to salvage the roots and a portion of the crown of a badly broken down molar through endodontic treatment. A periodontally involved molar, otherwise indicated for extraction, may sometimes be salvaged by periodontal and endodontic treatment accompanied with reduction of the clinical crown almost level with gingival tissues. An unopposed molar may have overly erupted to such an extent that even restoring the tooth with a crown is inadequate to develop a harmonious occlusion. Then too, it is not unusual to encounter a molar that is so grossly tipped anteriorly that it cannot serve as an abutment unless the clinical crown is reduced drastically.

Such teeth as described above should be considered for possible support for an otherwise distal extension denture base. Endodontic treatment and preparation of the coronal portion of the tooth as a slightly elevated dome-shaped abutment often offers an alternative to a distal extension base (Fig. 9-31). The student is referred to the Selected References (Textbooks; Abutment Retainers) for sources of information on overdenture abutments and overlay type prostheses.

SELF-ASSESSMENT AIDS

1. Forces are transmitted to abutment teeth and residual ridges by removable partial dentures. One of the factors of a force is its magnitude. Can you recall the other three factors of a force that a dentist must consider in designing removable partial dentures?
2. True or false—the design of a removable restoration requires a consideration of mechanics as well as biologic considerations?
3. There are six simple machines recognized today. What are they?
4. Can a simple machine impart a greater force (effort) than the effort expended to activate it?
5. Of the simple machines, which two are more likely to be encountered in the design of removable partial dentures?
6. What is a lever? A cantilever?
7. Can you name the three classes of levers and give an example of each?
8. Of the three classes of lever systems, which two are most likely to be encountered in removable partial prosthodontics?
9. Can you figure the mechanical advantage of a lever system, given dimensions of effort and resistance arms?
10. What class lever system is most likely to be encountered with a restoration on a Class II, modification 1, arch when a force is placed on the extension base?
11. What factor permits a distal extension denture to rotate when the denture base is forced toward the basal seat?
12. Is an abutment tooth better able to resist a force directed apically or directed horizontally? Why?
13. Where is the horizontal (tipping) axis of an abutment tooth located?
14. Where is the horizontal (tipping) axis of a fence post located?
15. If you had to shake a fence post out of the ground, where would you apply the force—at its top or at ground level?
16. Why should components of a direct retainer assembly be located as close to the tipping axis of a tooth as practical?
17. The text suggests at least nine considerations or factors that will influence the design of a removable partial denture. How many of these considerations can you jot down?
18. Do you feel that design of a denture is influenced by the classification of the arch being restored?
19. There are really only two types of removable partial dentures. What are they?
20. Since there are two basic types of removable partial dentures, it is evident that a dentist must consider (1) the manner in which each is supported, (2) the method of impression registration, (3) the need or lack of need for indirect retention, and (4) the use of a base material that can be readily relined. Could you write a meaningful essay of 100 words or less about each of these listed considerations?
21. What is a guiding plane?
22. What are the functions of guiding plane surfaces contacted by minor connectors? There are at least six functions.
23. Should guiding planes prepared on enamel surfaces of abutment teeth be rounded or flat? Why?
24. Can you give a rule of thumb for the dimensions of proximal guiding planes?
25. Direct retainers for tooth-borne dentures differ in design from those employed in extension type dentures to a great extent. What requirement, in relation to an undercut, exists for the direct retainer (clasp) on a terminal abutment of an extension denture when the denture base is forced in heavier contact with the residual ridge?
26. Name the components of a removable partial denture that must be rigid. Name the component(s) in which flexibility is desirable.
27. Would you agree that a fixed partial denture, where indicated, should be the restoration of choice in lieu of a removable partial denture?

28. What method should usually be used to replace single missing teeth or missing anterior teeth? Can you justify your answer?

29. You are confronted with a Class I arch in which all molars and first premolars are missing. Should you consider replacing the first premolars with fixed partial dentures rather than restoring the spaces with the removable restoration? Why?

30. What is a splint bar?

31. Can you draw a splint bar from a frontal, horizontal, and sagittal view?

32. What purposes are served by utilizing splint bars where indicated.

33. A decision has been made to utilize a splint bar from canine to canine. Will this decision influence the design of the framework?

34. Do you know what an internal clip attachment is? Have you ever seen one?

35. The internal clip attachment must be used in conjunction with some type of bar supported by abutment teeth. What is the cross-sectional shape of such a bar?

36. What advantages accrue from using such a design for a restoration?

37. For what reasons must a splint bar be convex rather than concave adjacent to the residual ridge?

38. You are confronted with a mandibular arch with only the six anterior teeth and two second molars remaining. The maxillary arch is edentulous. The anterior teeth are restorable individually and show no mobility or periodontal involvement. The molars, however, are grossly involved with caries; in fact most of the clinical crown is gone. They also show a Miller mobility classification of 1 and exhibit a 5 to 6 mm gingival crevicular depth. They can be treated periodontally and endodontically. In such a situation, if finances were not a factor, would you (1) extract both molars? (2) prepare the molars for an overlay prosthesis? (3) extract all the mandibular teeth and treat the patient with complete dentures?

40. If you elected to prepare the molars mentioned in the preceding section for an overlay prosthesis, state your reasons for so doing in terms of benefits to the patient.

10 SURVEYING

A dental surveyor has been defined as an instrument used to determine the relative parallelism of two or more surfaces of the teeth or other parts of the cast of a dental arch.

Any one of the several moderately priced surveyors on the market will adequately accomplish the procedures necessary to rationalize the design and construction of a partial denture. In addition, these surveyors may be used to parallel internal rests and intracoronal retainers. With handpiece holder added, they also may be used to machine internal rests and to parallel guiding plane surfaces of abutment restorations.

DESCRIPTION OF DENTAL SURVEYOR

Perhaps the most widely used surveyors are the Ney (Fig. 10-1) and the Jelenko (Fig. 10-2) surveyors. Both of these are precision-made instruments but differ principally in that the Jelenko arm swivels whereas the Ney arm is fixed. The technique for surveying and trimming blockout is therefore somewhat different. Other surveyors also differ in this respect, and the dentist may prefer one over another for this reason.

The principal parts of the Ney surveyor are as follows:

1. Platform on which the base is moved
2. Vertical arm that supports the superstructure
3. Horizontal arm from which the surveying tool suspends
4. Table to which the cast is attached
5. Base upon which the table swivels
6. Paralleling tool or guideline marker (This tool contacts the convex surface to be studied in a tangential manner. The relative parallelism of one surface to another may thus be determined. By substituting a carbon marker, the height of contour then may be delineated on the surfaces of the abutment teeth and also areas of interference requiring reduction on blockout.)
7. Mandrel for holding special tools (Fig. 10-3)

The principal parts of the Jelenko surveyor are essentially the same as those for the Ney surveyor except that by loosening the nut at the top of the vertical arm, the horizontal arm may be made to swivel. The objective of this feature, originally designed by Dr. Noble Wills, is to permit freedom of movement of the arm in a horizontal plane rather than to depend entirely on the horizontal movement of the cast. To some this is confusing because two horizontal movements must thus be coordinated. For those who prefer to move the cast only in a horizontal relationship to a fixed vertical arm, the nut may be tightened and the horizontal arm used in a fixed position. The jointed horizontal arm of the Williams surveyor (Fig. 10-4) differs from both the Ney and Jelenko surveyors. This feature permits the vertical arm to be moved to scribe the survey lines without moving the cast.

Another difference in the Ney and Jelenko surveyors is that the vertical arm on the Ney surveyor is retained by friction within a fixed bearing. The shaft may be moved up or down within this bearing but remains in any vertical position until again moved. The shaft may be fixed in any vertical position desired by tightening a set screw. In contrast, the vertical arm of the Jelenko surveyor is spring mounted and returns to the top position when released. It must be held down against spring tension while in use, which to some is a disadvantage. The spring may be removed, but the friction of the two bearings supporting the arm does not hold it in position as securely as does a bearing designed for that purpose. These minor differences in the two

Text continued on p. 148.

Fig. 10-1. Ney surveyor is widely used because of its simplicity and durability. Dental students should be required to own such a surveyor. By becoming familiar with and dependent on its use, they are more likely to continue using the surveyor in practice as a necessary piece of equipment toward more adequate diagnosis, effective treatment planning, and the performance of many other aspects of prosthodontic treatment. (Courtesy J. M. Ney Co., Hartford, Conn.)

Fig. 10-2. Jelenko surveyor. Note spring-mounted paralleling tool and swivel at top of vertical arm. Horizontal arm may be fixed in any position by tightening the nut at top of vertical arm. (Courtesy J. F. Jelenko & Co., Inc., New York, N.Y.)

Fig. 10-3. Various tools that may be used with a dental surveyor. **A,** Ney undercut gauges. **B,** Jelenko undercut gauge. **C,** Ney carbon marker with metal reinforcement sleeve. **D,** Jelenko carbon marker. **E,** Tapered tools, 2- and 6-degree, for trimming blockout when some nonparallelism is desired. **F,** Ney wax trimmer for paralleling blockout. **G,** Surveying blade being used for trimming blockout.

Fig. 10-4. Williams surveyor, which features a Gimbal stage table that is adjustable to any desired anterior, posterior, or lateral tilt. The degree of inclination can be recorded for repositioning of cast at any time. A distinct advantage of this table over the universal tilt table is that the center of rotation always remains constant. The superstructure of this surveyor consists of a jointed arm and spring-supported survey rod, all components of which can be locked in a fixed position if desired. This surveyor is perhaps best suited for placement of internal attachments, rather than for cast analyzing and other purposes. (Courtesy Williams Gold Refining Co., Buffalo, N.Y.)

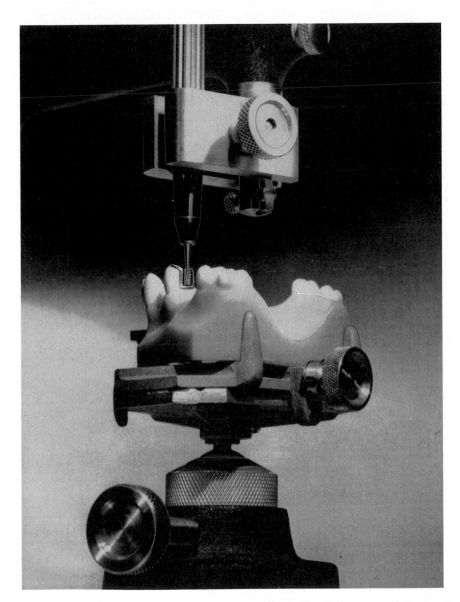

Fig. 10-5. Ney handpiece holder attached to vertical spindle of surveyor may be used as a drill press to cut internal rests and recesses in wax patterns and gold castings and to establish lingual surfaces above a ledge, which are parallel to path of placement in abutment restorations. (Courtesy J. M. Ney Co., Hartford, Conn.)

surveyors lead to personal preference but do not detract from the effectiveness of either surveyor when properly used.

Since the shaft on the Ney surveyor is stable in any vertical position, yet may be moved vertically with ease, it lends itself well for use as a drill press when a handpiece holder is added (Fig. 10-5). The handpiece may thus be used to cut recesses in gold restorations with precision by using burs or carborundum points of various sizes in a dental handpiece.

Several other types of surveyors have been designed and are in use today. Many of these are more elaborate and costly, yet possess little advantage over the more simple type of surveyors.

PURPOSES OF SURVEYOR

The surveyor may be used for surveying the diagnostic cast, recontouring abutment teeth on the diagnostic cast, contouring wax patterns, measuring a specific depth of undercut, surveying ceramic veneer crowns, placing the intracoronal retainers, placing internal rests, machining cast restorations, and surveying and blocking out the master cast.

Surveying the diagnostic cast. Surveying the diagnostic cast is essential to effective diagnosis and treatment planning. The objectives are as follows:

1. To determine the most acceptable path of placement that will eliminate or minimize interference to placement and removal (Fig. 10-6). *The path of placement is the direction in which a restoration moves from the point of initial contact of its rigid parts with the supporting teeth to the terminal resting position, with rests seated and the denture base in contact with the tissues.* The *path of removal* is exactly the reverse, since it is the direction of restoration movement from its terminal resting position of the last contact of its rigid parts with the supporting teeth. When the restoration is properly designed to have positive guiding planes, the patient may place and remove the restoration with ease in only one direction because of the guiding influence of tooth surfaces made parallel to that path of placement.

2. To identify proximal tooth surfaces that are or can be made parallel so that they act as guiding planes during placement and removal.

3. To locate and measure areas of the teeth that may be used for retention.

4. To determine whether tooth and bony areas of interference will need to be eliminated either by extraction or by selecting a different path of placement.

5. To determine the most suitable path of placement that will permit locating retainers and artificial teeth to the best esthetic advantage.

6. To permit an accurate charting of the mouth preparations to be made. This includes the disking of proximal tooth surfaces to provide guiding planes and the reduction of excessive tooth contours to eliminate interference and to permit a more acceptable location of reciprocal and retentive clasp arms. By marking these areas on the diagnostic cast with red pencil using an undercut gauge to estimate the amount of tooth structure that may safely (without exposing dentin) be removed, and then trimming the marked areas on the stone cast with the surveyor blade, the angulation and extent of tooth reduction may be established prior to preparing the teeth in the mouth (Fig. 10-7). With the diagnostic cast on the surveyor at the time of mouth preparations, disking and reduction of tooth contours may thus be accomplished with acceptable accuracy.

7. To delineate the height of contour on abutment teeth and to locate areas of undesirable tooth undercut that are to be avoided,

Path of placement

Fig. 10-6. Tilt of cast on adjustable table of surveyor in relation to vertical arm establishes path of placement and removal that partial denture will take. All mouth preparations must be made to conform to a previously determined path of placement, which has been recorded by scoring the base of cast or by tripoding.

Fig. 10-7. **A,** Solid line represents height of contour on an abutment at a selected orientation of diagnostic cast to vertical spindle of surveyor. Dotted line represents the desirable height of contour to optimally locate a component of direct retainer assembly. A 0.01-inch (0.25 mm) undercut gauge is used to mark location of tip of retentive arm of direct retainer. **B,** By reducing axial contour of stone tooth only 0.01 inch, the optimal height of contour can be achieved without exposing dentin. **C,** Stone tooth is trimmed with surveyor blade to desired height of contour. Trimmed area is marked in red pencil and serves as a blueprint for similar recontouring in the mouth. If we can safely assume that the enamel is 1 mm thick in area of contemplated reduction, only 0.25 mm of enamel need be removed to achieve an optimal height of contour.

Fig. 10-8. **A,** Wax patterns have been carved to meet requirements of occlusion. **B,** After cast has been oriented to surveyor at the predetermined path of placement, vertical surfaces of wax patterns are altered with surveyor blade to meet specific requirements for optimum placement of framework components.

eliminated, or blocked out. This will include areas of the teeth to be contacted by rigid connectors, the location of nonretentive reciprocal and stabilizing arms, and the location of retentive clasp terminals.

8. To record the cast position in relation to the selected path of placement for future reference. This may be done by locating three dots or parallel lines on the cast, thus establishing the horizontal plane in relation to the vertical arm of the surveyor (Fig. 11-2).

Contouring wax patterns. The surveyor blade is used as a wax carver during this phase of mouth preparation so that the proposed path of placement may be maintained throughout the preparation of cast restorations for abutment teeth (Fig. 10-8).

All proximal surfaces of wax patterns adjacent to an edentulous area should be made parallel to the previously determined path of placement. Similarly, all other tooth contours that will be contacted by rigid connectors should be made parallel whenever possible. The surfaces of restorations upon which reciprocal and stabilizing components will be placed should be contoured to permit their location well below occlusal surfaces and upon nonretentive areas. Those surfaces of the restoration that are to provide retention for clasp arms should be contoured so that retentive clasps may be placed in the cervical one third of the crown and to the best esthetic advantage. Generally a small amount of undercut (0.375 mm [0.015 in] or less) is sufficient for retentive purposes.

Surveying ceramic veneer crowns. Ceramic veneer crowns are often used to restore abutment teeth on which extracoronal direct retainers will be placed. The surveyor is used to contour all areas of the wax pattern for the veneer crown except the buccal or labial surface. It is unlikely that the ceramic veneer portion can be fabricated exactly to the form required for the planned placement of retentive clasp arms without some reshaping with stones. Before the final glaze is placed, the abutment crowns should be returned to the surveyor on a full arch cast to assure the correct contour of the veneered portions or to locate those areas that need recontouring (Fig. 10-9). The final glaze is accomplished after the crowns have been recontoured.

Fig. 10-9. Final glaze has not been placed on veneer crown. Cast has been reoriented to surveyor by indices or tripod marks on cast, and height of contour has been scribed on veneer crown. Alterations to surfaces to conform to ideal placement of components now can be performed by a machining operation. Final glaze is placed on veneer crown only after necessary recontouring is accomplished.

Placement of intracoronal retainers (internal attachments). In the placement of intracoronal retainers the surveyor is used as follows:

1. To select a path of placement in relation to the long axes of the abutment teeth that will avoid areas of interference elsewhere in the arch.

2. To cut recesses in the stone teeth on the diagnostic cast for estimating the proximity of the recess to the pulp (in conjunction with roentgenographic information as to pulp size and location). Also, to facilitate the fabrication of metal or resin jigs to guide the preparations of the recesses in the mouth.

3. To carve recesses in wax patterns, or to place internal attachment trays in wax patterns, or to cut recesses in the gold casting with the handpiece holder, whichever method is preferred.

4. To place the keyway portion of the attachment in the casting prior to investing and soldering, each located parallel to the other similar attachments elsewhere in the arch.

Placement of internal rests. The surveyor may be used as a drill press, with a dental handpiece attached to the vertical arm by means of a handpiece holder. Internal rests may be carved in the wax patterns and further refined with the handpiece after casting, or the entire rest may be cut in the cast restoration with the handpiece. It is best that the outline form of the rest be carved first in wax and merely refined on the casting with the handpiece.

An internal rest differs from an internal attachment in that some portion of the cast prosthesis is waxed and cast to fit into the rest rather than a matched key and keyway attachment being used. The former is usually nonretentive but provides a definite seat for a removable restoration or a cantilever rest for a broken-stress fixed partial denture. When used with fixed partial dentures, nonparallel abutment pieces may thus be placed separately.

The internal rest in partial denture construction provides a positive occlusal support that is more favorably located in relation to the rotational axis of the abutment tooth than is the conventional spoon-shaped occlusal rest. It also provides horizontal stabilization through the parallelism of the vertical walls, thereby serving the same purpose as stabilizing and reciprocal arms placed extracoronally. Due to the movement of a distal extension base, more torque may be applied to the abutment tooth by an interlocking type of rest, and for this reason its use in conjunction with a distal extension partial denture is contraindicated. The ball-and-socket, spoon-shaped occlusal, or noninterlocking rest should be used in distal extension partial denture designs. The use of the dovetailed or interlocking internal rest should be limited to tooth-borne removable restorations, except when it is used in conjunction with some kind of stressbreaker between the abutment pieces and the movable base. The use of stressbreakers has been considered in Chapter 8.

Internal rest seats may be made in the form of a nonretentive box, a retentive box fashioned after the internal attachment, or a semiretentive box. In the latter the walls are usually parallel and nonretentive, but a recess in the floor of the box prevents proximal movement of the male portion. These are cut with dental burs of various sizes and shapes. Tapered or cylindric fissure burs are used to form the vertical walls, and small round burs are used to cut recesses in the floor of the rest seat.

Machining cast restorations. With handpiece holder attached (Fig. 10-5), axial sur-

faces of cast and ceramic restorations may be refined by machining with a suitable cylindric carborundum point. Proximal surfaces of crowns and inlays, which will serve as guiding planes, and vertical surfaces above crown ledges may be improved by machining, but only if the relationship of one crown to another is correct. Unless the seating of removable dies is accurate and held in place with additional stone or plaster, cast restorations should first be tried in the mouth and then transferred by means of a plaster index impression to a reinforced stone cast for machining purposes. The new cast is then positioned on the surveyor, conforming to the path of placement of the partial denture, and vertical surfaces are machined with a true running cylindrical carborundum point.

Whereas machined parallelism may be considered ideal and beyond the realm of everyday application, its merits more than justify the additional steps required to accomplish it. When such parallelism is accomplished and reproduced in a master cast, it is essential that subsequent laboratory steps be directed toward the utilization of these parallel guiding plane surfaces.

Surveying the master cast. Since surveying the master cast follows mouth preparations, the path of placement, the location of retentive areas, and the location of remaining interference must be known before proceeding with the final design of the denture framework. The objectives are as follows:

1. To select the most suitable path of placement by following mouth preparations that satisfy the requirements of *guiding planes, retention, noninterference,* and *esthetics.*

2. To permit measurement of retentive areas and to identify the location of clasp terminals in proportion to the flexibility of the clasp arm being used. Flexibility will depend on many factors: (1) the alloy used for the clasp, (b) the design and type of the clasp, (c) whether its form is round or half-round, (d) whether it is of cast or wrought material, and (e) the length of the clasp arm from its point of origin to its terminal end. Retention will then depend on (a) the flexibility of the clasp arm, (b) the magnitude of the tooth undercut, and (c) the depth the clasp terminal is placed into this undercut.

3. To locate areas of undesirable remain-

Fig. 10-10. Only terminal portion of a retentive direct retainer arm of a metal framework may be located in an undercut. All other areas of involved teeth should be blocked out parallel to path of placement. Lingual interproximal spaces presenting undercuts must be blocked out parallel to path of placement when a linguoplate has been planned as major connector. The small carbon steel diagnostic stylus, warmed slightly with an alcohol torch, simplifies this blocking out procedure.

ing undercut that will be crossed by rigid parts of the restoration during placement and removal. These must be eliminated by blockout.

4. To trim blockout material parallel to the path of placement prior to duplication (Fig. 10-10).

• • •

The partial denture must be designed so that (1) it will not stress abutment teeth beyond their physiologic tolerance, (2) it can be easily placed and removed by the patient, (3) it will be retained against reasonable dislodging forces, and (4) it will not create an unfavorable appearance. It is necessary that the diagnostic cast be surveyed with these principles in mind. Mouth preparation should therefore be planned in accordance with certain factors that will influence the path of placement and removal.

FACTORS THAT DETERMINE PATH OF PLACEMENT AND REMOVAL

The factors that will determine the path of placement and removal are guiding planes, retentive areas, interference, and esthetics.

Guiding planes. Proximal tooth surfaces that bear a parallel relationship to one another must either be found or be created to act as guiding planes during placement and removal of the denture. Guiding planes may be compared to the valve guides in an engine and act to assure a definite path of placement as the rigid parts of the prosthesis contact parallel tooth surfaces.

Guiding planes are necessary to assure the passage of the rigid parts of the prosthesis past existing areas of interference. Thus the denture can be easily placed and removed by the patient without strain on the teeth contacted or on the denture itself and without damage to the underlying soft tissues.

Guiding planes are also necessary to assure predictable clasp retention. For a clasp to be retentive, its retentive arm must be forced to flex. Hence, guiding planes are necessary to give a positive direction to the movement of the restoration to and from its terminal position.

Retentive areas. Retentive areas must exist for a given path of placement, which will be contacted by retentive clasp arms that will be forced to flex over a convex surface during placement and removal. Satisfactory clasp retention is no more than the resistance of metal to deformation. For a clasp to be retentive, its path of escapement must be other than parallel to the path of removal of the denture itself; otherwise it would not be forced to flex and thereby generate the resistance known as retention. Clasp retention is therefore dependent on the existence of a definite path of placement and removal.

Retention at each principal abutment does not necessarily have to be balanced in relation to the tooth on the opposite side of the arch, that is, exactly equal and opposite in magnitude and relative location. This is, of course, assuming that positive reciprocation to retentive elements is present (which must be cross-arch). Retention should be sufficient only to resist reasonable dislodging forces. In other words, it should be the minimum acceptable for adequate retention against reasonable dislodging forces.

Fairly even retention may be obtained by one of two means. One is to change the path of placement to increase or decrease the angle of cervical convergence of opposing retentive surfaces of abutment teeth. The other is to alter the flexibility of the clasp arm by changing its design, its size and length, or the material of which it is made.

Interference. The prosthesis must be designed so that it may be placed and removed without encountering tooth or soft tissue interference. A path of placement may be selected that encounters interference only if the interference can be eliminated during mouth preparations or on the master cast by means of a reasonable amount of blockout. Interference may be eliminated during mouth preparations by surgery, extraction, disking of interfering tooth surfaces, or altering tooth contours with cast restorations.

Generally, interference that *cannot* be eliminated for one reason or another will take precedence over the factors of retention and guiding planes. Sometimes certain areas can be made noninterfering only by selecting a different path of placement at the expense of existing retentive areas and guiding planes. These must then be modified with restorations that are in harmony with the path dictated by the existing interference. On the other hand, if areas of interference *can* be eliminated by various reasonable means, they should be. By so doing, the axial contours of existing abutments may frequently be utilized with little or no alteration.

Esthetics. By one path of placement the most esthetic location of artificial teeth is made possible, and less clasp metal and less base material may be displayed.

The location of retentive areas may influence the path of placement selected, and therefore retentive areas always should be selected with the most esthetic location of clasps in mind. When restorations are to be made for other reasons, they should be contoured to permit the least display of clasp metal. Generally, less metal will be displayed if the retentive clasp is placed at a more distogingival area of tooth surface, made possible either by the path of placement selected or by the contour of cast restorations.

Esthetics also may dictate the choice of path selected when missing anterior teeth must be replaced with the partial denture. In such situations a more vertical path of placement is necessary so that neither the artificial teeth nor the adjacent natural teeth will have to be modified excessively (Fig. 10-11). In this instance esthetics may take precedence over other factors. This necessitates

Fig. 10-11. When anterior teeth must be replaced with a partial denture, a vertical path of placement may be necessary to avoid excessively altering abutment teeth and supplied teeth.

the preparation of abutment teeth to eliminate interferences and to provide guiding planes and retention in *harmony with* that path of placement dictated by esthetic factors.

Esthetics ordinarily should not be the primary factor in partial denture design. *Therefore the replacement of missing anterior teeth should be accomplished by means of fixed restorations whenever possible, rather than permit their replacement to influence the mechanical and functional effectiveness of the partial denture.* Since the primary consideration should be the preservation of the remaining oral tissues, esthetics should not be allowed to jeopardize the success of the partial denture.

STEP-BY-STEP PROCEDURES IN SURVEYING A DIAGNOSTIC CAST

Attach the cast to the adjustable surveyor table by means of the clamp provided. Position the adjustable table so that the occlusal surfaces of the teeth are approximately parallel to the platform (Fig. 10-12). (This is only a tentative, but practical, way to start considering the factors that influence the path of placement and removal.)

Guiding planes. Determine the relative parallelism of proximal tooth surfaces by contacting proximal tooth surfaces with the surveyor blade or diagnostic stylus. Alter the cast position anteroposteriorly until the prox-

Fig. 10-13. Relative parallelism of proximal tooth surfaces will determine anteroposterior tilt of cast in relation to vertical arm of surveyor.

Fig. 10-12. Recommended method for manipulating dental surveyor. Right hand is braced on horizontal arm of surveyor, and fingers are used, as illustrated, to raise and lower vertical shaft in its spindle. Left hand holding cast on adjustable table slides horizontally on platform in relation to vertical arm. Right hand must be used also to loosen and tighten tilting mechanism as a suitable anteroposterior and lateral tilt of cast in relation to surveyor is being determined.

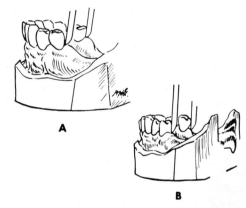

Fig. 10-14. In selecting the most desirable anteroposterior tilt of cast in relation to surveyor blade, a choice must be made between positions illustrated in **A** and **B**. In **A**, distal surface of left premolar abutment would have to be extended by means of a cast restoration. In **B**, right premolar could be disked slightly to provide an acceptably parallel guiding plane. Unless cast restorations are necessary for other reasons, tilt shown in **B** is almost always preferred.

imal surfaces are in a parallel relation to one another or near enough that they can be made parallel by disking. This will determine the *anteroposterior tilt* of the cast in relation to the vertical arm of the surveyor (Fig. 10-13). Although the surveyor table is universally adjustable, it should be thought of as having only two axes, thus allowing only anteroposterior and lateral tilting.

In making a choice between having contact with a proximal surface at the cervical area only or contact at the marginal ridge only, the latter is preferred because a plane may then be established by disking (Fig. 10-14). It is obvious that when only gingival contact exists, a cast restoration is the only means of

establishing a guiding plane. Therefore, if a tilt that does not provide proximal contact is accepted, the proximal surface must be established with some kind of restoration. In making a choice between having a good guiding plane on one proximal surface and one on another as against having a good plane on one and disking the other, the latter is preferred, and the need for disking is indicated on the diagnostic cast with red pencil. This holds true only when cast restorations are not otherwise necessary.

The end result of selecting a suitable anteroposterior tilt should be *to provide the greatest area of parallel proximal surfaces that may act as guiding planes.* Other axial surfaces of abutment teeth may also be utilized as guiding planes. However, this is realized most often by having the stabilizing component of the direct retainer assembly contacting in its entirety the axial surface of the abutment, which has been found or made parallel to the path of placement. Therefore a lateral tilt of the cast to the vertical arm of the surveyor must also be considered as well as the anteroposterior tilt to utilize guiding planes.

Retentive areas. By contacting buccal and lingual surfaces of abutment teeth with the surveyor blade, the amount of retention existing below their height of convexity may be determined. This is best accomplished by directing a small source of light toward the cast from the side away from the dentist. The *angle of cervical convergence* is best observed as a triangle of light between the surveyor blade and the apical portion of the tooth surface being studied.

Alter the cast position by tilting it laterally until not grossly different retentive areas exist on the principal abutment teeth. If only two abutment teeth are involved, as in a Kennedy Class I partially edentulous arch, they are both principal abutments. However, if four abutment teeth are involved, as in a Kennedy Class III, modification 1, arch, they are all principal abutments, and retentive areas should be located on all four. But if three abutment teeth are involved, as in a Kennedy Class II, modification 1, arch, the posterior abutment on the tooth-borne side and the abutment on the distal extension side are considered to be the principal abutments, and retention is somewhat equalized accordingly. The third abutment may be considered to be secondary, and less retention is expected from it than from the other two. An exception is when the posterior abutment on the tooth-borne side has a poor prognosis and the denture is designed to ultimately be a Class I. In such a situation the two stronger abutments are considered to be principal abutments.

In tilting the cast laterally to establish reasonable uniformity of retention, it is necessary that the table be rotated about an imaginary longitudinal axis without disturbing the anteroposterior tilt previously established. The resulting position is one that provides or makes possible parallel guiding planes and provides for acceptable retention on the abutment teeth. Note that possible interference to this tentative path of placement has not, as yet, been taken into consideration.

Interference. If a mandibular cast is being surveyed, check the lingual surfaces that will be crossed by a lingual bar major connector during placement and removal. Bony prominences and lingually inclined premolar teeth are the most common causes of interference to a lingual bar connector.

If the interference is bilateral, surgery or disking of lingual tooth surfaces, or both, may be unavoidable. If it is only unilateral, a change in the lateral tilt may be necessary to avoid an area of tooth or tissue interference. In changing the path of placement to avoid interference, previously established guiding planes and an ideal location for retentive elements may be lost. Then the decision must be made whether to remove the existing interference by whatever means necessary or to resort to restorations on the abutment teeth, thereby changing the proximal and retentive areas to conform to the new path of placement.

In like manner, bony undercuts that will offer interference to the seating of denture bases must be studied and the decision made to remove them surgically, to change the path of placement at the expense of guiding planes and retention, or to design denture bases to avoid such undercut areas. The latter may be done by eliminating buccal and labial flanges and distolingual extension of denture bases. *However, it should be remembered that the maximum area available for support of the denture base should be utilized whenever possible.*

Interference to major connectors rarely exists in the maxillary arch. Areas of interference are usually found on buccally inclined posterior teeth and those bony areas on the buccal aspect of edentulous spaces. As with the mandibular cast, the decision must be made whether to eliminate them, to change the path of placement at the expense of guiding planes and retention, or to design the connectors and bases to avoid them.

Other areas of possible interference to be studied are those surfaces of abutment teeth that will support or be crossed by minor connectors and clasp arms. While interference to vertical minor connectors may be blocked out, doing so may cause discomfort to the patient's tongue and may create objectionable spaces for the trapping of food. Also it is desirable that tooth surfaces contacted by vertical connectors be utilized as auxiliary guiding planes whenever possible. Too much relief is perhaps better than too little because of the possibility of irritation to soft tissues, but it is always better that the relief be placed intentionally rather than as a blockout of interference. If possible, a minor connector should pass vertically along a tooth surface that is either parallel to the path of placement (which is considered ideal) or tapered occlusally. If tooth undercuts that would necessitate the use of an objectionable amount of blockout exist, they may be eliminated or minimized by slight changes in the path of placement or eliminated during mouth preparations. The need for such alteration should be indicated on the diagnostic cast in red pencil after final acceptance of a path of placement.

Tooth surfaces upon which reciprocal and stabilizing clasp arms will be placed should be studied to see if sufficient areas exist above the height of convexity for the placement of these components. The addition of a clasp arm to the occlusal third of an abutment tooth adds to its occlusal dimension and therefore to the occlusal loading of that tooth. *Nonretentive and stabilizing clasp arms are best located between the middle third and gingival third of the crown rather than upon the occlusal third.*

Areas of interference to more ideal placement of clasp arms usually can be eliminated by reshaping tooth surfaces during mouth preparations, and this is indicated on the diagnostic cast. Gross areas of interference to the placement of clasps may necessitate minor changes in the path of placement or changes in the clasp design. For example, a bar clasp arm originating mesially from the major connector to provide reciprocation and

stabilization might be substituted for a distally originating circumferential arm.

Areas of interference frequently overlooked are the distal line angles of premolar abutment teeth and the mesial line angles of molar abutments. These areas frequently offer interference to the origin of circumferential clasp arms. If not detected at the time of initial survey, they are not included in the plan for mouth preparations. When such an undercut exists, three alternatives may be considered:

1. It may be blocked out the same as any other area of interference. This is by far the least satisfactory method because the origin of the clasp must then stand away from the tooth in proportion to the amount of blockout used. Although this is perhaps less objectionable than its being placed occlusally, it may be objectionable to the tongue and the cheek and may create a food trap.

2. It may be circumvented by approaching the retentive area from a gingival direction with a bar clasp arm. This is frequently a satisfactory solution to the problem if other contraindications to the use of a bar clasp arm are not present, such as a severe tissue undercut or a retentive area that is too high on the tooth.

3. It may be eliminated by reducing the tooth contour during mouth preparation. This permits the use of a circumferential clasp arm originating well below the occlusal surface in a satisfactory manner. If the tooth is to be modified during mouth preparations, it should be indicated on the diagnostic cast with red pencil.

When the retentive area is located objectionably high on the abutment tooth or the undercut is too severe, interference may also exist on tooth surfaces that are to support retentive clasps. Such areas of extreme or high convexity must be considered as areas of interference and should be reduced accordingly. These areas are likewise indicated on the diagnostic cast for reduction during mouth preparations.

Esthetics. The path of placement thus established must yet be considered from the standpoint of esthetics, both as to the location of clasps and the arrangement of artificial teeth.

Clasp designs that will provide satisfactory esthetics for any given path of placement usually may be selected. In some instances gingivally placed bar clasp arms may be used to advantage; in others circumferential clasp arms located cervically may be used. This is especially true when other abutment teeth located more posteriorly may bear the major responsibility for retention. In still other instances a tapered wrought-wire retentive clasp arm may be placed to better esthetic advantage than a cast clasp arm. The location of clasp arms for esthetic reasons does not ordinarily justify altering the path of placement at the expense of mechanical factors. It should, however, be considered concurrently with other factors, and if a choice between two paths of equal merit permits a more esthetic placement of clasp arms by one path than the other, that path should be given preference.

When anterior replacements are involved, the choice of path is limited to a more vertical one for reasons previously stated. In this instance alone esthetics must be given primary consideration even at the expense of altering the path of placement and making all other factors conform. This factor should be remembered when considering the other three factors, so that compromises can be made at the time other factors are being considered.

FINAL PATH OF PLACEMENT

The final path of placement will be the anteroposterior and lateral position of the cast in relation to the vertical arm of the surveyor that best satisfies all four factors, that is, *guiding planes, retention, interference,* and *esthetics.*

All proposed mouth changes should be indicated on the diagnostic cast in red pencil, with the exception of restorations to be done. These may also be indicated on an accompanying chart if desired. Extractions and surgery are given priority to allow for healing. The remaining red marks represent the actual modifications of the remaining teeth to be done, which consists of the disking of proximal surfaces, the reduction of buccal and lingual surfaces, and, last, the preparation of rest seats. Except when they are placed in the wax pattern for a cast restoration, the preparation of rest seats should always be deferred until all other mouth preparations have been completed.

The actual location of rests will be determined by the proposed design of the denture framework. Therefore the tentative design should be sketched on the diagnostic cast in pencil after the path of placement has been decided on. This is done not only to locate rest areas but also to record graphically the plan of treatment prior to mouth preparations. *In the intervening time between patient visits, other partial denture restorations may have been considered. The dentist should have the plan of treatment before him at each succeeding appointment to avoid confusion and to refresh his memory as to what is to be done and in what sequence.*

The plan for treatment should include (1) the diagnostic cast with the mouth preparations and the denture design marked upon it, (2) a chart showing the proposed design and the planned treatment for each abutment, (3) a working chart showing the total treatment involved that will permit a quick review and a checkoff of each step as the work progresses, and (4) a record of the fee quoted for each phase of treatment that can be checked off as it is recorded on the patient's permanent record.

Red pencil marks on the diagnostic cast are used to indicate the location of areas to be disked or otherwise modified, as well as the location of rests. Although it is not necessary that rest areas be prepared on the diagnostic cast, it is advisable for the beginning student to have done so before proceeding to alter the abutment teeth. Also this applies equally to crown and inlay preparations on abutment teeth. It is advisable, however, for even the most experienced dentist to have trimmed the stone teeth with the surveyor blade wherever tooth reduction is to be done. This identifies not only the *amount* to be removed in a given area but also the *plane* in which the tooth is to be prepared. For example, a proximal surface may need to be disked in only the upper third or the middle third to establish a guiding plane that will be parallel to the path of placement. This is not usually parallel to the long axis of the tooth, and if the disk is laid against the side of the tooth, the existing surface angle will be maintained rather than establishing a new plane that is parallel to the path of placement.

The surveyor blade representing the path of placement may be used to advantage to trim the surface of the abutment tooth when-

ever a red mark appears. The resulting surface represents the amount of tooth to be
removed in the mouth and indicates the
angle at which the handpiece must be held.
The cut surface on the stone tooth is not
again marked with red pencil but is *outlined*
in red pencil to positively locate the area to
be disked.

RECORDING RELATION OF CAST TO SURVEYOR

Some method of recording the relation of
the cast to the vertical arm of the surveyor
must be used so that it may be returned to
the surveyor for future reference, especially
during mouth preparations. The same applies to the need for returning any working
cast to the surveyor for shaping wax patterns,
trimming blockout on the master cast, or
locating clasp arms in relation to undercut
areas.

Obviously the trimmed base will vary with
each cast; therefore recording the position
of the surveyor table is of no value. If it were,
calibrations could be incorporated on the surveyor table, which would allow the same
position to be reestablished. Instead, the
position of each cast must be established separately, and any positional record applies
only to that cast.

Of several methods, two seem to be the
most convenient and accurate. One method
is to place three widely divergent dots on the
tissue surface of the cast with the tip of the
carbon marker, having the vertical arm of the
surveyor in a locked position. Preferably
these dots should not be placed on areas of
the cast involved in the framework design.
Then the dots should be encircled with a
colored pencil for easy identification. On returning the cast to the surveyor, it may be
tilted until the tip of the surveyor blade or
diagnostic stylus again contacts the three dots
in the same plane. This will produce the
original position of the cast and therefore the
original path of placement. This is known as
tripoding the cast (Fig. 11-2). Some dentists
prefer to make tiny pits in the cast at the location of the tripoding dots to preserve the
orientation of the cast and to transfer this
relationship to the refractory cast.

A second method is to score two sides and
the dorsal aspect of the base of the cast with
a sharp instrument held against the surveyor
blade (Fig. 11-2). By tilting the cast until all

three lines are again parallel to the surveyor
blade, the original cast position can be reestablished. Fortunately the scratch lines will
be reproduced in any duplication, thereby
permitting any duplicate cast to be related
to the surveyor in a similar manner. Whereas
a diagnostic cast and a master cast cannot
be made interchangeable, a refractory cast,
being a duplicate of the master cast, can be
repositioned on the surveyor at any time.
The technologist must be cautioned not to
trim the sides of the cast on the cast trimmer
and thereby lose the reference marks for
repositioning.

SURVEYING THE MASTER CAST

The master cast must be surveyed as a new
cast, but the prepared proximal guiding
plane surfaces will indicate the correct anteroposterior tilt. Some compromises may
be necessary, but the amount of guiding
plane surface remaining after blockout should
be the maximum for each tooth. Areas above
the point of contact with the surveyor blade
are not considered to be part of the guiding
plane area and neither are gingival undercut
areas, which will be blocked out.

The lateral tilt will be the position that provides equal retentive areas on all principal
abutments in relation to the planned clasp
design. Factors of flexibility and the need for
extra flexibility on distal extension abutments
must be considered in deciding what will
provide equal retention on all abutment
teeth. For example, cast circumferential or
cast bar retention on the tooth-borne side of
a Class II design will be balanced against the
18-gauge wrought-wire retention on a distal
abutment only if the more rigid cast clasp engages a lesser undercut than the wrought-
wire clasp arm. Therefore the degree of undercut alone does not assure relatively equal
retention unless clasp arms of equal length,
diameter, form, and material are used.

Gross interference will have been eliminated during mouth preparation. Thus, for a
given path of placement providing guiding
planes and balanced retention, any remaining interference must be eliminated with
blockout. If mouth preparations have been
adequately planned and executed, the undercuts remaining to be blocked out should
be minimal.

The base of the cast is now scored or the
cast is tripoded as described previously. The

Fig. 10-15. Worn carbon marker (left) should be discarded because it will invariably misleadingly mark other than the true height of contour for a given orientation of cast to vertical spindle of surveyor. An unworn carbon (right) with an angled end is preferable for marking heights of contour on abutment teeth and performing survey of soft tissue areas.

surveyor blade or diagnostic stylus then may be replaced with a carbon marker and the height of convexity of each abutment tooth and soft tissue contours delineated. Similarly, any areas of interference to the rigid parts of the framework during seating and removal should be indicated with the carbon marker to locate areas to be blocked out or relieved.

Carbon markers that become the slightest bit worn from use should be discarded. A worn (tapered) carbon marker will indicate heights of contour more occlusally located than actually exist. The carbon marker must be parallel to the vertical spindle of the surveyor (Fig. 10-15).

MEASURING RETENTION

The surveyor is used with the master cast for two purposes: (1) to delineate the height of convexity of the abutment teeth for locating clasp arms and to identify both the location and magnitude of retentive undercuts and (2) to trim blockout of any remaining interference to placement and removal of the denture. The areas involved are those that will be crossed by rigid parts of the denture framework.

The exact undercut that retentive clasp terminals will occupy must be measured and marked on the master cast (Fig. 10-16, *A* and *B*). Undercuts may be measured with the use of either an undercut gauge, such as those

provided with the Ney and Jelenko surveyors, or by a dial gauge, such as is incorporated in the Saddle-Lock Retentoscope, the Ticonium Stress-o-graph, or the Austenal Micro-Analyzer. Whether an undercut gauge or a dial gauge is used, the amount of undercut is measured in hundredths of an inch, the gauges allowing measurements up to 0.03 inch. Theoretically the amount of undercut used may vary with the clasp to be used up to a full 0.03 inch. However, undercuts of 0.01 inch are often adequate for retention by cast retainers, an amount that can be measured with practical accuracy, whereas tapered wrought-wire retention may safely utilize up to 0.02 inch without inducing undesirable torque on the abutment tooth, *provided the wire retentive arm is long enough. The use of 0.03 inch is rarely, if ever, justified with any clasp.* When greater retention is required, such as when abutment teeth remain on only one side of the arch, multiple abutments should be used rather than an increase of the retention on any one tooth.

When a source of light is directed toward the tooth being surveyed, a triangle of light is visible. This triangle is bounded by the surface of the abutment tooth on one side and the blade of the surveyor on the other, the apex being the point of contact at the height of convexity and the base of the triangle being the gingival tissues (Fig. 10-17). Retention will be determined by (1) the magnitude of the angle of cervical convergence below the point of convexity, (2) the depth at which the clasp terminal is placed in the angle, and (3) the flexibility of the clasp arm. The intelligent application of various clasp designs and their relative flexibility is of greater importance than the ability to measure an undercut with precise accuracy.

The final design may now be drawn on the master cast with a fine crayon pencil, preferably one that will not come off during duplication. Graphite is usually lifted in duplication, but some crayon pencil marks will withstand duplication without blurring or transfer.* Sizing or spraying the master cast to protect such pencil marks is usually not advisable unless done with extreme care to avoid obliterating the surface detail.

---

*Such as the Dixon Thinex pencil.

Fig. 10-16. A, Undercut gauge will measure depth of undercut below height of contour. Tip of an l-bar–type direct retainer will be placed at area being marked. The depth to which a retentive clasp arm can be placed depends not only on its length, taper, diameter, and alloy from which it is made but also on type of clasp. A circumferential clasp arm is more flexible than is a bar-type clasp arm of same length. (See Chapter 6.) **B,** A specific measurement of undercut gingival to height of contour may be ascertained by use of an undercut gauge attached to surveyor. Simultaneous contact of shank of undercut gauge at height of contour and contact of lip of a specific undercut gauge on tooth in an infrabulge area establishes a definitive degree and location of undercut. Therefore tip of a retentive arm of a direct retainer may be placed in a "planned depth of undercut."

Fig. 10-17. Tooth undercut is best viewed against a good source of light passing through a triangle, which is bounded by surface of abutment tooth, surveyor blade, and gingival tissues.

BLOCKING OUT THE MASTER CAST

After the establishment of the path of placement and the location of undercut areas on the master cast, any undercut areas that will be crossed by rigid parts of the denture (which is every part of the denture framework but the retentive clasp terminals) must be eliminated by blockout.

In the broader sense the term *blockout* includes not only the areas crossed by the denture framework during seating and removal but also (1) those areas not involved that are blocked out for convenience, (2) ledges on which clasp patterns are to be placed, (3) relief beneath connectors to avoid tissue impingement, and (4) relief to provide for later attachment of the denture base to the framework.

Ledges or shelves (shaped blockout) for locating clasp patterns may or may not be used (Fig. 10-18). However, this should not be confused with the actual blocking out of undercut areas that would offer interference to the placement of the denture framework. Only the latter is made on the surveyor, with the surveyor blade or diagnostic stylus being used as a paralleling device.

Blockout material may be purchased, or it

Fig. 10-18. Wax ledge on buccal surface of molar abutment will be duplicated in refractory cast for exact placement of clasp pattern. Note that ledge has been carved slightly below penciled outline of clasp arm. This will allow gingival edge of clasp arm to be polished and still remain in its planned relationship to tooth when denture is seated. It should also be noted that wax ledge definitively establishes planned placement of direct retainer tip into a measured undercut.

may be made up according to the following formula:

Melt and mix together:
　4½ sheets of baseplate wax
　4½ sticks of temporary gutta percha stopping
　3 sticks of sticky wax
　½ tsp. kaolin
Add ½ tube lipstick for color.

Some of the ready-made blockout materials contain a mixture of wax and clay. Hard inlay wax also may be used satisfactorily as a blockout material. It is easily applied and is easily trimmed with the surveyor blade. Trimming is facilitated by slightly warming the surveyor blade with an alcohol torch. Whereas it is true that any wax will melt more readily than a wax-clay mixture if the temperature of the duplicating material is too high, it should be presumed that the duplicating material will not be used at such an elevated temperature. If the temperature of the duplicating material is high enough to damage a wax blockout, other distortions resulting in an inaccurate duplication will also be likely.

Paralleled blockout is necessary cervical to guiding plane surfaces and over all undercut areas that will be crossed by major or minor connectors. Other areas that are to be blocked out for convenience and to avoid difficulties in duplication should be blocked out with hard baseplate wax or an oil-base modeling clay (artist's modeling clay). *A modeling clay that is water-soluble should not be used when duplication procedures are involved.* Such areas are the labial surfaces and labial undercuts not involved in the denture design and the sublingual and distolingual areas beyond the limits of the denture design. These are blocked out arbitrarily with hard baseplate wax or clay, but since they have no relation to the path of placement, they do not require the use of the surveyor.

Areas to be crossed by rigid connectors, on the other hand, should be trimmed with the surveyor blade or some other surveyor tool parallel to the path of placement (Fig. 10-19). This imposes a considerable responsibility on the technologist. Should he fail to trim the blockout sufficiently to expose guiding plane surfaces, the effect of these guiding planes, which were carefully established by the dentist, will be nullified. If, on the other

Wax
Blockout wax made parallel
to path of placement

Fig. 10-19. All guiding plane areas must be parallel to path of placement, and all other areas that will be contacted by rigid parts of denture framework must at least be free of undercut if not parallel.

hand, the technician is overzealous in paralleling the blockout, the stone cast may be abraded by heavy contact with the surveyor blade. Although the resulting cast framework would seat back onto the master cast without interference, interference to placement in the mouth would result. This would necessitate relieving the casting at the chair, which is not only an embarrassing and time-consuming operation but also one that may have the effect of obliterating guiding plane surfaces.

RELIEVING THE MASTER CAST

Tissue undercuts that must be blocked out are paralleled in much the same manner as tooth undercuts. The difference between *blockout* and *relief* must be clearly understood (Figs. 10-20 and 10-21). For example, tissue undercuts that would offer interference to the seating of a lingual bar connector are blocked out with blockout wax and trimmed parallel to the path of placement. This does not in itself necessarily afford relief to avoid tissue impingement. In addition to such blockout a relief of varying thickness must sometimes be used, depending on the location of the connector, the relative slope of the alveolar ridge, and the predictable effect of denture rotation. It must be assumed that indirect retainers, as such, or indirect retention is provided in the design of the denture to prevent rotation of the lingual bar inferiorly. A vertical downward rotation of the denture bases around posterior abut-

A

B

Fig. 10-20. Relationship of parallel blockout and relief to the partial denture framework. **A,** Interproximal spaces to be occupied by minor connectors are blocked out parallel to path of placement. In a like manner, tissue undercuts intimate to lingual bar and minor connectors are blocked out *parallel* to path of placement rather than using an arbitrary blockout. Arbitrary blockout in lingual bar region creates unnecessary spaces for entrapment of foods. Guiding planes have been prepared on distal of second premolar abutments. Blockout of tissue surface inferior to buccal surface of right second premolar is required. Since this slight undercut coincided with placement of a bar-type direct retainer arm, it was blocked out *parallel* to path of placement to avoid damaging tissue when denture rotated or when restoration was being removed or placed. Edentulous ridges have been covered with 20-gauge sheet wax to provide space for denture base to totally enclose denture base minor connector. A 20-gauge sheet-wax relief is preferable if residual ridges have undergone excessive vertical resorption and space available to place artificial teeth is adequate. **B,** Finished removable partial denture framework accurately fits blocked out master cast. Adjustment of framework by grinding to fit master cast is eliminated when blockout of cast has been meticulously carried out.

Fig. 10-21. Relief and blockout of a master cast before duplication. All undercuts involved in denture design (except tips of retentive clasp arms) have been blocked out *parallel* to path of placement. Residual ridges have been relieved with 20-gauge sheet wax. Small wax window has been created adjacent to distogingival surface of each posterior abutment. Framework will occupy this space and will definitively establish most anterior extent of denture bases in these regions. Severe undercuts in retromylohyoid regions of cast have been arbitrarily blocked out to prevent possible distortion of duplicating mold when master cast is removed.

Fig. 10-22. Sagittal section of cast and denture framework. Lingual alveolar ridge slopes inferiorly and posteriorly (upper figure). When a force is directed to displace denture base downward, lingual bar rotates upward but does not impinge on soft tissue of alveolar ridge (lower figure). Therefore in such instances adequate relief to avoid impingement is gained when tissue side of lingual bar is highly polished during finishing process.

ments places the bar increasingly farther from the lingual aspect of the alveolar ridge when this surface slopes inferiorly and posteriorly (Fig. 10-22). Adequate relief of soft tissues adjacent to the lingual bar is obtained by the initial finishing and polishing of the framework in these instances. However, excessive upward vertical rotation of a lingual bar will impinge lingual tissues if the alveolar ridge is nearly vertical or undercut to the path of placement (Fig. 10-23). The region of the cast involving the proposed placement of the lingual bar should, in this situation, be first relieved by parallel blockout and then by a 32-gauge wax strip. Low-fusing casting wax such as Kerr's green casting wax should not be used for this purpose, for it is too easily thinned during adapting and may be affected by the temperature of the duplicating material. Pink casting wax should be used, but it is difficult to adapt uniformly. A pressure-sensitive adhesive-coated casting wax is preferable because it adapts readily and adheres to the cast surface. Any wax, even the ad-

Fig. 10-23. Undercut alveolar ridge was blocked out parallel to path of placement in fabricating the lingual bar (upper figure). Application of a vertical force to create a rotation of lingual bar upward will cause impingement of lingual tissue on alveolar ridge (lower figure). To avoid impingement in these instances, master cast should not only be blocked out parallel to path of placement, but an additional relief of 32-gauge sheet wax should also be utilized in blocking out cast in such undercut areas.

Table 2. *Differentiations between parallel blockout, shaped blockout, arbitrary blockout, and relief*

Site	Material	Thickness
Paralleled blockout		
Proximal tooth surfaces to be used as guiding planes	Hard baseplate wax or blockout material	Only undercut remaining gingival to contact of surveyor blade with tooth surface
Beneath all minor connectors	Hard baseplate wax or blockout material	Only undercut remaining gingival to contact of surveyor blade with tooth surface
Tissue undercuts to be crossed by rigid connectors	Hard baseplate wax or blockout material	Only undercut remaining below contact of surveyor blade with surface of cast
Tissue undercuts to be crossed by origin of bar clasps	Hard baseplate wax or blockout material	Only undercut remaining below contact of surveyor blade with surface of cast
Deep interproximal spaces to be covered by minor connectors or linguoplates	Hard baseplate wax or blockout material	Only undercut remaining below contact of surveyor blade with surface of cast
Beneath bar clasp arms to gingival crevice	Hard baseplate wax or blockout material	Only undercut area involved in attachment of clasp arm to minor connector
Shaped blockout		
On buccal and lingual surfaces to locate plastic or wax patterns for clasp arms	Hard baseplate wax	Ledges for location of reciprocal clasp arms to follow height of convexity so that they may be placed as cervical as possible without becoming retentive Ledges for location of retentive clasp arms to be placed as cervical as tooth contour permits; point of origin of clasp to be occlusal or incisal to height of convexity, crossing survey line at terminal one fourth, and to include undercut area previously selected in keeping with flexibility of type of clasp being used
Arbitrary blockout		
All gingival crevices	Hard baseplate wax	Enough to just eliminate gingival crevice
Gross tissue undercuts situated below areas involved in design of denture framework	Hard baseplate wax or oil-base clay	Leveled arbitrarily with wax spatula
Tissue undercuts distal to cast framework	Hard baseplate wax or oil-base clay	Smoothed arbitrarily with wax spatula
Labial and buccal tooth and tissue undercuts not involved in denture design	Hard baseplate wax or oil-base clay	Filled and tapered to within upper third of crown of

Relief

Beneath lingual bar connectors or the bar portion of linguoplates when indicated (see text)	Adhesive wax sealed to cast; should be wider than width of major connector to be placed upon it	32-gauge wax if slope of lingual alveolar ridge is parallel to path of placement 32-gauge wax after parallel blockout of undercuts if slope of lingual alveolar ridge is undercut to path of placement
Areas in which major connectors will contact thin tissue, such as hard areas so frequently found on lingual of mandibular ridges and elevated median palatal raphes	Hard baseplate wax	Thin layer flowed on with hot wax spatula; however, if maxillary torus must be covered, the thickness of the relief must represent the difference in the degree of displacement of the tissues covering the torus and the tissues covering the residual ridges
Beneath framework extensions onto ridge areas for attachment of resin bases	Adhesive wax, well adapted and sealed to cast beyond involved area	20-gauge wax

hesive type, should be sealed all around its borders with a hot spatula to prevent its lifting when the cast is moistened prior to or during duplication.

Horizontal rotational tendencies of a lower distal extension denture probably account for many of the tissue irritations seen adjacent to a lingual mandibular major connector. These irritations can usually be avoided by blocking out all undercuts adjacent to the bar parallel to the path of placement, and then including adequate stabilizing components in the design of the framework to resist horizontal rotation. Judicious relief of the tissue side of the lingual bar with rubber wheels at the site of the irritation will most often correct the discrepancy, all other factors being equal. Under no circumstances should the rigidity of the major connector be jeopardized by grinding any portion of it.

Still other areas requiring relief are the gingival crossings and gingival crevices. All gingival areas should be protected from possible impingement due to rotation of the denture framework, and all gingival crevices should be bridged by the denture framework. Hard inlay wax may be used to block out gingival crevices (Fig. 10-20).

PARALLELED BLOCKOUT, SHAPED BLOCKOUT, ARBITRARY BLOCKOUT, AND RELIEF

Table 2 differentiates between *paralleled blockout, shaped blockout, arbitrary blockout,* and *relief.* The same factors apply to both the maxillary and mandibular arches, except that relief is ordinarily not used beneath palatal major connectors, as it is with mandibular lingual bar connectors, except when maxillary tori cannot be circumvented or when resistive median palatal raphes are encountered.

SELF-ASSESSMENT AIDS

1. How would you define a dental cast surveyor?
2. What are the basic parts of a surveyor?
3. Do you recall the term *height of contour* and can you relate it to a direct retainer assembly?
4. Since no component of a removable partial denture may engage an undercut except a portion of the retentive arm of a direct retainer, then both desirable and undesirable undercuts must be known in designing a restoration. True or false?

5. When planning the design of a partial denture, there are four factors that must be considered in determining the path of placement and removal. Two of these factors are retention and esthetics. Can you name the other two factors?

6. With the diagnostic cast securely clamped to the adjustable table and the diagnostic stylus in the vertical spindle, what orientation of the occlusal plane to the base of the surveyor is recommended as a provisional study position?

7. You are considering a design for a Class III, modification 1, arch. Which directional tilt of the cast will indicate the greatest area of parallel proximal surfaces to act as guiding planes—anteroposterior or lateral?

8. Suppose, in the above situation, that the diagnostic stylus touches only gingival areas of the proximal surfaces, what are your options to obtain guiding plane surfaces?

9. When possible retentive areas are being ascertained, the cast is tilted laterally. How do you avoid changing the established anteroposterior tilt of the cast?

10. Uniformity of retention bilaterally is desirable. In what manner does the angle of cervical convergence contribute to obtaining uniform retention?

11. What are the most common causes of interference to the placement of a mandibular major connector?

12. Why should soft tissue contours be surveyed as well as teeth?

13. What advantages accrue in having the tip of the carbon marker touch gingival areas intermittently when marking the heights of contour of abutment teeth?

14. After the diagnostic cast has been surveyed, how can you record the relationship of the cast to the vertical spindle of the surveyor in three dimensions?

15. What is the disadvantage of using a carbon marker that is even only slightly worn?

16. What is an undercut gauge? How can it be used to measure the depth of undercut in the angle of cervical convergence?

17. Heights of contour in many instances will be more optimally located for direct retainer assemblies if axial surfaces are recontoured. How may an undercut gauge assist you in determining whether they can be recontoured without exposing dentin?

18. Diagnostic casts are quite often altered during design on the surveyor or in other uses. Why is it a good idea to have duplicate diagnostic casts?

19. The designed diagnostic cast can readily serve as a blueprint to accomplish like contouring of abutment teeth during mouth preparation procedures. How may the contoured areas on the diagnostic cast be indicated to avoid overlooking these areas when preparing them in the mouth?

20. After mouth preparation procedures are completed and a master cast has been made, it must be surveyed to definitively locate components. What are your guides to relate the cast to the surveyor?

21. The terminal portion of the retentive arm of a direct retainer should engage a planned and measured undercut. Utilizing the same degree of undercut bilaterally will not necessarily assure relative equal retention. What factor other than the degree of undercut must be considered?

22. After the path of placement is established, undercut areas that will be crossed by rigid parts must be eliminated. Do you know how this is accomplished? With what materials?

23. By what means can the definitive locations of components of the framework be transferred from the master cast to the duplicate investment (cast) on which the pattern for the framework will be developed?

24. Can you explain the differences between shaped blockout, arbitrary blockout, relief of the master cast, and parallel blockout?

25. Why should undercuts on the master cast not involved with the framework be blocked out?

26. How do you handle the blockout of gingival crevices that will be crossed by a component of the framework?

27. What relief of a mandibular master cast is required for the lingual of the alveolar ridge that will be covered by a lingual bar or linguoplate when (1) the ridge slopes inferiorly and posteriorly, (2) the ridge is parallel to the path of placement, and (3) the ridge is undercut to the path of placement?

28. Why should a master cast be relieved at all?

29. What determines the amount of palatal relief required when a major connector must traverse the median palatal raphe in a Class I arch?

30. What are the requirements for relief on a master cast for minor connectors that will attach acrylic resin bases to the major connector?

31. What uses can you think of for a dental cast surveyor other than surveying casts for designs and preparation of master casts for duplication in a refractory investment?

32. How can a dental cast surveyor help you in developing optimal contour for crowns?

33. By what means can some dental cast surveyors be converted into a convenient "drill press" or machining tool?

34. Ceramometal restorations in many instances

require machining prior to the final glazing procedures to make sure that contours as originally planned are accomplished. How can this be done?

35. Internal rests on crowns may be machined using the surveyor as a drill press, or they may be made by another method involving the dental cast surveyor. Do you know this other method?

36. Why would a dental cast surveyor be required to place some types of manufactured internal attachments?

37. What are some sequelae of marring a master cast during surveying or blocking-out procedures?

38. Can you think of an application for use of the dental cast surveyor in planning for a fixed partial denture?

11 DIAGNOSIS AND TREATMENT PLANNING

The purpose of dental treatment is to respond to a patient's needs. Each patient, however, is unique and as singular as a fingerprint. Treatment, therefore, must be highly individualized for the patient as well as the disease entity.

Meaningful treatment embodies three fundamentally different processes: (1) ascertaining a patient's needs, (2) developing a treatment plan relevant to these needs, and (3) executing the treatment.*

Diagnosis and treatment planning for oral rehabilitation must take into consideration some or all of the following procedures: the restoration of individual teeth, the restoration of harmonious occlusal relationships, the replacement of missing teeth by fixed restorations, and the replacement of other missing teeth by means of removable partial dentures. Therefore selection of the type, amount, and chronology of treatment should be ascertained before irreversible procedures are undertaken.

The treatment plan for the partial denture, which is too frequently the final step in an extensive and lengthy sequence of treatment, should precede earlier treatment so that abutment teeth and other areas in the mouth may be properly prepared to support and retain the partial denture. *This means that diagnostic casts for designing and planning partial denture treatment must be made before definitive treatment is undertaken.* The design that is drawn on the diagnostic cast, along with a detailed chart of mouth conditions and proposed treatment, is the master plan for the mouth preparations and the partial denture to follow.

Failures of partial dentures, other than structural defects, can usually be attributed

*From Kabcenell, J. L.: Planning for individualized prosthetic treatment, J. Prosthet. Dent. 34:389-392, 1975.

to inadequate diagnosis, failure to properly evaluate the conditions present, and failure to prepare the patient and his mouth properly prior to construction of the master cast. The importance of the examination, the consideration of favorable and unfavorable aspects, and the importance of planning the elimination of unfavorable influences cannot be stressed too strongly.

VISUAL EXAMINATION

Visual examination will reveal many of the signs of dental disease. Consideration of *caries susceptibility* is of primary importance. The number of restored teeth present, signs of recurrent caries, and evidence of decalcification should be noted. Only those patients with demonstrated good oral hygiene habits and low caries susceptibility may be considered good risks without resorting to such prophylactic measures as the crowning of abutment teeth.

Evidence of periodontal disease, inflammation of gingival areas, and the degree of gingival recession should be observed at the time of initial examination. In addition the depths of periodontal pockets should be determined by instrumentation and the degree of mobility of the teeth by digital examination. Although evidence of periodontal disease is detectable visually, the *extent* of damage to the supporting structure by periodontal disease must be determined by roentgenographic interpretation and instrumentation.

The number of teeth remaining, the location of the edentulous areas, and the quality of the residual ridge will have a definite bearing on the proportionate amount of support that the partial denture will receive from the teeth and the edentulous ridges. Tissue contours may appear representative of a well-formed edentulous residual ridge. Palpation often indicates, however, that supporting bone has been resorbed and has been replaced by displaceable, fibrous connective tissue. Such a situation is common in maxillary tuberosity regions. The removable partial denture cannot be supported adequately by tissues that are easily displaced, and this tissue should be removed surgically, unless otherwise contraindicated, in preparing the mouth. A small but stable residual ridge is preferable to a larger unstable ridge to obtain support for the denture.

The presence of tori or other bony exostoses must be detected and an evaluation of their presence in relation to framework design must be made. Failure to palpate the tissue over the median palatal raphe to ascertain the difference in its displaceability as compared to the displaceability of the soft tissues covering the residual ridges will often lead to a "rocking," unstable, uncomfortable denture and dissatisfied patient. Adequate relief of palatal major connectors must be planned, and the amount of relief required is directly proportionate to the difference in displaceability of the tissues over the midline of the palate and the tissues covering the residual ridges.

During the oral examination not only must each arch be considered separately but also its occlusal relationship with the opposing arch. A situation that looks simple when the teeth are apart may be complicated when the teeth are in occlusion. For example, an extreme vertical overlap may complicate the attachment of anterior teeth to a maxillary denture. Extrusion of a tooth or teeth into an opposing edentulous area may complicate the replacement of teeth in the edentulous area, or it may create cuspal interference, which will complicate the location and design of clasp retainers and occlusal rests. When occlusal interference cannot be adequately determined by visual examination, the interposition of wax strips of varying thickness between the teeth may assist in determining the amount of interference or clearance present. Such findings subsequently will be evaluated further by a study of mounted diagnostic casts.

Need for determining type of mandibular major connector. As discussed in Chapter 4, one of the criteria for determining the use of the lingual bar or linguoplate was the height of the floor of the patient's mouth when the tongue is elevated. Since the inferior border of both the lingual bar and linguoplate are placed at the same vertical level and since subsequent mouth preparations depend in part on the selection of the mandibular major connector, determination of the type of major connector must be made during the oral examination. This determination is facilitated by measuring the height of the elevated floor of the patient's mouth in relation to lingual gingivae with a periodontal probe and recording the measurement for later transfer to diagnostic and master casts. It is most difficult to make a determination of the type of mandibular major connector to be used solely from a stone cast that may or may not accurately indicate the active range of movement of the floor of the patient's mouth. Too many mandibular major connectors are ruined, being made flexible because subsequent grinding of the inferior border is necessary to relieve impingement of the sensitive tissues of the floor of the mouth.

Need for reshaping remaining teeth. Many failures of partial dentures can be attributed to the fact that the teeth were not reshaped properly to receive clasp arms and occlusal rests before the impression for the master cast was made. Of particular importance are the paralleling of proximal tooth surfaces to act as guiding planes, the preparation of adequate rest areas, and the reduction of unfavorable tooth contours. To neglect to plan such mouth preparations in advance is inexcusable.

The design of clasps is dependent on the location of the retentive, reciprocal and supporting areas in relation to a definite path of placement and removal. Failure to reshape unfavorably inclined tooth surfaces and, if necessary, to place onlays and crowns with suitable contours not only complicates the design and location of clasp retainers but also frequently leads to failure of the partial denture because of poor clasp design.

A malaligned tooth or one that is inclined unfavorably may make it necessary to place certain parts of the clasp so that they interfere with the opposing teeth. Proximal tooth surfaces that are not parallel not only will fail to provide needed guiding planes during placement and removal but also will make excessive blockout necessary. This inevitably results in the connectors' being placed so far out of contact with tooth surfaces that food traps are created. To pass lingually inclined lower teeth, clearance for a lingual bar major connector may have to be so great that a food trap will result when the restoration is fully seated, and the lingual bar will be located so that it will interfere with tongue comfort and function. These are only some of the objectionable consequences of inadequate mouth preparations.

Reduction of unfavorable tooth contours. Slight reduction of unfavorable tooth contours will greatly facilitate the design of the partial denture framework. The need for modification of tooth contours must be established during the diagnosis and treatment planning phase of partial denture service.

The amount of reduction of tooth contours should be kept to a minimum, and all modified tooth surfaces should not only be repolished after reduction but also should be subjected to fluoride treatment to lessen the incidence of caries. If it is not possible to produce the contour desired without perforating the enamel, inlays or crowns must be used. The age of the patient, caries activity evidenced elsewhere in the mouth, and the ap-

parent oral hygiene habits all must be taken into consideration when deciding between reducing the enamel or modifying tooth contours with protective restorations.

Some of the areas frequently needing correction are the lingual surfaces of mandibular premolars, the mesial and lingual surfaces of mandibular molars, the distobuccal line angle of maxillary premolars, and the mesiobuccal line angle of maxillary molars. The actual degree of inclination of teeth in relation to the path of placement and the location of retentive and supportive areas are not readily interpretable during visual examination. These are established during a comprehensive survey of the diagnostic cast with a cast surveyor, which should follow the visual examination.

DENTAL CAST SURVEYOR

The cast surveyor (Fig. 11-1) is a simple enough instrument but *is most essential to planning partial denture treatment.* Its main working parts are the vertical arm and the adjustable table that holds the cast in a fixed relation to the vertical arm. This represents

Vertical spindle

Path of placement

Adjustable table

Fig. 11-1. Most essential parts of a dental surveyor (Ney Parallelometer), showing vertical arm in relation to adjustable table.

that path of placement that the partial denture will ultimately take in the mouth.

The adjustable table may be tilted in relation to the vertical arm of the surveyor until a path that best satisfies all the factors involved can be found. A cast in a horizontal relationship to the vertical arm represents a vertical path of placement; a cast in a tilted relationship represents a path of placement toward the side of the cast that is tilted upward. The vertical arm, when brought in contact with a tooth surface, will indicate the areas available for retention and those available for support, as well as the existence of tooth and other tissue interference to the path of placement.

If conditions are found that are not favorable for the particular path of placement being considered, the conditions produced by a different path of placement should be studied. The cast is merely tilted in relation to the vertical arm until the most suitable path is found. Then mouth preparations are planned with a definite path of placement in mind.

The path of placement also must take into consideration the presence of tissue undercuts that will interfere with the placement of major connectors, the location of vertical minor connectors, the origin of bar clasp arms, and the denture bases.

Recording the path of placement. Once the path of placement for all factors involved has been ascertained, the base of the cast can be scored or tripod marks can be placed on the cast to record the relation of the cast to the surveyor for future reference (Fig. 11-2, A to C). Then a guideline may be scribed on

Fig. 11-2. **A** and **B,** Path of placement having been determined, base of cast is scored to record its relation to surveyor for future repositioning. **C,** Alternate method to record relation of cast to surveyor is known as *tripoding.* A carbon marker is placed in vertical arm of surveyor, and arm is adjusted to a height by which cast can be contacted in three divergent locations. Vertical arm is locked in position, and cast is brought into contact with tip of carbon marker. Three resultant marks are encircled with a colored lead pencil for ease of identification. Reorientation of cast to surveyor is accomplished by tilting cast until plane created by three marks is at a right angle to vertical arm of surveyor. **D,** Height of contour is then delineated by a carbon marker.

the surfaces of the abutment teeth by means of a graphite marker, replacing the diagnostic stylus (Fig. 11-2, *D*). This guideline will graphically locate the division between retentive and supportive areas, as well as areas of interference. Modification of tooth contours and clasp designs then may be planned with accuracy, and mouth preparations planned accordingly. The cast surveyor is an indispensable instrument in surveying the cast of the mouth prior to preparing the mouth to receive a partial denture. Only by its use can the dentist ascertain the mechanical factors on which the success or failure of the partial denture will depend. The dental cast surveyor and its uses have been discussed in detail in Chapter 10.

ORAL EXAMINATION

A complete oral examination should precede any mouth rehabilitation procedures. An oral examination should be complete—not limited to only one arch. It should include, in addition to a visual and digital examination of the teeth and surrounding tissues with mouth mirror, explorer, and periodontal probe, a complete intraoral roentgenographic survey, a vitality test of critical teeth, *and an examination of casts correctly oriented on an adjustable articulator.*

During the examination the objective to be kept foremost in mind should be the consideration of the possibilities for maintaining the remaining oral structures in a state of health for the longest period of time. In addition to the elimination of infection the primary objectives should be the prevention of tooth migration and the correction of traumatic influences. Second should be the consideration of the best method for restoring lost function within the limits of tissue tolerance of the patient. Third, and not before, the decision should be made as to how best to maintain or improve on the appearance of the mouth. As the first two objectives are satisfied, so will the requirement of a comfortable and esthetically pleasing restoration also be satisfied.

Objectives of prosthodontic treatment. The objectives of any prosthodontic treatment may be stated as (1) the elimination of disease, (2) the preservation of the health and relationship of the teeth and the health of the remaining oral tissues, and (3) the selected replacement of lost teeth and the restoration of function in an esthetically pleasing manner.

Patients with missing teeth may specifically request their replacement, especially when anterior teeth are missing and the patients are concerned only with the cosmetic implications. On the other hand, they may seek diagnosis and advice, the result of which is frequently the recommendation that the missing teeth be replaced with either fixed or removable restorations. In many instances the patient is usually concerned only with the replacement of the missing teeth. The dentist's primary obligation to the patient is to emphasize the importance of restoring the total mouth to a state of health and of preserving the remaining teeth and surrounding tissues. Incident to this is the functional and esthetically acceptable replacement of missing teeth in a harmonious relation with the remaining teeth and surrounding structures.

In many instances, restoration of lost function must be modified and minimized to avoid overloading the supporting structures. The prevention of tooth migration, the healthful stimulation of oral tissues, and the preservation of the remaining teeth are of greater importance. The extent to which lost masticatory function can be restored depends on the tissue tolerance of the individual, as influenced by his age, his general health, and the health of his oral tissues.

Sequence for oral examination. An oral examination should be accomplished in the following sequence:

1. *A thorough and complete oral prophylaxis.* An adequate examination can be accomplished best with the teeth free of accumulated calculus and debris. Also, accurate diagnostic casts of the dental arches can be obtained only if the teeth are clean; otherwise the teeth reproduced on the diagnostic casts are not a true representation of tooth and gingival contours. Cursory examination may precede an oral prophylaxis, but a thorough oral examination should be deferred until the teeth have been thoroughly cleaned.

2. *The placement of individual temporary restorations.* This is advisable not only to relieve discomfort arising from tooth defects but also to determine as early as possible the extent of caries and to arrest further caries activity until definitive treatment can

be instituted. By restoring tooth contours with temporary restorations, the impression will not be torn in removal from the mouth, and a more accurate diagnostic cast may be obtained.

3. *A complete intraoral roentgenographic survey* (Fig. 11-3). The objectives of a roentgenographic examination are (a) to locate areas of infection and other pathosis that may be present; (b) to reveal the presence of root fragments, foreign objects, bone spicules, and irregular ridge formations; (c) to reveal the presence and extent of caries and the relation of carious lesions to the pulp; (d) to permit evaluation of existing restorations as to evidence of recurrent caries, marginal leakage, and overhanging gingival margins; (e) to reveal the presence of root canal fillings and to permit their evaluation as to future prognosis (the design of the partial denture may hinge on the decision to retain or extract an endodontically treated tooth); (f) to permit an evaluation of periodontal conditions present and to establish the need and possibilities for treatment; and (g) to evaluate the alveolar support of abutment teeth—the number, the supporting length, and the morphology of their roots, the relative amount of alveolar bone loss suffered through pathogenic processes, and the amount of alveolar support remaining.

4. *Vitality tests of remaining teeth*. Vitality tests of remaining teeth should be given particularly to teeth to be used as abutments and those having deep restorations or deep carious lesions. This may be done either by thermal or by electronic means, whichever the dentist has learned to interpret best.

5. *The exploration of teeth and investing structures*. These can be explored by instrumentation and visual means. This should include a determination of tooth mobility and an examination of occlusal relationships. At this time the presence of tori and other bony protuberances should be noted and their clinical significance evaluated. Also, history and diagnosis charts should be filled out at this time, as well as a simple working chart for future reference (Figs. 11-4 and 11-5). The latter does not become part of the patient's permanent record but registers the nature and sequence of treatment, and it can be used by the dentist as a checklist during treatment. A breakdown of the fee may be recorded on the back of this chart for easy reference if adjustments or substitutions become necessary by changes in the diagnosis as the work progresses.

6. *Determining the height of the floor of the mouth to locate inferior borders of lingual mandibular major connectors*. Mouth preparation procedures are influenced by a choice of the major connectors. This determination must precede altering contours of abutment teeth.

7. *Impressions for making accurate diagnostic casts*. The casts preferably will be articulated on a suitable instrument. The importance of accurate diagnostic casts and their use will be discussed later in this chapter.

The fee for examination, which should include the cost of the roentgenographic survey and the examination of articulated diagnostic casts, should be established prior to the examination and should not be related to

Fig. 11-3. Complete intraoral roentgenographic survey of remaining teeth and adjacent edentulous areas reveals much information vital to effective diagnosis and treatment planning. The response of bone to previous stress is of particular value in establishing prognosis of teeth that are to be used as abutments.

PARTIAL DENTURE DIAGNOSIS AND TREATMENT RECORD

Patient:_____ Reg. No._____

Student:_____ Date:_____

Pertinent Radiographic Findings:_____

	UPPER	LOWER
Kennedy Classification		
Initial	Class_____, Mod._____	Class_____, Mod._____
Final	Class_____, Mod._____	Class_____, Mod._____
Abutment Teeth		
Teeth to be Extracted and Reason		
Surgical Preparation of Ridges		
Abutment Restorations		
(Tooth No. & Type Restorations)		
Final Mouth Preparations:		
Guiding Planes		
Reduction of Tooth Contours		
Occlusal Rests		
Date above completed		
Impression Materials Used:		
For Master Cast		
For Correction of Supporting Ridges		
Denture Base Materials		
Tooth Selection		
Occlusal Registration; Methods Used		
Drawing of Partial Denture Design:		
Metal framework in blue,		
Resin bases or attachments in red,		
Wrought retentive clasp arms in red.	MAXILLARY OCCLUSAL VIEW	MANDIBULAR OCCLUSAL VIEW
Placement Date:		
Post-Placement Notes:		

Fig. 11-4. Diagnosis and treatment record chart for recording treatment plan and pertinent data.

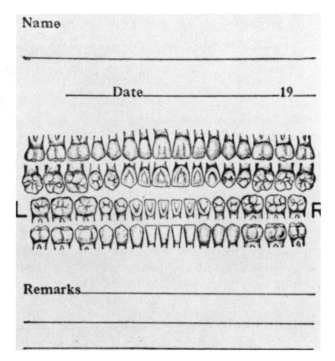

Fig. 11-5. Simple working chart. Restorations for individual teeth, crowns, and fixed partial dentures to be made may be marked on chart and checked off as completed during mouth preparations.

the cost of treatment. It should be understood that the fee for examination is based on the time involved and the service rendered and that the material value of the roentgenographs and diagnostic casts is incidental to the effectiveness of the examination.

The examination record should always be available in the office for future consultation. If consultation with another dentist is requested, modern respect for the hazards of unnecessary radiation justifies the dentist's loaning the roentgenograms for this purpose. Preferably, however, double-film packs should be used so that one copy may be retained in the dentist's files.

ROENTGENOGRAPHIC INTERPRETATION

Many of the reasons for roentgenographic interpretation during oral examination are outlined herein and are considered in greater detail in other texts. The aspects of such interpretation that are the most pertinent to partial denture construction are those rela-

tive to the prognosis of remaining teeth that may be used as abutments.

The quality of the alveolar support of an abutment tooth is of primary importance because the tooth will be called on to withstand greater stress loads when supporting a dental prosthesis. Abutment teeth providing total abutment support to the prosthesis, be it either fixed or removable, will have to withstand a greater load than before and especially greater horizontal forces. The latter may be minimized by establishing a harmonious occlusion and by distributing the horizontal forces among several teeth through the use of rigid connectors. Bilateral stabilization against horizontal forces is one of the attributes of a properly designed tooth-borne removable prosthesis. In many instances abutment teeth may be aided more than weakened by the presence of a bilaterally rigid partial denture.

In contrast, abutment teeth adjacent to distal extension bases are subjected not only to vertical and horizontal forces but to torque as well because of the movement of the tissue-supported base. Vertical support and stabilization against horizontal movement with rigid connectors are just as important as they are with a tooth-borne prosthesis, and the partial denture must be designed accordingly. In addition, the abutment tooth adjacent to the extension base will be subjected to torque in proportion to the design of the retainers, the size of the denture base, the tissue support received by the base, and the total occlusal load applied. With this in mind, each abutment tooth must be evaluated carefully as to the alveolar support present and the past reaction of that bone to occlusal stress.

Value of interpreting bone density. The quality and quantity of bone in any part of the body is often evaluated by roentgenographic means. A detailed treatise concerning the bone support of the abutment tooth should include many considerations not possible to include in this text because of space limitations. The reader should realize that subclinical variations in bone may exist but may not be observed because of the limitations inherent in technical methods and equipment.

Of importance to the prosthodontist when evaluating the quality and quantity of the alveolar bone are the height and the quality of the remaining bone. In estimating bone height, care must be taken to avoid interpretive errors resulting from angulation factors. Technically, when an exposure is being made, the central ray should be directed at right angles to both the tooth and the film. The most commonly used roentgenographic technique, that is, the short-cone technique, does not follow this principle; instead the ray is directed through the root of the tooth at a predetermined angle. This technique invariably causes the buccal bone to be projected higher on the crown than is the lingual or palatal bone. Therefore, in interpreting bone height, it is imperative to follow the line of the lamina dura from the apex toward the crown of the tooth until the opacity of the lamina materially decreases. At this point of opacity change a less dense bone extends farther toward the tooth crown. This additional amount of bone represents false bone height. Thus the true height of the bone is ordinarily where the lamina shows a marked decrease in opacity. At this point the trabecular pattern of bone superimposed on the tooth root

is lost. The portion of the root between the cementoenamel junction and the true bone height has the appearance of being bare or devoid of covering.

Roentgenographic evaluation of bone quality is hazardous but is often necessary. It is essential to emphasize that changes in bone calcification up to 25% often cannot be recognized by ordinary roentgenographic means. Optimum bone qualities are ordinarily expressed by normal-sized interdental trabecular spaces that usually tend to decrease slightly in size as examination of the bone proceeds from the root apex toward the coronal portion. The normal interproximal crest is ordinarily shown by a relatively thin white line crossing from the lamina dura of one tooth to the lamina dura of the adjacent tooth. Considerable variation in the size of trabecular spaces may exist within the limits of normal, and the roentgenographic appearance of crestal alveolar bone may vary considerably, depending on its shape and the direction that the x-ray takes as it passes through the bone.

Normal bone usually responds favorably to ordinary stresses. Abnormal stresses, however, may create a reduction in the size of the trabecular pattern, particularly in that area of bone directly adjacent to the lamina dura of the affected tooth. This decrease in size of the trabecular pattern (that is, *so-called bone condensation*) is often regarded as a favorable bone response, indicative of an improvement in bone quality. This is not necessarily an accurate interpretation. Such bone changes usually indicate stresses that should be relieved because if the resistance of the patient decreases, the bone may exhibit a progressively less favorable response in future roentgenograms.

An increased thickness of the periodontal space ordinarily suggests varying degrees of tooth mobility. This should be evaluated clinically. Roentgenographic evidence coupled with clinical findings may suggest to the prosthodontist the inadvisability of utilizing such a tooth as an abutment. Furthermore, an irregular intercrestal bone surface should make the prosthodontist suspicious of active bone deterioration.

It is essential that the prosthodontist realize that roentgenographic evidence shows the *result* of changes which have taken place and may not necessarily represent the present condition. For example, periodontal disease may have progressed beyond the stage visibly demonstrated in the roentgenograms. As was pointed out earlier, roentgenographic changes are not observed until approximately 25% of the calcific content has been depleted. On the other hand, bone condensations probably do represent the present situation.

Roentgenographic findings should serve the dentist as an adjunct to his clinical observations. Too often the roentgenographic appearance alone is used in arriving at a diagnosis. Roentgenographic interpretation also will serve an important function if used periodically *after* the prosthesis has been placed. Future bone changes of *any type* suggest traumatic interference from some source. The nature of such interference should be determined and corrective measures taken.

Index areas. Index areas are those areas of alveolar support that disclose the reaction of bone to additional stress. Favorable reaction to such stress may be taken as an indication of future reaction to an added stress load.

Teeth that have been subjected to abnormal loading due to the loss of adjacent teeth or that have withstood tipping forces in addition to occlusal loading may be better risks as abutment teeth than those that have not been called on to carry an extra occlusal load (Fig. 11-6). If occlusal harmony can be improved and unfavorable forces minimized by the reshaping of occlusal surfaces and the favorable distribution of occlusal loading, such teeth may be expected to support the prosthesis without difficulty. At the same time, other teeth, although not at present carrying an extra load, may be expected to react favorably because of the favorable reaction of alveolar bone to abnormal loading elsewhere in the same arch.

Such index areas are those around teeth that have been subjected to abnormal occlusal loading, that have been subjected to diagonal occlusal loading due to tooth migration, and that have reacted to additional loading, such as around existing fixed partial denture abutments. The reaction of the bone to additional stresses in these areas may be

Fig. 11-6. Reaction of bone adjacent to teeth that have been subjected to abnormal stress serves as an indication of probable reaction of that bone when such teeth are used as abutments for fixed or removable restorations. Such areas are called *index areas.*

either positive or negative, with evidence of a supporting trabecular pattern, a heavy cortical layer, and a dense lamina dura, or the reverse response. With the former the patient is said to have a *positive bone factor*, meaning the ability to build additional support wherever needed. With the latter he is said to have a *negative bone factor*, meaning inability to respond favorably to stress.

Alveolar lamina dura. The alveolar lamina dura is also considered in a roentgenographic interpretation of abutment teeth. The lamina dura is the thin layer of hard cortical bone that normally lines the sockets of all teeth. It affords attachment for the fibers of the periodontal membrane, and, as with all cortical bone, its function is to withstand mechanical strain. In a roentgenogram the lamina dura is shown as a *radiopaque* white line around the radiolucent dark line that represents the periodontal membrane.

When a tooth is in the process of being tipped, the center of rotation is not at the apex of the root but in the apical third. Resorption of bone occurs where there is pressure, and apposition occurs where there is tension. Therefore, during the active tipping process the lamina dura is uneven, with evidence of both pressure and tension on the same side of the root. For example, in a mesially tipping lower molar the lamina dura will be thinner on the coronal mesial and apical distal aspects and thicker on the apical mesial and coronal distal aspects because the axis of rotation is not at the root apex but above it. When the tooth has been tipped into an edentulous space by some change in the occlusion and becomes set in its new position, the effects of leverage are discontinued. The lamina dura on the side to which the tooth is sloping becomes uniformly heavier, which is nature's reinforcement against abnormal stresses. The bone trabeculations are arranged at right angles to the heavier lamina dura.

Thus it is possible to say that for a given individual, nature is able to build support where it is needed and on this basis to predict future reaction elsewhere in the arch to additional loading of teeth used as abutments. However, since bone is approximately 30% organic, and this mostly protein, and since the body is not able to store a protein reserve in large amounts, any change in body health may be reflected in the patient's abil-

Fig. 11-7. A, Prognosis for abutment service is more favorable for molar with divergent roots (shaded) than for same tooth if its roots were fused and conical. **B,** Evidence that a prospective abutment has conical and fused roots indicates the necessity for formulating a framework design that will minimize additional stresses placed on tooth by abutment service.

ity to maintain this support permanently. When systemic disease is associated with faulty protein metabolism and when the ability to repair is diminished, bone is resorbed and the lamina dura is disturbed. Therefore the loading of any abutment tooth must be kept to a minimum inasmuch as the patient's future health status and the eventualities of aging are unpredictable.

Root morphology. The morphologic characteristics of the roots determine, to a great extent, the ability of prospective abutment teeth to resist successfully additional rotational forces that may be placed on them. Teeth with multiple and divergent roots will resist stresses better than will teeth whose roots are fused and conical, since the resultant forces are distributed through a greater number of periodontal fibers to a larger amount of supporting bone (Fig. 11-7).

Fig. 11-8. First and second molars have been lost by this 18-year-old patient. A distal extension removable partial denture may be constructed until third molar erupts and is fully formed. A tooth-borne restoration can then be constructed.

Third molars. Unerupted third molars should be considered as prospective future abutments to eliminate the need for a distal extension removable partial denture (Fig. 11-8). The increased stability of a tooth-borne denture is most desirable to enhance the health of the oral environment.

DIAGNOSTIC CASTS

A diagnostic cast should be an *accurate* reproduction of the teeth and adjacent tissues. In a partially edentulous arch this must include the edentulous spaces, since these also must be evaluated in determining the type of denture base to be used and the extent of available denture-supporting area.

A diagnostic cast is usually made of dental stone because of its strength and the fact that it is less easily abraded than is dental plaster. Generally the improved dental stones (die stones) are not used for diagnostic casts because of their cost. Their greater resistance to abrasion does, however, justify their use for master casts.

The impression for the diagnostic cast is usually made with an irreversible hydrocolloid (alginate) in a perforated partial denture impression tray. The size of the arch will determine the size of the tray to be used. The tray should be sufficiently oversize to assure an optimum thickness of impression material to avoid distortion or tearing on removal from the mouth. The technique for the making of impressions will be covered in more detail in Chapter 14.

Purposes for which diagnostic casts are used. Diagnostic casts serve several purposes as an aid to diagnosis and treatment planning. Some of these are as follows:

1. Diagnostic casts are used to supplement the oral examination by permitting a view of the occlusion from the lingual as well as from the buccal aspect. Analysis of the existing occlusion is made possible when opposing casts are occluded, as well as a study of the possibilities for improvement either by occlusal adjustment or occlusal reconstruction, or both. The degree of overclosure, the amount of interocclusal space needed, and the possibilities of interference to the location of rests also may be determined.

As stated previously, possibilities for improvement of the occlusal scheme, either by occlusal adjustment or occlusal reconstruction or both, are made possible by the use of mounted diagnostic casts. Such procedures often include "diagnostic waxing" to determine the possibility of enhancing the occlusion before definitive treatment is begun (Fig. 11-9). In other words, diagnostic casts permit the dentist to "plan ahead" and avoid undesirable compromises in the treatment being given a patient.

2. Diagnostic casts are used to permit a topographic survey of the dental arch that is to be restored by means of a removable partial denture. The cast of the arch in question may be surveyed individually with a cast surveyor to determine the parallelism or lack of parallelism of tooth surfaces involved and to establish its influence on the design of the partial denture. The principal considerations in studying the parallelism of tooth and tissue surfaces of the dental arch are (a) proximal tooth surfaces, which can be made parallel to serve as guiding planes, (b) retentive and nonretentive areas of the abutment teeth, and (c) areas of interference to placement and removal. From such a survey a path of placement may be selected that will satisfy requirements for parallelism and retention to the best mechanical, functional, and esthetic advantage. Then mouth preparations may be planned accordingly.

3. Diagnostic casts are used to permit a logical and comprehensive presentation to the patient of his present and future restorative needs, as well as of the hazards of future neglect. Occluded and individual diagnostic casts can be used to point out to the

Fig. 11-9. A, Diagnostic casts have been mounted, and articulator has been adjusted by intraoral, eccentric, maxillomandibular records. **B,** Lower stone abutment teeth for prospective fixed partial dentures have been reduced so that diagnostic occlusal waxing may be performed. Maxillary artificial teeth have been arranged in conjunction with waxing of lower occlusal surfaces to satisfy the demands of the proposed occlusal scheme. **C,** Anterior stone teeth have also been altered to satisfy occlusal scheme. With such guides developed on diagnostic casts, similar oral preparatory procedures can be accomplished for a predetermined end result. (**C** from Morris, A. L., and Bohannon, H. M., editors: Dental specialties in general practice, Philadelphia, 1969, W. B. Saunders Co.)

patient (a) evidence of tooth migration and the existing results of such migration, (b) effects of further tooth migration, (c) loss of occlusal support and its consequences, (d) hazards of traumatic occlusal contacts, and (e) cariogenic and periodontal implications of further neglect.

Treatment planning actually may be accomplished with the patient present so that economic considerations may be discussed also. Such use of diagnostic casts permits a justification of the proposed fee through the patient's understanding of the problems involved and of the treatment needed. Inasmuch as mouth rehabilitation procedures are frequently protracted, there must be complete accord between dentist and patient before extensive treatment is begun, and financial arrangements must be consummated during the planning phase.

4. Individual impression trays may be fabricated on the diagnostic casts, or the diagnostic cast may be used in selecting and fitting a stock impression tray for the final impression. If wax blockout is to be used in the fabrication of individual trays, a duplicate cast made from an irreversible hydrocolloid (alginate) impression of the diagnostic cast should be used for this purpose. The diagnostic cast is too valuable for future reference to risk damage resulting from the making of an impression tray. On the other hand, if only a wet asbestos blockout is used, the diagnostic cast may be used without fear of damage.

Since essential areas will be known in advance of making the final impression, the tray

Fig. 11-10. Proposed mouth changes and design of partial denture framework are indicated in pencil on diagnostic cast in relation to a previously determined path of placement.

must be selected or made with these in mind. These areas as recorded in the final impression may then be examined critically for possible artifacts.

5. Diagnostic casts may be used as a constant reference as the work progresses. Penciled marks indicating the type of restorations, the areas of tooth surfaces to be modified, the location of rests, and the design of the partial denture framework, as well as the path of placement and removal, all may be recorded on the diagnostic cast for future reference (Fig. 11-10). Then these steps may be checked off the work sheet as they are completed.

Areas of abutment teeth to be modified may first be changed on the diagnostic cast by trimming the stone cast with the surveyor blade. A record is thus made of the location and degree of modification to be done in the mouth. This must be done in relation to a definite path of placement. Any mouth preparations to be accomplished with new cast restorations require that wax patterns be shaped in accordance with a previously determined path of placement. Even so, the shaping of abutment teeth on the diagnostic cast serves as a guide to the form of the abutment pattern. This is particularly true if the contouring of wax patterns is to be delegated to the technician, as it may be in a busy practice.

6. *Unaltered diagnostic casts should become a permanent part of the patient's record because records of conditions existing before treatment are just as important as are preoperative roentgenograms. Therefore diagnostic casts should be duplicated, one cast serving as a permanent record and the other cast being used in situations that may require alterations to it.*

Mounting diagnostic casts. Although some diagnostic casts may be occluded by hand, occlusal analysis is much better accomplished when casts are mounted on an adjustable articulator. By definition an articulator is "a mechanical device that represents the temporomandibular joints and jaw members, to which maxillary and mandibular casts may be attached." Since the dominant influence on mandibular movement in a partially edentulous mouth is the cusps of the remaining teeth, an anatomic reproduction of condylar paths is probably not obtainable. Still, movement of the casts in relation to one another as influenced by the cusps of the remaining teeth, when mounted at a reasonably accurate radius from the axis of condylar rotation, permits a relatively valid analysis of occlusal relationships. This is much better than a simple hinge mounting.

It is probably still better that the casts be mounted in relation to the axis-orbital plane to permit better interpretation of the plane of occlusion in relation to the horizontal plane. Whereas it is true that an axis-orbital mounting has no functional value on a non-arcon instrument, since that plane ceases to exist when opposing casts are separated, the value of such a mounting lies in the orientation of the casts in occlusion. (An *arcon* articulator is one in which the condyles are attached to the lower member as they are in nature, the term being a derivation coined by Bergström from the words *ar*ticulation and *con*dyle [Fig. 11-11]. All the more widely used articulators such as the Hanau [H series], Dentatus, and improved Gysi have the condyles attached to the upper member and are therefore *non-arcon* instruments.)

Mounting maxillary cast to axis-orbital plane. The face-bow is a relatively simple device used to obtain a transfer record for orienting a maxillary cast on an articulating instrument. Originally the face-bow was used only to transfer a *radius* from condyle reference points so that a given point on the cast

Fig. 11-11. A, Bergström arcon articulator showing condyle attached to lower arm of articulator and condyle path to upper arm. **B,** Bergström face-bow attached to articulator prior to mounting the upper cast. (Courtesy Dr. H. O. Beck.)

would be the same distance from the condyle as it is on the patient. The addition of an adjustable infraorbital pointer to the face-bow and the addition of an orbital plane indicator to the articulator make possible also the transfer of the *elevation* of the cast in relation to the axis-orbital plane. This permits the maxillary cast to be correctly oriented in the articulator space comparable to the relationship of the maxillae to the Frankfort horizontal on the patient. To accommodate a maxillary cast so oriented and still have room for the mandibular cast, the posts of the conventional articulator must be lengthened. The older Hanau model H articulator usually will not permit a face-bow transfer using an infraorbital pointer.

A face-bow may be used to transfer a comparable radius from arbitrary reference points, or it may be designed so that the transfer can be made from hinge axis points. The latter type of transfer requires that a hinge-bow attached to the mandible be used initially to determine the hinge axis points, to which the face-bow is then adjusted for making the hinge axis transfer.

A face-bow transfer of the maxillary cast, which is oriented to the axis-orbital plane, to a suitable articulator is an uncomplicated procedure. Hanau models S-M, S-M-X, and H-2 and the Dentatus model ARH will accept this transfer, since these models have the longer posts and orbital plane indicator necessary for such a transfer (Fig. 11-18). Both the Hanau face-bow model S-M and the Dentatus face-bow type AEB incorporate the infraorbital pointer which permits transfer of

Fig. 11-12. Location of an arbitrary axis 11 to 13 mm anterior to upper one third of tragus of ear from a line extending from upper margin of external auditory meatus to outer canthus of eye. The lowest point on inferior orbital margin is marked as third point of reference for establishing axis-orbital plane.

the infraorbital plane to the articulator. Neither of these is a hinge axis bow but is used instead at an arbitrary point.

The location of this arbitrary point or axis has long been the subject of some controversy. Gysi and others have placed it 11 to 13 mm anterior to the upper one third of the tragus of the ear on a line extending from the upper margin of the external auditory meatus to the outer canthus of the eye (Fig. 11-12). Others have placed it 13 mm anterior to the posterior margin of the center of the

Fig. 11-13. A, Base of cast has been prepared for mounting. **B,** Triangular grooves can be conveniently and quickly cut in base of cast by using a 3-inch (7.5 cm) stone mounted in a laboratory lathe.

tragus of the ear on a line extending to the corner of the eye. Bergström has located the arbitrary axis 10 mm anterior to the center of a spherical insert for the external auditory meatus and 7 mm below the Frankfort horizontal plane.

In a series of experiments reported by Beck it was shown that the arbitrary axis suggested by Bergström falls consistently closer to the kinematic axis than do the other two. It is, of course, desirable that an arbitrary axis be placed as close as is possible to the kinematic axis. Although most authorities agree that any of the three axes will permit a transfer of the maxillary cast with reasonable accuracy, it would seem that the Bergström point compares most favorably with the kinematic axis.

The lowest point on the inferior orbital margin is taken as the third point of reference for establishing the axis-orbital plane. Some authorities use the point on the lower margin of the bony orbit in line with the center of the pupil of the eye. For the sake of consistency the right infraorbital point is generally used and the face-bow assembled in this relationship. All three points (right and left axes and infraorbital point) are marked on the face with an ink dot before making the transfer.

Casts are prepared for mounting on an articulator by placing three index grooves in the base of the cast. Two V-shaped grooves are placed in the posterior section of the cast and one groove in the anterior portion (Fig. 11-13).

An occlusion rim should be utilized in face-bow procedures involving the transfer of casts representative of the Class I and II par-

tially edentulous situations. Without occlusion rims, such casts cannot be located accurately in the imprints of the wax covering the face-bow fork. Tissues covering the residual ridges may be displaced grossly when the patient closes into the wax on the face-bow fork. Therefore the wax imprints of the soft tissues are not true negatives of the edentulous regions of the diagnostic casts.

The face-bow fork is covered with a roll of softened baseplate wax with the wax distributed equally on the top and on the underneath side of the face-bow fork. Then the fork should be pressed lightly on the diagnostic cast with the midline of the face-bow fork corresponding to the midline of the central incisors (Fig. 11-14). This will leave imprints of the occlusal and incisal surfaces of the maxillary cast and occlusion rim on the softened baseplate wax and is an aid in correctly orienting the face-bow fork in the patient's mouth. The face-bow fork is placed in position in the mouth, and the patient is asked to close the lower teeth into the wax to stabilize it in position. It is removed from the mouth and chilled in cool water and then replaced in position in the patient's mouth. An alternative method of stabilizing the face-bow fork and record bases is to enlist the assistance of the patient (Fig. 11-15).

With the face-bow fork in position the face-bow toggle is slipped over the anterior projection of the face-bow fork and positioned so that the calibrations on the shaft on either side read the same as they rest lightly on the two dots located anterior to the external auditory meatuses. The calibrated shafts are then locked in this bilaterally equal position. The

Fig. 11-14. Orienting face-bow fork to maxillary cast and occlusion rims will avoid displacing occlusion rim in mouth when patient closes to maintain face-bow fork in position. Face-bow fork illustrated here is a Whipmix type. When an offset type of face-bow fork (Hanau) is used, offset handle must be on the patient's left.

Fig. 11-15. Whipmix face-bow has been adjusted on patient, and toggles have been tightened. Patient assisted in stabilizing face-bow fork and occlusion rim by holding them securely in position with her thumbs while dentist adjusted and locked instrument in position.

Fig. 11-16. Hanau S-M face-bow is positioned on face so that calibrations on shaft on either side read the same as they rest lightly on two dots located anterior to external auditory meatus. Infraorbital pointer is adjusted to rest lightly on infraorbital point previously marked on face.

With the infraorbital pointer on the extreme right side of the face-bow, it is angled toward the infraorbital point previously identified with an ink dot. It is then locked into position with its tip lightly touching the skin at the dot (Fig. 11-16). This establishes the *elevation* of the face-bow in relation to the axis-orbital plane. Extreme care must be taken to avoid any slip that might damage the patient's eye.

With all elements tightened securely the patient is asked to open, and the entire assembly is removed intact, rinsed with cold water, and set aside. The face-bow records not only the radius from the condyles to the incisal contacts of the upper central incisors but also the angular relationship of the occlusal plane to the axis-orbital plane.

face-bow may have to be removed to accomplish this. It is then returned to position and locked to the face-bow fork while being held with equal contact over the dots on either side of the face. This accomplishes the *radius* aspect of the face-bow transfer.

The face-bow must be positioned on the articulator in the same axis-orbital relation as on the patient (Figs. 11-17 and 11-18). The calibrated condyle rods of the face-bow ordinarily will not fit the condyle shafts of the articulator unless the width between the condyles just happens to be the same. With a Hanau model C face-bow the calibrations must be reequalized when in position on the articulator. For example, they might have read 74 (mm) on each side of the patient but must be adjusted to read 69 (mm) on each side of the articulator. With some later model articulators having adjustable condyle rods, these may instead be adjusted to fit the face-bow. It is necessary that the face-bow be centered in either case.

The third point of reference is the orbital plane indicator, which must be swung to the right so that it will be above the tip of the infraorbital pointer. The entire face-bow with maxillary cast in place must be raised until the tip of the pointer contacts the orbital plane indicator (Figs. 11-17 and 11-18). The elevation having thus been established, for all practical purposes the orbital plane indicator and pointer may now be removed because they may interfere with placing the mounting stone.

An auxiliary device called a *cast support* is available*; it is used to support the face-bow fork and the maxillary cast during the mounting operation (Fig. 11-19). With this device the weight of the cast and the mounting stone is supported separately from the face-bow, thus preventing possible downward movement resulting from their combined weight. The cast support is raised to supporting contact with the face-bow fork after the face-bow height has been adjusted to the level of the orbital plane. Use of some type of cast support is highly recommended as an adjunct to face-bow mounting. Fig. 11-21, *C*, demonstrates a simple and inexpensive method.

The keyed and lubricated maxillary cast is now attached to the upper arm of the articulator with mounting stone, thus completing the face-bow transfer (Fig. 11-20). Not only will the face-bow have permitted the upper cast to be mounted with reasonable accuracy, but it also will have served as a convenient means of supporting the cast during mounting. The ease and speed with which a face-bow transfer can be effected makes ridicu-

*Hanau Engineering Co., Buffalo, N.Y.

lous the frequently expressed objection to its use on the basis of time involved. Once mastered, its use becomes a great convenience rather than a time-consuming nuisance.

It is preferable that the upper cast be mounted while the patient is still present, thus eliminating a possible reappointment if the face-bow record is unacceptable for some reason. Not too infrequently the face-bow record has to be redone with the offset type face-bow fork repositioned to avoid interference with some part of the articulator.

An ear face-bow to orient the maxillary cast to an articulator is used by many dentists (Fig. 11-21). Its use, although described by Dalbey in 1914, had been rather limited until the early sixties.

In an investigation by Teteruck and Lundeen it was demonstrated that by the ear face-bow method the maxillary cast could consistently be oriented more accurately to the hinge axis than by the method utilizing an arbitrary mark on the tragus-canthus line. The ear face-bow is a simple instrument to use, does not require measurements or marks on the face, consumes less time for its use, and is as accurate, if not more so, than are other arbitrary methods of face-bow transfer.

Jaw relationship records for diagnostic casts. One of the first critical decisions that must be made in a removable partial denture service involves the selection of the horizontal jaw relation to which the removable partial denture will be constructed—centric relation or centric occlusion. All mouth preparation procedures depend on this analysis. Failure to make this decision correctly may result in the destruction of the residual ridges and supporting structures of the teeth.

Almost all dentists agree that deflective occlusal contacts in centric occlusion and eccentric positions must be corrected as a preventive measure. Not all dentists agree that centric relation and centric occlusion must be harmonious in the natural dentition. Apparently there are many dentitions that function satisfactorily with the opposing teeth maximally intercusped or interdigitated in an eccentric position without either diagnosable or subjective indications of temporomandibular joint dysfunction, muscle dysfunction, or disease of the supporting structures of the teeth. In many such situations no attempt should be made to alter the occlusion. It is not required to interfere with an occlusion simply

Fig. 11-17. **A,** Model H-2 Hanau articulator with S-M face-bow attached. Note orientation of face-bow to orbital plane indicator, supported by adjustable screw on face-bow. **B,** Hanau University articulator, model 130-28. An S-M face-bow is used on 130-28 in same manner as illustrated in **A.** (Courtesy Hanau Engineering Co., Buffalo, N.Y.)

Fig. 11-18. Hanau face-bow model S-M attached to articulator prior to mounting of maxillary cast. Note elevation of face-bow with orbital plane indicator. The handle of offset face-bow fork must be on patient's left side; otherwise the two face-bow toggles as used here would interfere with each other.

Fig. 11-19. Face-bow fork support attached to lower arm of Hanau H-2 articulator. This device is used to support face-bow fork and maxillary cast at determined elevation while it is being attached to upper arm of articulator with mounting stone. Orbital pointer and orbital plane indicator may then be removed to facilitate mounting of maxillary cast. (Courtesy Hanau Engineering Co., Buffalo, N.Y.)

Fig. 11-20. Maxillary diagnostic cast mounted by face-bow transfer. Note that cast has been keyed prior to mounting and may be removed for repositioning on surveyor.

Fig. 11-21. A, Whipmix ear face-bow and face-bow fork are assembled on patient. A *nasion* relator forms anterior third point of reference in establishing *axis-orbital plane*. **B,** Face-bow assembly and cast are transferred to Whipmix articulator (an arcon instrument). **C,** Two wedge-shaped, rubber door stops are used to support face-bow fork and cast during mounting procedures. **D,** Mounting of maxillary cast is completed. Plane of occlusion as observed on articulator is the same as that in mouth when Frankfort plane of patient is parallel to floor.

because it does not completely conform to a relationship that is considered ideal.

If most natural posterior teeth remain and there is no evidence of temporomandibular joint disturbances, neuromuscular dysfunction, or periodontal disturbances related to occlusal factors, the proposed restoration may safely be constructed in centric occlusion (maximum interdigitation of remaining teeth). The proposed restoration, however, should be constructed so that centric occlusion is in harmony with centric relation when most natural centric stops are missing. By far the greater majority of removable partial dentures should be constructed in the horizontal jaw relationship of centric relation. In most instances in which edentulous spaces have not been restored the remaining posterior teeth will have assumed malaligned positions through drifting, tipping, or extrusion. Correction of the natural occlusion to create a coincidence of centric relation and centric occlusion is indicated in such situations.

Regardless of the method employed in creating a harmonious functional occlusion, an evaluation of the existing relationships of the opposing natural teeth must be made. This evaluation is in addition to, and in conjunction with, other diagnostic procedures that contribute to an adequate diagnosis and treatment plan.

Diagnostic casts provide an opportunity to evaluate the relationship of remaining oral structures when correctly mounted on an adjustable articulator by using a face-bow transfer and interocclusal records. Diagnostic casts are mounted in centric relation (most retruded relation of the mandible to the maxillae) so that deflective occlusal contacts can be correlated with those observed in the mouth. Deflective contacts of opposing teeth are usually destructive to the supporting structures involved and should be eliminated. Diagnostic casts demonstrate the nature and location of such interfering tooth contacts and indicate the direction that must be followed for their correction. Necessary alteration of teeth to harmonize the occlusion can be performed initially on the mounted diagnostic casts to act as guides for similar necessary corrections in the mouth. In many instances the degree of alteration required will indicate the need for crowns or onlays to be fabricated or for the recontouring, re-

positioning, or the elimination of extruded teeth.

The maxillary cast is correctly oriented to the opening axis of the articulator by means of the face-bow transfer and becomes spatially related to the upper member of the articulator in the same relationship that the maxillae are related to the hinge axis and the Frankfort plane. Similarly, when a centric relation record is made at an established vertical dimension, the mandible is in its most retruded relation to the maxillae. Therefore, when the maxillary cast is correctly oriented to the axis of the articulator, the lower cast automatically becomes correctly oriented to the opening axis, with an accurate centric relation record.

It is necessary to prove that the relationship of the mounted casts is correct. This can be done simply by making another interocclusal record, fitting the casts into the record, and checking to see that the condylar elements of the articulator are snug against the condylar housings. If this is not seen, it can be assumed that the original record was incorrect or that the record was correct and the mounting procedure faulty, or that the last record made was incorrect. Since centric relation is the only jaw position that can be routinely assumed by the patient, mountings in this position can be verified for correctness.

A straightforward protrusive record is made to adjust the horizontal condylar inclines on the articulator. Lateral eccentric records are made so that the lateral condylar inclinations can be properly adjusted. All interocclusal records should be made as near the vertical relation of occlusion as possible. Opposing teeth or occlusion rims must not be allowed to contact when the records are made. A contact of the inclined planes of opposing teeth will invalidate an interocclusal record.

In some instances a mounting of a duplicate diagnostic cast in centric occlusion also may be desirable to definitively study this relationship on the articulator. Since articulators only simulate jaw movements, it is not unreasonable to assume that the relationship of the casts mounted in centric relation may differ minutely in the centric occlusion that is seen on the articulator and that is observed in the mouth. When diagnostic casts are hand related by maximum interdigitation for purposes of mounting on an articulator, it is essential that three (preferably four) positive contacts of opposing posterior teeth are present, having molar contacts on each side of the arch. If occlusion rims are necessary to correctly orient casts on an articulator, centric relation should usually be the choice of the horizontal jaw relationship to which the removable partial denture will be constructed.

Materials and methods for recording centric relation. Materials available for recording centric relation are (1) wax, (2) modeling plastic, (3) quick-setting impression plaster, and (4) metallic oxide impression paste. Of these, wax is the least satisfactory material because it may not be uniformly softened when introduced into the mouth and because it does not remain rigid and dimensionally stable after removal.

Modeling plastic is a satisfactory record medium because it can be flamed and tempered until uniformly soft before it is placed into the mouth. After chilling, it is sufficiently stable to permit the mounting of casts with accuracy. For these reasons it is a satisfactory medium for recording occlusal relations for either complete or partial dentures. It also can be used with opposing natural teeth.

Impression plaster has advantages of softness when introduced and rigidity when set, which makes it a satisfactory material for recording jaw relations. Its use is highly recommended when occlusion rims are indicated to mount casts correctly or to adjust articulators with interocclusal eccentric records.

Impression paste offers many of the advantages of plaster, with less friability. Although not strong enough to be used alone, when supported by a gauze mesh it is a satisfactory recording medium. Also it may be used with occlusion rims.

The adjustable frame* was devised for use with those materials that have the combined advantage of offering no resistance when the patient closes and of being firm and stable when set. It consists of an adjustable wire frame to which gauze bibs are added to support the impression paste (Fig. 11-22). Pastes that set rapidly to a hard state are the most satisfactory, although any metallic oxide impression paste may be used.

---

*Kerr Manufacturing Co., Detroit, Mich.

The frame is adjusted to fit the lower cast. Each gauze bib has incorporated into it a tube, which may be slid over the lingual extension on each side of the arch. These bibs are placed so that a space remains distal to the gauze so that the dentist can see to place the frame beyond the last tooth; otherwise the patient might close on the cross bar of the frame. The gauze is then attached to the buccal wing of the frame with sticky wax.

An impression paste is mixed according to the manufacturer's directions and is applied on both sides of the gauze bibs. The frame is then placed in the mouth while the patient is guided into centric relation. When edentulous bases with wax occlusion rims are being used to support the occlusion in those areas, the wax must have been trimmed and adjusted previously so that it does not contact either the opposing natural dentition or an opposing occlusion rim. The cross bar of the frame must be placed posterior to any occlusion rims or any remaining posterior teeth.

After the paste has set, the frame is removed from the mouth and the buccal side of the gauze released where it has been secured with sticky wax. The tube on the lingual side may then be slid off the lingual extension of the frame. The frame is not needed when mounting casts with this type of registration, since the tube alone lends sufficient support to the interocclusal record.

The lower cast should be mounted on the lower arm of the articulator with the articulator inverted. The articulator is first locked in centric position and the incisal pin is adjusted so that the anterior distance between the upper and lower arms of the articulator will be increased 2 to 3 mm greater than the normal parallel relationship of the arms. This is done to compensate for the thickness of the interocclusal record so that the arms of the articulator will again be nearly parallel when the interocclusal record is removed and the opposing casts contact. The projection of the pin on the Dentatus articulator serves most conveniently as the third leg of a tripod for supporting the articulator while the lower cast is being mounted, whereas the Hanau articulator, when inverted, must be supported by other means. A mounting stand for this purpose is available (Fig. 11-23).

The base of the cast should be keyed and lightly lubricated for future removal. With

Fig. 11-22. Adjustable frame may be used either bilaterally or unilaterally but is always used bilaterally in a removable partial denture procedure. Each gauze bib is made with a tube that is slid over open lingual portion of frame and attached to its buccal portion with sticky wax. For bilateral use, frame must be adjusted to mouth or cast to avoid interference distal to last teeth in occlusion. A metallic oxide impression paste is applied to both sides of gauze, frame is oriented in mouth, and patient's lower jaw is closed into a rehearsed horizontal jaw relation until paste hardens. After set record is removed from mouth, sticky wax is released from frame and tube is slid off the frame. Gross excess and any sharp projections into interproximal spaces and into deep sulci are trimmed with a sharp knife before record is placed between casts for mounting on articulator.

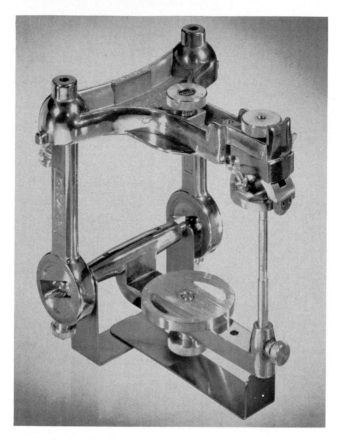

Fig. 11-23. Hanau stand is useful to support any model H or SMX articulator in an inverted position while mandibular cast is being mounted. (Courtesy Hanau Engineering Co., Buffalo, N.Y.)

the articulator inverted the dentist's thumbs should be pressed through the soft mounting stone onto the base of the cast to reseat it into the interocclusal record. This is done to prevent a faulty mounting if the angle of closure into the mounting stone has caused the cast to be displaced slightly. The articulator is then propped up in the inverted position until the stone has set.

An articulator mounting thus made will have related the casts in centric relation. The dentist then can proceed to make an occlusal analysis by observing the influence of cusps in relation to one another after the articulator has been adjusted by using eccentric interocclusal records.

After an occlusal analysis has been made the casts may be removed from their mounting for the purpose of surveying them individually and for other purposes as outlined previously. The indexed mounting ring rec-

ord also should be retained throughout the course of treatment in the event that further study should be needed. It is advisable that the mounting be identified with the articulator used, so that it may always be placed back onto the *same articulator*.

Factors involved in occlusal analysis. From the occlusal analysis made from mounted diagnostic casts the dentist must decide whether it is best to accept and maintain the existing occlusion or to attempt to improve on it by means of occlusal adjustment and the restoration of occlusal surfaces. *It must be remembered that the partial denture can only supplement the occlusion that exists at the time the prosthesis is constructed.* The dominant force dictating the occlusal pattern will be the cuspal harmony or disharmony of the remaining teeth and their proprioreceptal influence on kinematic movement. At best the supplied teeth can only be made to harmonize with the cause and effect of the existing occlusion.

Improvements in the natural occlusion must be accomplished prior to the construction of the denture, not subsequent to it. The objective of occlusal reconstruction by any means should be occlusal harmony of the restored dentition in relation to the natural forces already present or established. Therefore one of the earliest decisions in planning reconstructive treatment must be whether to accept or reject the existing occlusion. If occlusal adjustment is indicated, cuspal analysis always should precede any corrective procedures in the mouth by selective grinding. On the other hand, if reconstruction is to be the means of correction, the manner and sequence should be outlined as part of the overall treatment plan.

EXAMINATION DATA

As a result of the oral examination and diagnosis, certain data should be recorded, much of which is based on decisions that are the result of the diagnosis. These are as follows:

1. *Patient's present and predictable future health status.*

2. *Periodontal conditions that are present* throughout the mouth in general and around abutment teeth in particular. This includes the amount of alveolar support remaining and the past and predictable future reaction to additional occlusal stress. Evidence of tooth mobility should be noted, as well as suggestions as to its cause and the corrective measures to be employed. This may involve simple correction of occlusal disharmony, or it may involve extensive periodontal treatment and, in some instances, splinting of periodontally weakened teeth.

3. *Oral hygiene habits* of the patient and the likelihood of patient cooperation in this regard, as well as the likelihood that the patient will return periodically for maintenance after reconstruction. The teeth remaining will need attention no less after placement of a partial denture and perhaps even more so. Denture bases may need relining to compensate for changes in the supporting tissues. Therefore the patient must be willing to share with the dentist the responsibility for maintaining the health of the mouth after restorative treatment.

The most decisive evidence of oral hygiene

habits is the condition of the mouth prior to the initial prophylaxis. Good or bad oral hygiene is basic to the patient's nature, and although it may be influenced somewhat by patient education, the long-range view must be taken. It is reasonably fair to assume that the patient will do little better in the long-term future than he has done in the past. In making decisions as to the method of treatment based upon oral hygiene, *the future in years*, rather than in weeks and months, must be considered. Probably in this instance it is better not to give the patient the benefit of any doubt as to future oral hygiene habits. Rather, the benefit should come from protective measures where any doubt exists as to future oral hygiene habits.

4. *Caries activity* in the mouth, past and present, and the need for protective restorations. The decision to use full coverage is based upon the age of the patient, evidence of caries activity, and the patient's oral hygiene habits. Occasionally three-quarter crowns may be used where buccal or lingual surfaces are completely sound, but intracoronal restoration (inlays) is seldom indicated in any mouth with evidence of past extensive caries or precarious areas of decalcification, erosion, or exposed cementum.

5. *Need for surgery or extractions.* The same criteria apply to surgical intervention in the partially edentulous arch as in the completely edentulous arch. Grossly displaceable soft tissues covering basal seat areas and hyperplastic tissue should be removed to provide a firm denture foundation. Mandibular tori should be removed if they will interfere with the optimal location of a lingual bar connector or a favorable path of placement. Any other areas of bone prominence that will interfere with the path of placement should be removed also. The path of placement will be dictated primarily by the tooth guidance of the abutment teeth. Therefore some areas may present interference to the path of placement of the partial denture by reason of the fact that other unalterable factors such as retention and esthetics must take precedence in selecting that path.

Extraction of teeth may be indicated for one of the following three reasons:

　　a. If the tooth cannot be restored to a state of health, extraction may be unavoidable. Modern advancements in the treatment of periodontal disease and in restorative procedures, including endodontic therapy, have resulted in the saving of teeth that were once considered untreatable. *All avenues of treatment should be considered both from a prognostic and an economic standpoint before recommending extraction.*

b. A tooth may be removed if its absence will permit a more serviceable and less complicated partial denture design. Teeth that are in extreme malposition—lingually inclined mandibular teeth, buccally inclined maxillary teeth, and mesially inclined teeth posterior to an edentulous space—may be removed if an adjacent tooth is good alignment and with good support is available for use as an abutment. Justification for extraction lies in the decision that a suitable crown, which will provide satisfactory contour and support, cannot be fabricated or that orthodontic treatment to realign the tooth is not feasible. An exception to the arbitrary removal of a malposed tooth is when by so doing a distal extension partial denture base would have to be made rather than the more desirable tooth-supported base through the use of the tooth in question. If alveolar support is adequate, a posterior abutment should be retained if at all possible in preference to a tissue-supported extension base.

Teeth deemed to have insufficient alveolar support may be extracted if their prognosis is poor and if other adjacent teeth may be used to better advantage as abutments. The decision to extract such a tooth should be based on the degree of mobility and other periodontal considerations and upon the number, length, and shape of the roots contributing to its support.

c. A tooth may be extracted if it is so unesthetically located as to justify its removal to improve appearance. In this regard a veneer crown should be considered in preference to removal. If removal is advisable because of unesthetic tooth position,

the biomechanical problems involved in replacing anterior teeth with a removable partial denture must be weighed against the problems involved in making an esthetically acceptable fixed restoration. Admittedly the removable replacement is frequently the more esthetic of the two, despite modern advancements in retainers and pontics. Yet the mechanical disadvantage of the removable restoration frequently makes the fixed replacement of missing anterior teeth preferable.

6. *Need for fixed restorations for tooth-bounded spaces* rather than including them in the partial denture to the detriment of isolated abutment teeth. The advantage of splinting must be weighed against the total cost, with the weight of experience always in favor of utilizing fixed restorations for tooth-bounded spaces. One of the least successful of partial denture designs is where multiple tooth-bounded areas are replaced with the partial dentures in conjunction with isolated abutment teeth and distal extension bases. Biomechanical considerations and the future health of the remaining teeth should be given preference over economic considerations where such a choice is possible.

7. *Need for occlusal correction,* either by selective grinding of teeth or by occlusal restorations, or both.

8. *Need for periodontal consultation and treatment.*

9. *Need for orthodontic treatment of malposed and disarranged teeth.* Occasionally, orthodontic movement of teeth followed by retention through the use of fixed restorations makes possible a better partial denture design, mechanically and esthetically, than could otherwise be used.

10. *Need for restorations elsewhere in either arch,* including individual restorations, fixed partial dentures, and splinted abutments.

11. *Need for prospective or planned endodontic treatment.* This includes abutments for overlay type removable partial dentures.

12. *Selection of the type of mandibular major connector,* since the selection is influenced by the height of the floor of the patient's mouth during normal physiologic activity. The type of major connector selected (lingual bar or linguoplate) will certainly in-

fluence mouth preparations. A linguoplate should be supported at least by positive rests on canines occupying prepared rest seats. Additionally, lingual proximal surfaces contacted by a linguoplate must be recontoured in many instances to avoid excessive, enclosed interproximal spaces bridged by a linguoplate.

DIFFERENTIAL DIAGNOSIS: FIXED OR REMOVABLE PARTIAL DENTURES*

Total oral rehabilitation is the objective in treating the partially edentulous patient. The replacement of missing teeth by means of fixed restorations is the method of preference; a removable restoration should be used only where a fixed restoration is contraindicated.

Indications for use of fixed restorations

Tooth-bounded edentulous regions. Generally any unilateral edentulous space bounded by teeth suitable for use as abutments should be restored with a fixed partial denture cemented to one or more abutment teeth at either end. The length of the span and the periodontal support of the abutment teeth will determine the number of abutments required.

Lack of parallelism of the abutment teeth may be counteracted with copings or locking recesses to provide parallel sectional placement. Sound abutment teeth make possible the use of more conservative retainers such as inlays rather than full crowns. The age of the patient, evidence of caries activity, oral hygiene habits, and soundness of remaining tooth structure must be considered in any decision to use less-than-full coverage for abutment teeth.

Economics should not be allowed to dictate the use of a unilateral, tooth-supported removable restoration when a fixed partial is indicated. The dentist must follow the best procedure for the welfare of his patient. The patient is always free to seek more than one opinion if he so desires, but the responsibility for the choice of dental treatment becomes the patient's. In most in-

stances, when a removable unilateral restoration is made for such a patient, it should be considered primarily as a space maintainer and an interim denture until more permanent treatment is possible.

There are two specific contraindications for the use of unilateral fixed restorations. One is a long edentulous span and abutment teeth that would not be able to withstand the trauma of horizontal and diagonal occlusal forces. The other is abutment teeth, weakened by periodontal disease, that would benefit from cross-arch stabilization. In either situation a bilateral removable restoration can be used more effectively to replace the missing teeth.

Modification spaces. A removable partial denture for a Class III arch is better supported and stabilized when a modification area on the opposite side of the arch is present. Such an edentulous area need not be restored by a fixed partial denture, since it may be essential to the design of the removable partial denture. Additional modification spaces, however, particularly those involving single missing teeth, are better restored separately by means of a fixed denture. Not only is a lone-standing abutment thus stabilized by the splinting effect of a fixed restoration, but also a possible teeter-totter effect of the denture is avoided and the denture is made less complicated by not having to include other abutment teeth for the support and retention of an additional edentulous space or spaces.

When an edentulous space that is a modification of either a Class I or Class II arch exists anterior to a lone-standing abutment tooth, this tooth is subjected to trauma by the movements of a distal extension partial denture far in excess of its ability to withstand such stresses. The splinting of the lone abutment to the nearest tooth is mandatory. Splinting is best accomplished in such a situation by means of a fixed partial denture uniting the two teeth on either side of the edentulous space. The abutment crown should be contoured for support and retention of the partial denture, and in addition a means of supporting a stabilizing component on the anterior abutment of the fixed partial denture or on the occlusal surface of the pontic usually should be provided.

Anterior modification spaces. Usually any missing anterior teeth in a partially

---

*Paraphrased from McCracken, W. L.: Differential diagnosis; fixed or removable partial dentures, J. Am. Dent. Assoc. **63:**767-775, 1961.

edentulous arch, except in a Kennedy Class IV arch in which only anterior teeth are missing, are best replaced by means of a fixed restoration. There are exceptions. Sometimes a better esthetic result is obtainable when the anterior replacements are supplied by the removable partial denture. This is also true when excessive tissue and bone resorption necessitates the placement of pontics too far posteriorly for good esthetics and for an acceptable relation with the opposing teeth. However, in most instances, from both a mechanical and a biologic standpoint, anterior replacements are best accomplished with fixed restorations. The replacement of missing posterior teeth with a removable partial denture is then made much less complicated and gives more satisfactory results.

Nonreplacement of missing molars. Frequently the decision of whether to replace unilaterally missing molars must be made. To do so with a removable denture necessitates the making of a distal extension restoration with the major connector joining the edentulous side to retentive and stabilizing components located on the nonedentulous side of the arch. Leverage factors are always unfavorable, and the retainers that must be used on the nonedentulous side are frequently unsatisfactory. Several factors therefore will influence the decision to make a unilateral, distal extension partial denture.

First the opposing teeth must be considered. If they are to be prevented from extrusion and migration, some opposing occlusion must be provided. This would influence the replacement of the missing molars far more than any improvement in masticating efficiency that might result. The replacement of missing molars on one side is seldom necessary for reasons of mastication alone.

Second the future of a maxillary tuberosity must be considered. Left uncovered, the tuberosity frequently will seem to drop and increase in size. However, covering the tuberosity with a partial denture base, in combination with the stimulating effect of the intermittent occlusion provided, helps to maintain the normalcy of the tuberosity. This is of considerable importance in any future denture replacements. In such an instance it may be better to make a unilateral removable partial denture than to leave a maxillary tuberosity uncovered.

A third consideration is the condition of the opposing second molar. If this tooth is missing or can logically be ignored or eliminated, then only first molar occlusion need be supplied by utilizing a cantilever-type fixed restoration. Occlusion need be only minimal to maintain occlusal relations between the natural first molar in the one arch and the prosthetic molar in the opposite arch. Such a pontic should be narrow buccolingually and need not occlude with more than one half to two thirds of the opposing tooth. Frequently such a restoration is the preferred method of treatment. However, unless three abutments are used to support a cantilever molar opposed by a natural molar, only limited success should be anticipated.

Indications for removable partial dentures

Although a removable partial denture should be considered only when a fixed restoration is contraindicated, there are several specific indications for the use of a removable restoration.

Distal extension situations. Except in situations in which the replacement of missing second (and third) molars is either inadvisable or unnecessary, or in which unilateral replacement of a missing first molar can be accomplished by means of a multiple abutment, cantilevered fixed restoration, replacement of missing posterior teeth without the assistance of a posterior abutment must be accomplished with a removable partial denture. The most common partially edentulous situations are the Kennedy Class I and Class II. With the latter an edentulous space on the opposite side of the arch is often conveniently present, or can be effected, to aid in the required retention and stabilization of the partial denture. If no space is present, embrasure clasps or intracoronal retainers generally must be used. As previously stated, all other edentulous areas are best replaced with fixed partial dentures.

After recent extractions. The replacement of teeth after recent extractions cannot be accomplished satisfactorily with a fixed restoration. When relining will be required later or when a fixed restoration will be constructed later, a temporary removable partial denture must be used. If an all-resin denture is used rather than a more elaborate partial denture, the immediate cost to the patient is much less, and the resin denture lends itself best to future temporary modifications.

A tooth-bounded edentulous area in which, because of recent extractions, some change is anticipated in the residual ridge is also best restored with a removable partial denture. Although the relining of a tooth-supported resin denture base thus is made possible, this is usually done only to improve esthetics, oral cleanliness, or patient comfort. Support for such a restoration is supplied by occlusal rests on the abutment teeth at each end of the edentulous space.

Long span. A long span may be totally tooth supported if the abutments and the means of transferring the support to the denture are adequate and if the denture framework is rigid. There is little, if any, difference between the support afforded a removable partial denture and that afforded a fixed restoration by the adjacent abutment teeth. However, in the absence of cross-arch stabilization the torque and leverage on the two abutment teeth would be excessive. Instead a removable denture deriving retention, support, and stabilization from abutment teeth on the opposite side of the arch is indicated as the logical means of replacing the missing teeth.

Need for effect of bilateral stabilization. In a mouth weakened by periodontal disease, because of the lack of cross-arch stabilization, a fixed restoration may jeopardize the future of periodontically involved abutment teeth unless the splinting effect of multiple abutments is employed. The removable partial denture, on the other hand, may act as a periodontal splint through its effective cross-arch stabilizing of teeth weakened by periodontal disease. When abutment teeth throughout the arch are properly prepared and restored, the beneficial effect of a removable partial denture can be far greater than that of a unilateral fixed partial denture.

Esthetics in anterior region. When the replacement of missing anterior teeth is the primary consideration, it is sometimes advisable, for reasons of appearance, to use translucent artificial teeth on a removable restoration rather than often dull fixed partial denture pontics. This is particularly true when several anterior teeth are missing and when a better tooth arrangement, for support, contour, and phonetics, can be accomplished.

Excessive loss of residual bone. The pontic of a fixed partial denture must be related to the residual ridge in such a manner that the contact with the mucosa is gentle. Whenever excessive resorption has occurred, however, teeth supported by a denture base may be arranged in a more acceptable buccolingual position than is possible with a fixed partial denture.

Artificial teeth supported by a denture base can be located without regard to the crest of the residual ridge and more nearly in the position of the natural dentition for normal tongue and cheek contacts. This is particularly true of a maxillary denture.

Anteriorly, loss of residual bone occurs from the labial aspect. Often the incisive papilla lies at the crest of the residual ridge. Since the central incisors are normally located anterior to this landmark, any other location of artificial central incisors is unnatural. An anterior fixed partial denture made for such a mouth will have pontics resting on the labial aspect of this resorbed ridge and will be too far lingual to provide desirable lip support. Frequently the only way the incisal edges of the pontics can be made to occlude with the opposing lower anterior teeth is to use a labial inclination that is excessive and unnatural, and both esthetics and lip support suffer thereby. Because the same condition exists with a removable partial denture in which the anterior teeth are abutted on the residual ridge, a labial flange must be utilized to permit the teeth to be located more nearly in their natural position.

The same method of treatment applies to the replacement of missing lower anterior teeth. Sometimes a lower anterior fixed partial denture is made six or more units in length, in which the remaining space necessitates either leaving out one anterior tooth or using the original number of teeth but with all of them too narrow for esthetics. In either instance the denture is nearly in a straight line because the pontics follow the form of the resorbed ridge. A removable partial denture will permit the location of the replaced teeth in a favorable relation to the lip and opposing dentition regardless of the shape of the residual ridge. When such a removable prosthesis is made, however, positive support must be obtained from the adjacent abutments.

Unusually sound abutment teeth. Sometimes the excuse for making a removable restoration is the wish to see sound teeth preserved in their natural state and not prepared for abutment retainers. The reasons for the loss of the teeth being replaced must be considered. If loss is due to caries, then it is likely that caries will occur eventually in the abutment teeth. If the teeth were lost because of periodontal disease, then the periodontium of the remaining teeth must be evaluated. If the teeth were lost due to neglect of minimal caries and if the caries activity seems to be arrested, the utilization of existing tooth surfaces to support a removable restoration may be justified. If the oral hygiene habits of the patient are favorable and if the abutment teeth are sound with good periodontal support, unprotected abutments may be used to support and retain a removable restoration. When this condition exists, the dentist should not hesitate to reshape and modify existing enamel surfaces to provide proximal guiding planes, occlusal rest areas, optimal retentive areas, and surfaces on which nonretentive stabilizing components may be placed.

It is only in selected instances, then, that the making of a removable prosthetic restoration on unprotected abutments can be justified.

Economic considerations. Economics should not be the sole criterion in arriving at a method of treatment. When, for economic reasons, complete treatment is out of the question and yet replacement of missing teeth is indicated, the restorative procedures dictated by these considerations must be described clearly to the patient as being of an interim nature and not representative of the best that modern dentistry has to offer. Ordinarily a prosthesis that is made

to satisfy economic considerations alone is doomed to limited success, and both professional esteem and the patient suffer thereby.

THE CHOICE BETWEEN COMPLETE DENTURES AND REMOVABLE PARTIAL DENTURES

When the diagnosis preceding prosthodontic service is made, the probable length of service that can be expected from a partial denture must always be weighed against the patient's economic status. A decision may have to be made between a partial denture and a complete denture, in either arch or both. One patient may prefer complete dentures to the traumatic experience of complete oral rehabilitation, regardless of his ability to pay. Another may be so determined to keep his own teeth that he will make great financial sacrifices to do so if given a reasonable assurance of the success of oral rehabilitation.

The value of listening to the patient during the examination and the diagnostic procedures should not be disregarded nor treated lightly. During the presentation of pertinent facts, time should be allowed for the patient to express himself freely as to his desires in retaining and restoring his natural teeth. At this time a treatment plan may be influenced or even drastically changed to conform to the expressed and implied desires of the patient.

For example, there may be a reasonable possibility of saving teeth in both arches through the use of partial dentures. With only anterior teeth remaining, a partial denture can be made to replace the posterior teeth by utilizing good abutment support and, in the maxillary arch, utilizing full palatal coverage for retention and stability. If the patient expresses a desire to retain his anterior teeth "at any cost" and if the remaining teeth are esthetically acceptable and functionally sound, then the dentist should do his best to make successful removable dentures for both arches and thus fulfill his professional obligation to the patient.

On the other hand, if for economic or other reasons the patient believes that a complete maxillary denture would best satisfy his denture requirements but for fear of difficulty in wearing a complete mandibular denture he would prefer restoration of that arch with a partial denture, then, all factors being acceptable, his wishes should be respected and treatment planned accordingly.

Still another patient, for economic or other reasons, may prefer to have complete dentures made for both arches rather than undergo complete rehabilitation of the partially edentulous arches. It is frequently unwise to insist on the latter course with such a patient. *The professional obligation to present the facts and then do the best in accordance with the patient's expressed desires still applies.*

Still another patient may wish to retain the remaining teeth for an indefinite but relatively short period of time, with eventual complete dentures a foregone conclusion. In this instance the professional obligation may be to recommend interim partial dentures without extensive mouth preparations. Such dentures will aid in mastication and will provide esthetic replacements, at the same time serving as conditioning restorations, which will make the later transition to complete dentures somewhat easier. Such partial dentures should be designed and fabricated with care, but the total cost of partial denture service will be considerably less.

An expressed desire on the part of the patient to retain only six lower anterior teeth must be considered carefully before being agreed to as the planned treatment. The advantages to the patient are obvious: he may retain six esthetically acceptable teeth; he does not become totally edentulous; and he has the advantage of direct retention that would not be possible if he were completely edentulous. Retaining even the lower canine teeth would accomplish the latter two objectives. These advantages cannot be denied. Yet the disadvantages, which are less obvious to the patient, must also be considered and explained to him. These are mechanical and functional considerations; that is, the edentulous maxilla anteriorly is structurally not able to withstand the trauma of positive tooth contact against natural opposing teeth. The possible result is the loss of residual maxillary bone, loosening of the maxillary denture because of the tripping influence of the natural lower teeth, and the loss of basal foundation for the support of future prostheses. However, if the maxillary anteriors are arranged to contact in eccentric positions only and the patient appreciates periodic recall, these problems are certainly minimized. The presence of inflamed hyperplastic tissue is a frequent sequel to continued loss of support and denture movement.

The prevention of this sequence of events lies in the maintenance of positive occlusal support posteriorly and the continual elimination of traumatic influence from the remaining anterior teeth. Such support is sometimes impossible to maintain without frequent relining or remaking of the lower partial denture base. On the other hand, this may cause undesirable resorption of the posterior ridges because of overloading. The results in any event are undesirable, and the patient must be made aware of the hazards involved.

Whereas some patients are able to wear a lower partial denture supported only by anterior teeth against a complete upper denture, the odds are that undesirable consequences will result unless the patient faithfully follows the instructions of the dentist. In no other situation in treatment planning is the general health of the patient and the quality of residual alveolar bone as critical as it is in this situation.

In addition to considering the age and health of the patient and his ability to build bone is response to stress, it is well to consider why the teeth being replaced were extracted. In all probability any history of severe periodontal disease precludes the wearing of such combination dentures successfully. On the other hand, the loss of teeth because of caries or the premature loss of teeth that might have been saved justifies the conclusion that the residual bone is probably healthy and will be able to withstand stresses within reasonable limits. In such instances, combination dentures may be constructed if the patient is made aware of the need for periodic reexamination and is willing to make the transition to a complete lower denture upon the first signs of serious damage to supporting structures.

The final treatment plan should represent the best possible course for the patient after consideration has been given to all physical, mental, mechanical, esthetic, and economic factors involved.

FACTORS IN SELECTING METAL ALLOYS FOR REMOVABLE PARTIAL DENTURE FRAMEWORKS

Practically all cast frameworks for removable partial dentures are made either from a gold alloy (Type IV) or from a chromium-cobalt alloy. The choice of the alloy from which the framework of a removable partial denture will be constructed is logically made during the treatment planning phase. Inherent differences in the physical properties of alloys presently available to the dental profession must be considered in making this choice. For example, mouth preparation procedures, especially the recontouring of abutment teeth for the optimal placement of retentive elements, depend to a large extent on the modulus of elasticity (stiffness) of a particular alloy.

It is estimated that the chromium-cobalt alloys are utilized many times more than are the gold alloys in removable partial prosthodontics. The popularity of the chromium-cobalt alloys has been attributed to their low density (weight), high modulus of elasticity (stiffness), low material cost, and resistance to tarnish in comparison with that of gold alloys.

Use of the chromium-cobalt alloys in preference to the gold alloys continues to be somewhat controversial among members of the dental profession. This controversy stems, in part, from the necessity of using specialized equipment and techniques in the application of the chromium-cobalt alloys, which has restricted the fabrication of frameworks almost entirely to commercial dental laboratories.

Successful removable restorations may be made from either the gold or chromium-cobalt alloys. Because the cost of the alloy used for a framework is only a part of the total cost for the service, cost alone should not justify the substitution of a base alloy for a noble alloy. The alloy chosen should show a definite superiority or an important saving in cost to justify its use for a particular patient.

Each of the alloys has advantages under certain conditions. Obviously, then, the material that is considered capable of rendering the best overall service to the patient over a period of years is the one that should be used. The choice of alloy is based on several factors: (1) weighed advantages or disadvantages of the physical properties of the alloy, (2) the dimensional accuracy with which the alloy can be cast, (3) the availability of the alloy, (4) the versatility of the alloy, and (5) the individual clinical observation and experiences with alloys in respect to quality control and service to the patient.

The following are comparable characteristics of gold alloys and chromium-cobalt alloys: (1) each is well tolerated by oral tissues; (2) they are equally acceptable esthetically; (3) enamel abrasion by either alloy is insignificant on vertical tooth surfaces; (4) a low-fusing chrome-cobalt alloy or gold alloy can be cast to wrought wire, and wrought-wire components may be soldered to either gold or chrome-cobalt alloys. (These characteristics are important in overcoming the objection by some dentists to the increased stiffness of chromium-cobalt alloys for the portions of direct retainers that must engage an undercut of the abutment tooth); (5) the accuracy obtainable in casting either alloy is clinically acceptable under strictly controlled investing and casting procedures; and (6) soldering procedures for the repair of frameworks can be performed on each alloy.

Comparative physical properties. Chromium-cobalt alloys generally have a lower *yield strength* than do the gold alloys used for removable partial dentures (Table 3). Yield strength is the greatest amount of stress an alloy will withstand and still return to its original shape in an unweakened condition. Possessing a lower proportional limit, the chromium-cobalt alloys will deform permanently at lower loads than will gold alloys. Therefore the dentist must design the chromium-cobalt framework so that the degree of deformation expected in a direct retainer is less than a comparable degree of deformation for a gold component.

The *modulus of elasticity* refers to stiffness of an alloy. Gold alloys have a modulus of elasticity approximately one half of that for chromium-cobalt alloys for similar uses. The greater stiffness of chromium-cobalt alloy is advantageous but at the same time offers disadvantages. Greater rigidity can be obtained with the chromium-cobalt

Table 3. *Mechanical properties of representative stellite alloys**

Properties	Stellite alloys[†]					Hardened partial denture gold alloys
	A	B	D	E	21	
Yield strength (psi)	64,500	61,000	56,000	62,400	82,300	65,000-90,000
Tensile strength (psi)	180,500	107,500	84,500	102,500	101,300	107,000-120,000
Elongation (%)	3.4	3.2	6.0	1.9	8.2	1.5-8.0
Modulus of elasticity (psi × 10^{-6})	28.0	29.5	27.5	28.5	36.0	13-15
Hardness (R[30N])[‡]	53.0	60.0	51.0	55.0	—	—

*From Peyton, F. A.: Dent. Clin. North Am., pp. 759-771, Nov., 1958.
[†]Data for lettered alloys from Taylor, D. F., Liebfritz, W. A., and Adler, A. G.: J. Am. Dent. Assoc. **56**:343-351, 1958; for Stellite No. 21 from Metals Handbook, 1948 ed., p. 579; for gold alloys from manufacturers property charts.
[‡]Rockwell 30N hardness scale.

alloy in reduced sections in which cross-arch stabilization is required, thereby eliminating an appreciable bulk of the framework. Its greater rigidity is also an advantage when the greatest undercut that can be found on an abutment tooth is in the nature of 0.005 inch. A gold retentive element would not be as efficient in retaining the restoration under such conditions as would the chromium-cobalt clasp arm.

A high yield strength and a low modulus of elasticity produce higher *flexibility*. The gold alloys are approximately twice as flexible as the chromium-cobalt alloys, which is a distinct advantage in the optimal location of retentive elements of the framework in many instances. The greater flexibility of the gold alloys usually permits location of the tips of retainer arms in the gingival third of the abutment tooth. As mentioned earlier, this problem, because of the stiffness of the chromium-cobalt alloys, can be overcome by including wrought-wire retentive elements in the framework.

The bulk of a retentive clasp arm for a removable partial denture is often reduced for greater flexibility when chromium-cobalt alloys are used as opposed to gold alloys. This, however, is inadvisable, since the grain size of the chromium-cobalt alloys is usually larger and is associated with a lower proportional limit, and so a decrease in the bulk of cast clasps increases the likelihood of fracture or permanent deformation. The retentive clasp arms for both alloys should be approximately the same size, but the depth of undercut used for retention must be reduced by one half when

chromium-cobalt is the choice of alloys. Chromium-cobalt alloys are reported to work-harden more rapidly than gold alloys, and this, associated with coarse grain size, may lead to failure in service. When adjustments by bending are necessary, they must be executed with extreme caution and limited optimism.

Chromium-cobalt alloys have a lower *density* than do gold alloys in comparable sections and are therefore about one half as heavy as the gold alloys. Weight of the alloy in most instances in not a valid criterion for selection of one metal over another, since after placement of a partial denture the patient seldom notices the weight of the restoration. The comparable lightness of the chromium-cobalt alloys, however, is an advantage when full-palatal coverage is indicated for the bilateral distal extension denture. Weight is a factor that must be considered when the force of gravity must be overcome so that usually passive direct retainers will not be activated constantly to the detriment of abutment teeth.

The hardness of chromium-cobalt alloys offers a disadvantage when a component of the framework, such as a rest, is opposed by a natural tooth or one that has been restored. We have observed what is believed to be excessive wear of natural teeth opposed by some of the various chromium-cobalt alloys as contrasted to the type IV gold alloys.

It has been observed that gold frameworks for removable partial dentures are more prone to produce uncomfortable galvanic shocks to abutment teeth restored with silver amalgam than are frameworks

Fig. 11-24. A, Photomicrograph of a type IV gold alloy. (×200.) Grain structure appears in form of a crystalline aggregate. **B,** Internal structure of a gold wrought wire appears to be fibrous. (×200.) Original crystals have become entangled and elongated as a result of being drawn from an ingot.

made of chromium-cobalt alloy. This may not be a valid criterion for the selection of a particular alloy when the dentist has complete control over the choice of restorative materials. It may, however, be a consideration in some institutional dental services in which silver amalgam restorations must, of necessity, be placed rather than gold restorations.

Wrought wire: selection and quality control. Wrought-wire direct retainer arms may be attached to the restoration by embedding a portion of the wire in an acrylic resin denture base, by soldering to the fabricated framework, or by casting the framework to the wire. The physical (mechanical) properties of available wrought wires are most important considerations in selecting a proper wire for the desired method of attachment. These properties are yield strength or proportional limit, percentage elongation, tensile strength, and fusion temperature. After selection of the wire the procedures to which the wire is subjected in fabricating the restoration become critical in maintaining quality control for service, or putting it another way, improper laboratory procedures can diminish certain desirable physical properties of the wrought structure so as to render it relatively useless for its intended purpose.

All alloys solidify in crystalline form when they cool from the molten state. The properties of wrought structures are different from cast structures in mechanical charac-

teristics and in microstructure (Fig. 11-24). It is considered that many mechanical properties of the wrought structure are superior to those of the cast structure. Craig* has suggested that the tensile strength of the wrought structure is approximately 25% greater than that of the cast alloy from which it was made. The wrought structure's hardness and strength are also greater. This means that a wrought structure having a smaller cross-section that a cast structure may be used as a retainer arm (retentive) to perform the same function.

Craig has also suggested that a minimum yield strength of 60,000 psi is required for the retentive element of a direct retainer. A percentage elongation of less than 6% is indicative that a wrought wire may not be amenable to contouring without attendant undesirable changes in microstructure.

When wrought wire is heated, its physical properties and microstructure may be considerably altered depending on the temperature, heating time, and cooling operation. In a cast-to process, wrought wire is subjected to a one-half hour heat-soaking period of burnout at 1250° F when a Type IV gold is used for the framework. When a low-fusing (2350° F) chrome-cobalt alloy (Ticonium) is selected for the framework, the burnout subjects the invested wire to a heat-soaking period of two hours at 1300° F. When

---

*Craig, R. G.: Restorative dental materials, ed. 6, St. Louis, 1980, The C. V. Mosby Co.

Fig. 11-25. A, Internal structure of a gold wrought wire subjected to 1400° F for one hour. (×200.) Recrystallization has been initiated, although evidence of the once fibrous structure of wire is still apparent. Useful strength (yield strength) of wire and other physical properties have been reduced because of recrystallization. **B,** Piece of wrought wire (from same specimen as in **A** and Fig. 11-24) subjected to 1500° F for one hour. (×200.) Grain growth has occurred, and useful physical properties of wire have been further reduced. Internal structure of this wire probably renders it unfit for adequate service as a retentive portion of direct retainer assembly.

wrought wire is soldered to frameworks by electric soldering, it is subjected to a momentary temperature of about 1500° F—of course depending on the solder used. The yield strength of both gold and base metal alloy (Ticonium) wrought wires can be drastically reduced simply by subjecting the wire to too much heat. If the heat is high enough and long enough, the fibrous microstructure of the wrought wire disappears and is replaced by a grain or crystalline microstructure. The process is known as recrystallization or grain growth and is a most undesirable occurrence in wrought-wire retainer arms (Fig. 11-25).

To avoid recrystallization of wrought wire, high fusing wires should be selected, and temperatures must be rigidly controlled when either using the cast-to or soldering methods. Each manufacturer of wrought forms for dental applications furnishes charts listing their products and the physical properties of each product. Two examples of such information are demonstrated in Fig. 11-26. Note that the percentage of nobility metals is given. Additionally most manufacturers designate those wires that may be cast-to.

A.D.A. Specification No. 7 addresses itself to wrought gold wire both as to content and minimum physical properties. This specification recognizes two types of wire, namely a Type I (high precious metal alloy) and a Type II (low precious metal alloy). Table 4 compares the minimum mechanical properties. A knowledge of A.D.A. Specification No. 7 and reference material furnished by dental manufacturers will enhance the proper selection of wrought wire for specific methods of attachment to the framework or removable restoration.

Our laboratory experiments involving soldering procedures and casting alloys to various gold alloy wrought wires under controlled conditions, indicates that gold wrought wires having a proportional limit of 70,000 psi in the semihardened condition, a fusion temperature above 1800° F and a nobility gold and platinum group content of at least 61% are satisfactory for such operations. None of the wires tested having at least the above physical properties showed recrystallization in photomicrographs. All the gold wires, including the platinum, gold, and palladium type wire, were heat soaked for two hours at 1300° F in a refractory investment. The furnace in which this was carried out was accurately calibrated.

When a Type IV gold alloy was cast against the selected gold wrought wires and a PGP wrought wire, there was no evidence of recrystallization. A low fusing chrome-cobalt alloy (Ticonium) was cast against the PGP wire without recrystallization's occurring.

It was noted upon examination of only

NEY WIRE PROPERTIES

ALLOY	Condition	Ultimate Tensile Strength		Proportional Limit		Elongation Percent	Hardness		Fusion Temp.		Density		Nobility Gold & Platinum Group Metals
		Lbs/in.²	Kg/cm²	Lbs/in.²	Kg/cm²	2 in. or 5.1 cm	BHN	HV	°F	°C	dwt./in.³	gm/cm³	
ELASTIC #4*	S	117,500	8,260	86,500	6,080	15	190	215	1925	1050	164	15.6	79.5%
	H	173,000	12,160	131,000	9,170	7	270	305					
ELASTIC #12	S	125,000	8,790	88,000	6,190	20	175	200	2010	1150	127	12.1	61.0%
	H	178,000	12,510	135,000	9,490	15	275	310					
PALINEY #7**	S	120,000	8,440	89,000	6,260	24	180	205	1985	1085	125	11.9	55.0%
	H	180,000	12,650	148,000	10,400	9	280	315					
PALINEY #6**	S	110,000	7,730	63,500	4,460	24	150	170	1970	1075	115	10.9	45.0%
	H	170,000	11,950	127,000	8,930	15	270	305					
NEYLASTIC H.F.**	S	110,000	7,730	75,000	5,270	20	215	245	1830	1000	183	17.4	76.0%
	H	145,000	10,190	85,000	5,980	6	260	295					
GOLD COLOR ELASTIC*	S	120,000	8,440	73,000	5,130	14	200	225	1675	915	160	15.2	73.0%
	H	165,000	11,600	135,000	9,490	1	290	330					
DENTURE CLASP (GOLD COLOR)	S	100,000	7,030	52,000	3,660	22	160	180	1650	900	145	13.8	61.5%
	H	157,000	11,040	122,000	8,580	1	265	300					
PGP***		125,000	8,790	80,000	5,620	15	200	225	2790	1535	185	17.6	100%
P & I***		120,000	8,440	115,000	8,080	2	180	200	3250	1790	226	21.5	100%

* This product appears on The American Dental Association List of Certified Dental Material.
** This wire recommended for Crozat Technic.
*** This wire recommended for cast-to applications.

A

Fig. 11-26. Physical properties and nobility gold and platinum group metal content of various wires are furnished in chart form by manufacturers. Such information is necessary to select a wrought wire for a particular purpose and attachment method. (**A** courtesy J. M. Ney Company, Bloomfield, Conn.; **B**, courtesy J. F. Jelenko and Company, New Rochelle, N.Y.)

JELENKO GOLD WIRES		Solders Recommended	Hardness: Brinell D.P.H.	U. T. S. lbs./sq. in. (kg./cm.²)	% Elong. in 2 in. (5 cm.)	Yield Strength lbs./sq. in. (kg./cm.²)	No. of Cold Bends	Fusion Temperature (Approx.)
EXTRA HIGH FUSING (All Gold Alloys Can Be Cast To It, Including Jelenko "O")	† **NO. 12 WIRE** (Plat. Color)	Jelenko "O" Ortho Solder Can Be Used With All Others	Q 183 Q 200 H 204 H 225	88,500 (6,220) 103,000 (7,240)	11 9	66,500 (4,675) 70,000 (4,920)	6 5	2225°F. 1218°C.
HIGH FUSING (Can be Cast Against) For Clasps, Bars, Pins Including Jelenko "O"	**SUPER WIRE*** (Plat. Color)	Orthoflex H.F.	Q 200 Q 220 H 255 H 280	132,000 (9,280) 175,000 (12,303)	20 12	89,000 (6,260) 127,000 (8,930)	6.5 3.5	1845°F. 1007°C.
	THRIFT WIRE (Plat. Color)	Alboro H.F.	Q 200 Q 220 H 250 H 275	126,000 (8,860) 170,000 (11,950)	20 4	78,000 (5,485) 118,000 (8,295)	6.0 3.5	1890°F. 1032°C.
MEDIUM HIGH FUSING (Can Be Cast Against) For Clasps, Bars and Wrought Structures	**STANDARD WIRE** (Gold Color)	708 650 615	Q 165 Q 180 H 260 H 285	110,400 (7,760) 165,000 (11,600)	22 8	54,000 (3,795) 112,000 (7,875)	6.0 3.5	1735°F. 946°C.
MEDIUM FUSING (Not to be Cast Against) For Clasps, Bars and Dowels	**NO. 25 WIRE** (Gold Color)	650 615 585	Q 145 Q 160 H 230 H 250	93,200 (6,550) 147,000 (10,330)	26 9	53,000 (3,725) 112,000 (7,875)	6.0 3.5	1615°F. 879°C.
	NO. 2 WIRE (Gold Color)	650 615 585	Q 140 Q 155 H 250 H 275	95,000 (6,680) 155,000 (10,900)	27 5	48,000 (3,375) 110,000 (7,735)	5.0 1.5	1620°F. 882°C.
For PARALLEL PIN WORK	**PONTO WIRE** (Plat. Color)		230 250	136,000 (9,560)	20	105,000 (7,380)	5.5	2732°F. 1500°C.

† Hardens in a manner similar to Jelenko "O" Cast Gold. (After casting, slow cool from approximately 1800°F. (982°C.) in flask.)

NOTE: Ponto wire is knurled. "Q" is quenched or softened and "H" is hardened.

Heat treatment instructions included with each wire.

Jelenko Wires are immunized, Calor-Ohmically Heat Hardened, and furnished in straight 1 ft. (0.3m) lengths unless otherwise specified.

MADE IN THESE GAUGES

12 13 14 15 16 17 18 19 20 21 22 23 24 25 26

AVAILABLE IN THESE STYLES

Round   Half Round   Half Round "Bevelled"

Anterior   Posterior   Oval

B

Fig. 11-26, cont'd. For legend see opposite page.

Table 4. *Comparative specifications contained in A.D.A. Specification No. 7*

	Type I	Type II
Content of metals of the gold, platinum group (minimum)	75%	65%
Minimum fusion temperature	1742° F	1898° F
Minimum yield point value (hardened or oven cooled)	125,000 psi	95,000 psi
Minimum elongation (hardened)	4%	2%
Minimum elongation (softened)	15%	15%

heat-soaked invested wires that all wires appeared to be surface oxidized. Since such oxidation will likely prevent interface wetting of the wire and cast alloy, mechanical retention of the wire in the cast framework should be provided. This can be accomplished simply by having the portion of the wrought wire embedded in the framework contoured to lie in two planes (Fig. 11-27).

Matching color gold solders may be used to solder wrought retainers to any type alloy framework by electric soldering. Recrystallization of gold wrought wires and PGP wire has been noted in specimens when a triple thick 19K gold solder with a melting temperature of 1675° F was used. However, a 650 fine gold solder with a melting temperature of 1420° to 1490° F produced no recrystallization of the wrought structures. Since color matching gold solders with a melting range of 1400 to 1500° F are available and can be used for soldering both gold alloys and gold to chrome-cobalt alloys and are entirely adequate for the job, it seems prudent to employ the lower-fusing solder.

Electric soldering is preferred to torch soldering to attach wrought wires to a framework because of the rapid localization of heat at the electrode. Triple thick, color-matching gold solder should be used. The additional bulk of triple thick solder will retard melting momentarily while the carbon electrode conducts heat to the area being soldered. Use of a flux is essential to prevent oxidation of the parts being joined and the solder itself. A borax type flux is recommended for soldering gold alloys to gold alloys. However, a fluoride type flux must be employed when chromium-cobalt alloys are soldered to alloys containing chromium. A fluoride type flux should also be used when a gold alloy is soldered to a chromium-cobalt alloy. Electric soldering for repair of removable partial dentures is described in Chapter 21.

Gold wrought wires are usually furnished in a semihardened condition by their manufacturer and may be safely contoured without annealing. Additionally the application of heat in the cast-to and soldering processes suggests that some annealing may occur. Therefore it is recommended that gold alloy wrought wires be given a hardening heat treatment after either being soldered or cast-to just prior to beginning final finishing procedures on the metal framework. A harden-

Fig. 11-27. Wrought-wire retainer arm has been contoured to design on a duplicate stone cast of blocked-out master cast. It will be transferred to refractory cast and will become an integral part of framework pattern and will be cast-to. Wire is contoured in two planes and will be mechanically retained in casting.

ing heat treatment will increase the proportional limit, tensile strength, and hardness of a wrought, cast to or soldered gold wire. An acceptable hardening heat treatment for most gold alloys consists of placing the framework in a furnace at 840° F for about five minutes and then uniformly cooling the oven to 480° F in thirty minutes and immediately quenching the framework in water upon removal from the furnace. It should be mentioned here that PGP wire and the base metal wrought wire (Ticonium) are not affected by the above hardening heat treatment.

Regardless of the method of attaching the wrought wire retainer either by embedding, soldering, or cast-to, tapering the wrought arm seems most rational. A retainer arm is in essence a cantilever and can be made more serviceable and efficient by tapering. Tapering permits more uniform distribution of service stresses throughout the length of the arm, being readily demonstrated by photoelastic stress analysis. Uniform tapering of an 18-gauge, round wire arm can be accomplished, as illustrated in Fig. 11-28, before the retainer arm is contoured. The dimensions of the taper we prefer are illustrated in Fig. 11-29.

It should be mentioned here that our clinical experience with one base metal wrought wire suggests that it is applicable to the three different methods of attaching wire

Fig. 11-28. A, Round, 18-gauge wrought wire is uniformly tapered the length of retainer arm contacting abutment. This is conveniently accomplished by rapidly spinning wire in angled contact with a fast-running, abrasive cut-off disk in a dental lathe. **B,** Tapered wire is polished by spinning wire in angled contact with a fast-running, mildly abrasive rubber disk in a dental lathe.

Fig. 11-29. Round, 18-gauge wrought wire for retentive component of direct retainer assembly (clasp) is uniformly tapered from its full diameter to one-half diameter at its terminus. Tapering should precede contouring wire for a retainer arm.

retainers. This wrought wire is Ticonium 18-gauge round wire. Its composition consists primarily of cobalt, chrome, tungston, and nickel. Physical properties of the wire furnished by the manufacturers are tensile strength, 200,000 psi; yield strength, 133,000 psi; and percentage elongation, 19%.

Summary. In making a selection of materials it must be remembered that fundamentals do not change. These are inviolable. It is only methods, procedures, and substances—by which the dentist effects the best possible end result—that change. The responsibility of decision still rests with the dentist, who must *evaluate all factors* in relation to the *results* that he hopes to achieve. In any instance, therefore, the dentist must weigh the problems involved, compare and evaluate the characteristics of different potential materials, and then choose the road leading to the greatest possible service to the patient.

After the dentist makes his choice of alloys to be used in rendering a service to his patient, he should prescribe only those alloys that conform to the specifications set forth by the American Dental Association for the particular type of alloy.

It is to the lasting credit of those interested in biomaterials that continual research is being conducted to incorporate as many desirable characteristics in the chromium-cobalt alloys used in prosthodontics as possible. Efforts are being made to simplify casting procedures while obtaining greater accuracy and to make these alloys available to the professsion at reasonable cost. There is little doubt in our mind but that a chromium-cobalt alloy will be developed, retaining the desirable characteristics that these alloys presently possess— plus many of the physical characteristics of Type IV gold alloys. Such an alloy could surely be made universally available to the dental profession and within the economy of all nations to utilize. Unfortunately this is not presently true of precious metal alloys.

SELF-ASSESSMENT AIDS

1. State in your own words the purpose of dental treatment.
2. Meaningful treatment of a patient embodies three fundamentally different processes. Can you name these processes in chronological order of accomplishment?

3. What are the objectives of prosthodontic treatment for a partially edentulous patient?

4. Do you feel that ascertaining the past dental experiences of a patient you are treating for the first time would contribute to patient management?

5. Do you most always review the present health status of the patient before conducting an oral examination?

6. A complete oral examination is not limited to a visual and digital examination of teeth and surrounding structures but should also include three more entities; these are _____, _____, and _____.

7. It is not unusual for a patient to be primarily concerned with the cosmetic implications of a missing tooth. What are the obligations of the dentist to broaden the concern of total treatment?

8. A logical sequence of a thorough oral examination includes at least seven different procedures accomplished in order. Two of the six procedures are a thorough prophylaxis and the placement of individual temporary restorations. Can you list the other five factors?

9. For what reason should the definitive location of the inferior border of a mandibular major connector be ascertained as a part of an oral examination?

10. Rationalize the importance of the following areas which must be ascertained by radiographic interpretation:
    a. Quality of alveolar support of prospective abutment teeth
    b. Interpretation of relative bone density
    c. Increased width of the periodontal space
    d. Index areas
    e. Lamina dura
    f. Root morphology
    g. Unerupted third molars

11. What is a diagnostic cast?

12. Can you describe a diagnostic cast of a partially edentulous arch that may be considered a quality cast?

13. Diagnostic casts serve several purposes as aids in diagnosis and treatment planning. Can you think of six different uses for them?

14. Two sets of diagnostic casts (one a duplicate set) should be made for a patient requiring treatment. Why?

15. What can be gained from a study of accurately mounted diagnostic casts on a programmed, semiadjustable articulator?

16. The base of a diagnostic cast should be prepared in a certain way prior to any mounting on the articulator. Can you describe the preparation and tell why it is important?

17. What is a record base? An occlusion rim?

18. Are record bases usually necessary to correctly orient diagnostic casts of partially edentulous arches to an articulator? Why?

19. What four maxillomandibular records are necessary to orient casts to an arcon type articulator and to program the articulator?

20. What is meant by "proving the articulator," and how is it accomplished?

21. Can you name and describe the use of at least four different media used for recording maxillomandibular relations?

22. In relation to occlusion, one of the earliest decisions to be made in diagnosis is whether to accept or reject the existing occlusion as demonstrated by the correctly oriented and articulated diagnostic casts. True and false?

23. Improvements in the natural occlusion must be accomplished prior to construction of the denture, not subsequent to it. True or false?

24. The decision-making process in planning the restoration of a partially edentulous mouth must include a differential diagnosis of fixed or removable restorations or a combination of both as a means of restoration. Most always, where indicated, a fixed restoration is preferred to a removable restoration. True or false?

25. What are the indications for the use of fixed restorations in (a) tooth-bounded edentulous regions, (b) posterior modification spaces, and (c) anterior modifications spaces?

26. Although a removable partial denture should be considered as the means of treatment only when a fixed partial denture is contraindicated, there are several specific indications for the use of a removable restoration. Please briefly discuss these indications related to (a) distal extension situations, (b) postextraction periods, (c) long tooth-bounded edentulous spans, (d) need for bilateral stabilization, (e) excessive loss of residual bone, (f) esthetics in the anterior region of the mouth, and (g) economic considerations.

27. In many instances the dentist is confronted with the decision of treating the partially edentulous patient with removable partial dentures or complete dentures. Please discuss the following factors that certainly have a bearing on the decision-making process; (a) economics, (b) patient preference or desires of patient, (c) age, (d) health, (e) present periodontal status, and (f) dental I.Q. or prospective I.Q.

28. As a result of oral examination and diagnosis, certain data should be recorded, much of which is based on decisions that are the result of diagnosis, patient's attitudes, and economics. Some of these data are present and predictable health status, periodontal conditions present, oral hygiene habits, caries activity, need for extractions or surgery, need for fixed restorations, and a need for orthodontic treatment. There are at least four more areas of

treatment that should be recorded at this time. Can you think what they are?

29. Most frameworks for removable partial dentures today are made of some type of chromium-cobalt alloy rather than with an extra hard gold alloy. Four reasons are usually projected for this wide variation. What are they?

30. The choice of an alloy(s) is based on what factors?

31. Compare the physical properties of yield strength (proportional limit) and percentage elongation of chrome-cobalt alloy and partial denture gold alloy.

32. Which alloy is the sitffest in comparable sections—gold alloy or chrome-cobalt alloy? What are the advantages and disadvantages of comparable stiffness?

33. The retentive clasp arms for both chromium-cobalt and gold alloys should be dimensionally the same. Why or why not?

34. Many dentists prefer to use wrought-wire retentive arms in certain instances. Wrought wire may be attached to the denture by being cast-to, soldered, or embedded in the resin base. Does the method of attachment have a bearing on the selection of framework alloy and wrought wire? Why?

35. Excessive heat can alter the physical characteristics of any alloy. Discuss the precautions that must be taken in cast-to and soldering processes when wrought wire is used.

36. In the cast-to process using wrought wire, what phenomenon takes place which requires that the portion of the wire covered by the casting alloy be contoured in at least two planes for positive retention.

37. Discuss choice of solders and soldering procedures for wrought wire.

38. How would you go about selecting a wrought wire for a specific application of the wire?

39. Why should certain alloys be given a hardening heat treatment? Can you describe a hardening heat treatment for alloys described as precious metal alloys?

40. A wrought wire consisting of only platinum, gold, and paladium (is) (is not) affected by a hardening heat treatment after being cast-to with a Type IV gold alloy.

12 PREPARATION OF MOUTH FOR REMOVABLE PARTIAL DENTURES

The preparation of the mouth is fundamental to a successful removable partial denture service. Thorough mouth preparation, perhaps more than any other single factor, contributes to the philosophy that the prescribed prosthesis must not only replace what is missing but, of perhaps even greater importance, must also preserve what is remaining.

Mouth preparation follows the preliminary diagnosis and the development of a tentative treatment plan. Final treatment planning may be deferred until the response to the preparatory procedures can be ascertained. In general, mouth preparation includes procedures in three categories: oral surgical preparation, periodontal preparation, and preparation of abutment teeth. The objectives of the procedures involved in all three areas are to return the mouth to optimum health and to eliminate any condition that would be detrimental to the success of the partial denture.

Naturally, mouth preparation must be accomplished prior to the impression procedures that will produce the master cast upon which the denture will be constructed. Oral surgical and peridontal procedures should precede abutment tooth preparation and should be completed far enough in advance to allow for the necessary healing period. If at all possible, a period of *at least* six weeks and preferably three months should be provided between surgical and restorative dentistry procedures.

ORAL SURGICAL PREPARATION*

As a rule all surgical treatment for the removable partial denture patient should be completed as early as possible. By their very nature the surgical procedures generally indicated include the manipulation of both hard and soft tissues, which introduces the necessity for adequate healing time prior to the fabrication of the prosthesis. When possible, necessary endodontic surgery, periodontal surgery, and oral surgery should be planned so that they can be completed during the same time frame. The longer the interval between the surgery and the impression procedure, the more complete the healing and consequently the more stable the denture bearing area.

A variety of oral surgical techniques can prove beneficial to the clinician in preparing the patient for prosthetic replacements. However, it is not the purpose of this section to present the details of surgical correction. Rather, attention is called to some of the more common oral conditions or changes in which surgical intervention is indicated as an aid to denture design and construction and as an aid to the restoration's successful function in contributing further to the health and well-being of the patient. Additional information concerning the actual techniques employed is available in a standard oral surgery text.* It is important to emphasize, however, that the dentist providing the partial denture treatment bears the responsibility for seeing that the necessary surgical procedures are accomplished. Measures to control apprehension, including the use of intravenous and inhalation agents, have made the most extensive surgery acceptable to patients. Whether the dentist chooses to perform these procedures himself or elects to refer the patient to someone else, perhaps more qualified, is immaterial.

---

*Revision by Emmett R. Costich, Professor, Department of Oral Surgery, College of Dentistry, University of Kentucky, Lexington, Ky., and Raymond P. White, Jr., Dean, School of Dentistry, University of North Carolina, Chapel Hill, N.C.

---

*See Costich, E. R., and White, R. P., Jr.: Fundamentals of oral surgery, Philadelphia, 1971, W. B. Saunders Co.

The important consideration is that the patient not be deprived of any treatment that would enhance the success of the partial denture.

Extractions

Planned extractions should occur early in the treatment regimen but not before a careful and thorough evaluation of each remaining member of the dental arch is completed. Regardless of its condition, each tooth must be evaluated concerning its strategic importance and its potential contribution to the success of the removable partial denture. With the knowledge and technical capability available in dentistry today, *almost any tooth may be salvaged* if its retention is sufficiently important to warrant the procedures necessary. On the other hand, heroic attempts to salvage seriously involved teeth or those of doubtful nature whose retention would contribute little if anything, even if successfully treated and maintained, are contraindicated.

The extraction of *nonstrategic* teeth that present complications or those whose presence may be detrimental to the design of the partial denture thus becomes not an admission of defeat but a valuable asset to treatment and an integral part of the overall treatment plan.

Removal of residual roots

Generally all retained roots or root fragments should be removed. This is particularly true if they are in close proximity to the tissue surface or, of course, if there is evidence of associated pathology. Residual roots adjacent to abutment teeth may contribute to the progression of periodontal pockets and compromise the results to be expected from subsequent periodontal therapy. The removal of root tips can be accomplished from the facial or palatal surfaces without resulting in a reduction of alveolar ridge height or endangering adjacent teeth (Figs. 12-1 and 12-2).

Fig. 12-1. Retained root with associated bone resorption. (From Costich, E. R., and White, R. P., Jr.: Fundamentals of oral surgery, Philadelphia, 1971, W. B. Saunders Co.)

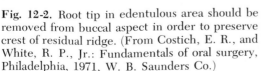

Fig. 12-2. Root tip in edentulous area should be removed from buccal aspect in order to preserve crest of residual ridge. (From Costich, E. R., and White, R. P., Jr.: Fundamentals of oral surgery, Philadelphia, 1971, W. B. Saunders Co.)

Fig. 12-3. Lateral oblique roentgenogram showing unerupted maxillary third molar and impacted mandibular second and third molars. Maxillary third molar and mandibular second molar could be contacted by a periodontal probe. (From Costich, E. R., and White, R. P., Jr.: Fundamentals of oral surgery, Philadelphia, 1971, W. B. Saunders Co.)

Impacted teeth

All impacted teeth should be considered for removal. This applies equally to impactions in edentulous areas as well as to those adjacent to abutment teeth. The periodontal implications of the latter are similar to those for retained roots. These teeth are often neglected until there are serious periodontal implications.

The skeletal structure of the body changes with age. Alterations that affect the jaws frequently result in minute exposures of impacted teeth to the oral cavity via sinus tracts. Resultant infections cause much bone destruction and serious illness for persons who are elderly and not physically able to tolerate the debilitation. Early elective removal of impactions prevents later serious acute and chronic infection with extensive bone loss. Any impacted teeth that can be reached with a periodontal probe must be removed to treat the periodontal pocket and prevent more extensive damage (Fig. 12-3).

Malposed teeth

The loss of individual teeth or groups of teeth may lead to supraeruption, mesial drifting, or combinations of malpositioning of remaining teeth. In most instances the alveolar bone supporting overly erupted teeth will be carried occlusally as the teeth continue to erupt, providing good support for the teeth that are out of harmony with the dental arches (Fig. 12-4, A). Orthodontics may be useful in correcting many occlusal discrepancies. But for some patients, such treatment may not be practical due to lack of teeth for anchorage of the orthodontic appliances or for other reasons. In such situations, individual teeth or groups of teeth and their supporting alveolar bone can be surgically repositioned. This type of surgery can be accomplished in an outpatient setting and should be given serious consideration before condemning additional teeth or compromising the design of removable partial dentures (Fig. 12-4, B).

Cysts and odontogenic tumors

Panoramic roentgenograms of the jaws are recommended to survey the jaws for unsuspected pathology. When a suspicious area appears on the survey film, a periapical radiograph should be taken to confirm or deny the presence of a lesion. All radiolucencies or radiopacities observed in the jaws should be investigated by biopsy. Although the diagnosis may appear obvious from clinical and radiographic examinations, the dentist should confirm his impression through submission of biopsy specimens to the pathologist for microscopic study. The patient should be assured of the diagnosis as well as the successful resolution of the abnormality as confirmed by the pathologist's report.

Exostoses and tori

The existence of abnormal bony enlargements should not be allowed to compromise the design of the removable partial denture. Although modification of denture design can, at times, accommodate for exostoses, more frequently this results in additional stress to the supporting elements and compromised function. The removal of exostoses and tori is not a complex procedure, and the advantages to be realized from such removal are great in contrast to the deleterious effects their continued presence can create (Fig. 12-5).

Fig. 12-4. A, Sequelae of unrestored partial edentulism. Maxillary premolars and first molar, unopposed for an extended period, have moved inferiorly to such an extent that little space remains between their occlusal surfaces and mandibular residual ridge at vertical dimension of occlusion. B, Results obtained by surgically repositioning supraerupted teeth and their supporting bone. Adequate space now exists between residual ridge and opposing teeth to construct a removable partial denture without compromising occlusal harmony. Maxillary first premolar will be replaced with fixed partial denture.

Fig. 12-5. A, Maxillary torus extending to junction of hard and soft palates. If torus is inoperable, its presence would require an undesirable horseshoe design major connector for the removable partial denture. B, Torus is exposed and readily visible and accessible for surgical removal. Design of major connector for removable restoration will not be compromised. C, Mandibular, lingual tori that should be surgically removed to avoid compromises in design of major connector for Class I removable partial denture. D, Sharp, mandibular lingual tuberosity. Removal of this bony projection should be accomplished three to four weeks prior to final impression procedures for a removable partial denture. Patient comfort during impression procedures and later use of the restoration are justifications for surgical removal of the sharp bony projection.

Ordinarily the mucosa covering bony protuberances is extremely thin and friable. Partial denture components in proximity to this type of tissue may cause irritation and chronic ulceration. Also, exostoses approximating gingival margins may complicate the maintenance of periodontal health and lead to the eventual loss of strategic abutment teeth.

The air-turbine handpiece is ideal for removing bony irregularities and is much easier to control than a mallet and chisel. The lower speeds (20,000 to 50,000 rpm) provide more torque and thus a better sense of feel for what is being cut. All handpieces used in surgery should be vented outside the mouth to prevent the complication of emphysema. In addition the assistant should provide copious irrigation to assure against thermal damage to the bone.

Hyperplastic tissue

Hyperplastic tissues are seen in the form of fibrous tuberosities, soft flabby ridges, folds of redundant tissue in the vestibule or floor of the mouth, and as palatal papillomatosis (Fig. 12-6). All these forms of excess tissue should be removed to provide a firm base for the denture. This will produce a more stable denture and reduce stress and strain on the supporting teeth and tissues. The appropriate surgical approaches should not reduce vestibular depth. Hyperplastic tissue can be removed with any preferred combination of scalpel, curette, or electrosurgery. Some form of surgical stent should always be considered for these patients so that the period of healing will be more comfortable for the patient. An old denture modified properly can serve as a surgical stent. Although hyperplastic tissue has no great malignant propensity, all such excised tissue should be sent to an oral pathologist for microscopic study.

Muscle attachments and freni

As a result of the loss of alveolar bone height, muscle attachments may insert on or near the alveolar crest. The mylohyoid, buccinator, mentalis, and genioglossus muscles are those most likely to introduce problems of this nature. In addition to the problem of the attachments of the muscles themselves, the mentalis and genioglossus muscles occasionally produce bony protuberances at their attachments that may also interfere with denture design. Appropriate ridge extension procedures can reposition attachments and remove bony spines, which will enhance the comfort and function of the removable partial denture.

Repositioning of the mylohyoid muscle is successfully achieved by several methods. The genioglossus muscle is more difficult to reposition, but careful surgery can reduce the prominence of the genial tubercles, as well as provide some sulcus depth in the anterior lingual area.

A

B

Fig. 12-6. **A,** Fibrous, unsupported maxillary tuberosities should be vertically reduced to provide supportive basal seat for denture. Stability and longevity of restoration will be enhanced by surgical procedures. **B,** Inflamed palatal papillary hyperplasia. Removal of palatal papillomatosis early in mouth preparation procedures is indicated so that complete healing can take place before final impressions are made in treatment of patient.

Surgical procedures using skin or mucosal grafts have largely replaced secondary epithelialization procedures for the facial aspect of the mandible. Mucosal grafts using the palate as a donor site offer the best possibility for success; transplanted skin can be used when large areas must be grafted.

The maxillary labial and mandibular lingual freni are probably the most frequent sources of frenum interference with denture design. These can be modified easily with any of several surgical procedures. Under no circumstances should a frenum be allowed to compromise the design or comfort of a removable partial denture.

Bony spines and knife-edge ridges

Sharp bony spicules should be removed and knifelike crests gently rounded. These procedures should be carried out with a minimal amount of bone loss. If, however, the correction of a knife-edge alveolar crest results in insufficient ridge support for the denture base, then the dentist should resort to vestibular deepening for correction of the deficiency or insertion of rib grafts.

Polyps, papilloma, and traumatic hemangiomas

All abnormal soft tissue lesions should be excised and submitted for pathologic examination prior to the fabrication of a removable partial denture. Even though the patient may relate a history of the condition's having been present for an indefinite period, its removal is indicated. New or additional stimulation to the area introduced by the prosthesis may produce discomfort or even malignant changes in the tumor.

Hyperkeratoses, erythroplasia, and ulcerations

All abnormal, white, red, or ulcerative lesions should be investigated, regardless of their relationship to the proposed denture base or framework. Incisional biopsy of areas larger than 5 mm should be completed, and if the lesions are large (over 2 cm in diameter), multiple biopsies should be taken. The biopsy report will determine whether the margins of the tissue to be excised can be wide or narrow. The lesions should be removed and healing accomplished before the denture is constructed. On occasion the denture design will have to be radically modified to avoid areas of possible sensitivity such as after irradiation for malignancy or the excoriations of erosive lichen planus.

Dentofacial deformity

Patients with a dentofacial deformity often have multiple missing teeth as part of their problem. Correction of the jaw deformity can simplify the dental rehabilitation. Before specific problems with the dentition can be corrected, the patient's overall problem must be evaluated thoroughly. Several dentists (prosthodontist, oral surgeon, periodontist, orthodontist, general dentist) may play a role in the patient's treatment. These individuals must be involved in producing the diagnostic data base and in planning treatment for the patient. Information obtained from a general patient evaluation to determine the patient's health status, a clinical evaluation directed toward facial esthetics and the status of the teeth and oral soft tissue, and an analysis of appropriate diagnostic records produce a data base. From this data base the patient's problems can be enumerated with the most severe problem being placed at the top of the list. Other identified problems would follow in the order of their severity. It is only after this step that input from several dentists can provide a final treatment plan for a patient.

Surgical correction of a jaw deformity can be made in horizontal, sagittal, or frontal planes. Mandibles and maxillae may be positioned anteriorly or posteriorly, and their relationship to the facial planes may be surgically altered to achieve improved appearance (Fig. 12-7). Replacement of missing teeth and development of a harmonious occlusion are most always a major problem in treating these patients.

PERIODONTAL PREPARATION*

The periodontal preparation of the mouth usually follows, or is performed simultaneously with, the oral surgical procedures employed in the treatment of the conditions described in the previous discussion. Ordinarily tooth extraction and removal of impacted teeth or retained roots or fragments are accomplished prior to definitive peri-

---

*Revision by Samuel B. Low, Department of Periodontics, College of Dentistry, University of Florida, Gainesville, Florida.

Fig. 12-7. **A,** Maxillary dental and skeletal deficiency leaves upper lip unsupported. **B,** Pretreatment dental relationships. **C,** Postsurgical relationship of opposing arches after maxillae were repositioned anteriorly and inferiorly. **D,** Profile of patient three years after surgery. Prosthodontic treatment consisted of both fixed and removable restorations.

odontal therapy. The elimination of exostoses, tori, hyperplastic tissue, muscle attachments, and freni, on the other hand, can be incorporated with periodontal surgical techniques. In any situation, periodontal therapy should be completed before restorative dentistry procedures are begun for any dental patient. This is particularly true when a removable partial denture is contemplated because the ultimate success of this restoration rests directly on the health and integrity of the supporting structures of the remaining teeth. The periodontal health of the remaining teeth then, especially those to be utilized as abutment teeth, must be evaluated carefully by the dentist and corrective measures instituted prior to partial denture construction.

This discussion will attempt to demonstrate how periodontal procedures affect diagnosis and treatment planning in a denture service rather than how the procedures are actually accomplished. For technical details the reader is referred to any of several excellent textbooks on periodontics.

Objectives of periodontal therapy

The overall objective of periodontal therapy is the return of health to the supporting and investing structures of the teeth so that the remaining dentition may be maintained in health, function, and comfort. The specific criteria by which the satisfaction of this objective is measured are as follows:

1. Removal of all etiologic factors responsible for periodontal changes

Fig. 12-8. **A,** Michigan-0 periodontal probe graduated in millimeters (top figure) and Nabers furcation probe (bottom figure). **B,** Periodontal probe inserted parallel to long axis of tooth on labial surface. **C,** Periodontal probe inserted parallel to long axis of tooth interproximally. **D,** Furcation probe detecting buccal furcation involvement.

2. Elimination of all pathologic pockets with the establishment of gingival sulci free of inflammation
3. Restoration of a physiologic gingival and osseous architecture
4. Establishment of a harmonious, functional occlusion
5. Maintenance of the result achieved by oral physiotherapy procedures and periodic recall visits to the dentist

At the very least the dentist considering partial denture construction should be certain that these criteria have been satisfied prior to proceeding with impression procedures for the master cast.

Periodontal diagnosis and treatment planning

Diagnosis. The diagnosis of periodontal disease results from a *clinical* procedure in which the dentist systematically and carefully inspects the periodontium for deviations from normal. It follows the procurement of the health history of the patient and is performed using direct vision, palpation, periodontal probe, mouth mirror, and other auxiliary aids such as curved explorers, diagnostic casts, and roentgenograms.

In the diagnostic procedure nothing is so important as the careful exploration of the gingival sulcus with a suitably designed instrument—the periodontal probe (Fig. 12-8). Under no circumstances should partial denture construction begin without an accurate appraisal of sulcus depth and health as provided by the use of the probe. The probe is inserted gently but firmly between the gingival margin and the tooth surface, and the depth of the sulcus is explored circumferentially around each tooth. A critical assessment of sulcular health by judging the amount of hemorrhage on probing is considered more important than the depth itself, for it is the recognition of the inflammatory disease process which mainly concerns the clinician.

Dental roentgenograms are used to supplement the clinical examination but cannot be used as a substitute for it. The extent and pattern of bone loss can be estimated

Fig. 12-9. Mobility can be visualized best when pressure is exerted on tooth through instrument handles. If fingers are used for this purpose, movement of soft tissue may mask accurate determination of mobility.

from roentgenograms, and this information serves to substantiate the impression gained from the clinical diagnosis.

Each tooth should be tested carefully for mobility (Fig. 12-9). The degree of mobility present coupled with a determination of the etiologic factor responsible provides additional information, which is invaluable in planning for the removable partial denture. If the etiologic factor can be removed, many mobile teeth will become stable and can be used successfully to help support and retain the partial denture. Mobility is not in itself an indication for extraction unless the mobile tooth cannot aid in the stability of the partial denture. In general a tooth that is important to the design of the partial denture and that has a mobility greater than 2 mm in a buccolingual direction requires immobilization via splinting.

Treatment planning. Depending on the extent and severity of the periodontal changes present, a variety of therapeutic procedures ranging from simple to relatively complex may be indicated. As was the case with the oral surgical procedures discussed, it is the responsibility of the dentist rendering the removable partial denture service to see that the required periodontal care is accomplished for his patient. Periodontal treatment planning can usually be divided into three phases. The first phase is considered disease control or initial therapy, for its objective is to essentially eliminate or reduce all the local etiologic factors and environ-

mental influences prior to periodontal surgery and restorative dentistry. These procedures include oral hygiene instruction, scaling and planing (curettage), occlusal adjustment, and so forth.

During the second phase, general therapy is administered as periodontal surgery and restorative dentistry. All procedures for maintaining periodontal health are provided in the third phase of therapy considered as the recall or maintenance phase.

Initial disease control therapy (phase 1)

Oral hygiene instruction. Ordinarily dental treatment should be introduced to the patient through instruction in a carefully devised oral hygiene regimen. The cooperation witnessed by the patient's acceptance and compliance with the prescribed procedure, as evidenced by improved oral hygiene, will provide the dentist with a valuable means of evaluating his interest and the long-term prognosis of treatment.

For the oral physiotherapy routine to be successful, the patient must be motivated to follow the prescribed procedure regularly and conscientiously. The most effective motivation is based on the patient's understanding of dental disease and the benefits to be derived from the procedures advocated. Hence an explanation of dental disease, its etiology, initiation, and progression, is an important component of oral physiotherapy instruction. After this discussion the patient should be instructed in the use of disclosing wafers, soft nylon toothbrush, and unwaxed dental floss (Fig. 12-10). At subsequent appointments oral hygiene can be evaluated carefully, and further treatment should be withheld until a satisfactory level has been achieved (Fig. 12-11). This is a particularly critical point for the patient requiring extensive restorative dentistry or a removable partial denture. Without good oral hygiene any dental procedure, regardless of how well it is performed, is ultimately doomed to failure. The wise dentist insists that acceptable oral hygiene be demonstrated and maintained prior to embarking on an extensive restorative dentistry treatment plan.

Scaling and root planing. One of the most important services rendered to the patient is the removal of calculus and plaque deposits from the coronal and root surfaces of the teeth. Scaling and root planing compromise

Fig. 12-10. Standard oral hygiene armamentarium prescribed includes disclosing wafers; soft nylon toothbrush; and unwaxed dental floss. Supplementary hygiene aids may be recommended for those patients with special needs.

Fig. 12-11. Tissue response to poor oral hygiene procedures. Note bulbous papillae in interproximal areas of mandibular anterior teeth. Favorable tissue response in same patient to effective oral hygiene procedures only (one month). Especially noticeable is reduction of inflamed and edematous interdental papillae.

Fig. 12-12. Basic set of curettes for calculus removal and root planing. **A,** 3-4 Gracey for anterior teeth. **B,** 11-12 Gracey for mesial surfaces of posterior teeth. **C,** 13-14 Gracey for distal surfaces of posterior teeth. **D,** Columbia 4R-4L as a universal instrument.

the definitive treatment for periodontal disease. Without meticulous calculus, plaque, and necrotic cementum removal no other form of periodontal therapy can be successful.

Although some of the new ultrasonic instruments may be helpful in calculus removal, hand instrumentation remains the treatment of choice for definitive debridement. The curette is the best designed hand instrument for scaling and root planing (Fig. 12-12). Thorough calculus removal precedes other forms of periodontal therapy that must be completed prior to impression procedures for the removable partial denture.

Elimination of local irritating factors other than calculus. Overhanging margins (of amalgam alloy and inlay restorations), overhanging crown margins, and open contacts leading to food impaction should be corrected before definitive prosthetic treatment is begun. Although periodontal health predisposes to a much better environment for restorative correction, it is not always possible to delay all restorative procedures until complete periodontal therapy and healing have occurred. This is especially true for patients with deep-seated carious lesions, for whom pulpal exposures are a possibility. Excavation of these areas and placement of adequate restorations must be incorporated early in treatment. Amalgam restorations are far superior to the cements in treating these patients, since the margins can be controlled and the possibility of washouts is eliminated. The placement of temporary or treatment fillings must not, in itself, become a local etiologic factor.

Elimination of gross occlusal interferences. Oral accretions and poor restorative dentistry cause damage to the periodontium, as also may poor occlusal relationships. Although occlusal interferences may be eliminated by a variety of techniques, at this stage of treatment selective grinding is the procedure generally applied. Particular attention is directed to the occlusal relationships of mobile teeth. Traumatic cuspal interferences are removed by a judicious grinding procedure. An attempt is made to establish a positive centric occlusion that coincides with centric relation. Deflective contacts in the centric path of closure are removed, eliminating mandibular displacement from the closing pattern. After this the relationship of the teeth in the various excursive movements of the mandible are observed, with special attention to cuspal contact, wear, mobility, and radiographic changes in the periodontium. Interferences on both the working and nonworking sides should be observed and, if present, removed.

The mere presence of occlusal abnormalities in the absence of demonstrable pathologic change associated with the occlusion does not necessarily constitute an indication for the grinding procedure. The indication for occlusal adjustment is based on the presence of pathology rather than on a preconceived articular pattern. In the natural dentition the attempt to create bilateral balance, in the prosthetic sense, has no place in the occlusal adjustment procedure. Balanced occlusion not only is impossible to obtain on natural dentition but also is apparently unnecessary in view of its absence in most normal healthy mouths. Occlusion on natural teeth needs to be perfected only to a point at which cuspal interference within the patient's functional range of contact is eliminated and normal physiologic function can occur.

Guide to occlusal adjustment. Schuyler has provided the following guide to occlusal adjustment by selective grinding:

In the study or evaluation of occlusal disharmony of the natural dentition, accurately mounted diagnostic casts are extremely helpful, if not essential, in determining static cusp to fossae contacts of opposing teeth and as a guide in the correction of occlusal anomalies in both centric and eccentric functional relations. Occlusion can be coordinated only by selective spot grinding. Ground tooth surfaces should be subsequently smoothed and polished.

1. A static coordinated occlusal contact of the maximum number of teeth when the mandible is in centric relation to the maxillae should be our first objective.

    a. A prematurely contacting cusp should be reduced only if the cusp point is in premature contact in both centric and eccentric relations. If a cusp point is in premature contact in the centric relation only, the opposing sulcus should be deepened.

    b. When anterior teeth are in premature contact in centric relation, or in both centric and eccentric relations, corrections should be made by grinding the incisal edge of the lower teeth. If premature contact occurs only in the eccentric relation, correction must be made by grinding the lingual incline of the upper teeth.

c. Usually, premature contacts in the centric relation are relieved by grinding the buccal cusps of the lower teeth, the lingual cusp of upper teeth, and the incisal edges of the lower anterior teeth. In deepening the sulcus of a posterior tooth or the lingual contact area in centric relation of an upper anterior tooth, we change and increase the steepness of the eccentric guiding inclines of the tooth; although we relieve trauma in the centric relation, we may predispose the tooth to trauma in eccentric relations.

2. After establishing a static, even distribution of stress over the maximum number of teeth in the centric relation, we are ready to evaluate opposing tooth contact or lack of contact in eccentric functional relations. Our attention is directed first to balancing side contacts. In extreme cases of pathologic balancing contacts, relief may be needed even before the corrective procedures in the centric relation. Where balancing contacts exist, it is extremely difficult to differentiate the harmless from the destructive because we cannot visualize the influence of these fulcrum contacts on the functional movements of the condyle in the articular fossa. Subluxation, pain, lack of normal functional movement of the joint, or loss of alveolar support of the teeth involved may be evidence of excessive balancing contacts. Balancing side contacts receive less frictional wear than working side contacts, and premature contacts may develop progressively with wear. A reduction in the steepness of the guiding tooth inclines on the working side will increase the proximity of the teeth on the balancing side and may contribute to destructive prematurities. In all corrective grinding to relieve premature or excessive contacts in eccentric relations, care must be exercised to avoid the loss of a static supporting contact in the centric relation. This static support in centric relation may exist between the lower buccal cusp fitting into the central fossae of the upper tooth or between the upper lingual cusp fitting into the central fossae of the lower tooth or may exist in both cases. While both the upper lingual cusp and the lower buccal cusp may sometimes have a static centric contact in the sulcus of the opposing tooth, often only one of these cusps has this static contact. In such instances the contacting cusp must be left untouched to maintain this essential support in centric occlusion, and all corrective grinding to relieve premature contacts in eccentric positions would be done on the opposing tooth inclines. The lower buccal cusp is in a static central contact in the upper sulcus more often than the upper lingual cusp is in a static contact in its opposing lower sulcus. Therefore corrective grinding to relieve premature balancing contacts is more often done on the upper lingual cusps.

3. To obtain maximum function and the distribution of functional stress in eccentric positions on the working side, necessary grinding must be done on the lingual surfaces of the upper anterior teeth. Corrective grinding on the posterior teeth at this time should always be done on the buccal cusp of the upper premolars and molars and on the lingual cusp of the lower premolars and molars. The grinding of lower buccal cusps or upper lingual cusps at this time would rob these cusps of their static contact in the opposing central sulci in centric relation.

4. Corrective grinding to relieve premature protrusive contacts of one or more anterior teeth should be accomplished by grinding the lingual surface of the upper anterior teeth. Anterior teeth should never be ground to bring the posterior teeth into contact in either protrusive position or on the balancing side. In the elimination of premature protrusive contacts of posterior teeth, neither the upper lingual cusps nor the lower buccal cusps should be ground. Corrective grinding should be done on the surface of the opposing teeth on which these cusps function in the eccentric position, leaving the centric contact undisturbed.

5. Any sharp edges left by grinding should be rounded off.*

Temporary splinting. Teeth that are mobile at the time of the initial examination frequently present a diagnostic problem for

---

*Courtesy Dr. C. H. Schuyler, Montclair, N.J.

Fig. 12-13. An **A** splint used to stabilize a mobile anterior segment. Markley pins embedded in plastic filling material in dovetail preparations on lingual surfaces. (Courtesy Dr. Daniel R. Trinler, Lexington, Ky.)

Fig. 12-14. Removable acrylic resin splint with flat occlusal plane can be used effectively as a form of temporary stabilization and as a means of eliminating excessive lateral forces created by clenching and grinding habits.

the dentist. Their response to temporary immobilization may be helpful in establishing a prognosis for them and may lead to a rational decision as to whether they should be retained or sacrificed. Mobility due to the presence of an inflammatory lesion may be reversible if the disease process has not destroyed too much of the attachment apparatus. Mobility caused by occlusal interference also may disappear after selective grinding. In some cases, however, the teeth must be stabilized because of loss of supporting structure from the periodontal process.

Teeth may be immobilized during periodontal treatment by interdental wiring with acrylic resin splints, with cast removable splints, or with intracoronal attachments (Fig. 12-13). The latter, an example of which is the **A** splint, necessitates cutting tooth surfaces and embedding a ridge connector between adjacent teeth.

After periodontal treatment, splinting may be accomplished with cast removable restorations or cast cemented restorations. The preferred form of permanent splinting is with two or more cast restorations soldered or cast together. They may be cemented with either permanent (zinc oxyphosphate or resin) cements or temporary (zinc oxide–eugenol) cements. A properly designed removable partial denture can also stabilize mobile teeth if provision for such immobilization is planned as the denture is designed.

Use of nightguard. The removable acrylic resin splint, originally designed as an aid in eliminating the deleterious effects of nocturnal clenching and grinding, has been used to advantage for the removable partial denture patient. The nightguard may be helpful as a form of temporary splinting if worn at night when the partial denture has been removed. The flat occlusal surface prevents the interdigitation of the teeth, which eliminates lateral occlusal forces (Fig. 12-14).

The nightguard is particularly useful prior to the fabrication of a partial denture when one of the abutment teeth has been unopposed for an extended period of time. The periodontium of a tooth without an antagonist undergoes deterioration characterized by a loss of orientation of periodontal ligament fibers, loss of supporting bone, and narrowing of the periodontal membrane space. If such a tooth is suddenly returned to full function when it is carrying an increased burden, pain and prolonged sensitivity may result. If, however, a nightguard is used to return some functional stimulation to the tooth, the periodontal changes are reversed and an uneventful course is experienced when the tooth is returned to full function.

Minor tooth movement. The increased utilization of orthodontic procedures in conjunction with restorative and prosthetic dentistry has contributed to the success of many restorations by altering the periodontal climate in which they are placed. Malposed teeth that were once doomed to extraction

Fig. 12-15. Tooth movement used to upright a tilted molar tooth to prepare the segment for receipt of a pontic. **A,** Placement of orthodontic appliance. **B,** Space gained after three months' active movement.

should be considered now for repositioning and retention. The additional stability provided for a removable partial denture from uprighting a tilted or drifted tooth may mean much in terms of comfort to the patient. The techniques employed are not difficult to master, and the rewards in terms of a better restorative dentistry service are great (Fig. 12-15).

General therapy (phase 2)

Periodontal surgery. After initial therapy subsides, the patient is reevaluated for the general treatment phase. If oral hygiene is at an optimum level, yet sulcular depth and inflammation have not resolved, then a variety of periodontal surgical techniques can be employed to advantage in satisfying the objectives of periodontal therapy for the removable partial denture patient. These are largely directed at the elimination of the periodontal pocket, the lesion pathognomonic of

periodontal disease, and at a return of physiologic architecture to the area.

Pocket elimination may be achieved by shrinkage, surgical excision, and new attachment procedures. Of these, surgical excision presents the therapist with the most predictable result. Surgical procedures also afford the opportunity for recreating a physiologic architectural pattern, and hence much periodontal therapy is surgical in nature. However, one must keep in mind that elimination of the inflammatory disease process, not just sulcular depth, is the major objective of periodontal surgery.

Gingivectomy. This form of surgical therapy is one of the oldest excision-type procedures and is one that has been used widely for years. When the gingivectomy is indicated, it satisfies the objectives previously stated for periodontal therapy. However, as periodontics has experienced greater refinement in recent years and as the requirements for successful treatment have expanded, situations in which the gingivectomy alone will suffice have been greatly reduced to a minimum.

The gingivectomy is indicated when the following conditions are present (Fig. 12-16):
1. Suprabony pockets of fibrotic tissue
2. Absence of deformities in the underlying bony tissue
3. Pocket depth confined to the band of attached gingiva

If osseous deformities are present or if pocket depth traverses or approximates the mucogingival junction, the gingivectomy is *not* the procedure of choice. The gingivectomy technique is best accomplished with appropriate cutting instruments. However, gingivoplasty or reshaping of the gingiva can also be performed with electrosurgery and assorted diamond stones.

Because most patients with moderate to advanced periodontal disease have experienced various degrees of bone loss, the gingivectomy alone can only rarely reestablish the desired physiologic architecture. For that reason more complex forms of treatment, including osseous and mucogingival surgery, have been developed as periodontics has entered an era of plastic and reconstructive surgery.

Periodontal flap. Today the apically repositioned flap is the periodontal surgical procedure of greatest versatility and, conse-

Fig. 12-16. A, Preoperative photograph of patient with pocket depth in anterior segment. Tissue is fibrotic, and pocket depth is confined within band of attached gingiva. **B,** Roentgenograph confirms clinical impression of minimal bone loss and acceptable bony topography. **C,** Immediate gingivectomy view of mandibular anterior segment. Frenectomy is included in operative procedure. **D,** Appearance of maxillary and mandibular anterior segments approximately three months after gingivectomy procedures.

Fig. 12-17. A, Preoperative condition with pocket depth traversing mucogingival junction, osseous deformities and carious lesions extending beneath gingival margin. **B,** Gingival flap repositioned after osseous correction and crown-lengthening procedure on mandibular right canine tooth. **C,** Permanent splint with provision for removable partial denture. (Courtesy Dr. Keith Brooks, Lexington, Ky.)

Fig. 12-18. A, Preoperative view of mandibular second premolar with inadequate zone of attached gingiva and pocket depth traversing mucogingival junction. **B,** Pedicle graft sutured into position. **C,** Postoperative view showing new zone of attached gingiva with no pocket depth present.

quently, is widely applied in the treatment of periodontal disease (Fig. 12-17). Several healing studies have contributed to a greater understanding of periodontal therapy, and because of these, emphasis is currently placed on closure of the surgical area by various flap techniques.

Indications for the repositioned flap are as follows:

1. Pocket depth traversing the mucogingival junction
2. Presence of osseous deformities that must be corrected to eliminate the

Fig. 12-19. **A,** Preoperative condition showing patient with no attached gingiva on buccal of mandibular secondar premolar. **B,** Operative site with free gingival graft in place. **C,** New zone of attached gingiva nine weeks postoperatively.

pocket and restore physiologic architecture
3. Muscle or frenum attachment at the gingival margin

Adjunctive procedures. In addition to the apically repositioned flap, other adjunctive mucogingival surgical techniques have added to the armamentarium of the therapist in eliminating periodontal disease and in the preparation of the mouth for restorative and

prosthetic dentistry. Among these are lateral sliding flaps, pedicle grafts (Fig. 12-18), and free gingival grafts (Fig. 12-19). These procedures have particular application in the reestablishment of an adequate zone of attached gingiva around abutments for the removable partial denture and require at least 2 mm of attached gingiva to preserve gingival health.

Recall maintenance (phase 3)

Several longitudinal studies have now demonstrated the increasing importance of maintenance for all patients who have undergone any periodontal therapy. This not only includes reinforcement of plaque control measures, but also thorough debridement of all root surfaces of supragingival and subgingival calculus and plaque by the dentist or his auxiliary.

The frequency of recall appointments should be customized for the patient depending on susceptibility and severity of periodontal disease. It is now conceivable that patients with previous moderate to severe periodontitis should be placed on a 3- to 4-month recall system.

Advantages of periodontal therapy

Periodontal therapy prior to the fabrication of a removable prosthesis has several advantages. First the elimination of periodontal disease removes a primary etiologic factor in tooth loss. The long-term success of dental treatment is dependent on the maintenance of the remaining oral structures, and periodontal health is mandatory if further loss is to be avoided. Second a periodontium free of disease presents a much better environment for restorative correction. The elimination of periodontal pockets with the associated return of a physiologic architectural pattern establishes a normal gingival contour at a stable position on the root surface. Thus the optimum position for gingival margins of individual restorations can be established with accuracy. The coronal contours of these restorations also can be developed in correct relationships to the gingival margin, assuring the proper degree of protection and functional stimulation to the gingival tissues. Third the response of strategic but questionable teeth to periodontal therapy provides an important opportunity for reevaluating their prognosis before the final decision is made to include (or exclude) them in the partial den-

Fig. 12-20. A, Fractured first premolar tooth after endodontic therapy. **B,** Periodontal partial thickness flap retracted for access and apical repositioning of gingival margin. **C,** Appearance of tooth after healing and preparation to receive crown. **D,** Restoration in place, splinted to canine tooth, to act as abutment for removable partial denture.

ture design. And last the overall reaction of the patient to periodontal procedures provides the dentist with an excellent indication of the degree of cooperation to be expected in the future.

Even in the absence of periodontal disease, periodontal procedures may be an invaluable aid in partial denture construction. Through periodontal surgical techniques the environment of potential abutment teeth may be altered to the point of making an otherwise unacceptable tooth a most satisfactory retainer for a partial denture. The lengthening of a clinical crown through the removal of gingival tissue and bone is a common example of the application of periodontal surgical techniques as an aid in partial denture construction (Fig. 12-20).

ABUTMENT TEETH

Abutment restorations. Equipped with the diagnostic casts on which a tentative partial denture design has been drawn, the dentist is able to accomplish preparation of abut-

ment teeth with accuracy. The information at hand should include the proposed path of placement, the areas of teeth to be disked and tooth contours to be changed, and the location of rests.

During examination and subsequent treatment planning, in conjunction with a survey of diagnostic casts, each abutment tooth is considered individually as to whether full coverage is indicated. Abutment teeth presenting sound enamel surfaces in a mouth in which good oral hygiene habits are evident may be considered a fair risk for use as partial denture abutments. One should not be misled, however, by a patient's promise to do better as far as oral hygiene habits are concerned. Good or bad oral hygiene is a habit of long standing and is not likely to be changed appreciably because a partial denture is being worn. Therefore one must be conservative in evaluating the oral hygiene habits of the patient in the future. It is well to remember that clasps as such do not cause teeth to decay, and if the individual will keep the teeth and the partial denture clean, one need not condemn clasps from a cariogenic standpoint. On the other hand, more partial dentures have been condemned as cariogenic because the dentist did not provide for the protection of abutment teeth than because of inadequate care on the part of the patient.

The full cast gold crown is objectionable from an esthetic standpoint, and therefore the veneer type of full crown must be resorted to when a canine or premolar abutment is to be restored or protected. Less frequently does the molar have to be treated in such a manner, and except for maxillary first molars the full gold crown is usually acceptable.

When there is proximal caries on abutment teeth with sound buccal and lingual enamel surfaces, in a mouth exhibiting average oral hygiene and low caries activity, a gold inlay is usually indicated. Silver amalgam for the restoration of proximal caries should not be condemned, however, although one must admit that an inlay cast of a hard-type gold will provide the best possible support for occlusal rests, at the same time giving an esthetically pleasing restoration. But an amalgam restoration, properly condensed, is capable of supporting an occlusal rest without appreciable flow over a long period of time.

The most vulnerable area on the abutment tooth is the proximal gingival area, which lies beneath the minor connector of the partial denture framework and is therefore subject to the lodgment of debris in an area most susceptible to caries attack. Even when the partial denture is removed for cleaning the teeth, these areas, especially those on the distal surface of an anterior abutment, are often missed by the toothbrush, and bacterial plaques and debris are allowed to remain for long periods of time. Except in a caries-immune mouth or in a mouth in which the teeth are subjected to meticulous brushing, decalcification and caries frequently occur in this region. It is therefore necessary that this area of the tooth be fully protected by whatever restoration is used. When an inlay restoration is used, the preparation should be carried to or beneath the gingival margin and well out onto the buccal and lingual surfaces to afford the best possible protection to the abutment tooth. Even the full crown can be deficient in this most vulnerable area, which lies at and just above the gingival mar-

gin. The full crown, which is cast short of this area, will not afford protection where it is most needed.

All proximal tooth surfaces that are to serve as guiding planes for the partial denture should be disked so that they will be made as nearly as possible parallel to the path of placement. This is accomplished on sound enamel or on existing restoration by disking those tooth surfaces parallel to the path of placement, and the same can be done for the recently placed full crown or inlay.

Contouring wax patterns. Modern indirect techniques using hydrocolloid or rubber base impression materials permit the contouring of wax patterns on the stone abutments with the aid of the surveyor blade. All abutment teeth to be restored with castings can be prepared at one time and an impression made that will provide an accurate stone replica of the prepared arch. Wax patterns may then be refined on separated individual dies or removable dies. All tooth surfaces facing edentulous areas should be made parallel to the path of placement by the use of the surveyor blade. This will provide proximal tooth surfaces that will be parallel without any further disking in the mouth, will permit the most positive seating of the partial denture along the path of placement, and will provide the least amount of undesirable space beneath minor connectors for the lodgment of debris.

Rest seats. After the proximal surfaces of the wax patterns have been made parallel and buccal and lingual contours have been established, which will satisfy the requirements of retention with the best possible esthetic placement of clasp arms, the occlusal rest seats should be prepared in the wax pattern rather than in the finished gold restoration. The placement of occlusal rests should be considered at the time the teeth are prepared to receive cast restorations so that there will be sufficient clearance beneath the floor of the occlusal rest seat. Too many times we see a completed gold restoration cemented in the mouth for a partial denture abutment without any provision for the occlusal rest having been made in the wax pattern. The dentist then proceeds to cut an occlusal rest seat in the gold restoration, being ever conscious of the fact that he may perforate the gold during the process of forming the rest seat. The unfortunate result is usually a poorly formed rest seat that is too shallow and does not incline toward the center of the tooth in the desired manner.

If tooth structure has been removed to provide for the placement of the occlusal rest seat, it may be ideally placed in the wax pattern by using a No. 8 round bur to lower the marginal ridge and to establish the outline form of the rest and then using a No. 6 round bur to deepen slightly the floor of the rest seat inside this lowered marginal ridge. This provides for an occlusal rest that best satisfies the requirements that the rest be placed so that any occlusal force will be directed axially and that there will be the least possible interference to occlusion with the opposing teeth.

Perhaps the most important function of a rest is the division of stress loads to the partial denture to provide for greatest efficiency with the least damaging effect to the abutment teeth. For a distal extension partial denture the rest must be able to transmit occlusal forces to the abutment teeth in a vertical direction only, thereby permitting the least possible lateral stresses to be transmitted to the abutment tooth.

For this reason the floor of the rest seat should incline toward the center of the tooth so that the occlusal forces, insofar as possible, are centered over the root apex. Any other form but that of a spoon shape permits a locking of the occlusal rest and the transmission of tipping forces to the abutment tooth. A ball-and-socket type of relationship between occlusal rest and abutment tooth is the most desirable. At the same time, the marginal ridge must be lowered so that the angle formed by the occlusal rest with the minor connector will stand above the occlusal surface of the abutment tooth as little as possible and avoid interference with the opposing teeth. Simultaneously, sufficient bulk must be provided for to prevent a weakness in the occlusal rest at the marginal ridge. The marginal ridge must be lowered and yet not be the deepest part of the rest preparation. To permit occlusal stresses to be directed toward the center of the abutment tooth, the angle formed by the floor of the occlusal rest with the minor connector should be less than 90 degrees. In other words, the floor of the occlusal rest should incline slightly from the lowered marginal ridge toward the center of the tooth.

This proper form can be readily accomplished in the wax pattern if care is taken during crown or inlay preparation to provide for the location of the rest. If an amalgam restoration is used, sufficient bulk must be present in this area to allow proper occlusal rest seat form without weakening the restoration. When the rest seat is placed in sound enamel, it is best accomplished by the use of round diamond points of approximately No. 4, 6, and 8 sizes in the following sequence. First the larger of the diamonds is used to lower the marginal ridge and at the same time create the relative outline form of the rest seat. The result is a rest seat preparation with marginal ridge lowered and gross outline form established but without sufficient deepening of the rest seat preparation toward the center of the tooth. The smaller diamond points or a carbide bur of approximately No. 4 or 6 size may then be used to deepen the floor of the rest seat to a gradual incline toward the center of the tooth. Enamel rods are then smoothed by the planing action of a round bur revolving with little pressure. Abrasive rubber points, followed by the use of wet flour of pumice on a stiff bristle brush, are sufficient to complete the polishing of the rest seat preparation.

Rest seat preparations in existing restorations or on abutment teeth where no restorations are to be placed should always follow, not precede, the disking of proximal tooth surfaces. The disking of proximal tooth surfaces should be done first because if the occlusal portion of the rest seat is placed first and the proximal tooth surface is disked later, the outline form of the rest seat is sometimes irreparably altered.

The success or failure of a removable partial denture may well depend on how well the mouth preparations were accomplished. It is only through intelligent planning and competent execution of mouth preparations that the denture can satisfactorily restore lost dental functions and contribute to the health of the remaining oral tissues.

SELF-ASSESSMENT AIDS

1. A prescribed prosthesis not only must replace what is missing but also, of even greater importance, must _____ what is remaining.
2. Preparation of oral structures most often involves three categories. One of these categories is oral surgical preparation. What are the other two?
3. Which treatment should be accomplished first—oral surgery or preparation of abutment teeth? Why?

4. Generally all retained roots or root fragments should be removed as a mouth preparation procedure. True or false?

5. All impacted teeth should be considered for removal. However, any impacted tooth that can be reached with a periodontal probe must be removed. True or false?

6. Unapposed posterior teeth quite often overly erupt, severely limiting space for a prosthesis and the opportunity to create a harmonious occlusion. Name different methods by which these discrepancies may be corrected, depending of course on the severity of the malpositions.

7. You are viewing a panoramic radiograph of a patient and you see a suspicious radiopaque area. What procedures, listed in chronologic order, would you undertake to resolve the possible problem?

8. Visual examination, carefully conducted, reveals undesirable bony exostoses or tori in some patients. Unless these are removed, the design of the restoration will be compromised. In what areas are these various protuberances likely to be found?

9. Why should hyperplastic tissues seen in the form of fibrous tuberosities, flabby ridges, folds of redundant tissue in vestibular regions, and palatal papillomatosis be surgically removed prior to the construction of a removable restoration?

10. Discuss the influence of muscle attachments and freni that are inserted on the crest of residual ridges in relation to denture stability.

11. Should all abnormal soft tissue lesions be excised and submitted for pathologic examination prior to fabrication of a removable restoration?

12. Periodontal therapy should be completed before restorative procedures are undertaken. True or false?

13. What is the overall objective of periodontal therapy for the partially edentulous patient?

14. The indication for occlusal adjustment is based on the presence of pathology rather than on a preconceived articular pattern. Can you support and explain this statement?

15. What procedure(s) is most often used to eliminate gross occlusal interferences initially as a phase of periodontal considerations?

16. What is a nightguard and what purpose does it serve?

17. Teeth that demonstrate mobility at the time of the initial examination may be temporarily splinted. How does this help to establish a prognosis?

18. Under what clinical circumstances should minor tooth movement by orthodontic means be considered to enhance treatment?

19. Can you give at least four distinct advantages of performing periodontal therapy (when indicated) prior to fabricating a removable prosthesis?

20. It is only through intelligent planning and competent execution of mouth preparations that the denture can satisfactorily restore lost dental functions and contribute to the health of the remaining oral tissues. True or false?

13 PREPARATION OF ABUTMENT TEETH

After surgery, periodontal treatment, and any endodontic treatment of the arch involved, the abutment teeth then may be prepared to provide support, stabilization, reciprocation, and retention for the partial denture.

Endodontic treatment of any teeth elsewhere in the arch, as well as abutment teeth, should precede the making of the partial denture, so that the success of treatment can be reasonably well established before proceeding. Similarly, favorable response to any deep restorations and the results of periodontal treatment should be established prior to construction of the denture, since if the prognosis of a tooth under treatment becomes unfavorable, its loss can be compensated for by a change in the denture design. The condemned tooth or teeth may then be included in the original denture design, whereas if they are lost subsequently, the partial denture must be added to, remade, or replaced. Many partial denture designs do not lend themselves well to later additions, although this eventuality should be considered in the design of a denture.

Particularly when the tooth in question will be used as an abutment, every diagnostic aid should be used to determine the success of previous treatment. It is usually not so difficult to add a tooth or teeth to a partial denture as it is to add a retaining unit when the original abutment is lost and the next adjacent tooth must be used for that purpose.

It is sometimes possible to design a removable partial denture so that a single posterior abutment about which there is some doubt can be retained and utilized as one end of a tooth-supported base. Then, if that posterior abutment is lost, it can be replaced with a distal extension base. Such a design will include provision for future indirect retention and flexible clasping on the future

terminal abutment. Anterior abutments, which are considered to be poor risks, may not be so freely used because of the problems involved in adding a new abutment retainer when the original one is lost. It is rational that such questionable teeth be condemned in favor of a better abutment, even though the original treatment plan must be modified accordingly.

CLASSIFICATION OF ABUTMENT TEETH

The subject of abutment preparations may be grouped as follows: (1) those abutment teeth that are to be used in their present state, (2) those that are to have cast inlays, and (3) those that are to have cast crowns. The latter group includes abutments for fixed partial dentures, since inlay retainers are not commonly used for such restorations.

Abutment teeth to be used in their present state include teeth with sound enamel, those having small restorations not involved in the denture design, those having acceptable restorations that will be involved in the denture design, and those having existing crown restorations. The latter may exist either as an individual crown or as the abutment of a fixed restoration.

The use of unprotected abutments has been discussed previously. Although full protection of all abutments is desirable, it is not always possible or practical to do so. The decision to use unprotected abutments involves certain risks of which the patient must be advised, including his own responsibility for maintaining oral hygiene and caries control. The making of crown restorations to fit existing denture clasps is an art in itself, which will be covered later in this chapter, but the fact that it is possible to do so may influence the decision to use uncrowned but otherwise sound teeth as abutments.

Preferably, silver amalgam alloy should not be used for the support of occlusal rests because of its tendency to flow. Although cast gold will provide the best possible support for occlusal rests, an amalgam alloy restoration, properly condensed, is capable of supporting an occlusal rest without appreciable flow over a long period of time. If the patient's economic status or other factors beyond the control of the dentist prevent the use of cast restorations, any existing silver amalgam alloy fillings about which there is any doubt should be replaced with new amalgam restorations. This should be done far enough in advance of disking and the preparation of occlusal rest seats to permit aging and polishing of the restoration.

SEQUENCE OF ABUTMENT PREPARATIONS ON SOUND ENAMEL OR EXISTING RESTORATIONS

Abutment preparations on either sound enamel or existing restorations should be done in the following order:

1. The disking of proximal surfaces parallel to the path of placement to provide guiding planes (Fig. 13-1, *A*). The term *disking* is used in a broad sense and refers to the paralleling of proximal surfaces by the use of abrasive instruments. With ultra speeds, parallelism can frequently be accomplished as well or better by the use of cylindric diamond points moved buccolingually across the proximal surface. The term disking may ultimately be replaced by terminology descriptive of modern cutting methods.

2. The reduction of excessive tooth contours (Fig. 13-1, *B* and *C*), thereby lowering the height of contours so that (a) the origin of circumferential clasp arms may be placed well below the occlusal surface, preferably at the junction of the gingival and middle thirds; (b) retentive clasp terminals may be placed in the gingival third of the crown, for better esthetics and better mechanical advantage; and (c) reciprocal clasp arms may be placed on and above a height of contour that is no higher than the cervical portion of the middle third of the crown of the abutment tooth.

3. *After alterations of axial contours are believed accomplished and before rest seat preparations are instituted, an impression of*

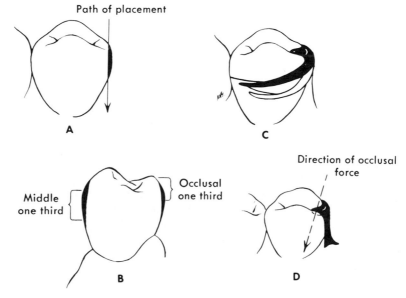

Fig. 13-1. Abutment contours should be altered during mouth preparations in the following sequence. **A,** Proximal surface is disked parallel to path of placement to create a guiding plane. **B,** Height of contour on buccal and lingual surfaces is lowered when necessary to permit retentive clasp terminus to be located within gingival third of crown and reciprocal clasp arm on opposite side of tooth to be placed no higher than cervical portion of middle third of crown. **C,** Area of tooth at which a retentive clasp arm originates should be altered if necessary to permit more direct approach to gingival third of tooth. **D,** An occlusal rest preparation that will direct occlusal forces along long axis of tooth should be final step in mouth preparations.

the arch should be made in irreversible hydrocolloid and a cast poured in a fast-setting stone. This cast can be returned to the surveyor to determine the adequacy of axial alterations before proceeding with rest seat preparations. If axial surfaces require additional axial recontouring, it can be performed during the same appointment and without compromise.

4. The preparation of occlusal rest areas that will direct occlusal forces along the long axis of the abutment tooth (Fig. 13-1, *D*).

Mouth preparation should follow a plan that was outlined on the diagnostic cast in red pencil at the time the cast was surveyed and also follow the design of the partial denture outlined. Better still, proposed changes to abutment teeth actually may be made on the diagnostic cast and *outlined* in red pencil to indicate not only the area but also the *amount* and *angulation* of the disking to be done (Chapter 11). Although occlusal rest seats also may be prepared on the diagnostic cast, indication of their *location* in red pencil is usually sufficient for the experienced dentist, since rest preparations follow a definite pattern (Chapter 5).

ABUTMENT PREPARATIONS USING CAST INLAYS

Inlay preparations on teeth to be used as removable partial denture abutments differ from conventional inlay preparations in the amount of protection afforded the tooth, the width of the preparation at the occlusal rest, and the depth of the preparation beneath the occlusal rest.

Conventional inlay preparations are permissible on the proximal surface of the tooth not to be contacted by a minor connector of the partial denture. On the other hand, proximal and occlusal surfaces supporting minor connectors and occlusal rests require somewhat different treatment than the conventional inlay preparation. The extent of occlusal coverage (that is, whether or not cusps are capped) will be governed by the usual factors, such as the extent of caries, the presence of unsupported enamel walls, and the extent of occlusal abrasion and attrition.

Of primary consideration in the preparation of proximal inlays that will lie beneath minor connectors is the amount of protection afforded vulnerable areas by the inlay. The most vulnerable area on the abutment tooth is the proximal gingival area lying beneath

the minor connector of the partial denture because of accumulation of debris and difficulty in keeping the area clean.

Except in a caries-immune mouth or in a mouth in which the teeth are kept meticulously clean, some decalcification and caries attack in this region is inevitable. Even the most conscientious toothbrushing may miss the distal surfaces of abutments because they cannot be seen. It is always important that the patient be instructed, with casts and before a mirror, in the significance of brushing these areas and the correct use of dental floss.

It is necessary that these areas be fully protected by the cast restoration, whether it be an inlay or a partial or full crown. Even the full crown can be deficient in this most vulnerable area, which lies at or just above the gingival margin. A full crown that is short or becomes short because of gingival recession does not afford protection where it is most needed.

When an inlay is the restoration of choice for an abutment tooth, certain modifications of the outline form are necessary. To prevent the buccal and lingual proximal margins from lying at or near the minor connector or the occlusal rest, these margins must be extended well beyond the line angles of the tooth. This additional extension may be accomplished by slicing the conventional box preparation. However, the gold margin produced by such a preparation may be quite thin and may be damaged by the clasp during placement or removal of the partial denture. This hazard may be avoided by extending the outline of the box beyond the line angle, thus producing a strong gold-to-tooth junction. (See Fig. 13-2.)

In this type of preparation the pulp is particularly vulnerable unless the axial wall is curved to conform with the external proximal curvature of the tooth. When caries is of minimal depth, the gingival seat should have an axial depth at all points about the width of a No. 559 fissure bur. It is of utmost importance that the gingival seat be placed below the free gingival margin. The proximal contour necessary to produce the proper guiding plane surface and the close proximity of the minor connector render this area particularly vulnerable to future caries attack. Every effort should be made to provide the restoration with maximum resistance and retention as well as clinically imperceptible gold margins. The first requisite can be satis-

Fig. 13-2. MOD inlay preparation for lower left second premolar to be used as a partial denture abutment. **A,** View of distal surface showing broad extension of box, well beyond area that will be covered by minor connector of partial denture. **B,** Occlusal view showing that axial wall is curved to conform with external proximal curvature of tooth. **C,** View of mesial surface where normal tooth contact occurs, being extended into a free-cleansing area but not as broadly as the distal surface.

Fig. 13-3. MO inlay preparation on lower left first premolar to be used for support of mesially placed occlusal rest. Weak lingual cusp is protected by an extension of inlay margin lingually.

fied by preparing opposing cavity walls 5 degrees or less from parallel and producing flat floors and sharp, clean line angles. Through the use of modern impression materials and casting technique the second requisite is not nearly as difficult as it was a few years ago.

The extended box provides the broad occlusoproximal area necessary to accommodate an occlusal rest. Care should be exercised to place the rest area in such a manner that an adequate amount of gold is allowed in both buccal and lingual directions. The proposed depth of the rest must be determined prior to preparing the tooth to ensure an adequate thickness of gold in the axiopulpal area. Additional depth in this area may be obtained by rounding the axiopulpal line angle of the preparation. In most instances, if the preparation is well into dentin at this point, adequate thickness of gold will be ensured. However, in problem situations a careful study of the roentgenogram will give some indication regarding the depth to which the pulpal floor can be carried with safety.

It is sometimes necessary to use an inlay on a lower first premolar for the support of an indirect retainer. The narrow occlusal

width buccolingually and the lingual inclination of the occlusal surface of such a tooth often complicate the two-surface inlay preparation. Even the most exacting occlusal cavity preparation often leaves a thin and weak lingual cusp remaining.

Fig. 13-3 illustrates a modification of the two-surface extended-box inlay preparation, which lends support to a weak lingual cusp. Enough of the tip of the lingual cusp must be removed to allow for sufficient thickness of gold to withstand occlusal forces. Tooth structure should be removed in the direction of the enamel rods, and the cut is terminated with a bevel just lingual to the proximal embrasure. A short bevel is then placed along the lingual surface of the reduced cusp. A modified inlay preparation such as this permits adequate coverage of a potentially weak cusp and eliminates the necessity of resorting to some type of more extensive restoration such as an MOD inlay or three-quarter crown.

An inlay preparation should be wide enough that the margins will be well beyond the occlusal rest area (Fig. 13-4). Since the rest seat will be carved in the wax pattern, the margins of the inlay should not be jeopardized by their proximity to the rest seat. Generally there should be at least 1 to 1.5 mm of gold between the occlusal rest and the inlay margin. The refinement of the margins, which is the final step in creating an inlay wax pattern, should not infringe on the outline form of the rest seat. The depth of the

Fig. 13-4. Occlusal view of Class II inlay properly designed to support an occlusal rest. Inlay preparation has been made with sufficient width to accommodate occlusal rest without jeopardizing inlay margins.

Fig. 13-5. Full arch with removal dies for five abutment crowns. Note depressions in preparations to accommodate occlusal rests.

occlusal rest seat should be provided for in the preparation. If there is any doubt, the axiopulpal line angle should be beveled or made concave to accommodate the occlusal rest.

One of the advantages of making cast restorations for abutment teeth is that mouth preparations that would otherwise have to be done in the mouth may be done on the surveyor with far greater accuracy. It is extremely difficult, and many times impossible, to make several proximal surfaces parallel to one another by disking them intraorally. The opportunity of paralleling and contouring wax patterns on the surveyor in relation to a path of placement should be utilized to the fullnest advantage whenever cast restorations are being made.

Although it is not always possible, it is best that all wax patterns be made at the same time. A cast of the arch with removable dies may be used if they are sufficiently keyed for accuracy (Fig. 13-5). If preferred, the paralleling and contouring of wax patterns may be done on a solid cast of the arch, using supplementary individual dies to refine margins. Modern impression materials and indirect techniques make either method equally satisfactory.

The same sequence for preparing teeth in the mouth applies to the contouring of wax patterns, differing only in that it may be done with greater accuracy and precision when indirect methods are used. After the cast has been placed on the surveyor to conform to the selected path of placement, and the wax patterns have been carved for occlusion and contact, proximal surfaces that are to act as guiding planes then may be carved parallel to the path of placement with a surveyor blade. This usually will be extended to the junction of the middle and gingival thirds of the tooth surface involved but not to the gingival margin, since the minor connector must be relieved when it crosses the gingivae. A guiding plane that includes the occlusal two thirds or even one half of the proximal area is usually adequate without endangering gingival tissues.

After the paralleling of guiding planes and any other contouring, occlusal rest seats are carved in the wax pattern. This has been outlined in Chapter 5.

It should be emphasized that critical areas

thus prepared in wax should not be destroyed by careless spruing or polishing. The wax pattern should be sprued to preserve paralleled surfaces and rest areas. Polishing should consist of little more than burnishing. Rest areas should need only refining with round finishing burs. If some interference by spruing is unavoidable, the casting must be returned to the surveyor for the refinement of proximal surfaces. However, this can only be done accurately with the aid of a handpiece holder attached to the vertical arm of the surveyor or some similar machining device. Need for later corrections to the casting can be avoided by carving the wax pattern with care and spruing and polishing with equal care.

ABUTMENT PREPARATIONS USING CAST CROWNS

Much that has been said in the preceding paragraphs about the preparation of inlays for partial denture abutments applies equally to cast-crown restorations. These may be in the form of three-quarter or full cast gold crowns or procelain veneer crowns. The latter are, of course, used for esthetic reasons only, but consideration for esthetics must not be allowed to jeopardize the success of the partial denture design. Retentive contours therefore must be provided on veneer crowns the same as on full cast crowns.

The ideal crown restoration for a partial denture abutment is the full cast gold crown, which can be carved to satisfy ideally all requirements for support, stabilization, and retention without compromise for cosmetic reasons. Porcelain veneer crowns can be made equally satisfactory but only by the added step of contouring the veneered surface on the surveyor prior to the final glaze. If this is not done, retentive contours may be excessive or inadequate. The full cast crown is preferable as an ideal abutment piece whenever esthetics will allow its use.

The three-quarter crown does not permit the creating of retentive areas as does the full crown. However, if buccal or labial surfaces are sound and retentive areas are acceptable or can be made so by slight modification of tooth surfaces, the three-quarter crown is a conservative restoration of merit. The same criteria apply in the decision to leave a portion of an abutment unprotected, as in the decision to leave any tooth unprotected that is to serve a partial denture abutment.

Regardless of the type of crown used, the preparation should be made to accommodate the depth of the occlusal rest seat. This is best accomplished by creating a depression in the prepared tooth at the occlusal rest area (Fig. 13-6). Since the location of any occlusal rests will have been established previously during treatment planning, this will be known in advance of any crown preparations. If, for example, double occlusal rests are to be used, this will be known so that the tooth can be prepared to accommodate the depth of both rests. It is almost as bad to find, when waxing a pattern, that a rest seat has to be made more shallow than is desirable because of lack of foresight as it is to have to make a rest seat shallow in an existing crown or inlay because its thickness is not known. Here the

Fig. 13-6. Close-up view of full crown abutment preparation with depression to accommodate depth of occlusal rest.

opportunity for creating an ideal rest seat depends only on the few seconds it takes to create a space for it.

Ledges on abutment crowns

In addition to providing abutment protection, more nearly ideal retentive contours, definite guiding planes, and optimal occlusal rest support, crown restorations on teeth used as partial denture abutments offer still another advantage not obtainable on natural teeth. This is the crown ledge or shoulder, which provides effective reciprocation and stabilization (Fig. 13-7).

The functions of the reciprocal clasp arm have been stated in Chapter 6. Briefly, these are reciprocation, stabilization, and auxiliary indirect retention. Any rigid reciprocal arm may provide horizontal stabilization. To a large extent, since it is placed about the height of convexity, a rigid reciprocal arm may also act as an auxiliary indirect retainer. However, its function as a reciprocating arm against the action of the retentive clasp arm is limited only to stabilization against possible orthodontic movement when the denture framework is in its terminal position. Only when the retentive clasp produces an active orthodontic force, because of acci-

Fig. 13-7. Axial surfaces of abutment crown patterns requiring parallelism are readily contoured with a surveyor and carving accessory. Three fourths of lingual surface of molar pattern has been carved with surveyor blade, parallel to path of placement, for a crown ledge preparation. Reciprocal element of direct retainer will occupy prepared lingual surface, thus restoring contour of crown when removable partial denture is seated.

dental distortion or improper design, is such reciprocation needed. Reciprocation is most needed when the restoration is being placed or when a dislodging force is applied, to prevent transient horizontal forces that may be detrimental to abutment stability. Perhaps the term *orthodontic force* is incorrect, since the term signifies a slight but continuous influence that would logically reach equilibrium as soon as the tooth is orthodontically moved. Instead, the transient forces of placement and removal lead to periodontal destruction and eventual instability rather than to orthodontic movement followed by consolidation.

True reciprocation is not possible with a clasp arm that is placed upon an occlusally inclined tooth surface because it does not become effective until the prosthesis is fully seated. Immediately, when a dislodging force is applied, the reciprocal clasp arm, along with the occlusal rest, breaks contact with the supporting tooth surfaces, and they are no longer effective. Thus, as the retentive clasp flexes over the height of contour, thereby exerting a horizontal force on the abutment, reciprocation is nonexistent just when it is needed most. (See Fig. 13-8.)

True reciprocation can be obtained only by creating a path of placement for the reciprocal clasp arm that is parallel to other guiding planes. In this manner the inferior border of the reciprocal clasp makes contact with its guiding surface before the retentive clasp on the other side of the tooth begins to flex (Fig. 13-9). Thus reciprocation exists during the entire path of placement and removal. The presence of a ledge on the abutment crown acts as a terminal stop for the reciprocal clasp arm, as well as augmenting the occlusal rest and providing some indirect retention for a distal extension partial denture.

A ledge on an abutment crown has still another advantage. Although the usual reciprocal clasp arm is half-round, and therefore convex, and is superimposed upon an already convex surface, a reciprocal clasp arm built on a crown ledge is actually inlayed into the crown and reproduces more nearly normal crown contours (Fig. 13-9). The patient's tongue then contacts a continuously convex surface rather than the projection of a clasp arm. Unfortunately the enamel cap is neither thick enough nor is the tooth so shaped that an effective ledge can be created on an un-

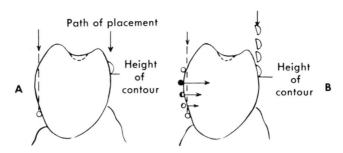

Fig. 13-8. A, Relationship of a retentive and a reciprocal clasp arm to each other when partial denture framework is fully seated. As retentive clasp arm flexes over height of contour during placement and removal, reciprocal clasp arm cannot be effective because it is not in contact with tooth until denture framework is fully seated. **B,** Horizontal forces applied to an abutment tooth as a retentive clasp flexes over height of contour during placement and removal. Open circle at top and bottom illustrates that retentive clasp is only passive at its first contact with tooth during placement and when in its terminal position with denture fully seated. During placement and removal a rigid clasp arm placed on opposite side of tooth cannot provide resistance against these horizontal forces.

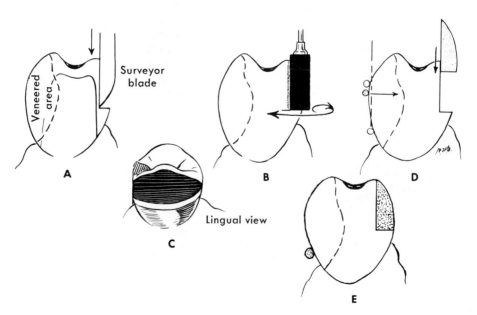

Fig. 13-9. A, Preparation of a ledge on a wax pattern with surveyor blade parallel to path of placement. **B,** Refinement of ledge on a gold casting, using a suitable carborundum stone in handpiece attached to dental surveyor or a specialized drill press for the purpose. **C,** Approximate width and depth of ledge formed on an abutment crown, which will permit a reciprocal clasp arm to be inlayed within normal contours of tooth. **D,** True reciprocation throughout full path of placement and removal that is possible when a reciprocal clasp arm is inlayed onto a ledge on an abutment crown. **E,** Direct retainer assembly is fully seated. Reciprocal arm restores lingual contour of abutment.

crowned tooth. Narrow enamel shoulders are sometimes used as rest seats on anterior teeth, but these do not provide the parallelism that is essential to reciprocation during placement and removal.

The crown ledge may be used on any full or three-quarter crown restoration that covers the nonretentive side of an abutment tooth. It is used most frequently on premolars and molars but also may be used on canine restorations. It is not ordinarily used on buccal surfaces for reciprocation against lingual retention because of the excessive display of metal, but it may be used just as effectively on posterior abutments when esthetics is not a factor.

The fact that a crown ledge is to be used should be known in advance of crown preparation to assure sufficient removal of tooth structure in this area. Although a shoulder or ledge is not included in the preparation itself, adequate space must be provided so that the ledge may be made sufficiently wide and the surface above it may be made parallel to the path of placement. The ledge should be placed at the junction of the gingival and middle third of the tooth, curving slightly to follow the curvature of the gingival tissues. On the side of the tooth at which the clasp arm will originate, the ledge must be kept low enough to allow the origin of the clasp arm to be wide enough for sufficient strength and rigidity.

In forming the crown ledge, which is usually located on the lingual surface, the wax pattern of the crown is completed except for refinement of the margins before the ledge is carved. After the proximal guiding planes and the occlusal rests and retentive contours are formed, the ledge is carved with the surveyor blade so that the surface above is parallel to the path of placement. Thus a continuous guiding plane surface will exist from the proximal around the lingual surface, the dif-

Fig. 13-10. A, Faro laboratory handpiece attached to Ney surveyor by means of handpiece holder. With a bur or stone, lingual surface and ledge are machined in relation to previously established path of placement. **B,** Austenal Micro-Drill used to mill internal rest seats and lingual grooves and ledges in cast gold restorations. Such a device permits more precise milling than is possible with a dental handpiece attached to a dental surveyor. To be effective, cast must be positioned on Micro-Drill in such a manner that previously established path of placement is maintained. Movable stage or base therefore should be adjustable until relation of cast to axis of drill has been made the same as that obtained when cast was on dental surveyor. (**B** courtesy Austenal, Inc., Chicago, Ill.)

ference being only that the lingual portion ends in a definite ledge and the proximal does not.

The full effectiveness of the crown ledge cannot be had with a crown that is not returned to the surveyor for refinement after casting. To afford true reciprocation, the crown casting must have a surface above the ledge that is parallel to the path of placement. This can be accomplished with precision only by machining the casting parallel to the path of placement with a handpiece holder in the surveyor or some other suitable machining device (Fig. 13-10). Similarly, the parallelism of proximal guiding planes needs to be perfected after casting and polishing. Although it is possible to *approximate* parallelism and, at the same time, form the crown ledge on the wax pattern with a surveyor blade, some of its accuracy is lost in casting and polishing. The use of suitable burs such as No. 557, 558, and 559 fissure burs and true

Fig. 13-11. Lingual ledges on cast gold crowns are machined with a No. 558 dental bur. Experience has shown that in absence of a rigid jig for holding the cast, a bur is difficult to use. Therefore it is best that ledge be formed as accurately as possible in wax pattern and that machining of finished casting be done with a cylindric carborundum point. Note scratch line on left posterior portion of cast, indicating path of placement.

Fig. 13-12. Lingual ledges after machining and polishing. Note that embrasures for clasping are also machined parallel to path of placement and that occlusal rests are used in addition to supporting ledges. These are to prevent tooth separation and to shunt food away from interproximal areas.

cylindric carborundum stones in the hand-piece holder permits the paralleling of all guiding planes on the finished casting with the accuracy necessary for the effectiveness of those guiding plane surfaces (Figs. 13-11 to 13-13).

The reciprocal clasp arm is ultimately waxed on the investment cast so that it is continuous with the ledge inferiorly and contoured superiorly to restore the crown contour including the tip of the cusp. It is obvious that polishing must not be allowed to destroy the form of the shoulder that was prepared in wax nor destroy the parallelism of the guiding plane surface. It is equally vital that the denture casting must be polished with great care so that the accuracy of the counterpart is not destroyed. Modern investments, casting alloys, and polishing techniques make this degree of accuracy possible. Only the human element, by carelessness or lack of understanding, may fail to produce a crown and counterpart with the desired accuracy. It is just as necessary for the technician to understand the purpose of the crown ledge as it is for the dentist who designs and plans for its use.

Veneer crowns for support of clasp arms

Resin and porcelain veneer crowns are used for cosmetic reasons on abutment teeth that would otherwise display an objectionable amount of metal. They may be in the form of porcelain veneers retained by pins and cemented to the crown, porcelain fused directly to a cast crown, or acrylic resin processed directly to a cast crown.

The retentive clasp terminal should rest on metal when an acrylic resin veneer crown is utilized as an abutment restoration (Fig. 13-14). In this instance the crown is contoured to be retentive in the desired area, and that area is not included in carving the space for the resin veneer. Whereas the suprabulge portion of the clasp arm crosses the surface of the veneer, the portion that crosses the height of contour and engages an undercut in which abrasion could occur is supported by the metal of the crown itself. The only disadvantage of a veneer crown so prepared is the display of metal, which more often than not is on the mesial side of the abutment tooth and therefore is cosmetically objectionable. Ceramic-gold crowns do not present this problem.

Fig. 13-13. Buccal and lingual views of abutment crowns designed to accept embrasure clasps and lingual reciprocal arms resting on prepared ledges. All surfaces above ledges are made parallel with path of placement. Note size and form of occlusal rests on either side of embrasure ledges.

Fig. 13-14. Close-up view of relation of surveyor blade to distal surface of an abutment crown. Note that this guiding plane is made parallel to path of placement.

Fig. 13-15. Porcelain veneer crown is resurveyed prior to glazing. At this stage, veneered portion can be recontoured by grinding to achieve optimal height of contour to place the reciprocal and retentive portion of planned clasp assembly.

If the veneer crown is not contoured to provide retention on metal, suitable retention does not exist until the veneer has been added. This means that the veneer must be slightly overcontoured and then shaped to provide the desired undercut for the location of the retentive clasp arm (Fig. 13-15). If the veneer is of porcelain, this procedure must precede glazing, and if of resin, before final polishing. If this most important step in the making of veneered abutments is neglected or omitted, excessive or inadequate retentive contours may result, to the detriment of effective clasp design.

The flat underside of a cast clasp makes sufficient contact with the surface of the veneer so that abrasion of a resin veneer may result. Although the underside of the clasp may be polished (with some loss in accuracy of fit), abrasion results from the trapping and holding of food debris against the tooth surface as the clasp moves during function. *Therefore, unless the retentive clasp terminal rests on metal, glazed porcelain should be used to assure the future retentiveness of the veneered surface.* Present-day acrylic resins, being cross-linked copolymers, are much harder than formerly and will withstand abrasion for considerable time but not nearly to the same degree as porcelain. Therefore acrylic resin veneers are used best in conjunction with exposed metal supporting the half-round clasp terminal.

SPLINTING OF ABUTMENT TEETH

Frequently a tooth is deemed too weak to use alone as a partial denture abutment because of the short length or excessive taper of a single root or because of bone loss resulting in an unfavorable crown-root ratio. In such instances, splinting of weak abutment teeth to the adjacent tooth or teeth is utilized as a means of gaining *multiple abutment support*. Thus two single-rooted teeth may be used as a multirooted abutment.

Splinting should not be used to retain a tooth that would otherwise be condemned for periodontal reasons, in the futile hope that by doing so the tooth may be retained. Such a gamble may be justified when, if successful, the need for a prosthetic restoration would be avoided. However, when the length of service of a restoration may depend on the serviceability of an abutment, any periodontally questionable tooth should be condemned in favor of using an adjacent healthy tooth as the abutment, even

Fig. 13-16. Six remaining mandibular anterior teeth are splinted with pin onlays. Lingual rest seats on canines and lateral incisors will qupport a linguoplate major connector. Teeth were prepared for onlays following healing from periodontal surgery. All teeth were slightly mobile.

though the span is increased one tooth by doing so.

The most frequent application of the use of multiple abutments is the splinting of two premolars or a first premolar and a canine. Mandibular premolars generally have round and tapered roots, which are easily loosened by rotation as well as by tipping. They are the weakest of posterior abutments. But maxillary premolars also often have tapered roots, which make them also poor risks as abutments, particularly when they will be called on to resist the leverage of a distal extension base. Such teeth are best splinted by casting or soldering two crowns or inlays together. When a first premolar to be used as an abutment has poor root form or support, it is best that it be splinted to the stronger canine in a similar manner.

Anterior teeth upon which lingual rests are to be placed frequently need to be splinted together to avoid orthodontic movement of individual teeth. Mandibular anterior teeth are seldom so used, but if they are, splinting of the teeth involved is advisable (Fig. 13-16). When such splinting is impossible for one reason or another, individual lingual rests on cast restorations may be inclined slightly apically to avoid possible tooth displacement, or lingual rests may be used in conjunction with incisal rests, engaging slightly the labial surface of the teeth.

Lingual rests should always be placed as low on the cingulum as possible, and single anterior teeth, other than canines, should not ordinarily be used for occlusal support.

Where lingual rests are employed on central and lateral incisors, as many teeth as possible should be included to distribute the load over several teeth, thereby minimizing the force on any one tooth. Even so, some movement of individual teeth is likely to occur, particularly when they are subjected to the forces of indirect retention. This is best avoided by splinting several teeth with united cast restorations. The condition of the teeth and cosmetic considerations will dictate whether full veneer crowns, three-quarter crowns, or pinledge inlays will be used for this purpose.

Splinting of molar teeth for multiple abutment support is less frequently used, because they are generally multirooted teeth to begin with and a two- or three-rooted tooth that is not strong enough alone is probably a poor abutment risk. There may be exceptions, however, that are notable when, because of fused and conical roots, the abutment would benefit from the effect of splinting.

USE OF ISOLATED TEETH AS ABUTMENTS

Although splinting is advocated for any abutment teeth that are considered too weak to risk using alone, a single abutment standing alone in the dental arch anterior to a distal extension basal seat generally requires the splinting effect of a fixed partial denture (Fig. 13-17). Even though the form and length of the root and the supporting bone seem to be adequate for an ordinary abutment, the fact

Fig. 13-17. Lone standing premolar should be splinted to canine with a fixed partial denture. Not only will design of removable partial denture be simplified but longevity of abutment service by premolar will be greatly extended.

that the tooth lacks proximal contact endangers the tooth when it is used to support a distal extension base.

The average abutment tooth is subjected to some distal tipping, to rotation, and to horizontal movement, all of which must be held to a minimum by the design of the denture and the quality of tissue support for the distal extension base. The isolated abutment tooth, however, is subjected also to mesial tipping because of lack of proximal contact. Despite indirect retention, some lifting of the distal extension base is inevitable, causing torque to the abutment as the fulcrum of a teeter-totter.

In a tooth-borne prosthesis an isolated tooth may be used as an abutment by using a fifth abutment for additional support. Thus rotational and horizontal forces are resisted by the additional stabilization obtained from the fifth abutment. When two such isolated abutments exist, that is, two second premolars with first premolars missing, the sixth abutment should be used. Thus the two canines, the two isolated premolars, and two posterior teeth are used as abutments.

In contrast, an isolated anterior abutment adjacent to a distal extension base usually should be splinted to the nearest tooth by means of a fixed partial denture. The effect is twofold: (1) the anterior edentulous segment is eliminated, thereby creating an intact dental arch anterior to the space, and (2) the isolated tooth is splinted to the other abutment of the fixed partial denture, thereby providing multiple abutment support. Here, also, splinting should be used only to gain multiple abutment support rather than

to support an otherwise weak abutment tooth.

The economic aspect of using fixed restorations as part of the mouth preparations for a partial denture is essentially the same as that for any other splinting procedure: the best design of the partial denture that will assure the longevity of its service makes the additional procedure and expense necessary. Although it must be recognized that economic considerations, combined with a particularly favorable prognosis of an isolated tooth, may influence the decision to forego the advantages of using a fixed partial denture, the original treatment plan should include this precautionary measure even though the alternative method is accepted for economic reasons.

A second factor may also influence the decision to use an isolated tooth as an abutment; this is the esthetic consideration for an otherwise sound anterior tooth that would have to be used as an abutment for a fixed restoration. However, neither esthetics nor economics should deter the dentist from recommending to the patient that an isolated tooth that will be used as a terminal abutment be given the advantage of splinting by means of a fixed partial denture. Then, if compromises are necessary, the patient must share a measure of the responsibility for using the isolated tooth as an abutment.

MISSING ANTERIOR TEETH

When a partial denture is to replace missing posterior teeth, especially in the absence of distal abutments, any additional missing teeth anteriorly are best replaced by means of fixed restorations rather than by being added to the denture. In any distal extension situation some teeter-totter action will inevitably result from the adding of an anterior segment to the denture. Here again the ideal treatment plan that treats the anterior edentulous space separately comes in conflict with economic and esthetic considerations. Each situation must be treated according to its own merits. Frequently the best esthetic result can be obtained by replacing missing anterior teeth with the partial denture rather than with a fixed restoration. From a biomechanical standpoint, however, a partial denture should replace only the missing posterior teeth *after* the remainder of the arch has been made intact by fixed restorations.

Although the occasional need for compromises is recognized, the decision to include an anterior segment on the denture will depend largely on the support available for that part of the denture. The greater the number of natural anterior teeth remaining, the better the support that will be available for the edentulous segment.

If definite rests are obtainable, the anterior segment may be treated as any other tooth-bounded modification space. Sound principles of rest support apply just as much as elsewhere in the arch. *Inclined tooth surfaces should not be used for occlusal support, nor should rests be placed upon unprepared lingual surfaces.* The best possible support for an anterior segment is multiple support extending, if possible, posteriorly across prepared lingual rest seats on the canine teeth to mesial occlusal rest seats on the first premolars. Such support will permit the missing anterior teeth to be included in the denture, frequently with some cosmetic advantages over fixed restorations.

In some instances the replacement of anterior teeth by means of a partial denture cannot be avoided. However, without adequate tooth support any such prosthesis will lack the stability that would exist from replacing only the posterior teeth with the partial denture and the anterior teeth with fixed restorations. When anterior teeth have been lost through accident or have been missing for some time, resorption of the anterior ridge may have progressed to the point that neither fixed nor removable pontics may be butted to the residual ridge. In such instances, for esthetic reasons, the missing teeth must be replaced with a denture base supporting teeth that are more nearly in their original position, considerably forward from the residual ridge. Although such teeth may be positioned to better cosmetic advantage, the contouring and coloring of a denture base to be esthetically pleasing requires the maximum artistic effort of both the dentist and the technologist. Such a partial denture, both from an esthetic and a biomechanical standpoint, is one of the most difficult of all prosthetic restorations. *However, a splint bar, connected by abutments on both sides of the edentulous space, will provide much-needed support to the anterior segment of the removable partial denture.* Since the splint bar will act as an occlusal rest, rest seats on abutments adjacent to the edentulous area need not be prepared, thus simplifying an anterior restoration to some extent.

TEMPORARY CROWNS AND TEMPORARY FIXED PARTIAL DENTURES

Each time a tooth is prepared for a full crown, a temporary crown must be placed for the protection and comfort of the exposed dentin. Ideally this crown will restore occlusion and contact, although not necessarily so.

Most inlay preparations may be filled with a thick mix of white WondrPak cement. Occasionally this may suffice also for a three-quarter crown preparation when only the deeper grooves need to be filled. However, for most three-quarter crown preparations and for large inlay preparations a temporary acrylic resin crown is used in preference to the WondrPak alone. In any case, WondrPak is the preferred cementing medium.

Individual full crown preparations, when esthetics does not prevent their use, may be satisfactorily covered with fitted aluminum crowns. Contact and occlusion may be less than ideal, but the length of time the crown will be worn is usually short. Temporary crowns should be trimmed short of the gingival tissues and should be smoothed and contoured to eliminate rough edges. The temporary crown should protect the tooth, yet should not interfere with gingival healing nor induce inflammation that might cause gingival pathology or recession.

For esthetic reasons, anterior temporary crowns should be made of a rapid-curing acrylic resin of a matching tooth shade, or polycarbonate crowns should be used. Anterior temporary fixed partial dentures may also be made of resin, and even posterior fixed partial dentures when better esthetics or occlusion is desirable. Single acrylic resin crowns may be made by filling a contoured copper band with the tooth-shade resin and pressing the resin onto the prepared tooth that has been coated with petrolatum (Fig. 13-18). On anterior teeth the copper band may be pinched labliolingually to form a more natural tooth contour. *In any direct application of tooth-shade resin for temporary purposes the crown must be removed and reseated while the material is still plastic, to make sure that the hardened crown will withdraw.* After hardening, the crown is removed

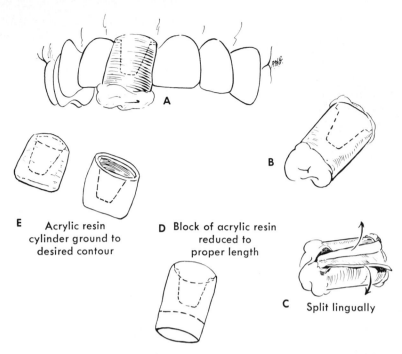

Fig. 13-18. Making of a single anterior resin temporary crown. **A,** Contoured copper band that has been flattened labiolingually is filled with acrylic resin of correct shade and pressed onto prepared tooth that has been coated with petrolatum. **B,** When acrylic resin has reached a leathery consistency, copper band is removed from tooth momentarily and then reseated onto tooth until resin has hardened. This is necessary to assure withdrawal of hardened acrylic resin without difficulty. **C,** As soon as acrylic resin has hardened, copper band is slit longitudinally with a carborundum disk and peeled off. **D,** Acrylic resin coping, which will be shaped in form of a temporary crown, is placed back onto tooth and marked with a pencil where excess thickness and occlusal interference is to be reduced. This is repeated until a temporary crown of acceptable contours has been formed. At the same time, any flash extending beyond abutment shoulders must be removed. **E,** Acrylic resin crown is then polished and temporarily cemented to abutment tooth.

and the copper band is slit on the lingual side and stripped away. The crown may then be ground to resemble the tooth being restored, polished, and cemented with temporary cement. Such a temporary crown provides excellent esthetics and fit and will serve for an indefinite period if necessary.

Individual acrylic resin crowns may also be made by the same methods as those used for making a temporary fixed partial denture. Once a technique has been adopted, acrylic resin temporary crowns are quickly made and are preferable because of their appearance and the fact that their natural contours are much more comfortable to the patient. Several methods for making acrylic resin temporary crowns and temporary fixed restorations are outlined as follows:

1. a. An impression is made of the mouth before the tooth or teeth are prepared. This impression may be made in alginate hydrocolloid or with baseplate wax in a fixed partial denture impression tray. The use of baseplate wax is expedient, inexpensive, does not require special handling during the interlude, and is rigid enough to permit compression molding. It is easily carved to create teeth to be added and is easily trimmed to increase the thickness of temporary crowns when little tooth structure has been removed, such as in the gingival one third.

Before this impression is made, missing tooth contours should be restored with inlay wax so that an impression of intact tooth surfaces can be made. If missing teeth are to be replaced, they may be waxed into the space or an artificial tooth may be fitted into each space before the impression is made. An alternate method is to carve the tooth form of the tooth or teeth to be replaced into the impression, which is then filled and shaped along with adjacent crowns. By placing some of the impression material on the opposite side of the tray and having the patient close into it, a means of stabilizing the tray in the mouth later is established. The patient then may close into the impression, thus making it unnecessary for the dentist to hold it while the plastic resin material is setting.

b. Rather than making an impression of the mouth before the preparations are begun, the dentist or assistant may make an impression or a previous diagnostic cast, after artificial tooth replacements have been waxed in to form the temporary pontics.

Whether method a or b is used, the impression should be trimmed to eliminate undercut areas and projections into interproximal spaces, which would interfere with reseating. If the impression is of alginate hydrocolloid, it must be wrapped in a wet towel and set aside while the teeth are being prepared. A baseplate wax impression may be set aside without any special precautions.

2. a. After the preparations are completed and impressions for working casts and jaw relations have been made, the prepared teeth are dried and coated with petroleum jelly. If the original impression was made with alginate hydrocolloid, it is now removed from the wet towel and dried with compressed air.

The portion of the impression involving the crowns is now filled with a self-curing acrylic resin of the desired shade. Although powder and liquid may be mixed to form a dough, a sprinkling method is preferred. At the time of this writing a material known as Jet repair acrylic resin is available in New-Hue shades and has proved to be a nearly ideal material for making temporary crowns and temporary fixed partial dentures. The powder is packaged in a flexible container that permits dispensing without waste and is therefore both economical and convenient to use for filling tooth molds by sprinkling. Sprinkle some powder into the mold first and then wet with liquid from a medicine dropper. Repeat this until the mold is filled, tapping the impression on the bench each time to facilitate absorption. After the crown area

is filled, any excess that has flowed into other areas should be removed with a pledget of cotton. The material must then be allowed to reach a soft, rubbery state before it is seated onto the petrolatum-coated teeth.

Using the unprepared teeth as a guide, the impression is reseated into the mouth and held until sufficient time has elapsed for the material to reach a stiff rubbery consistency. Unfortunately this must come from experience with the particular resin material being used. It is necessary that the crowns be removed once before the material has hardened, to assure their withdrawal. Preferably the rubbery plastic will remain in the impression at this time. It then may be removed from the impression, excess material trimmed away from the crowns with fine scissors, and the crowns reseated in the impression. The impression is then reseated in the mouth to finish compression molding of the plastic resin while it hardens. After time has elapsed for hardening, the impression is removed. This time the hardened resin will remain on the teeth, but having been removed once, it may easily be tapped off, and the crowns trimmed and polished. Parallelism of abutment teeth is an absolute necessity when temporary fixed partial dentures are made by this method. Otherwise, serious difficulty may be encountered in attempting to remove the rigid, temporary resin restoration. To avoid this hazard the rubbery plastic resin may be allowed to harden in the impression out of the mouth. If the material has reached a stiff rubbery state before removal from the mouth, this does not seem to materially affect its accuracy. (Even a well-fitting temporary crown should be reamed slightly to accommodate the temporary cement and make its subsequent removal less difficult.) After the material has hardened, it is removed from the impression, the excess is trimmed away, and the crown is then polished, taking care to preserve the accuracy of the gingival margins.

b. Rather than forming the temporary crowns or temporary fixed partial denture in the mouth, the following alternate method may be used: As soon as the preparations are completed, an alginate hydrocolloid impression of the prepared teeth is made and poured immediately in stone. The making of this impression should precede the making of other impressions, which may then be made while the stone cast is hardening. Retraction of tissues is not necessary for this impression, and if some of the alginate hydrocolloid is first smeared onto the prepared teeth with the finger, the impression will be relatively free of defects.

As soon as the cast can be separated from the hydrocolloid impression of the prepared teeth, any small air bubbles are removed and the cast is then painted with a tinfoil substitute. The original impression is filled with tooth-shade resin as in 2a, but rather than being placed back into the mouth, it is seated onto the cast of the prepared teeth. It is removed while rubbery, as before, the excess is trimmed with scissors, and the impression is then reseated until it hardens. This method differs from method 2a only in that the prepared teeth are made more accessible and the danger of damage to the mouth during removal of the hardened resin is avoided. If the stone teeth fracture during removal, no harm has been done, and the stone may be removed from the hardened resin crowns.

The alginate hydrocolloid impression of the prepared teeth may be poured in low-fusing metal rather than stone and thus separated immediately rather than waiting for the stone to set. Although some cooling shrinkage of the metal occurs, temporary crowns made on such a die can be reamed slightly if necessary. This usually should be done anyway to allow for the thickness of the temporary cement and to make removal of the crowns easier. The impression should be dried thoroughly with compressed air before pouring the low-fusing metal (such as Dialoy) into it. The molten metal should be poured from the ladle when just slightly above the congealing point rather than immediately after removal from the flame. This avoids sizzling and results in a more accurate cast.

Low-fusing metal may also be used to advantage in other ways when an immediate cast is desired. For example, during the preparation of abutment teeth there may be some question as to the parallelism of the preparation or of two or more fixed partial denture abutments. An alginate hydrocolloid impression of the prepared and adjacent teeth may be poured in low-fusing metal and separated immediately. In this way the dentist may see what further modifications are necessary before proceeding. Since the low-fusing metal is reusable, little time and mate-rial are used, and the possibility of making final impressions of inadequate preparations is thus eliminated.

TEMPORARY CROWNS WHEN A PARTIAL DENTURE IS BEING WORN

Occasionally an existing removable partial denture must remain serviceable while the mouth is being prepared for a new denture. In such situations, temporary crowns that will support the old denture and not interfere with its placement and removal must be made. Only rarely can an aluminum crown be made to serve this purpose. Instead, an acrylic resin temporary crown that duplicates the original form of the abutment tooth must be made (Fig. 13-19).

The technique for making temporary crowns to fit the inside of direct retainers is similar to that given for other types of acrylic resin temporary crowns. The principal difference is that an alginate hydrocolloid impression must be made of the entire arch with the existing partial denture in place. This is wrapped in a wet towel and set aside while the tooth or teeth are being prepared for new crowns.

After the preparations are completed and the impressions and jaw relation records have been made, the prepared teeth are dried and coated with petroleum jelly. The original alginate hydrocolloid impression is trimmed to eliminate any excess, undercuts, and interproximal projections that would interfere with its replacement in the mouth.

The tooth-shade resin is sprinkled into the impression in those areas that are to be temporary crowns, and any excess is removed with a pledget of cotton. When the material reaches a soft rubbery state, the impression is seated into the mouth, where it is held by the dentist until sufficient time has elapsed for it to reach a stiff rubbery stage. This again must be based on experience with the particular plastic material being used. At this time the impression is removed, the crowns remaining in the impression. These are then stripped out of the impression; all excess is trimmed away with scissors, and the crowns are reseated on the prepared abutments. The partial denture is then removed from the alginate impression and reseated in the mouth onto the plastic crowns, which are at this time in a stiff rubbery state. The patient

Fig. 13-19. Sequence of mouth preparations with temporary crowns formed to support an existing partial denture while new one is being made. **A,** Several abutment teeth have been prepared to receive full coverage crowns. **B,** Acrylic resin temporary crowns duplicating original tooth contour. An impression of teeth before preparation was begun was used to establish shape of temporary crowns. **C,** Existing partial denture, seated onto temporary crowns. These are then removed as often as necessary during succeeding appointments. **D,** Gold castings are tried in, prior to soldering and adding veneers. Temporary crowns and existing partial denture are then returned to mouth until abutment pieces are ready for cementation.

may bring the teeth into occlusion to reestablish the former position and occlusal relationship of the existing partial denture.

After the plastic crown or crowns have hardened, the partial denture is removed, the crowns remaining on the teeth. These are then tapped off, trimmed, polished, and temporarily cemented. The result is a temporary crown that restores the original abutment contours and allows the partial denture to be placed and removed without interference, at the same time providing the same support temporarily to the denture that existed before the teeth were prepared. This service, made possible by modern materials, should be routine for all patients requiring such service.

Cementation of temporary crowns. Cementation of acrylic resin temporary crowns differs from the cementation of aluminum crowns in that the plastic crowns fit closely and do not require cementation for reten-

tion. Since little or no space exists for the temporary cement, the crowns may need to be reamed slightly to accommodate the temporary cement and to facilitate removal. The temporary cement should be thin and applied only to the inside rim of the crowns to assure complete seating. As soon as the temporary cement has hardened, the occlusion may be checked and relieved accordingly.

Regardless of the type of temporary cement used, any excess that might be irritating to the gingivae should be removed. Too frequently the final act before dismissing the patient is the cementation of the temporary crowns. Instead, two considerations are necessary. One is the removal of excess cement after it has hardened. The second is the application of some medication to the slightly abused gingivae to facilitate healing and to prevent discomfort to the patient. Topical application of some antibacterial agent is, at best, a transient treatment that does little to prevent discomfort. Hydrocortisone acetate, 0.5%, in a denture adhesive powder, when applied topically to a freshly lacerated surface, both facilitates healing and prevents afterpain. It should be applied to the lacerated gingivae around each temporary crown and the patient dismissed without further rinsing of the mouth. Tissue response to this treatment has been so favorable that it is included here as a specific treatment. Apparently it is effective only on fresh wounds and is of little value as a follow-up treatment.

THE MAKING OF CROWNS AND INLAYS TO FIT EXISTING DENTURE RETAINERS

It is frequently necessary that an abutment tooth be restored with a full crown (and occasionally with an inlay) that will fit the inside of the clasp of an otherwise serviceable partial denture. The technique for doing so is simple enough but requires that an indirect-direct-indirect pattern be made and therefore justifies a fee for service above that for the usual full crown.

The technique for making a crown to fit the inside of a clasp is as follows: An alginate hydrocolloid impression of the mouth is made with the partial denture in place. This impression, which is used to make the plastic temporary crown, is wrapped in a wet towel and set aside while the tooth is being prepared. Even though several abutment teeth are to be restored, it is usually necessary that each one be completed before the next one is begun. This is necessary so that the original support and occlusal relationship of the partial denture can be maintained as each new crown is being made.

The abutment tooth is then prepared, during which time the partial denture is replaced frequently enough to ascertain that sufficient tooth structure is being removed to allow for the thickness of the gold casting. When the preparation is completed, a copper band impression of the tooth is obtained, from which a stone die is made.

An acrylic resin temporary crown is then made in the original alginate hydrocolloid impression as outlined in the preceding paragraphs. It is trimmed, polished, and temporarily cemented, and the denture is returned to the mouth. The patient is dismissed after the excess cement has been removed and the traumatized gingiva treated, as mentioned previously.

On the stone die made from the copper band impression a thin self-curing resin coping will be formed with a brush technique. The stone die should first be trimmed to the finishing line of the preparation, which is then delineated with a pencil, and the die painted with a tinfoil substitute. A material such as Al-Cote tinfoil substitute should be used, which will form a thin film on a cold, dry surface. Not all tinfoil substitutes are suitable for this purpose.

With self-curing acrylic resin powder and liquid in separate dappen dishes and a fine sable brush, a coping of acrylic resin of uniform thickness is painted onto the die. This should extend not quite to the pencil line representing the limit of the crown preparation. After hardening, the resin coping may be removed, inspected, and trimmed if necessary. The thin film of foil substitute should be removed before the coping is reseated onto the die.

The wax pattern is usually not begun until the patient returns, at which time it is built up at the chair. First the occlusal portion of the wax pattern is established by having the patient close and carve excursive paths in the wax (Fig. 13-20, *A*). Dull areas are added to until a smooth occlusal registration has been obtained. Except for narrowing the occlusal surface and the carving of grooves and spillways, this will be the occlusal anatomy of the finished restoration.

The second step is the adding of sufficient wax to establish contact relations with the adjoining tooth. At this time the occlusal relation of the marginal ridges also must be established.

Next, wax is added to buccal and lingual surfaces where the clasp arms will contact the crown, and the pattern is again reseated in the mouth. The clasp arms, minor connectors, and occlusal rests involved on the partial denture are warmed with a needle-point flame, being careful to avoid flaming any adjacent resin, and the denture is positioned in the mouth and onto the wax pattern (Fig. 13-20, *B*). Several attempts may be necessary until the denture is fully seated and the components of the clasp clearly recorded in the wax pattern. Each time the denture is removed, the pattern will draw with it and must be teased out of the clasp.

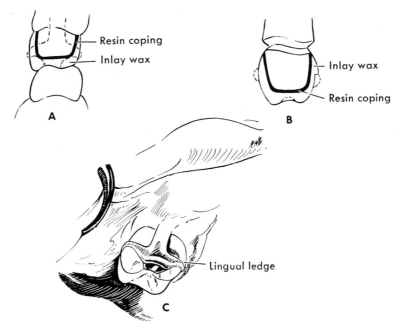

Fig. 13-20. Making of a cast crown to fit an existing partial denture clasp. **A,** Thin resin coping is first made on an individual die of prepared tooth. Inlay wax is then added and coping placed onto prepared tooth when occlusal surfaces and contact relations are established directly in mouth. Clasp assembly is warmed with a needle-point flame only enough to soften inlay wax, and partial denture is placed in mouth where it is guided gently to place by opposing occlusion. This step must be repeated several times and excess wax removed or wax added until full supporting contact with underside of clasp assembly has been established, with denture fully seated. Usually wax pattern withdraws with denture and must be gently teased out of clasp each time. **B,** Wax pattern is then placed back onto individual die to complete occlusal anatomy and refine margins. Excess wax remaining below impression of retentive clasp arm must be removed, but a wax ledge may be left below reciprocal clasp arm. **C,** Finished casting in mouth. Terminus of retentive clasp is then readapted to engage an undercut. It is frequently necessary to remove some interference from casting, as indicated by articulating paper placed between clasp and crown, until clasp is full seated.

When contact with the clasp arms and the occlusal relation of the denture have been established satisfactorily, the temporary crown may be replaced and the patient dismissed. The crown pattern is completed on the die by narrowing the occlusal surface buccolingually, adding grooves and spillways, and refining the margins.* Any wax ledge remaining below the reciprocal clasp arm may be left to provide some of the advantages of a crown ledge described earlier in this chapter. Excess wax remaining below the retentive clasp arm, however, must be removed to permit the adding of a retentive undercut later (Fig. 13-20, *C*).

If an acrylic resin veneer is to be added, the veneer space must now be carved in the wax pattern. In such cases the contour of the veneer may be recorded by making a stone matrix of the buccal surface, which can later be replaced onto the completed casting for waxing in the veneer. This stone matrix is then invested with the casting when the acrylic resin veneer is being processed.

The wax pattern must be sprued with care so that essential areas on the pattern are not destroyed. After casting, the crown should be subjected to a minimum of polishing, since the exact form of the axial and occlusal surfaces must be maintained.

Since it is impossible to withdraw a clasp arm from a retentive undercut on the wax pattern, the casting must be made without any provision for clasp retention. After the crown has been tried in the mouth with the denture in place, the location of the retentive clasp terminal is identified by scoring the crown with a sharp instrument. Then the crown may be ground and polished slightly in this area to create a retentive undercut. The clasp terminal then may be carefully adapted into this undercut, thereby creating clasp retention on the new crown.

The technique for making inlay patterns to fit the inside of denture clasps is essentially the same as for full crowns, except that it may be done entirely in wax. However, patterns for larger inlays that might be distorted during placement of the denture are best supported also by an acrylic resin foundation. In such cases the pattern is started by brushing in the acrylic resin until a supporting frame has been established. The wax pattern is then completed in the mouth as for a full crown.

Ideally all abutment teeth would best be protected with full crowns before the partial denture is constructed. Except for the possibility of recurrent caries because of defective crown margins or gingival recession, abutment teeth so protected may be expected to give many years of satisfactory service in the support and retention of the partial denture. Economically a policy of insisting on full coverage for all abutment teeth may well be justified from the long-term viewpoint. It must be recognized, however, that in practice full coverage of all abutment teeth is not always possible at the time indicated. Many factors act to influence the future health status of an abutment tooth, some of which cannot be forseen. It is necessary therefore that the dentist be able to treat abutment teeth that become defective at some later date in such a manner that their service as abutments may be restored and the serviceability of the partial denture maintained. Although it is not part of the original mouth preparations, this service accomplishes much the same objective by providing the denture with support, stability, and retention, and the dentist must be technically equipped to provide this service when it becomes necessary.

CEMENTATIONS FOR FIXED RESTORATIONS

Final cementation of fixed restorations should be deferred until evidence of the success of the restoration can be evaluated. Single crowns may be cemented permanently more often than fixed partial dentures. It seems that nonpermanent cementation of fixed restorations has many advantages and few disadvantages. Zinc oxide and eugenol temporary cements will adequately retain the restoration and protect the abutment teeth, yet may be removed without difficulty for future inspection of the abutments and the adjacent tissues. The restoration then may be cemented permanently or again only semipermanently. Restorations have been

---

*Margins on all crown and inlay wax patterns are refined with S. S. White red casting wax, which contrasts with the blue or green wax used for the pattern and permits the carving of delicate margins with accuracy. The preferred wax for the body of crown and inlay patterns is Maves inlay wax. This wax is available in both cone and stick form and has excellent carving properties and color.

removed after intervals as long as five years without evidence of leakage of deterioration of zinc oxide–eugenol cements.

Advantages of semipermanent cementation of fixed restorations. Some of the advantages of semipermanent cementation are as follows:

1. By cementing the restoration temporarily at first, the dentist can be sure that the crowns are fully seated and that the margins are satisfactory.

2. Less postoperative discomfort generally results from cementation with a temporary cement. Temporary cements are sedative, while zinc oxyphosphate cements are irritating to a pulp already suffering from trauma caused by operative procedures.

3. Restorations may be removed to inspect the tooth beneath and to take roentgenograms. The hazard of a single leaking abutment piece causing destruction of the tooth before it is detected can thus be eliminated.

4. Restorations may be removed to inspect and treat gingival and subjacent tissues. Future periodontal treatment is thus facilitated.

5. If root canal therapy becomes necessary, treatment may be accomplished without cutting through a cemented restoration.

6. Porcelain or acrylic resin pontics may be extended when needed to compensate for changes in the residual ridge.

7. Acrylic resin veneers may be replaced if they are lost or if they have become discolored or the shade no longer matches the aging enamel on adjacent teeth.

8. Fractured porcelain veneers or pontics may be more satisfactorily replaced.

9. Solder joints may be reinforced if they become weakened by attrition.

10. Future addition of another abutment for increased support is made possible.

11. Patient is encouraged to return at recommended intervals for inspection and maintenance. In this way the dentist has an opportunity at reasonable intervals to inspect both the fixed restorations and any removable partial dentures present and to recommend relining or the reestablishment of occlusion of partial dentures when needed. Also oral hygiene habits may be noted and the patient advised accordingly.

Patients seem quick to appreciate the value of semipermanent cementation, particularly for fixed partial dentures, and are prone to request a continuation of the practice. To the patient, as to the dentist, permanent cementation appears to be an irrevocable act that has fewer advantages than cementation with a reliable, semipermanent material.

SELF-ASSESSMENT AIDS

1. What does utilization of a terminal abutment contribute to a removable partial denture?
2. Endodontic treatment of any tooth in the arch (when indicated) should be performed prior to making a final impression for a removable restoration. Why?
3. If you are faced with a single posterior abutment (second molar) about which you have some doubt that it can be retained and utilized as one end of a tooth-supported base, what options do you have relative to design of the denture?
4. Abutment preparations on sound enamel should be accomplished in a definite order with the altered and designed diagnostic cast used as a blueprint. Give the order of preparation, including a method to check your preparation.
5. What is the danger of preparing an occlusal rest seat prior to recontouring the adjacent axial surface?
6. Inlay preparations on teeth to be used as removable partial denture abutments differ from conventional inlay preparations in three requirements. What are they?
7. Where is the most vulnerable area on an abutment tooth related to cleanliness?
8. Can you give a sequence of contouring wax patterns for abutment restorations to obtain ideal contours for optimal location of components by using a dental cast surveyor?
9. A rest seat is carved on the occlusal surface of a full gold crown pattern for a posterior abutment. The occlusal morphology has been carved to satisfy occlusal requirements, and axial contours have also been accomplished. The rest seat preparation, however, is inadequate because of its shallowness, created by insufficient room between the preparation and opposing occlusion in the area of the rest seat. What are your options to avoid a compromised result?
10. Crown ledges, parallel to the path of placement, are often carved on the lingual surfaces of abutment crowns. How does this enhance the direct retainer assembly?
11. Contrast the quality of reciprocation afforded by a crown ledge on a molar abutment and that offered by the lingual surface of an unrestored molar abutment.

12. Explain the method of preparing a lingual ledge on the wax pattern for an abutment crown. Include its depth, width, extent, and definitive location.

13. How may the crown ledge be refined after the crown has been cast?

14. Describe the contouring of the component of the direct retainer assembly that occupies the crown ledge preparation.

15. It is rare that the ceramic surface of a ceramo-metal crown can be fabricated and finished free-hand to exhibit the exact planned height of contour for a retentive clasp arm. How may a surveyor be used to assure that the planned location of the height of contour is established? At what stage in the fabrication of the crown should the procedure be undertaken?

16. Splinting of adjacent teeth is sometimes indicated as a means of gaining multiple abutment support. What examination data would indicate that splinting should be performed?

17. Where is the most frequent application of the use of multiple abutments by splinting found in an arch?

18. Quite often the design of a restoration requires lingual rests on lower anterior teeth. How can orthodontic movement of these teeth be minimized?

19. Isolated abutments adjacent and anterior to extension residual ridges usually have a poor prognosis utilized "as is." What is the reason for this?

20. An isolated anterior abutment adjacent to a distal extension base, when splinted to the nearest tooth, provides two beneficial effects. Can you tell what these desirable effects are?

21. An isolated abutment adjacent to an extension base may be splinted to the nearest tooth by either a fixed partial denture or by a _____?

22. Missing anterior teeth should be replaced with fixed partial dentures rather than including them in a removable restoration. What are the contraindications for the preceding treatment?

23. On rare occasions an abutment tooth supporting a removable partial denture will have to be restored with an inlay or crown. Can you describe a procedure whereby an abutment crown can be fabricated to an existing direct retainer?

14 IMPRESSION MATERIALS AND PROCEDURES FOR REMOVABLE PARTIAL DENTURES

Impression materials used in the various phases of partial denture construction may be classified as being rigid, thermoplastic, or elastic substances. Rigid impression materials are those that set to a rigid consistency. Thermoplastic impression materials are those that become plastic at higher temperatures and resume their original form when the temperature has again been lowered. Elastic impression materials are those that remain in an elastic or flexible state after they have been removed from the mouth.

Most impression materials used in prosthetic dentistry may be included in the following classification:

Rigid materials
    Plaster of Paris
    Metallic oxide pastes
Thermoplastic materials
    Modeling plastic
    Impression waxes and resins
Elastic materials
    Reversible hydrocolloids (agar-agar)
    Irreversible hydrocolloids (alginate)
    Mercaptan rubber-base impression materials
      (Thiokol)
    Silicone impression materials

Although rigid impression materials may be capable of recording tooth and tissue details accurately, they cannot be removed from the mouth without fracture and reassembly. Thermoplastic materials cannot record minute details accurately because they undergo distortion during withdrawal from tooth and tissue undercuts. Elastic materials are the only ones that can be withdrawn from tooth and tissue undercuts without permanent deformation and are therefore the only ones suitable for impressions of irregular contours of oral tissues. Whereas the rigid and thermoplastic impression materials are most frequently used in various combinations in the making of impressions for complete dentures, the elastic impression materials are most generally used for the making of impressions for removable partial dentures, immediate dentures, and crowns and fixed partial dentures when tooth and tissue undercuts and surface detail must be recorded with accuracy.

RIGID MATERIALS*

Plaster of Paris. One type of rigid impression material is plaster of Paris, which has been used in dentistry for over 200 years. Although all plaster-of-Paris impression materials are handled in approximately the same manner, the setting and flow characteristics of each manufacturer's product will vary. Some are pure, finely ground plaster of Paris with only an accelerator added to expedite setting within reasonable working limits. Others are modified impression plasters in which binders and plasticizers have been added to permit limited border molding while the material is setting. These do not set as hard or fracture as clean as pure plaster of Paris and therefore cannot be reassembled with as much accuracy if fracture occurs. However, they are preferred by some dentists because of their setting characteristics.

Plaster of Paris was once the only material that could be used for partial denture impressions, but now elastic materials have completely replaced the impression plasters is this phase of prosthetic dentistry. It is still widely used for making accurate trans-

*Much of this discussion has been quoted or paraphrased from McCracken, W. L.: Impression materials in prosthetic dentistry, Dent. Clin. North Am., pp. 671-684, Nov., 1958.

fers of abutment castings or copings in the fabrication of fixed restorations and internal attachment dentures and for making rigid indexes and matrices for various purposes in prosthetic dentistry.

Metallic oxide pastes. A second type of rigid impression material is that classified as metallic oxide pastes, these usually being some form of a zinc-oxide–eugenol combination. A number of these pastes are available today, and they are probably more widely used than any other secondary impression material. They are not used as primary impression materials and are not used in stock impression trays.

Metallic oxide pastes are manufactured with a wide variation of consistencies and setting characteristics. For convenience, most of them are dispensed from two tubes, an arrangement that enables the dentist to mix the correct proportion from each tube onto a glass or paper mixing slab. The previously prepared tray is loaded and positioned in the mouth with or without any attempt at border molding. Generally, border molding of metallic oxide impression pastes is not advisable, as wrinkles will occur if movement is permitted at the time the material reaches its setting state. Therefore, as in most modern impression techniques, the accuracy of the primary impression and of the impression tray has a great influence on the final impression. Some metallic oxide pastes remain fluid for a longer period of time than do others, and some manufacturers claim that border molding is possible. In general, however, all metallic oxide pastes have one thing in common with plaster-of-Paris impression materials: they all have a setting time during which they should not be disturbed and after which no further border molding is effective.

Although metallic oxide pastes, being rigid substances, are widely used as secondary impression materials for complete dentures, they are also used for secondary impressions in removable partial denture techniques. One widely used removable partial denture impression technique utilizes a paste impression of the edentulous ridge made in a resin or shellac impression tray, which is then finger-loaded through an opening in a stock perforated tray while an overall alginate hydrocolloid impression is made of the entire arch. This technique attempts to relate the zinc oxide impression of the edentulous ridge to the rest of the arch in a relationship similar to that which will be assumed when an occlusal load is applied. (See Chapter 15.)

Metallic oxide pastes are also used as an impression material for relining denture bases and may be used successfully for this purpose if the original denture base has been relieved sufficiently to allow the material to flow without displacement of either the denture or the underlying tissues.

THERMOPLASTIC MATERIALS*

Modeling plastic. Like plaster of Paris, modeling plastic is among the oldest of the impression materials used in prosthetic dentistry. It is manufactured "in several different colors, each color being an indication of the temperature range at which the material is plastic and workable. A common error in the use of modeling plastic is that it is subjected to higher temperatures than intended by the manufacturer. It then becomes too soft and loses [some of] its favorable working characteristics. If a controlled water bath is not used, a thermometer should be used routinely to maintain a temperature within limits that will not cause a weakening of the material or influence its working characteristics. If modeling plastic is softened at a temperature above that intended by the manufacturer, the material becomes brittle and unpredictable. Also there is the ever-present danger of burning the patient when the temperature used in softening the modeling plastic is too high."

The most commonly used modeling plastic is the red material that, in cake form, softens at about 132° F. It should never be softened at temperatures much above this. Niether it nor any other modeling plastic should be immersed in the water bath for an indefinite period of time. Rather, it should not leave the dentist's fingers during the softening period for more than a few seconds. It should be dipped and kneaded until soft, and it should be subjected to no more heat than necessary before loading the tray and positioning it in the mouth. Then it may be flamed with an alcohol torch for the purpose of border molding but should always be tem-

---

*Much of this discussion has been quoted or paraphrased from McCracken, W. L.: Impression materials in prosthetic dentistry, Dent. Clin. North Am., pp. 671-684, Nov., 1958.

pered by being dipped back into the water bath before its return to the mouth to avoid burning the patient. The modeling plastic then may be chilled before removal from the mouth, although this is not necessary if care is used in removing the impression. During sectional flaming and border molding it should be chilled in ice water after each removal from the mouth. Then it may be trimmed with a sharp knife without danger of fracture or distortion.

The red, gray, and green modeling plastics are obtainable in stick form for use in border molding an impression or an impression tray. The green material is the lowest fusing of the modeling plastics. The red and gray sticks have a higher and broader working range than do the cakes of like color so that they may be flamed without harming the material. Because of its contrasting lighter color, the gray material in stick form is preferred by some dentists for border molding. The choice between the use of green and gray sticks is purely optional and entirely up to the dentist.

Although modeling plastic had been used in past years as an impression material for diagnostic casts, it has now been replaced by the elastic materials. Some dentists still prefer to use modeling plastic as a secondary impression material for the recording of edentulous ridges in partial denture construction, but when this is done, the limitations and disadvantages are the same as for making a full modeling plastic impression for complete dentures. Similarly, modeling plastic is sometimes used as a reline impression material for partial denture bases. It is generally used, however, only as a means of building up the underside of the denture prior to recording the tissues with some secondary impression material. (See Chapter 15.)

Impression waxes and resins. A second group of thermoplastic impression materials are those impression waxes and resins commonly spoken of as "mouth-temperature waxes." The most familiar of these have been the Iowa wax and the Korecta waxes, both of which were developed for specific techniques. One must be cognizant of the characteristics of mouth-temperature waxes and use them knowingly. Manufacture of Korecta wax has now been discontinued by the Kerr Company.

The Iowa impression wax, for example, was designed to be used as a wax impression over a modeling plastic correction in an acrylic resin tray. The Korecta waxes were developed to record the supporting form of the edentulous areas, which provide support for a distal extension partial denture base. The No. 4 wax was the most fluid and was quite similar to the Iowa formula in most respects. In fact the two waxes may be used interchangeably without any detectable difference in results. The No. 1 Korecta wax was not an impression wax, but was instead a supporting wax that was unaffected by mouth temperature. Therefore it was used as a means for supporting the impression of the border during the making of fluid wax impressions. Kerr ivory inlay wax is an acceptable substitute for the Korecta No. 1 wax. The No. 2 and 3 Korecta waxes, although developed to provide a broader range of flow characteristics, have not been available for some time.

The Iowa wax was developed for use in recording the functional or supporting form of an edentulous ridge. It may be used either as a secondary impression material or as an impression material for relining the finished partial denture to obtain support from the underlying tissues. "The mouth-temperature waxes lend themselves well to all relining techniques as they will flow sufficiently in the mouth to avoid overdisplacement of tissues. As with any relining technique, it is necessary that sufficient relief be provided. In addition, escapement slots or holes in the original base must be used, to avoid locking the impression material against the tissues without opportunity for escape." Given an opportunity to flow, the fluid waxes record the tissues without overdisplacement and assure uniformity of support for the partial denture base.

The difference between impression wax and modeling plastic is that the impression waxes have the ability to flow as long as they are in the mouth and thereby permit equalization of pressure and prevent overdisplacement; whereas the modeling plastics flow only in proportion to the amount of flaming and tempering that can be done out of the mouth, and this does not continue after the plastic has approached mouth temperature. The principal advantage of mouth-temperature waxes is that given sufficient time they permit a rebound of those tissues that have been overdisplaced.

The impression waxes also may be used to correct the borders of impressions made of more rigid materials, thereby establishing optimal contact at the border of the denture. All mouth-temperature wax impressions have the ability to record border detail accurately and at the same time establish the correct width of the denture border. They have the advantage of being correctable, and if the dentist will take sufficient time in the making of the correction, he may record accurately not only surface detail but also all border areas that are available for support and retention of the denture.

Some mouth-temperature waxes vary in their working characteristics from those mentioned herein. Among these are the Jelenko Adaptol impression material and the Stalite impression material. Both of these seem to have a more resinous base. They are designed primarily for impression techniques that attempt to record the tissues under an occlusal load. In such techniques the occlusion rim or the arrangement of artificial teeth is completed first. Mouth-temperature wax is then applied to the tissue side of the denture base, and the final impression is made under functional loading, using various movements simulating functional activity. However, these mouth-temperature materials also may be used successfully in open-mouth impression techniques.

The Iowa wax will not distort after removal from the mouth at ordinary room temperatures, but the more resinous waxes must be stored at much lower temperatures to avoid flow out of the mouth. Resinous waxes are not ordinarily used in partial denture impression techniques, being limited to specific techniques for complete denture impressions.

ELASTIC MATERIALS*

Reversible hydrocolloids. Reversible (agar) hydrocolloids, which are fluid at higher temperatures and gel on a reduction in temperature, are used primarily as impression materials for fixed restorations. They are

*Much of this discussion has been quoted or paraphrased from McCracken, W. L.: Impression materials in prosthetic dentistry, Dent. Clin. North Am., pp. 671-684, Nov., 1958.

unsurpassed for accuracy when properly used. However, the reversible hydrocolloid impression materials offer few advantages over the irreversible or alginate hydrocolloids when used as a partial denture impression material. Present-day alginate hydrocolloids are sufficiently accurate for the making of master casts for partial dentures. However, border control of impressions made with these materials is difficult.

Irreversible hydrocolloids. The irreversible (alginate) hydrocolloids are used for the making of diagnostic casts, orthodontic treatment casts, and master casts for removable partial denture procedures. Since they are a colloidal material, an alginate hydrocolloid impression cannot be stored for any length of time but must be poured immediately. The same precautions in handling apply equally to both the reversible and irreversible hydrocolloid impression materials.

Mercaptan rubber-base impression materials. The mercaptan rubber-base (Thiokol) impression materials are used for removable partial denture impressions and especially for secondary or altered cast impressions. To be accurate the impression must have a uniform thickness not exceeding 3 mm (⅛ in). This necessitates the use of a carefully made individual impression tray of acrylic resin or some other material possessing adequate rigidity and stability. It is doubtful that the accuracy of a mercaptan rubber-base impression exceeds that of a properly made alginate hydrocolloid impression, and as with the hydrocolloid impression materials, certain precautions must be taken to avoid distortion of the impression. The mercaptan rubber-base impression materials do have an advantage over the hydrocolloid materials in that the surface of an artificial stone poured against them is of a smoother texture and therefore appears to be smoother and harder than one poured against a hydrocolloid material. This is probably due to the fact that the rubber material does not have the ability to retard or etch the surface of the setting stone. Despite their accuracy, this has always been a disadvantage of all hydrocolloid impression materials. A cast made from a mercaptan rubber or silicone impression possesses a smoother surface that may possibly lead to a more accurate dental casting. The fact that a smoother surface results does not, however, preclude the possibility of a grossly inaccurate impression and stone cast resulting from other causes. Rubber-base impression materials, possessing a longer setting time than the irreversible hydrocolloid materials, lend themselves better to border molding in adequate supporting trays.

Silicone impression materials. The silicone impression materials are similar in their accuracy and convenience to the rubber-base impression materials. They are used primarily as impression materials for crown and fixed partial denture procedures and require the same precautions as do the rubber-base materials. They are more delicate to handle in the laboratory, and because of their cost and delicate nature they are not widely used as impression materials for removable partial denture master casts. In general, however, they possess many of the same advantages and disadvantages of rubber-base materials and may be similarly used when handled with care.

IMPRESSIONS OF THE PARTIALLY EDENTULOUS ARCH

An impression of the partially edentulous arch must record accurately the anatomic form of the teeth and surrounding tissues. This is necessary so that the prosthesis may be designed to follow a definite path of placement and removal and also that support and retention on the abutment teeth may be precise and accurate.

Materials that could be permanently deformed by removal from tissue undercuts may not be used. This excludes the use of the thermoplastic impression materials for recording the anatomic form of the dental arch. The rigid materials such as plaster of Paris are capable of recording tissue detail accurately, but they must be sectioned for removal and subsequently reassembled.

Before the advent of the elastic hydrocolloid materials, plaster of Paris and modeling plastic were the only impression materials available for impressions of the partially edentulous arch. Modeling plastic was used for making preliminary impressions for diagnostic casts, despite its distortion on removal from undercuts. Such diagnostic casts were grossly inaccurate and permitted only approximate evaluation of tooth contours. Impressions for master casts were made of plaster of Paris, which was scored and sectioned for removal and then reassembled. This was time consuming and discomforting to the patient.

Plaster of Paris is accurate and dimensionally stable, is inexpensive, and requires no special equipment for its use. Its main disadvantages are its inflexibility and the fact that some separating medium must be used prior to pouring the cast to prevent the cast material, which is usually also a gypsum product, from adhering to it. Damage to the resulting cast can easily occur during removal of the impression from the cast. Since it must be removed from the mouth sectionally, small pieces from essential areas may be lost, and reassembly of the pieces may take considerable time.

The introduction of hydrocolloids as impression materials was a long step forward in dentistry. For the first time impressions could be made of undercut areas with a material that was elastic enough to be withdrawn from those undercuts without permanent distortion. It permits the making of a one-piece impression, which does not require the use of a separating medium, and it is an extremely accurate material when handled properly.

Phillips has reduced the complicated chemistry of the hydrocolloid impression materials to its simplest form in the following paragraphs:

Hydrocolloids can be classified into two general types: reversible and irreversible. These materials are suspensions of aggregates of molecules in a dispersing medium of water, the water being held by capillary action. Gelation of the reversible hydrocolloids is primarily a physical change in which a latticework of fibrils forms as the temperature is lowered. This gel can be readily dispersed by merely heating the material—thus the term reversible. An example of a reversible hydrocolloid is ordinary gelatin. When gelatin is dissolved in boiling water, it forms a colloidal sol which gels upon cooling. This gel can be returned to the liquid sol by heating, formed again by cooling, etc.

The base for dental reversible hydrocolloids is agar-agar, a material that can be liquefied at temperatures compatible to oral tissues and then solidified to a firm, yet elastic, gel at temperatures slightly above 100° F. This gelation is accomplished by means of water-cooled impression trays. Such factors as ability to secure routinely accurate reproductions of cavity preparation with one impression, reproductions of minor undercuts without rupture or distortion, and actual saving in chair time have been instrumental in the successful adaptation of this material for use in the indirect inlay technique. It is unexcelled when used in this procedure.

The irreversible hydrocolloids, or alginates, are not thermally reversible and their gelation is induced by an actual chemical reaction rather than by physical means. The powder is essentially sodium alginate and calcium sulphate which when mixed with water react to form a latticework of fibrils of insoluble calcium alginate. These materials have been used extensively in prosthetics and orthodontia. . . .

In general it can be said that the alginates approach the accuracy of reversible hydrocolloid but, due to the greater number of variables both in their manufacture and use, they are not routinely quite as accurate.*

The principal differences between agar and alginate hydrocolloids are as follows:

1. Agar converts from the gel form to a sol by the application of heat. It may be reverted to gel form by a reduction in temperature. This physical change is reversible.

2. Alginate hydrocolloid becomes a gel via a chemical reaction as a result of mixing alginate powder with water. This physical change is irreversible.

Agar hydrocolloid does have some disadvantages. It must be introduced into the mouth while warm enough to be a sol, converting to an elastic gel on cooling. Therefore there is an ever-present danger of burning the tissues of the mouth, a burn that is painful and slow to heal. It requires warming and tempering equipment that is thermostatically controlled and necessitates the use of water-jacketed impression trays for cooling.

All hydrocolloids are dimensionally stable only during a brief period after removal from the mouth. If exposed to the air, they rapidly lose water content, with a resulting shrinkage and other dimensional changes. If immersed in water, they imbibe water, with an accompanying swelling and dimensional changes. All hydrocolloid impressions should be poured immediately, but if they must be stored for a brief period of time, it should be in a saturated atmosphere rather than in water. This is accomplished simply by wrapping the impression in a damp towel.

*From Phillips, R. W.: The physical properties of hydrocolloids and alginates and factors influencing their work qualities and accuracy, Fortn. Rev. Chic. Dent. Soc. **26:**9-12, 1953.

All hydrocolloids also exhibit a phenomenon known as syneresis, which is associated with the giving off of a mucinous exudate. This mucinous exudate has a retarding effect on any gypsum material, which results in a soft or chalky cast surface. Sometimes this is less obvious and only detected by a close examination of the impression after removal from the cast. Nevertheless, such a cast surface is inaccurate, and an inaccurate denture casting ultimately results in proportion to the inaccuracy of the master cast. This can only be prevented by pouring the cast immediately and using some chemical accelerator such as potassium sulfate to counteract the retarding effect of the hydrocolloid.

Agar hydrocolloid impressions should be immersed in a 2% solution of potassium sulfate for five to ten minutes before the cast is poured, even though some accelerator may have been incorporated by the manufacturer. Almost all modern alginate hydrocolloid impression materials have an accelerator incorporated into the powder and no longer need to be treated with a "fixing solution" unless one is supplied by the manufacturer. However, an alginate hydrocolloid impression material that is compounded to require a "fixing solution" consistently gives a smoother cast surface than those that do not require immersion in such a solution. It is probably because of the popular demand for alginate impression materials that do not require fixing that the suppliers have all but abandoned the manufacture of those requiring a fixing solution.

Since no heat is employed in the preparation of alginate hydrocolloid, there is no danger of burning the patient. For this reason the patient will be more relaxed and cooperative during the positioning of the tray. However some disadvantages are associated with the use of alginate hydrocolloid. This material gels by means of a chemical reaction that is accelerated by the warmth of the tissues; whereas agar hydrocolloid gels from the tray in toward the tissues, because of the colling action of the water circulating through the tray. In the former, gelation takes place first next to the tissues, and any movement of the tray during gelation of the remote portions results in internal stresses that are released on removal of the impression from the mouth. A distorted and therefore inaccurate impression results from an alginate hydrocolloid impression that is not held immobile during gelation.

Another disadvantage of alginate hydrocolloid is that is must be introduced into the mouth at approximately 70° F, which causes an immediate increase in the viscosity and surface tension of the saliva. Air bubbles are therefore harder to dispel, and it is inevitable that more air will be trapped in an alginate impression than in an agar impression. Every precaution must be taken to avoid the entrapment of air in critical areas.

Important precautions to be observed in the handling of hydrocolloid. Some important precautions to be observed in the handling of hydrocolloid are as follows:

1. Impression should not be exposed to air because some dehydration will inevitably occur, resulting in shrinkage.

2. Impression should not be immersed in water because some imbibition will inevitably result, with an accompanying expansion.

3. Impression should be protected from dehydration by placing it in a humid atmosphere or wrapping it in a damp towel until a cast can be poured. To avoid volume change, this should be within fifteen minutes after removal from the mouth.

4. Exudate from hydrocolloid has a retarding effect on the chemical reaction of gypsum products and results in a chalky cast surface. This can be prevented by pouring the cast immediately and by first immersing the impression in a solution of accelerator.

Step-by-step procedure for making a hydrocolloid impression. The step-by-step procedure and important points to observe in the making of a hydrocolloid impression are as follows:

1. Select a suitable perforated impression tray that is large enough to provide a 4 to 5 mm border thickness of the impression material.

2. If the maxillary arch has a high palatal contour, build up the tray with beeswax to prevent the hydrocolloid from sagging away from the palatal surface (Fig. 14-1, A). If gelation occurs next to the tissues while the deeper portion is still fluid, a distorted impression of the palate may result, which cannot be detected in the finished impression. This may result in the major

Fig. 14-1. **A,** Maxillary impression tray with palatal portion built up with beeswax to prevent impression material from sagging away from palatal surface. Beeswax is also added across posterior border of tray to cover maxillary tuberosities and to prevent impression material from being expelled posteriorly when impression is made. **B,** Mandibular impression tray with beeswax added to lingual flanges to prevent tissues of floor of mouth from rising inside tray. Posterior end of tray is extended with beeswax to cover retromolar pad regions.

connector of the finished casting not being in contact with the underlying tissues. The maxillary tray frequently has to be extended posteriorly to include the tuberosities and vibrating line region of the palate. Such an extension also aids in correctly orienting the tray in the patient's mouth when the impression is being made.

3. The lingual flange of the mandibular tray may need to be lengthened with beeswax in the retromylohyoid area or to be extended posteriorly, but rarely ever needs to be lengthened elsewhere. Beeswax may need to be added *inside* the distolingual flange to prevent the tissues of the floor of the mouth from rising inside the tray (Fig. 14-1, *B*).

4. Place the patient in an upright position, with the involved arch nearly parallel to the floor.

5. When using alginate hydrocolloid, place the measured amount of water (at 70° F) in a clean, dry, rubber mixing bowl (600 ml capacity). Add the correct measure of powder. Spatulate rapidly against the side of the bowl with a short, *stiff* spatula. This should be accomplished in less than one minute. The patient should rinse his mouth with cool water to eliminate excess saliva while the impression material is being mixed and the tray is being loaded.

6. In placing the material in the tray, try to avoid entrapping air. Have the first layer of material lock through the perforations of the tray to prevent any possible dislodgment after gelation.

7. After loading the tray, quickly place (rub) some material with the finger on any critical areas such as rest preparations and abutment teeth. If a maxillary impression is being made, place material in the highest aspect of the palate and over the rugae.

8. Use a mouth mirror or index finger to retract the cheek on the side away from you as the tray is being rotated into the mouth from the near side.

9. Seat the tray first on the side away from you, next on the anterior area while reflecting the lip, and then on the near side, using the mouth mirror or finger for cheek retraction. Finally make sure that the lip is draping naturally over the tray.

10. Be careful not to seat the tray too deeply, leaving room for a thickness of material over the occlusal and incisal surfaces.

11. Hold the tray immobile for three minutes with light finger pressure over left and right premolar areas. Do not allow the tray to move during gelation to avoid internal stresses in the finished impression. Do not allow the patient or the assistant to hold the tray in position. Some movement of the tray is inevitable during the transfer, and at a critical time of gelation, movement will produce an inaccurate impression.

12. After releasing the surface tension, remove the impression quickly in line with the long axis of the teeth to avoid tearing or other distortion.

13. Rinse the impression free of saliva with gently running, room temperature tap water and examine critically. Cover the impression immediately with a damp towel.

A cast should be poured immediately into a hydrocolloid impression to avoid dimensional changes and syneresis. Circumstances often necessitate some delay, but this time lapse should be kept to a minimum. A fifteen-minute delay is not deleterious if the impression is kept in a humid atmosphere.

Step-by-step procedure for making a stone cast from a hydrocolloid impression. The step-by-step procedure for making the stone cast from the impression is as follows:

1. Have the measured dental stone at hand, along with a measured quantity of water, as recommended by the manufacturer. For most laboratory stones, 28 ml of water for each 100 g is recommended; for improved stones the proportion is 24 ml of water for each 100 g. A clean 600 ml mixing bowl, a stiff spatula, and a vibrator complete the preparations. A No. 7 spatula also should be within reach.

2. First pour the measure of water into the mixing bowl and then add the measure of stone. Spatulate thoroughly for one minute, remembering that a weak and porous stone cast may result from insufficient spatulation. *Mechanical spatulation or vacuum spatulation if such facilities are available may be used to advantage.* After any spatulation other than in a vacuum, place the mixing bowl on the vibrator and knead the material to permit the escape of any trapped air.

3. The hydrocolloid impression material used may require a fixing solution. If so, follow the manufacturer's instructions. Any fixing is done just prior to pouring the cast and is not meant to be used as a storing medium. After removing the impression from the damp towel or fixing solution, gently shake out surplus moisture and hold the impression in the left hand over the vibrator with the impression side up. The impression material must not be placed in contact with the vibrator because of possible distortion of the impression.

4. With a small spatula add the first cast material to the distal area away from you. Allow this first material to be vibrated around the arch from tooth to tooth toward the anterior part of the impression (Fig. 14-2). Continue to add small increments of material at this same distal area, each portion of added stone pushing the mass ahead of it. This avoids the entrapment of air. The weight of the material causes any excess

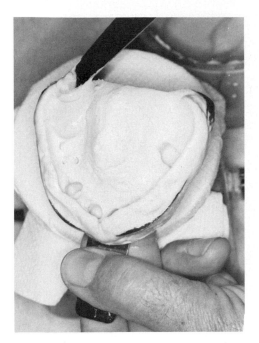

Fig. 14-2. Small portions of mechanically spatulated stone are applied at a posterior section of impression and vibrated around arch, pushing moisture and diluted stone ahead of mass. Stone is applied at this point only until impressions of teeth are filled and diluted stone is discarded at opposite end. Only then is remainder of impression filled with larger portions, using a larger spatula. Only handle of impression tray should be allowed to touch vibrator so that distortion of impression material will be avoided. (Note that vibrator is protected with a paper towel as impression is being filled.)

water to be pushed around the arch and to be expelled ultimately at the opposite end of the impression. Discard this fluid material. When the impressions of all teeth have been filled, continue to add artificial stone in larger portions until the impression is completely filled.

5. Then the filled impression should be placed on a supporting jig and the base of the cast completed with the same mix of stone (Fig. 14-3). The base of the cast should be 16 to 18 mm (⅔ to ¾ in) at its thinnest portion and should be extended beyond the borders of the impression so that buccal, labial, and lingual borders will be recorded correctly in the finished cast. *A distorted cast may result from an inverted impression.*

6. As soon as the cast material has developed sufficient body, trim the gross excess from the sides of the cast. Wrap the

impression and cast in a wet paper towel or place it in a humidor until the initial set of the stone has taken place. The impression is thus prevented from losing water by evaporation, which might in turn deprive the cast material of sufficient water for crystallization. Chalky cast surfaces around the teeth are often the result of the hydrocolloid's acting as a sponge and robbing the cast material of its necessary water for crystallization.

7. After the cast and impression have been in the humid atmosphere for thirty minutes, separate the impression from the cast. Thirty minutes is sufficient for initial setting. Any stone interfering with separation must be trimmed away with a knife.

8. Clean the impression tray immediately while the used impression material is still elastic.

9. The trimming of the cast should be deferred until final setting has occurred. The sides of the cast then may be trimmed to be parallel, and any blobs or defects due to air bubbles in the impression may be removed. If this is a cast for a permanent record, it may be trimmed to orthodontic specification to present a neat appearance for demonstration purposes. Master casts and other working casts are ordinarily trimmed only to remove excess stone.

Possible causes of an inaccurate cast of a dental arch. The possible causes of an inaccurate cast are as follows:

1. Distortion of the hydrocolloid impression (a) by partial dislodgment from tray, (b) by shrinkage due to dehydration, (c) by expansion due to imbibition (this will be toward the teeth and will result in an undersize rather than an oversize cast), (d) by attempting to pour the cast with stone that is too resistant.

2. A ratio of water to powder that is too high. While this may not cause volumetric changes in the size of the cast, it will result in a weak cast.

3. Improper mixing. This also results in a weak cast or one with a chalky surface.

4. Trapping of air, either in the mix or in pouring, because of insufficient vibration.

5. Soft or chalky cast surface due to the retarding action of the hydrocolloid or the absorption of necessary water for crystalization by the dehydrating hydrocolloid.

6. Premature separation of the cast from the impression.

7. Failure to separate the cast from the impression for an extended period of time.

Fig. 14-3. A, Homemade plastic jigs are used to support impressions. Handle of tray is placed in slotted portion, and posterior end of tray is supported by elevated cross-members. Jig used to support mandibular impression is on left. **B,** Note that impression trays are elevated and contact jigs at only three points. **C,** An impression could be easily distorted when cast is being poured if tray was placed on laboratory bench. Since impression is elevated by jig, distortion of impression is minimized. **D,** After impression is filled with stone, as previously demonstrated, it is placed in jig and additional stone is added to form base of cast. **E,** Mandibular impression placed in jig to demonstrate support by jig. Note that impression is supported by contact of tray only at handle and on either side posteriorly. **F,** Impression is returned to supporting jig after being filled with stone. Wet paper is placed in tongue space to support stone base in this region and to avoid locking impression tray to cast. **G,** Additional stone is added to impression to form a base for cast.

Pouring of working casts upon which abutment restorations are to be fabricated. The pouring of casts into hydrocolloid, mercaptan rubber, or silicone impressions to make removable dies is adequately covered in crown and fixed partial denture textbooks. However, a method will be given here for the making of a working cast upon which the contours of wax patterns may be refined to satisfy the requirements of *noninterference to placement, parallelism,* and *retention* for the partial denture.

Use of a double-pour technique, with separation of removable dies by means of a fine jeweler's saw blade has proven most adequate. The removable portion of the die must have keyed dowel pins for handling and for accuracy in seating back in the cast (Fig. 14-4, *A*). If a metal die surface is preferred, mercaptan and silicone impressions may be electroplated prior to dies being poured, which are then separated by sawing (Fig. 14-4, *B* and *C*).

The electroformed dies may be replaced in the original mercaptan rubber or silicone impression before the remainder of the cast is

Fig. 14-4. **A,** Placement of dowel pins in an impression of prepared teeth is guided by indelible pencil or pen lines previously drawn buccally and lingually at center of long axis of those teeth. After impression is filled above level of prepared teeth, it is supported between two pieces of clay, dowel pins are placed between and parallel to pencil lines. Lock washers then may be partially embedded into portions where separation is not desired. If impression is of prepared fixed partial denture abutments, a lock washer is also placed in edentulous space between abutments. After stone has set, areas to be separated are treated with a solution of sodium silicate or a commercial separating fluid such as Super-Sep. Impression may be boxed with wax if desired, and ends of dowel pins should be covered with a piece of utility wax so that they may be located after pouring remainder of cast. **B,** After remainder of cast is poured, preferably in stone of a different color, sides of cast should be trimmed and then allowed to dry overnight. With a No. 2 jeweler's saw blade in a saw frame, cast is cut throughout interproximal spaces, down to junction with second pour of stone. Saw cuts are made vertical unless a single die is involved; in such case, they are made converging. Dowel pin will not be encountered if it was placed perpendicular in center of prepared tooth. Utility wax is removed from ends of dowel pins, and each die is gently tapped out of its seat. **C,** Dies are now removed and are trimmed to expose precise gingival margins. Margins are lightly marked with pencil to facilitate accurate waxing and later finishing operations. Gingival thickness below margins should be as in die on left rather than too close to margin as on right. (Courtesy Kerr Manufacturing Co., Detroit, Mich.)

Scratch line indicating
path of placement

Fig. 14-5. Trimmed removable die for an abutment crown. Working cast is placed on surveyor in relation to path of placement and wax pattern formed with proximal guiding plane and with retentive and nonretentive contours in conformity with this path of placement.

poured. Although this may not be done with hydrocolloid impressions, if the careful person can reseat electroformed dies with accuracy, it is an acceptable method for making removable dies.

The method for making an electroformed die is as follows: After the impression is electroplated with silver or copper, the inside of the plated impression of each tooth involved is painted with a flux made of equal parts of concentrated hydrochloric acid, water, and glycerine. Into this fluxed concavity, low-fusing metal alloy (Dialoy or Cerrosafe metal) is poured to the top of each impression. A keyed dowel pin for each tooth is fluxed and dipped into the ladle of low-fusing alloy to tin the portion to be embedded in the impression. The metal in the impression is then melted on the surface with a needle-point flame and the tinned dowel pin inserted and held until the metal has solidified. Then each die may be removed and trimmed without fear of separation of the electroformed surface from the core of the die.

Regardless of the method used, the individual die, whether or not it is a removable die, must be trimmed to expose all margins of the preparation (Fig. 14-5). This is done to facilitate the waxing of precise gingival margins. If the die is not so trimmed, the location of gingival margins will be less exact, resulting in an overextended or, more often, an underextended restoration.

INDIVIDUAL IMPRESSION TRAYS

This chapter has dealt previously with the making of an impression in a stock tray of the anatomic form of a dental arch for making either a diagnostic cast, a working cast for restorations, or a master cast. There are times, however, when a stock tray is not suitable for the making of the final anatomic impression of the dental arch. Most tooth-borne partial dentures may be made upon a master cast from such an impression. Some maxillary distal extension partial dentures with broad palatal coverage, particularly those for a Kennedy Class I arch, may also be made upon an anatomic cast, but usually these necessitate the use of an individually made tray.

Unless a stock tray can be found that will fit the mouth with about 6 mm (¼ in) clearance for the impression material, yet without interference with bordering tissues, an individual tray made of some resin tray material should be used for the final anatomic impression.

Most partial denture trays are either of the rim-lock or perforated varieties. Both are made in a limited selection of sizes and shapes. One manufacturer in particular has gone to considerable length to provide a wide selection of perforated trays, including trays for both bilateral and unilateral edentulous areas, trays with built-in occlusal stops, and trays for particular techniques.* (See Fig. 14-6.)

All these trays have reinforced borders. Although a complete denture impression tray is, or should be, made of material that permits trimming and shaping to fit the mouth, the existence of a beaded border and the rigidity of a stock partial denture tray allow no trimming and little shaping. *The resulting impression is often a record of border tissues distorted by an ill-fitting tray rather than an impression of tissues draping naturally over a slightly underextended impression tray.*

An individual acrylic resin tray, on the other hand, can be made with sufficient clearance for the impression material and can be trimmed just short of the vestibular reflections to allow the tissues to drape naturally without distortion. The partial denture borders may then be made as accurate as complete denture borders with equal advantages.

Although techniques have been proposed for the making of individual impression trays that incorporate plastic tubing for water-cool-

*Nevin, J. J.: Tray selection for partial denture impressions, Cal **26:**10-16, July, 1963.

Fig. 14-6. Impression tray cabinet with doors open, exposing a wide selection of perforated impression trays for alginate hydrocolloid impressions. Beginning at top can be seen trays for completely edentulous mouths, depressed anterior trays, trays with unilateral occlusal stops, Hindel trays for use with a double impression technique, and the more commonly and regularly used perforated trays.

ing agar hydrocolloid impressions, the final anatomic impression usually will be made with alginate hydrocolloid, mercaptan rubber, or silicone impression materials.

Technique for making individual acrylic resin impression trays. The diagnostic cast is often adequate for the preparation of the individual tray. However, if extensive surgery or extractions were performed after the making of the diagnostic cast, a new impression in a stock tray and a new cast must be made. The procedures for making the new cast are identical to those described previously.

A duplicate of the diagnostic cast should be made upon which the individual tray can be fabricated. The cast upon which an individual tray is made is often damaged or must

be mutilated to separate the tray from the cast. Obviously the original diagnostic cast must be retained as a permanent record in the patient's file.

The technique for making an individual, maxillary acrylic resin tray is as follows:

1. Outline the extent of the tray on the cast with a pencil. The tray must include all teeth and tissues that will be involved in the removable partial denture. Adequate space must be provided for frenal attachments. Mark the area of the posterior palatal seal on the upper cast and cut a 1 mm × 1 mm groove following the line designating the posterior extent of the tray (Fig. 14-7, *A*).

2. Adapt one layer of baseplate wax over the tissue surfaces and teeth of the cast to serve as a spacer for impression material. The

Fig. 14-7. For legend see opposite page.

wax spacer should be trimmed to the outline drawn on the diagnostic cast. Wax covering the posterior palatal seal area should be removed so that intimate contact of the tray and tissue in this region may serve as an aid in correctly orienting the tray when making the impression. (See Fig. 14-7, *B*.)

3. Adapt an additional layer of baseplate wax over the teeth if the impression is to be made in irreversible hydrocolloid (alginate). This step is not necessary if the choice of impression material is a rubber-base or silicone type of material.

4. Expose portions of the incisal edges of the central incisors to serve as anterior stops when placing the tray in the mouth. Bevel the wax so that the completed tray will have a guiding incline that will help position the tray on the anterior stop.

5. Paint the exposed surfaces of the cast that may be contacted by the acrylic resin tray material with a tinfoil substitute (Alcote) to facilitate separation of the cured tray from the cast.

6. Mix the correct proportions of quick-setting acrylic resin monomer and polymer (8 ml of monomer to 24 ml of polymer) in a mixing jar or paper cup. When the resin mix is no longer stringy and can be handled without adhering to the fingers, form it into a wafer the size and thickness of a cake of modeling plastic or use special stone templates to form the wafer. (See Fig. 14-7, *C* to *E*.) A wooden roller and wafer-forming block are also available from dental supply houses in kit form.

7. Carefully transfer the resin wafer to position on the cast and adapt the resin with the fingers, covering the wax spacer and palatal seal area and maintaining a uniform thickness. Remove the gross excess with a sharp knife while the resin is still soft.

8. Form a handle with the excess resin. The handle should be about 12 mm (½ in) in width, about 6 mm (¼ in) in thickness, and about 5 cm (2 in) long.

9. Attach the handle to the tray over the region of the central incisors and shape it to extend 12 mm (½ in) downward and 2.5 cm (1 in) outward. (See Fig. 14-7, *F*.) It is usually necessary to place additional monomer on the handle and the tray to provide a satisfactory union.

10. Allow the resin to cure and remove the tray from the cast. The wax spacer can be removed from the tray with any suitable instrument.

11. Perfect the borders of the tray with rotary instruments (vulcanite burs, acrylic resin trimmers) and roughly polish the external surface of the tray (Fig. 14-7, *G*).

12. Place perforations (No. 8 bur size) in the resin tray at 4.5 mm (³/₁₆ in) intervals, with the exception of the alveolar groove areas, if an irreversible hydrocolloid impression material is to be used (Fig. 14-8).

Fig. 14-7. A, Desired outline of tray is drawn on a duplicate diagnostic cast. Post palatal seal region and a portion of incisal edges of central incisors are outlined. **B,** One thickness of baseplate wax is adapted to cast and is trimmed to penciled outline. Postpalatal seal region is not covered by wax but will be incuded in finished tray. Two thicknesses of baseplate wax cover teeth. A window is created in wax spacer over incisal edges. A tinfoil substitute is painted on stone surfaces of cast that will be contacted by autopolymerizing acrylic resin. **C,** Stone templates are used to form uniform wafers of acrylic resin dough about 3 mm (⅛ in) thick. The left template is used in making mandibular impression trays. These templates may be made by embedding a double thick shellac baseplate form in a 12 mm (½ in) thick patty of stone. They are lightly lubricated with petroleum jelly so that soft tray material will not adhere to stone when acrylic resin wafer is being made. **D,** Tray resin is mixed in a paper cup with a wooden tongue depressor. Tray material is spatulated onto stone template when it reaches a "nontacky" stage. **E,** A uniform acrylic resin wafer is made on stone template by using tongue depressor as a trowel to fill mold and to remove excess tray material. **F,** Resin wafer is carefully removed from template and adapted over cast with fingers. Excess tray material is removed from borders of cast with a sharp knife while resin is still doughy. Excess material is used to shape a handle, which is attached over incisal edges of anterior teeth. It is supported by a piece of baseplate wax until resin has become hard. **G,** As soon as tray material has hardened, tray is removed from cast, and wax spacer is removed from rough tray. An acrylic resin trimmer in a lathe is used to rough finish the tray.

Fig. 14-8. A, Holes are drilled through tray, being spaced approximately 4.5 mm (³/₁₆ in) apart. These holes will serve to lock impression material in tray. In addition, excess impression material is forced out of holes when impression is made, thereby minimally displacing soft oral tissues. **B,** Note elevated posterior palatal seal region of tray and incisal stop. These two features will assist in correctly orienting individualized impression tray in mouth.

13. The tray must be tried in the mouth so that any necessary corrections to the tray can be accomplished before the impression is made.

The technique for making an individual, mandibular acrylic resin tray follows the same procedures. The buccal shelf regions on the lower cast are left uncovered by the wax spacer to serve as posterior stops in orienting the tray in the patient's mouth and at the same time will permit selective placement of tissues in the mandibular stress-bearing areas (Fig. 14-9).

Perforations in a resin tray are not easily made with a round bur because after a few revolutions the bur becomes clogged. Instead a bi-beveled surgical drill is used, which will make the holes rapidly without clogging (Fig. 14-10). These are available in various sizes No. 100 through 106, the higher number being the smaller size. The size of the perforations should be slightly larger than those in a stock tray, and only about one third as many are used. This will be sufficient to lock the impression material in the tray

and thereby avoid distortion of the impression on removal from the mouth.

If mercaptan rubber or silicone is to be used, perforations are not usually necessary to lock the material in the tray, as the adhesive provided by the manufacturer provides reliable retention, and some confinement of these materials is desirable. However, a series of perforations are placed in the median palatal raphe and incisive papilla areas of the maxillary tray so that excess impression material will escape through them, thus providing relief of the tissues in this area. For the same reasons, perforations are placed in the alveolar groove of the mandibular tray. With the use of adhesives the impression material is not easily removed from the tray should a faulty impression have to be remade, but this is an inconvenience common to all newer elastic materials and does not prevent reuse of the impression tray.

The pouring of a cast in an alginate impression made in an individual tray presents a minor problem, since it is usually covered with the elastic material and is delicate to

Fig. 14-9. A, Outline of tray is penciled on a duplicate lower diagnostic cast. Buccal shelf region is outlined on each side of cast (dotted portion). **B,** A single sheet of baseplate wax is adapted to outline of tray, and another sheet of baseplate wax is adapted over teeth. Buccal shelves are uncovered, and a window is cut in spacer to expose incisal edges of lower central incisors. **C,** An acrylic resin wafer is formed in a stone template as described in Fig. 14-7. **D,** Tray material wafer is adapted over cast and spacer, and a handle is formed with excess tray material as previously described. **E** and **F,** Multiple holes are placed throughout tray with the exception of buccal shelf regions of tray and also the elevated incisal stop in tray. Buccal shelf region of tray on either side and incisal stop will assist in correctly orienting tray in patient's mouth.

Fig. 14-10. Bi-beveled drill used for making holes in resin impression trays. Such a drill will not clog and facilitates the making of a perforated impression tray for use with alginate hydrocolloid, mercaptan rubber, or silicone impression materials. They can be readily made with shank portion of a straight handpiece bur.

handle. Some of the excess material in the handle area may have to be cut away to expose enough of the rigid tray to make contact with the vibrator. The impression may then be vibrated while being filled, as with any other hydrocolloid impression.

Master casts made from impressions in individual resin trays are generally more accurate than are those made in stock trays. The use of individual trays should be considered a necessary step in the making of the majority of removable partial dentures when a secondary impression technique is not to be used. Reasons and methods for the making of a secondary impression will be considered in Chapter 15.

Final impressions for maxillary tooth-borne removable partial dentures often may be made in carefully selected and recontoured stock impression trays. However, an individual acrylic resin tray is preferred in those situations in the mandibular arch in which the floor of the mouth closely approximates the lingual gingiva of remaining anterior teeth. Recording the floor of the mouth at the elevation it assumes when the lips are licked is important in selecting the type of major connector to be used (Chapter 4). Modification of the borders of an individual tray to fulfill the requirements of an adequate tray is much easier than is the modification of a metal stock tray.

SELF-ASSESSMENT AIDS

1. Impression materials used in various phases of partial denture construction may be classified as rigid, thermoplastic, or elastic. Give two examples for each of the three categories.
2. Which type of impression material has been used the longest in prosthodontics?
3. Why should the metallic oxide paste types of impression material not be used for primary impressions of partially edentulous arches?
4. Modeling plastic (compound) may be used effectively in making secondary impressions of Class I and II partially edentulous arches. Why is it not used for primary impression for the partial denture patient?
5. What is an impression wax? Do its characteristics make it appropriate for use as a primary impression or for a secondary impression?
6. There are two types of hydrocolloid impression materials used in dentistry. What are the two types?
7. Are the hydrocolloid impression materials elastic or thermoplastic?
8. What is the advantage in using an elastic material versus a rigid material in making impressions of partially edentulous arches?
9. Briefly compare reversible and irreversible hydrocolloid impression materials from the standpoints of composition, gelation mechanism, trays, and relative accuracy.
10. Mercaptain rubber-base impression material may be used for primary or secondary impressions. Its characteristics make it best suited, however, for the _____ impression.

11. Does the use of mercaptan rubber-base material and silicone impression material require the use of a stock tray or an individualized tray? Why?

12. There are many different artificial stones used in dentistry and equally as many impression materials. Are these varied materials necessarily compatible with each other when used to make casts? What precautions should be taken to ensure compatibility?

13. What is syneresis? What effect will this phenomenon have on a cast poured in a hydrocolloid impression?

14. What is meant by the word "imbibition" in relation to hydrocolloid impressions? What effect does it have on a hydrocolloid impression?

15. How long should you wait to pour a cast into a hydrocolloid impression after it is removed from the mouth? Why?

16. What would be the quality of a cast poured in a hydrocolloid impression that had been exposed to air for thirty minutes?

17. The thickness of impression material when rubber-base type material is used should be about 3 mm (⅛ in) for accuracy and stability. Does this equally apply to a hydrocolloid impression material? If not, can you give a rule of thumb for the desirable thickness of the hydrocolloid material in the impression?

18. What are the advantages of using perforated stock trays vs. nonperforated stock trays when making impressions of partially edentulous arches with an irreversible hydrocolloid?

19. Inaccuracies of a cast made from a hydrocolloid impression may result from many causes. Can you think of at least six causes of such inaccuracy?

20. Why should impressions into which stone casts have been poured not be inverted until the initial set of the stone has taken place?

21. Can you describe a laboratory procedure by which removable dies or crown or inlay preparations can be recovered from an impression?

22. What are several advantages of a removable die-type cast?

23. An individual acrylic resin impression tray has two distinct advantages over any type of stock tray. Can you think of these two advantages?

24. Describe the procedures for making individual maxillary and mandibular impression trays, paying special attention to relief of the casts with wax spacers.

25. Holes about 3 mm (⅛ in) in diameter should be placed at strategic locations in both maxillary and mandibular individualized trays. Give the location of the holes and what is accomplished by so doing.

26. What is the advantage of drilling holes in acrylic resin trays with a bi-bevel drill rather than with fissure or round burs?

27. Under what circumstances would you use a stock tray in preference to an individual acrylic resin tray?

CHAPTER

15 SUPPORT FOR THE DISTAL EXTENSION DENTURE BASE

In a tooth-supported removable partial denture a metal base or the framework supporting a resin base is connected to and is part of a rigid framework that permits the direct transfer of occlusal forces to the abutment teeth through the occlusal rests. Even though the base of a tooth-supported (Kennedy Class III) partial denture supports the supplied teeth, the residual ridge beneath the base is not called on to aid in the support of the denture. Therefore the resiliency of the ridge tissues and the conformation and type of bone supporting these tissues are not factors in denture support. Regardless of the length of the span, if the framework is rigid, the abutment teeth are sound enough to carry the additional load, and the occlusal rests are properly formed, support comes entirely from the abutment teeth at either end of that span. Support may be augmented by splinting and by the use of additional abutments, but in any event the abutments are the sole support of the removable restoration.

An impression (and resulting reproduction in stone) that records faithfully the anatomic form of the teeth and their surrounding structures and the residual ridges of a dental arch is the only impression needed in the making of a tooth-borne removable partial denture. The impression also should record the moving tissues that will border the denture in an unstrained position so that the relationship of the denture base to those tissues may be as accurate as possible, being neither overextended nor underextended. Although underextension of the denture base in a tooth-supported prosthesis is the lesser of two evils, an underextended base may lead to food impaction and inadequate contours, particularly on the buccal and labial sides. For this reason, and also to record faithfully the moving tissues of the floor of the mouth in the

mandibular arch, an individual impression tray should be used rather than an ill-fitting or overextended stock tray. This has been discussed at length in Chapter 14.

DISTAL EXTENSION REMOVABLE PARTIAL DENTURE

The distal extension denture does not have the advantage of total tooth support, since one or more bases are extensions onto the residual ridge from the last available abutment. It therefore is dependent on the residual ridge for a portion of its support.

The distal extension partial denture not only must depend on the residual ridge for some *support* but also should obtain *retention* from its base, aided by indirect *retention* to prevent the denture's lifting away from the residual ridge. Whereas the tooth-supported base is secured at either end by the action of a direct retainer and supported at either end by a rest, this degree of support and direct retention are lacking in the distal extension restoration. *For this reason a distal abutment should be preserved whenever possible.* In event of the loss or absence of a distal abutment tooth, the patient must be made aware of the movements to be expected with a distal extension partial denture and the limitations imposed on the dentist when the residual ridge must be used for both support and retention for that part of the prosthesis.

FACTORS INFLUENCING THE SUPPORT OF A DISTAL EXTENSION BASE

Support from the residual ridge becomes greater as the distance from the last abutment increases and will depend on several factors:
1. Quality of the residual ridge
2. Extent of residual ridge coverage by the denture base

274

3. Type and accuracy of the impression registration
4. Accuracy of the denture base
5. Design of the partial framework
6. Total occlusal load applied

Quality of the residual ridge. The ideal residual ridge to support a denture base would consist of cortical bone covering relatively dense cancellous bone, a broad flat crest, and high vertical slopes and would be covered by firm, dense, fibrous connective tissue. Such a residual ridge would optimally support vertical and horizontal stresses placed on it by denture bases. Unfortunately this ideal is seldom encountered.

Easily displaceable tissue will not adequately support a denture base, and tissues that are interposed between a sharp, bony residual ridge and a denture base will not remain in a healthy state. Not only must the nature of the bone of the residual ridge be considered in developing optimal support for the denture base, but also its positional relationship to the direction of forces that will be placed upon it.

The crest of the bony mandibular residual ridge is most often cancellous in nature. Pressures placed on tissues overlying the crest of the mandibular residual ridge usually result in inflammation of these tissues, accompanied by the sequelae of chronic inflammation. Therefore the crest of the mandibular residual ridge cannot become a primary stress-bearing region. The buccal shelf region (bounded by the external oblique line and crest of alveolar ridge) seems to be more ideally suited for a primary stress-bearing role because it is covered by relatively firm, dense, fibrous connective tissue supported by cortical bone. In most instances this region bears more of a horizontal relationship to vertical forces than do other regions of the residual ridge (Fig. 15-1). The slopes of the residual ridge then would become the primary stress-bearing region to resist off-vertical directed forces.

The immediate crest of the bone of the maxillary residual ridge may consist primarily of cancellous bone. Oral tissues overlying the maxillary residual alveolar bone are usually of a firm, dense nature or can be surgically prepared to support a denture base. The topography of a partially edentulous maxillary arch imposes a restriction on selection of a primary stress-bearing area. In spite of impres-

Fig. 15-1. Dotted portion outlines crest of residual ridge, which should be recorded in its anatomic form in impression procedures. Similarly, retromolar pads should not be displaced by impression. Buccal shelf regions are outlined by herringbone pattern, and selected additional pressures may be placed on these regions for vertical support of denture base. Lingual slopes of residual ridge (cross-hatched) may furnish some vertical support to restoration; however, these regions principally resist horizontal rotational tendencies of denture base and should be recorded by impression in an undisplaced form.

sion procedures the crestal area of the residual ridge will become the primary stress-bearing area to vertically directed forces. Some resistance to these forces may be obtained by the immediate buccal and lingual slopes of the ridge. Palatal tissues lying between the median palatal raphe and the lingual slope of the edentulous ridge posteriorly are readily displaceable and cannot be considered as primary stress-bearing sites (Fig. 15-2). The tissues covering the crest of the maxillary residual ridge must be less displaceable than are the tissues covering palatal areas, or relief of palatal tissues must be provided either in the denture bases or for palatal major connectors.

Extent of residual ridge coverage by the denture base. The broader the coverage, the greater the distribution of the load, thereby resulting in less load per unit area. Most prosthodontists agree that a denture base should cover as much of the residual ridge as possible and be extended the maximum amount within the physiologic tolerance of the limiting border structures or tissues (Fig. 15-3). A knowledge of these border tissues and the structures that influence their move-

Fig. 15-2. Crest of maxillary residual ridge (herringbone pattern) is primary supporting region for maxillary distal extension denture base. Buccal and lingual slopes may furnish a limited amount of vertical support to denture base. It seems logical that their primary role is to counteract horizontal rotational tendencies of denture base. Dotted portion outlines incisive papilla and median palatal raphe. Relief must be provided these regions, especially if tissues covering palatal raphe are less displaceable than those covering crest of residual ridge.

Fig. 15-3. **A,** Denture base is extended posteriorly to cover maxillary tuberosities, ending in pterygomaxillary notches. Posterior border of denture is located at junction of hard and soft palate but is not extended onto soft palate. Buccal borders of denture are extended as much as possible but within the physiologic tolerance of bordering structures. **B,** Fully extended mandibular bases. Lingual flange extended into retromylohyoid space. S curve of lingual flange permits unrestricted contraction of mylohyoid muscle. Buccal portions of bases are supported by buccal shelves.

ment is paramount to developing broad coverage denture bases. In a series of experiments Kaires has shown that "maximum coverage of denture-bearing areas with large, wide denture bases is of the utmost importance in withstanding both vertical and horizontal stresses."

It is not within the scope of this text to review the anatomic considerations related to denture bases. The student is referred to several articles concerning this subject that are listed in Selected References.

Type of the impression registration. The residual ridge may be said to have two forms (Figs. 15-4 and 15-5, *A*). One is the *anatomic form,* which is the surface contour of the ridge when it is not supporting an occlusal load. It is this resting form that is recorded by a soft impression material such as plaster

of Paris or a metallic oxide impression paste *if the entire impression tray is uniformly relieved.* Depending on the viscosity of the particular impression material used and the impression tray, it is also the form recorded by mercaptan rubber, silicone, and hydrocolloid impression materials. Distortion and tissue displacement by pressure may result from confinement of the impression material within the tray and from insufficient thickness of impression material between the tray and the tissues, as well as from the viscosity of the impression material, but none of these factors is selective or physiologic in its action. These are accidental distortions of the tissues occurring through faulty technique.

Some dentists utilize the anatomic form of the residual ridge in constructing complete dentures, believing this is the most physio-

Fig. 15-4. Comparison of anatomic and functional ridge forms. **A,** Original master cast with edentulous area recorded in its anatomic form, using an elastic impression material. **B,** Same cast after edentulous area has been repoured to its functional form as recorded by a secondary impression.

Fig. 15-5. Comparison of functional and anatomic forms of same edentulous ridge. **A,** Master cast with edentulous area reproduced in its anatomic form from a hydrocolloid impression. **B,** Same master cast after edentulous areas have been repoured in their functional or supporting form, as recorded with a secondary impression. Note not only difference in surface anatomy but also that functional impression has recorded the width available for support of denture base. A new acrylic resin base may now be made by a sprinkling method to establish occlusal relationship on a base almost identical with that of finished denture.

logic form for support of the dentures. Such dentures are said to be made from anatomic impressions. However, many other dentists believe that certain regions of the residual ridge are more capable of supporting dentures than are other regions. Their impression methods are directed to placing more stress on primary stress-bearing regions with specially constructed individual trays and at the same time recording the anatomic form of other basal seat tissues, which cannot assume a stress-bearing role. Of the two rationalizations, the latter seems to be more logical.

Since there is no tooth support with which the denture base must be made compatible

and since the basal seat tissues are recorded with a predominantly anatomic impression, the complete denture fits the resting form of those tissues. When it may be presumed that occlusion is harmonious throughout the dental arch, the complete denture may move tissueward under function until the tissues beneath assume a supporting form or a compactness that will support an occlusal load. The same principle would apply to a removable partial denture made without abutment support, differing only in that the area of tissue support is less and the tissues adjacent to the remaining teeth would be impinged by tissueward movement of the denture. Without occlusal support from the natural teeth, occlusion on the tissue-supported partial denture would be negative, leaving only the remaining natural teeth to carry the masticatory load.

Several years ago, McLean and others recognized the need for recording the tissues supporting a distal extension partial denture base in their functional form or supporting state and then relating them to the remainder of the arch by means of a secondary impression. This was called a *functional impression* because it recorded the ridge relation under simulated function (Fig. 15-5, *B*).

The technique consisted of making an impression of the edentulous areas in a vulcanite or denture base tray, which was provided with modeling plastic occlusion rims. Impression paste was used to record the ridge areas while they were under biting stress. This impression was then related to the remainder of the arch by making a hydrocolloid impression with the original impression seated in the mouth. On removal of the impression from the mouth, a master cast was poured in the composite impression, with the edentulous areas recorded under functional loading. Although the tray used for the overall impression was in contact with the occlusion rims, finger pressure was necessary to hold the original impression in its functional position while the hydrocolloid material gelled. Finger pressure thus applied could at best be only an approximation of the occlusal loading under which the original impression was recorded. This variable tended to nullify the advantage of making the original impression under occlusal loading.

A variation of this technique eliminated the occlusion rims as such but provided stops of modeling plastic against the underside of the hydrocolloid impression tray for finger loading the original impression. In this method, also, the impression of the edentulous areas was made with impression paste but with the tissues in their resting form. A finger load was then applied to the hydrocolloid tray for relating the edentulous areas under some loading to the remainder of the arch as the hydrocolloid gelled. The resulting master cast recorded the anatomic or resting form of the ridge in a pseudofunctional relationship to the rest of the arch.

Hindels and others have used with apparent success a method of finger loading the anatomic impression through a hole in the hydrocolloid impression tray. These trays are available for use with the technique and eliminate the possibility of error arising from ineffective or incorrectly placed modeling plastic stops. It does not eliminate the variable of the dentist's individual interpretation of what constitutes functional loading. The occlusal loading of McLean was unquestionably a more accurate and less variable method of recording the residual ridge beneath a distal extension base, but it became a variable finger-loading relationship in the final impression. That such methods are better than making a partial denture from a one-piece anatomic impression cannot be denied, because they recognize the need for adequate support of the distal extension base.

Any method, whether it accomplishes the recording of the *functional relationship* of the ridge to the remainder of the arch or the recording of the *functional form* of the ridge itself, may provide acceptable support for the partial denture. On the other hand, those who use the static ridge form or ridge relationship for the partial denture should seriously consider the need for some mechanical stressbreaker to avoid the possible cantilever action of the distal extension base against the abutment teeth.

The one-piece colloidal or plaster impression will produce a cast that represents not a functional relationship between the various supporting structures of the mouth but only the hard and soft tissues at rest. With the partial denture in position in the dental arch the occlusal rest will fit the rest seat of the abutment tooth, while the denture base will fit the surface of the mucosa at rest. When a masticatory load is applied to the extension base, the rest will act as a definite stop, which will prevent the part of the base near the abutment tooth from transmitting the load to the underlying anatomic structures. The distal end of the base, however, being able to move freely, will transmit the full masticatory load.

It is obvious that the soft tissues covering the ridge cannot by themselves carry any load applied to them. They act as a protective padding for the bone, which in the final analysis is the structure that receives and carries the masticatory load. Distribution of this load over a maximum area of bone is a prime requisite in preventing trauma.

A denture constructed from a one-piece

impression, only recording the anatomic form of basal seat tissues, places the masticatory load only on the abutment teeth and that part of the bone that underlies the distal end of the extension base. The balance of the bony ridge will not function in carrying the load. The result will be a traumatic load to the bone underlying the distal end of the base and to the abutment tooth, which in turn will result in bone loss and loosening of the abutment tooth. Yet the use of a properly prepared individualized impression tray can be a means to record the primary stress-bearing areas in a functional form and the non-stress-bearing areas in an anatomic form, just as is often accomplished by many dentists in making impressions for complete dentures.

Some believe that every partial denture should be relined before its final placement in the mouth. Some believe that tissue can be evenly displaced and use impression materials of heavy consistency. This process introduces traumatic stresses to the underlying tissues. Some use easy-flowing pastes that produce an impression of the soft tissues at rest. During the functioning of a partial denture so relined the sequence of events will be similar to that of a partial denture constructed from a one-piece impression. The occlusal rest will act as a stop, preventing an even distribution of the masticatory load by the base to the edentulous ridge.

An impression technique as given by Hindels is as follows:

An acrylic resin tray is processed on a cast made from an impression that should include all areas of future tissue support of the partial denture. The tray is selectively relieved and, when checked in the mouth, should cover the edentulous areas up to the border tissue attachments and should include the retromolar pads. The bases of the tray should be connected with each other by means of an acrylic resin lingual bar. The bar should cover the area between the muscle attachments of the floor of the mouth and the lingual gingivae of the anterior teeth. The tray should clear the free gingivae around the abutment teeth to prevent future impingement and stripping.

This tray is loaded with an easy-flowing zinc oxide–eugenol paste and is brought into position in the mouth, care being taken that the soft tissues are left in their passive state.

After the material has hardened, the tray is removed and the impression examined. In a successful impression the tissue side of the tray is fully covered with impression material, and no part of the tray itself is visible. The material that has flowed from the tray onto the abutment teeth should now be cut away and the tray reinserted in the mouth and tested for stability.

The next step is to make an impression of the teeth and to establish a relationship between the teeth and the mucosa in a displaced state. For this purpose a perforated tray that has been provided with two circular openings of approximately 18 mm (¾ in) diameter in the region of the first molars is used. The impression of the soft tissue areas is placed in the mouth. Then, while the tray is being loaded with an alginate impression material, some of this material is used to fill in the space between the soft tissue impression and the remaining teeth. The loaded metal tray is then inserted over both the teeth and the acrylic resin tray. The index fingers are passed through the openings in the perforated tray until they contact the underlying tray; then pressure is exerted upon it. This pressure should be maintained until the alginate impression material has hardened. The completed impression is then removed as one unit. The cast made in this impression will be a reproduction of both the surface of the teeth and the undistorted surface of the mucosa, but the two will be related to each other with the mucosa in a functional state as it would be found under the partial denture base during mastication. While the base is related to the occlusal rest with the mucosa in a functional state, the tissue surface of the base is actually a reproduction of the passive and undistorted mucosa as obtained with zinc oxide–eugenol paste in the individual impression tray.*

The form of the residual ridge recorded under some loading, whether by occlusal loading, finger loading, specially designed individual trays, or the consistency of the recording medium, is called the *functional form*. This is the surface contour of the ridge when it is supporting a functional load. How much it will differ from the anatomic form

---

*Paraphrased from Hindels, G. W.: Load distribution in extension saddle partial dentures, J. Prosthet. Dent. 2:92-100, 1952.

will depend on the thickness and structural characteristics of the soft tissues overlying the residual bone. It will also differ from the anatomic form in proportion to the total load applied to the denture base.

The objective of any functional impression technique is to provide maximum support for the removable partial denture base, thereby maintaining occlusal contact to distribute the occlusal load over both natural and artificial dentition and at the same time minimize movement of the base, which would create leverage on the abutment teeth. While some tissueward movement of the distal extension base is unavoidable and dependent on the six factors listed previously, it can be minimized by providing the best possible support for the denture base.

Steffel has classified advocates of the various methods for treating the distal extension partial denture as follows:

1. Those who believe that ridge and tooth supports can best be equalized by the use of stressbreakers or resilient equalizers
2. Those who insist on bringing about the equalization of ridge and tooth support by physiologic basing, which is accomplished by a pressure impression or by relining the denture under functional stresses
3. Those who uphold the idea of extensive stress distribution for stress reduction at any one point

It would seem that there is little difference in the philosophy behind methods 2 and 3 as given by Steffel, for both the equalization of tooth and tissue support and stress distribution over the greatest area are objectives of the functional type of impression. Many of the requirements and advantages that may be given for the distributed stress denture apply equally well to the functionally or physiologically based denture. Some of these requirements are (1) positive occlusal rests; (2) an all-rigid, nonflexible framework; (3) indirect retainers, wherever practical, to add stability; and (4) well-adapted, broad-coverage bases.

Those who do not accept the theory of physiologic basing, for one reason or another, should use some form of stressbreaker between the abutment and the distal extension base. The advantages and disadvantages of doing so have been given in Chapter 8.

Accuracy of the denture base. Support of the distal extension base is enhanced by intimacy of contact of the tissue surface of the base and the tissues covering the residual ridge. The tissue surface of the denture base must optimally represent a true negative of the basal seat regions of the master cast. Denture bases have been discussed in Chapter 8.

In addition the denture base must be related to the partial denture framework the same as the basal seat tissues were related to the abutment teeth when the impression was made. Every precaution must be taken to ensure this relationship when the altered-cast technique of making a master cast is used.

Design of the partial denture framework. Some rotation movement of a distal extension base around posteriorly placed direct retainers is inevitable under functional loading. The greatest movement takes place at the most posterior extent of the denture base. The retromolar pad region of the mandibular residual ridge and the tuberosity region of the maxillary residual ridge therefore are subjected to the greatest movement of the denture base (Fig. 15-6). *As the rotational axis (fulcrum line) of the denture is moved anteriorly, more of the residual ridge is utilized to support the denture base, thereby distributing stresses over a proportionally greater area.* Steffel and Kratochvil have excellently demonstrated this concept in dental periodical literature (Fig. 15-7). In many instances, occlusal rests may be moved anteriorly to better utilize the residual ridge for support without jeopardizing either vertical or horizontal support of the denture by occlusal rests and guiding planes (Fig. 15-8).

Total occlusal load applied. The total occlusal load applied is influenced by the number of supplied teeth, the width of their occlusal surfaces, and their occlusal efficiency. Kaires conducted an investigation under laboratory conditions and concluded that "the reduction of the size of the occlusal table reduces the vertical and horizontal forces acting on the partial dentures and lessens the stress on the abutment teeth and supporting tissues."*

---

*From Kaires, A. K.: Effect of partial denture design on bilateral force distribution, J. Prosthet. Dent. 6:373-389, 1956.

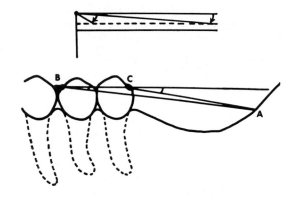

Fig. 15-6. Acute dip of a short denture base is compared with that of a long one in upper figure. In lower figure, when point of rotation is changed from *C* to *B*, it can be seen that a proportionally greater area of residual ridge is utilized to support denture base than occurs when fulcrum line passes through *C*. Line *AC* represents length of denture base.

Fig. 15-7. Assuming that rotation of a distal extension base occurs around nearest rest, as rest is moved anteriorly, more of residual ridge will be utilized to resist rotation. Compare the more nearly vertical arcs of "long-dash" broken line with arcs of solid line.

Fig. 15-8. A, Occlusal rest is placed on mesio-occlusal surface of lower first premolar to move point of rotation anterior to a conventionally placed distocclusal rest. Occlusal rest is connected to lingual bar by a minor connector, which contacts a small mesiolingual prepared guiding plane. Note vertical extension of denture base minor connector contacting a guiding plane surface also. Lingual guiding plane is prepared to extend from occlusal surface inferiorly to approximately one fifth the height of lingual surface and is as broad as contacting minor connector. Distal guiding plane extends from distal marginal ridge gingivally to about two thirds the height of distal surface. Such preparations will not lock tooth in a viselike grip when denture base rotates toward residual ridge. **B,** Buccal view of **A.** Direct retainer assembly is completed by a bar-type clasp with only retentive tip engaging an undercut. It is possible that rotation toward basal seat will occur around anterior portion of direct retainer retentive arm located occlusally to height of contour. In any event, rotation will occur around some portion of direct retainer assembly.

METHODS FOR OBTAINING FUNCTIONAL SUPPORT FOR THE DISTAL EXTENSION BASE

A thorough understanding of the characteristics of each of the impression materials leads to the obvious conclusion that no single material of itself can record both the anatomic form of the teeth and tissues in the dental arch and, at the same time, the functional form of the residual ridge. Therefore some secondary impression method must be used.

This may be accomplished by several methods. Each of them seems to satisfy the two requirements for providing adequate support to the distal extension partial denture base, which are (1) that it records and relates the tissues under some loading and (2) that it distributes the load over as large an area as possible.

FUNCTIONAL RELINING METHOD

Although there are hazards to be overcome in any relining procedure of a distal extension base, the *functional relining* method is used satisfactorily in competent hands. The principal hazard is that unless an open-mouth technique is used whereby the original relationship of the denture framework to the supporting teeth can be positively maintained, indirect retainers may not be seated when the functional impression is made. Because any settling of the denture base will have influenced the occlusion, restoring the denture framework to its original position with indirect retainers seated will result in an elevated occlusion. For this reason, readjustment of the occlusion must be anticipated when an open-mouth relining method is used. In extreme instances the teeth on the prosthesis will have to be reoccluded to the opposing dentition after relining of the denture base.

On the other hand, if a closed-mouth impression method is used, particularly with a bilateral distal extension denture, stops of self-curing resin or modeling plastic against resilient tissue may not be adequate to keep the distal extension base from settling tissueward under occlusal loading. In such an event the denture inevitably rotates about its fulcrum line, and the indirect retainers lift from their terminal position. Although occlusal harmony on the relined prosthesis will have been maintained by this method, the relationship of the denture framework to the supporting teeth will not be the same as it was on the original master cast.

A second hazard of any relining procedure is the possibility of occlusal discrepancies occurring during the reprocessing of an acrylic resin base. Relining of an acrylic resin base frequently results in an increase in vertical dimension. Although this can be minimized by careful laboratory procedures (Chapter 17), by the use of a free-flowing resin, by confirming that there is sufficient space inside the original base for the resin to flow, and by the employment of some space in the land area, some increase in dimension is always possible. Any such increase will result in a faulty relationship between the denture framework and the supporting natural teeth as well as changes in occlusal relationships.

When a relining method for functional basing is to be used, the original denture base may be processed over a spacer of metal (No. 7 Ash's metal) that has been adapted to the anatomic ridge form. This is the form of the ridge as reproduced on the master cast from a hydrocolloid impression. The relief metal is then stripped away from the resin base, leaving a space on the tissue side for the placement of the impression material and, later, the resin reline.

If this is not done, the underside of the denture base must be relieved by removing sufficient resin to accommodate the impression material. Clearance also should be adequate to assure freedom for the flow of the impression material. It should be remembered that thermoplastic impression materials are sluggish and that greater space for their flow is needed than when an impression paste or other easy flowing material is used. It also should be remembered that impression wax will not overdisplace tissue *if given sufficient space and time in which to flow.*

Following is Steffel's procedure for making a functional reline impression.

If there is an indirect retainer or additional points of contact of the framework to make tripoding or stabilization possible, it is preferable to reharmonize the positional relationship of the partial denture to teeth and tissues first, and also to correct the occlusion before you proceed with the reline impression. The procedure is as follows: Low-fusing modeling plastic is placed in excess on the distal one third to one half of the tissue surface of the bases. The denture is now mass heated in the 140° F water, quickly carried to the patient's mouth while the impression material is still readily moldable, and seated with firm pressure against only the framework. The material at the distal ends of the bases will have contacted the tissues and hardened so that the restoration is now reoriented in relation to its own arch, but out of harmony with the opposing arch (Fig. 15-9, *A*). With the modeling plastic for support distally and accurate metal-to-tooth support anteriorly, the partial denture is stabilized and positioned, and the occlusion altered and balanced in accordance with our judgment for this specific location.

After the occlusion has been corrected with the denture's being supported at its proper relative elevation, the impression substance, which has now served its purpose, is removed, undercuts are eliminated, and some material is cut away from the tissue surfaces and from the borders of the denture bases to make more room for, and provide better workability of, the impression materials (Fig. 15-9, *B*).

An excess amount of low-fusing modeling plastic (low-fusing to prevent overdisplacement of tissues) is now applied to the bases. Excess is used so that there will always be some present wherever needed. The restoration is mass heated in the water bath and placed part way toward the tissues but not seated. The patient is not allowed to close for contact. Seating all the way at the first placement might result in too severe pressures against supporting tissues, flowing of the moldable materials into the direct retainers, and the lack of occlusal contacts in the finished denture due to overclosure. Usually about four mass heatings and placements, progressively, are necessary before allowing the patient to close natural teeth to light centric occlusion contact. For the final closure the patient should be instructed to proceed just to the point of faint facet-to-facet or interdigitative contact, not asked to close with great force. Force might result in an upward displacement of the condyloid processes. At this juncture the bases will be at their correct vertical position, occlusion will be reestablished, and because correct occlusal contacts were provided beforehand, the metal work will have accurate adaptation to the natural teeth.

The border limits are now formed by heating and tempering short sections with the torch, then manipulating the cheeks and lips for border outline.

The reline impression at this point looks acceptable, has adequate tissue coverage, rounded smooth borders, smooth impression surfaces, and a stabilized, properly repositioned composite partial denture (Fig. 15-9, *C*). However, the borders are really not physiologically molded, and there will be small inaccuracies in surface detail, excessive stress against the crest of the ridge, and probably against the mylohyoid ridge.

Impression substance, and even base material if necessary, is now removed all along the crest of the ridge, and usually along the mylohyoid ridge. Also, if the distal extension bases are long, escape holes are bored completely through the base material at these areas requiring relief; if they are short, their open ends provide sufficient escapeways (Fig. 15-9, *D*). No impression bulk is removed along the normal slopes of the ridges.

Impression wax (Iowa) is now painted over the entire impression surface, the partial denture is placed, and the patient is instructed to gradually force it to place and then to continue with the functional movement of chewing. In contrast to modeling plastic, the wax must always be well chilled before removal for examination. After a short period in the mouth, five minutes, for example, excess wax is removed and the restoration is replaced (with wax additions, if necessary). The patient is again instructed to go through the functional movements of chewing together with facial and oral gymnastics for about ten minutes. The wax flows so readily that there is no danger of its remaining on any surface where its contour will not be tolerated later. Limited movement of the base extensions under the functional stresses will mold the soft wax for relief of vulnerable areas. Also, in the completed restoration the slight movement allowed by the passive retainers will preclude the possibility of tissue strangulation.

This final step in the reline impressions (the relieving of areas and the addition of wax) does not change the previously reestablished position of the partial denture in the arch, but merely refines the impression and specializes the fit with reference to the different types of supporting tissues. At this point the impression is ready for accurate conversion into a permanent material (Fig. 15-9, *E*). It presents (1) a surface that is smooth and tissue adapted, (2) a surface outline that will

Fig. 15-9. A, Modeling plastic placed to support distal extension bases during correction of occlusion. **B,** Ridge surfaces of bases prepared to receive modeling plastic. **C,** Smooth, accurate, border-molded impression in modeling plastic. **D,** Bases prepared for application of impression wax (Iowa formula). **E,** Finished impression made of modeling plastic and wax. Note escape of wax through holes in denture bases.

place additional stresses on tissues that can tolerate them, giving relief to others, and (3) borders that have a functional outline molded by physiologic muscular action and not by excessive manual manipulation.*

In the execution of a relining procedure three objectives generally must be remembered: (1) the repositioning of the displaced metal framework, (2) the reestablishing of lost occlusal contacts, and (3) the making of an impression that will ensure intimate tissue adaptation of the basal seat.

By this method of securing a new impression for the support of extension bases, as little or as much displacement of soft tissues as is desired can be achieved by a greater or lesser degree of heating of the impression plastic or wax and thereby controlling its flow. Additionally the partial denture is placed accurately into its functional position by the *light* closure of the opposing arch of teeth into occlusion and not by questionable finger placement.

In the reline impression as advocated by Steffel the impression wax is used as a final correction material. Iowa formula impression wax is used in much the same manner as for a complete denture impression, except that the impression for a partial denture is coordinated with the terminal position of the cast framework.

SELECTIVE TISSUE PLACEMENT IMPRESSION METHOD

Soft tissues covering basal seat areas may be either *placed, displaced,* or recorded in their *resting* or *anatomic form.* Placed and displaced tissues differ in degree of alteration from their resting form and in their physiologic reaction to the amount of displacement. For example, the palatal tissues in the vicinity of the vibrating line can be slightly displaced to develop a posterior palatal seal for the maxillary complete denture and will remain in a healthy state for extended periods of time. On the other hand, these tissues develop an immediate inflammatory response when they have been overly displaced in developing the posterior palatal seal.

Oral tissues that have been overly displaced attempt to regain their anatomic form.

---

*Paraphrased from Steffel, V. L.: Relining removable partial dentures for fit and function, J. Prosthet. Dent. 4:496-509, 1954.

When not permitted to do this by the denture bases, the tissues become inflamed and their physiologic functions become impaired, accompanied by bone resorption. Tissues that are minimally displaced (placed) by impression procedures respond favorably to the additional pressures placed on them by resultant denture bases if these pressures are intermittent rather than continuous.

The selective tissue placement impression method is based on the previously stated clinical observations, the histologic nature of tissues covering the residual alveolar bone, the nature of the residual ridge bone, and its positional relationship to the direction of stresses that will be placed on it. It is further believed that by use of specially designed individual trays for impressions, denture bases can be developed that will utilize those portions of the residual ridge that can withstand additional stress and at the same time relieve the tissues of the residual ridge that cannot withstand functional loading and remain healthy.

There are only minor variations in techniques in recording the basal seat tissues with the "functional reline method" and the "selective tissue placement impression method." The latter method is illustrated in Fig. 15-10 and is the predominant impression procedure for lower distal extension dentures in our practices.

There should be no difference philosophically in the requirement of support and coverage by bases of distal extension removable partial dentures and complete dentures, either maxillary or mandibular (Fig. 15-11). The tray is unquestionably the most important part of an impression. A tray must, however, be so formed and modified that the impression philosophy of the dentist can be carried out. The making of individualized acrylic resin impression trays is illustrated in the preceding chapter.

An impression for a lower distal extension partially edentulous arch may adequately be made in an individualized, full-arch tray. To do so, not only must the tray be formed to provide proper space for the particular impression material, but provision must also be made so that the functional form of primary stress-bearing areas may be recorded. Such an impression procedure, properly executed, can be used when metal bases are to be incorporated in the design of the restora-

Fig. 15-10. For legend see opposite page.

Fig. 15-10. Selective tissue placement impression method. **A,** Individual acrylic resin impression trays are attached to framework (Chapter 18). Holes are placed in tray along alveolar groove to allow escape of excess impression material. **B,** Framework and attached trays are tried in patient's mouth. Borders of tray are adjusted so that they are 2 to 3 mm short of all reflections but cover retromolar pads. **C,** Thin layer of red stick modeling plastic is "painted" on tissue sides of impression trays by first softening modeling plastic in a flame. **D,** Modeling plastic has been softened by a flame, tempered in 135° F water, and placed in patient's mouth. This procedure is repeated (usually three times) until basal seat tissues are not displaced and framework is correctly positioned. Impression trays will be stable at this time and border-molding procedures can begin. **E,** Borders are perfected by heating individual areas, placing tempered tray in mouth, manipulating cheeks, and having patient form lingual borders by tongue movements. Note that lingual flanges have assumed an S shape. This S shape has been formed by action of mylohyoid muscle. Note also that lingual flange has been extended into the retromylohyoid fossa. There would be *no difference* in the form of the impression of edentulous regions at this stage from a complete denture impression of same regions if patient was edentulous. **F,** Borders of compound impression are shortened 1 to 1.5 mm, and whole inside of impression, *with the exception of the buccal shelf region,* is relieved approximately 1 mm. **G,** Modeling plastic is removed from holes in tray. **H,** Final impression is completed with a rubber-base impression material wash. The framework must be perfectly seated and maintained in position while impression material is setting. **I,** Edentulous regions of cast are eliminated. Cut surfaces are grooved for additional retention of stone poured to make altered cast. **J,** Framework and impression are returned to cast and are luted with sticky wax to avoid displacement during boxing and pouring procedures. **K,** A utility wax is used to box the impression. **L,** Altered master cast with framework in position. Buccal shelf regions have been recorded in a functional form. Other regions of basal seats have been recorded in an anatomic form.

Fig. 15-11. A, Impression of a mandibular edentulous arch utilizing an individualized tray and a rubber-base impression material. Tray was so constructed and the impression so made that buccal shelves of mandible could assume a primary stress-bearing role. **B,** Rubber-base "secondary" impression of a Class I partially edentulous arch made in individualized trays attached to framework. Just as in **A,** buccal shelves will assume a primary stress-bearing role. Note similarity of two impressions. In each instance, individualized acrylic resin impression trays permitted dentist to carry out his philosophy of impression-making for support of denture bases. **C,** Impression of edentulous maxillary arch made with impression plaster in an individualized tray. **D,** Impression of a Class I partially edentulous arch made with an irreversible hydrocolloid material in an individualized tray. Again, without an individualized tray, properly constructed, a philosophy of impression making is most difficult to carry out.

tion. There is little difference, if any, between recording the basal seats in the partially edentulous arch and recording like areas for complete dentures on an edentulous arch. A secondary impression made in trays attached to the framework only makes definitive border control and tissue placement a bit easier compared to the individualized full arch tray. Both methods have produced desired and similar end results in our hands.

FLUID-WAX FUNCTIONAL IMPRESSION METHOD

One must differentiate between the wax "wash," or correction impression, as originally developed by Earl S. Smith of the University of Iowa, and the fluid-wax impression, as developed by O. C. Applegate of the University of Michigan and S. G. Applegate of the University of Detroit. The latter method used an impression wax (Korecta wax No. 4) that is slightly more fluid than the Iowa wax. Border extension was established by the impression wax and then reinforced by backing it up with a special hard wax (Korecta wax No. 1).*

---

*Korecta waxes are no longer available. Iowa wax is a suitable substitute for Korecta No. 4 wax, and Kerr Ivory Inlay wax may be used in lieu of Korecta No. 1 wax.

The Applegate method may be used for making a reline impression or for the correction of the original master cast. In either application the thickness of wax permits a greater flow of material and therefore less tissue displacement than does the wax "wash." However, if adequate space (1 to 2 mm) exists in the tray, the Iowa wax is most acceptable. The fluid-wax impression is used with an open-mouth procedure; therefore there is less danger of overdisplacement of tissues by the application of vertical forces. If adequate space for the flow of the material is provided and sufficient time is allowed for the escape of excess material, the fluid-wax impression will not overdisplace tissues. Only those soft tissues that can readily be displaced or made more compact by the consistency of the wax itself will be recorded in a different form from that recorded by the anatomic impression.

In addition to less displacement of tissues, the fluid-wax technique records the moving border tissues physiologically, resulting in an accurate denture border. Both the length and the width of the border are thus established in wax and reproduced in the denture base. The harder wax (Kerr Ivory Inlay wax) is used only to back up the impression and should not be allowed to influence the impression record.

Fig. 15-12. Armamentarium for making a secondary, functional impression of mandibular residual ridges with mouth temperature wax: heavy metal crucible for melting the wax, impression wax of Iowa formula, brush for applying wax, scalpel used for bisecting impression wax at borders prior to adding Kerr Ivory inlay wax for reinforcement, stick of Ivory inlay wax, and a No. 7 wax spatula for applying reinforcing wax.

Fig. 15-13. Nine steps in the making of a fluid-wax functional impression. **A,** Fluid Iowa wax is painted evenly over impression base. **B,** Denture framework is placed in mouth and held in its terminal position with three fingers, one on each principal occlusal rest and a third in between, holding framework forward in its terminal position with any indirect retainers fully seated. Chin is supported with other hand. **C,** While you are holding framework down, cheek on each side is pulled vertically against border of impression. This limits buccal extension to extreme positions of limiting structures. **D,** Again while you keep framework fully seated, patient is asked to place tongue forcibly into each cheek. This records extreme movement of sublingual tissues on opposite side. **E,** While you are still holding framework down, patient is asked to press tongue forward against lingual surface of anterior teeth. This limits distolingual extension of impression on both sides. After this movement, patient is asked to open wide, to make pterygomandibular raphe taut and to limit extreme distal portion of impression. **F,** Impression is removed and examined for a glossy surface, which is evidence of tissue contact. Once this has been checked, border is reinforced by bisecting the impression wax at border with a No. 11 Bard-Parker blade, leaving unsupported the impression wax extending beyond impression base. **G,** Hard Kerr Ivory Inlay wax is applied with a hot No. 7 spatula to reinforce impression wax at border. This must be applied hot enough to effect good attachment to impression base. Sufficient hard wax is used to act as a reinforcing extension of impression base and to prevent any undesirable shifting of impression wax at border. **H,** More Iowa wax is brushed on, just inside border, to provide an excess that will then be turned at border by a repetition of the previous movements. Wax must be fluid enough that it can be brushed on with broad sweeping strokes free of brush marks. **I,** Completed functional impression. Note border extension buccally and lingually and thickness of border permissible with this particular patient. This varies widely with each patient, but border recorded by this method should always be reproduced in finished denture.

Fig. 15-13, cont'd. For legend see opposite page.

O. C. Applegate has named this method the *fluid-wax functional impression*. Although it may be used for relining purposes, it is designed primarily for the making of a secondary impression for the correcting of a master cast. The anatomic ridge form, as recorded in hydrocolloid, is thus replaced with the functional form, as recorded in fluid wax, and the denture base is processed to the latter form. The fluid-wax functional impression is a rather time-consuming procedure but will produce desired results when properly executed.

Objectives in the making of a fluid-wax impression. Three objectives must be considered in the making of a fluid-wax impression, as in other impression procedures. These objectives are recording primary stress-bearing areas in their functional form, recording other basal seat or nonbearing areas in their anatomic form, and maximum extension of borders within the physiologic tolerance of bordering structures.

Armamentarium and procedures in making a fluid-wax impression and pouring a cast are illustrated in Figs. 15-12 to 15-14.

Fig. 15-14. For legend see opposite page.

ASSEMBLED METAL BASES

There has been some demand for removable partial dentures that combine the advantages of metal bases with the opportunity of replacing those bases in the event of changes in tissue support. The solution lies in replaceable metal bases attached to the denture framework with resin rather than by soldering. (See Fig. 15-15.)

In this method the denture framework is designed and cast as for a resin-base denture, except that an open retentive framework, which will fit inside the finishing line of the future metal base, is made. If, because of recent extractions or the possibility of changes due to disuse atrophy, any change in the supporting ridge is anticipated, the denture may be made first with a resin base. Such a base is preferably made to functional form, even though it is to be replaced later with a metal base. Better support and better stimulation of the residual ridge will result if the functional form is used to support reasonable occlusion. Under such conditions the amount of change in ridge forms will be held to a minimum.

Although artificial teeth are usually added, the resin base alone may be used, permitting stimulation as an exercise prosthesis as advocated by Applegate, who has this to say about the reconditioning of alveolar bone:

One of the most difficult situations with which the prosthodontist must deal is that existing when disuse atrophy (osteoporosis) has occurred in the edentulous area. Frequently, the missing teeth may have been extracted many years before their prosthetic replacement is accomplished. Bone is maintained only in response to the stimulation associated with its functional use. Of this, Weinmann and Sicher say, "If the loss of teeth is extensive or if the teeth bordering the edentulous area have lost their function, for instance, through the elimination of their antagonists, the osteoporosis is much more severe and the loss of bone substance at the alveolar ridge is much greater." One of the most common errors in prosthodontics is to assume that, because the bone is being maintained normally in the area of remaining teeth which have received greater than normal function the

Fig. 15-14. A, After the making of resin impression base attached to partial denture framework, ridge areas recorded in their static or anatomic form are removed from master cast by sawing with a spiral saw blade in two planes. One cut is made at right angles to longitudinal axis of ridge, 1 mm distal to abutment tooth. Second cut is made just lingual and parallel to lingual sulcus as recorded in original impression. The two are joined anteriorly, and anatomic reproduction of ridge is removed. At this time, if saw cuts are not rough enough, cut surfaces of cast should be scored with a knife to provide mechanical retention for attachment of new stone to old. **B,** Completed fluid-wax functional impression. **C,** Completed wax functional impression is seated on remainder of cast after anatomic ridges have been removed. Note scored surface for added retention. Cast metal framework is secured to dry cast with sticky wax after you have first made sure that no debris interferes with seating and that all occlusal rests and indirect retainers are seated. Utility wax is placed on original cast just anterior to saw cut and sealed anteriorly with a hot spatula. Sheet wax of adhesive type is placed lingually and sealed to cast and along side of impression base. It must be sealed anteriorly, but hot spatula must not come in contact with impression. Surface of cast anteriorly is then painted with sodium silicate or some other separator, such as Microfilm. Just prior to pouring new ridge areas, base of cast is immersed in 12 mm (½ in) of water for five minutes to provide saturation of the dry stone. **D,** Wax functional impression attached to master cast. Anatomic ridge form has been removed, and cut portion of cast has been undercut to assure attachment of new stone to old. Cast has been saturated by placing it base downward in 12 mm (½ in) of water for ten minutes prior to pouring. The only vibrating necessary in adding new mix of stone is to prevent trapping air at junction of wax impression with cut surfaces of stone cast. **E,** Ridge areas are poured with a stone of a different color, using no more vibration than necessary, and then are inverted into additional stone on a glass or ceramic slab immediately after new stone has lost its surface sheen. Stone must be brought up well around distal ends of impression. After stone has hardened, excess is trimmed away until margins of impression wax are exposed. Sticky wax is chilled with ice or cast is chilled and sticky wax flaked off. Cast is then immersed in water at 110° F, just sufficient to soften mouth-temperature wax, and framework with attached impression base is lifted. Usually, impression wax remains on impression base, leaving a clean cast as shown.

Fig. 15-15. Five steps in making of replaceable metal bases for a bilateral distal extension partial denture. **A,** Wax patterns for metal bases are formed on investment cast duplicate of corrected master cast. **B,** Original metal framework is placed over wax pattern, and the two are relieved or re-formed as needed to eliminate interference and provide retention and finishing lines for resin attachment. **C,** Cast bases are returned to master cast. **D,** Three pieces are assembled on master cast. This should be done by laboratory, at which time any remaining interference is eliminated. **E,** Pieces have been assembled with self-curing acrylic resin. Final jaw relations may now be established on this assembled denture, or this may be deferred until patient and tissues have become accustomed to the wearing of the prosthesis for a period of time before adding artificial teeth to denture base.

edentulous ridge in the same mouth also will furnish stable support immediately.

Frequently, the replacement of teeth is done in a manner to restore a nearly normal functional load to such edentulous areas, only to have a rapid resorptive change occur beneath the denture base. I make a plea for the preconditioning of the residual alveolar ridge, where there has been long disuse, before the normal stress load is restored. This can be done by one of the following procedures:

1. Supply a temporary exercise prosthesis for use over a period of a few months.

2. Construct the appliance with the base adapted to functional form and extended to maximum area, but do not replace the teeth until later.

In addition, have the patient exercise the ridge area with finger massage prior to the prosthetic service, while restorative and other mouth preparation is being done. Be certain also that the diet and vitamin intake are proper and that the physical condition of the patient is such as to assure the best possible metabolic function. . . .

To be of value, the ridge surfaces of the exercise bases should not only be maximum in area, but they should be related to the basal structures exactly as the bases of the finished partial denture will be. The daily two or three exercise periods of intermittent biting pressure will then direct stimuli through the base into the substructures in the same manner that work stimuli will later be induced by tooth surface contacts. Under this method of bone reconditioning, the edentulous ridge may be expected to undergo a process of reorganization which will prepare it to accept a reasonable occlusal load, at a later time, with much less resorptive change.*

Adding metal bases to the partial denture. When it may be presumed that the residual ridge has undergone its initial changes under the load of supporting a denture, the metal bases may be added in the following manner.

The original resin base may be relieved and used as an impression tray, or it may be removed entirely and replaced with a resin impression tray, as outlined previously in this chapter. A new functional impression is made and the original master cast or a new master cast is corrected to the existing functional ridge form as though for a resin base. The corrected master cast is then duplicated and an investment cast made.

Upon the investment cast a metal base or

basis is waxed, using 24-gauge wax over the ridge (Fig. 15-15). The borders are reinforced using 14-gauge round wax and freehand waxing. Before the finishing line for the resin attachment is located, the cast framework must be tried on the investment cast to see if the retentive frame will interfere. Any extension loops that were added to support resin bases are removed, leaving only the ladderlike retentive frame. The cross pieces should have been made originally far enough apart to accommodate nailhead retention on the metal base.

An undercut finishing line is added, forming a recess for the resin attachment beyond the limits of the retentive frame. The original cast framework may have to be warmed slightly to assure its seating into the wax pattern for the metal base. Within the boundaries of the retentive frame, two or more nailhead retention elements are added to secure the metal base to the resin attachment, which in turn will be attached to the retentive frame. Some care must be taken in waxing around the major connector to form a neat junction without interfering with separation of the cast framework from the wax pattern.

The cast framework now may be lifted and the metal base or bases sent to the laboratory for casting and polishing. The original framework and the master cast also must be sent to the laboratory so that the separate pieces may be fitted together on the master cast. On return from the laboratory there must be no definite contact between the separate pieces. Rather the metal base or bases must seat easily and the original framework go to its terminal position with clearance to spare. Since the attachment between the pieces will be with a self-curing acrylic resin, there is no need for their making contact, which could lead to errors in positioning.

Each piece should be tacked separately to the master cast with sticky wax. With the use of a brush technique first and then sprinkling, the pieces are secured to each other with sufficient acrylic resin to assure stability. Then occlusal relations may be established on this assembled denture.

Since the teeth will be attached to the metal base with resin, it is preferable that there be no line of junction between the acrylic resin attaching the separate pieces and the resin supporting the teeth. For this

*From Applegate, O. C.: The removable partial denture in the general practice of tomorrow, J. Prosthet. Dent. 8:609-622, 1958.

reason, before the teeth are arranged in wax, the original resin should be cut back short of the finishing line. In this way the only resin visible will be that supporting the artificial teeth.

The principal advantage of this method is that the metal base or bases may be easily removed at some future date by point flaming the underside of the metal base enough to soften the resin attachment. The original metal base then may be separated from the original framework, leaving the denture framework intact to support a new metal base and new occlusion.

By this method it is possible to replace metal bases when it becomes necessary because of changes in support, accomplishing much the same objective as with the relining of resin bases but with all desirable advantages of using metal bases.

SELF-ASSESSMENT AIDS

1. Support for a tooth-borne removable partial denture is provided by what oral structures?
2. Support for a distal extension denture is provided by what oral structures?
3. Residual ridges may be recorded by an impression in their anatomic form or functional form. A Class III arch may be recorded in its _____ form; however, the residual ridges in Class I or II arches should be recorded in their _____ form.
4. There are at least six important factors that influence the support of a distal extension denture base by the residual ridges. You should be able to state them without omission.
5. Describe what you would consider to be an ideal residual ridge to support a distal extension denture base.
6. What areas of the residual ridge are considered to be the primary stress-bearing areas for a mandibular distal extension base? A maxillary distal extension base?
7. Why can the crest of the mandibular residual ridge not assume a stress-bearing role?
8. Which type of tissue interposed between a denture base and the underlying bone would probably afford a more favorable reaction to stress—firm, dense, fibrous connective tissue or easily displaceable connective tissue?
9. The space that is available for a distal extension denture base is controlled by the structures that surround the space. True or false?
10. A denture base should cover as much of the residual ridge as possible and be extended the maximum amount within the physiologic tolerance of the limiting border structures. True or false?
11. The objective of any functional impression technique is to provide maximum support for the removable partial denture base. When this objective is attained, what advantages accrue to the denture environment?
12. How does accuracy or inaccuracy of the denture base influence the quality of support by the residual ridge?
13. Since some rotational movement of the extension denture is bound to occur and since utilization of as much of the primary stress-bearing areas as possible is desirable, in what manner may the design of the framework (location of rests) influence the greatest use of the primary stress-bearing areas? Can you illustrate your answer by a simple diagram?
14. Total occlusal load applied to a denture base certainly influences the quality of support for the base. What can be done to lessen the total occlusal load applied in relation to the prosthetically supplied teeth?
15. There are many approaches to recording the functional form of residual ridges in Class I and II arches and relating this form accurately to the rest of the dental arch. The various methods are only means to an end. A basic understanding of anatomy, histology, physiology, materials, and principles will permit each dentist to develop his own philosophy and a technique of impression making to carry out his philosophy. Therefore you should be able to rationalize the functional relining method and the selective tissue placement method, whether with fluid waxes or other materials, or to relate the anatomic form under functional loading to the rest of the arch (Hindel's approach).
16. Describe a functional reline impression procedure.
17. What are the risks involved in using a closed-mouth method when performing a functional reline impression procedure? How does this differ from an open-mouth functional reline procedure?
18. You will note in some of the various methods of making functional impressions of residual ridges that a series of holes are placed in the alveolar groove of the "trays." What is accomplished by such a procedure?
19. In executing any type of relining procedure of a fabricated denture to record the functional form of the ridge, three objectives must be met. Can you name them? They are very important.
20. What is the most important part of an impression? If you said the *tray*, you are correct. Can you rationalize why this must be true in

relation to what you are trying to accomplish in an impression procedure?

21. In your opinion, should there be any difference in the support characteristic, extension, and form of a removable partial denture extension base and a complete denture base occupying the same area?

22. One method discussed in the text is the selective tissue placement of impression making. What is meant by "tissue placement"?

23. Can you fully describe a selective tissue placement procedure for making impressions of mandibular extension residual ridges?

24. What is meant by a secondary impression?

25. What is meant by an "altered cast" in relation to impression making?

26. Some dentists prefer to use mouth temperature waxes in trays attached to the framework to record the functional form of mandibular residual ridges. Two dental pioneers stand out in the development of wax as an impression material. Can you recall their names?

27. Try describing a fluid-wax functional impression method.

28. Would you anticipate any gross differences in the form of a residual ridge on a cast made from a selective tissue placement impression method and the same ridge recorded by a fluid-wax functional impression method?

CHAPTER

16 OCCLUSAL RELATIONSHIPS FOR REMOVABLE PARTIAL DENTURES

The fourth phase* in the treatment of patients with removable partial dentures is the establishment of a functional and harmonious occlusal relationship between the opposing dentitions. This has long been one of the most neglected aspects of partial denture treatment.

Failure to provide and maintain adequate occlusion on the partial denture is primarily due to (1) lack of support for the denture base and (2) the fallacy of establishing occlusion to a single static jaw relation record only. Support for the jaw relation record base must be the same as for the finished prosthesis, either through occlusal rests or through a combination of occlusal and tissue support. The establishment of functional occlusal records will be covered later in this chapter.

Balanced occlusion is desirable on complete dentures because occlusal stresses may cause instability of the dentures or trauma to the supporting structures. And yet these stresses can reach a point beyond which movement of the dentures takes place. The stresses therefore are eliminated at the expense of denture stability and retention.

In partial dentures, however, because of the fixation to abutments, occlusal stresses are transmitted directly to the abutment teeth and other supporting structures, resulting in sustained stresses, which may be more damaging than those transient stresses found in complete dentures. *Therefore occlusal harmony between a partial denture and the remaining natural teeth is a major factor in the preservation of the health of their surrounding structures.*

In the treatment of patients with complete dentures, only one factor, which is the inclination of the condyle path, is not within the control of the dentist. All other factors may be altered to obtain occlusal balance and harmony in eccentric positions to conform to the dentist's particular concept and philosophy of occlusion.

In establishing occlusion on a partial denture the influence of the remaining natural teeth is usually such that the occlusal forms of the teeth on the denture must conform to an already established occlusal pattern. This pattern may have been improved on by occlusal adjustment or reconstruction, but the pattern present at the time the partial denture is made dictates the occlusion on the partial denture. The only exceptions are those in which an opposing complete denture can be made to harmonize with the partial denture or in which only anterior teeth remain in both arches and the incisal relationship can be made noninterfering. In these situations the recording of jaw relations and the arrangement of the teeth may proceed in the same manner as with complete dentures, and the same general principles apply.

With all other types of partial dentures the remaining teeth must dictate the occlusion, unless the dentist is willing to accept nothing more than centric occlusal contacts and ignore interference in lateral movement or has reason to believe that he can achieve occlusal harmony on the partial denture by adjusting the occlusion in the mouth. Although some claim that a functional relationship of the partial denture to the natural dentition may be adjusted satisfactorily in the mouth, it is doubtful that this is or ever can be done ade-

---

*See Chapter 2, under discussion on the six phases of partial denture service.

quately. Partial denture occlusion thus established can at best only perpetuate malocclusions that existed previously and help to maintain the existing vertical relationship, however inadequate it may be.

The establishment of a satisfactory occlusion for the partial denture patient should include the following: (1) an analysis of the existing occlusion, (2) the correction of existing occlusal disharmony as a necessary step in preparing the mouth for the partial denture, (3) the recording of centric relation or an adjusted centric occlusion, (4) the recording of eccentric jaw relationships or functional eccentric occlusion, and (5) the correction of occlusal discrepancies created in processing of the denture. An adjusted and corrected occlusion on the natural teeth is the occlusion that the dentist transfers to an instrument in such a manner that occlusal harmony on the partial denture is made possible.

Two methods are commonly used to develop an acceptable occlusion for the removable partial denture patient. The first and most common method involves the use of a semiadjustable articulator. Casts are oriented to the articulator by a face-bow and a static jaw relation record. The instrument is programmed by additional static jaw relation records. Articulators can simulate but not duplicate jaw movement. A realization of the limitations of a specific instrument and a knowledge of the procedures that can overcome these limitations are necessary if an adequate occlusion is to be created. For example, if an occlusal discrepancy is noted in the mouth due to Bennett movement, which was not reproduced by the articulator when the occlusion was being formulated, the dentures are reoriented on the articulator in the eccentric position causing the difficulty. The discrepancy is corrected in that position, using the articulator as a simple hinge instrument.

A second method is preferred by some dentists. This method involves creating functionally generated paths of opposing teeth in a wax recording medium placed on a denture base. A positive of this record is recovered in stone and forms a template to which the artificial teeth are oriented. The template and opposing denture framework may be mounted on an articulator, using the instrument as a simple hinge. Opposing frames

that slide vertically are also used to relate the casts, thus eliminating the need for an articulator in developing the final occlusion. The quality of the occlusion developed by this method is dependent on the stability of the denture base when the paths of opposing cusps are being generated. Design of the denture framework and the quality of the support of the denture bases are factors that influence stability.

A harmonious relationship of opposing occlusal and incisal surfaces, in itself, is not adequate to assure stability of distal extension removable partial dentures. In addition, the relationship of the teeth to the residual ridges must be considered. Bilateral eccentric contact of the lower distal extension denture need not be formulated to stabilize the denture. The buccal cusps may be favorably placed over the buccal turning point of the crest of the residual ridge, and in such positions the denture is not subjected to excessive tilting forces. On the other hand, the artificial teeth of the bilateral, distal extension, maxillary denture often must be placed laterally to the crest of the residual ridge. Such an unfavorable position is conducive to tipping the denture, restrained only by direct retainer action on the balancing side. To enhance the stability of the denture, it seems logical to provide simultaneous balancing and working contacts in these situations if possible.

Desirable contact relationships for removable partial dentures

The following occlusal arrangements, in different situations, are recommended to develop a harmonious occlusal relationship of partial dentures and to enhance stability of the dentures:

1. Simultaneous bilateral contacts of opposing posterior teeth must occur in centric occlusion.

2. Occlusion for tooth-borne dentures may be arranged similar to the occlusion seen in a harmonious natural dentition. Stability of the dentures is assured by direct retainers at both ends of the denture base.

3. Balanced occlusion in eccentric positions should be formulated when the partial denture is opposed by a maxillary complete denture. This is accomplished primarily to promote the stability of the complete denture. However, simultaneous contacts in a

protrusive relationship do not receive priority over appearance, phonetics, and a favorable occlusal plane.

4. Working side contacts should be obtained for the mandibular distal extension denture. These contacts should occur simultaneously with working side contacts of the natural teeth to distribute the stress over the greatest possible areas. Masticatory function of the denture is improved by such an arrangement, especially if the patient chews in a teardrop or elliptical pattern.

5. Simultaneous balancing and working contacts should be formulated for the maxillary bilateral distal extension partial denture whenever possible. Such an arrangement will compensate in part for the unfavorable position the maxillary artificial teeth must occupy in relation to the residual ridge, which is usually lateral to the crest of the ridge. This desirable relationship often must be compromised, however, when the patient's anterior teeth have an excessively steep vertical overlap with little or no horizontal overlap. Even in this situation, working side contacts can be obtained without resorting to excessively steep cuspal inclinations.

6. Only working contacts need to be formulated for the maxillary unilateral distal extension denture. Balancing side contacts would not enhance the stability of the denture, since it is entirely tooth supported by the framework on the balancing side.

7. In the Class IV removable partial denture situation, contact of opposing anterior teeth in centric occlusion is desirable to prevent a continuous eruption of the opposing natural incisors. Contact of the opposing anterior teeth in eccentric positions should not be developed. Such contact would be detrimental to the residual ridge and in no way enhances the stability of the denture.

8. Contact of opposing posterior teeth in a straightforward protrusive relationship is not desirable in any situation except when an opposing complete denture is placed.

9. Artificial posterior teeth should not be arranged farther distally than the beginning of a sharp upward incline of the lower residual ridge or over the retromolar pad. To do so would have the effect of shunting the denture anteriorly.

Five methods of establishing interocclusal relations for removable partial dentures will be briefly described. Before describing any

of these, it is necessary that the use of a face-bow mounting of the maxillary cast and the pertinent factors in partial denture occlusion be considered. The technique for applying the face-bow has been described briefly in Chapter 11.

Whereas a hinge axis mounting may be desirable for complete oral rehabilitation procedures, any of the common arbitrary type of face-bow will facilitate mounting of the maxillary cast in relation to the condylar axis of the articulating instrument with reasonable accuracy. As suggested in Chapter 11, it is still better that in addition to mounting the casts at a comparable radius, the plane of occlusion be related to the orbital-axis plane. Since the dominant factor in partial denture occlusion is the remaining natural teeth and their proprioceptor influence on occlusion, a comparable radius at the oriented plane of occlusion on an acceptable instrument will allow reasonably valid mandibular movements to be reproduced. Such instruments are the Hanau models S-M and H-2, the Dentatus model ARH, the Whip-Mix articulator, and similar instruments.

METHODS FOR ESTABLISHING OCCLUSAL RELATIONSHIPS

The recording of occlusal relationships for the partially edentulous arch may vary from the simple apposition of opposing casts by occluding sufficient remaining natural teeth to the recording of jaw relations in the same manner as for a completely edentulous patient. As long as there are natural teeth remaining in contact, however, some consideration must be given the cuspal influence that those teeth will have on functional jaw movements.

The horizontal jaw relation (centric occlusion or centric relation) in which the restoration is to be constructed should have been determined during diagnosis and treatment planning. Mouth preparations also should have been accomplished based on this determination, including occlusal adjustment of the natural dentition, if such was indicated. Therefore one of the following conditions should exist: (1) centric relation and centric occlusion coincide; (2) centric relation and centric occlusion do not coincide but the decision has been made to construct the restoration in centric occlusion; (3) posterior teeth do not contact and the restoration is to be constructed in centric relation; and (4) posterior teeth are not present in one or both arches and the denture will be constructed in centric relation.

Then occlusal relationships may be established by utilizing the most apropos of the following methods to fit a particular partially edentulous situation.

Direct apposition of casts. The *first method* is used when there are sufficient opposing teeth remaining in contact to make the existing jaw relationship obvious and when only a few teeth are to be replaced on short denture bases. In this method, opposing casts may be occluded by hand. The occluded casts should be held in apposition with 2 wire nails attached with sticky wax to the bases of the casts until they are securely mounted on the articulator.

At best, this method can only perpetuate the existing vertical dimension and any existing occlusal disharmony present between the natural dentition. *Occlusal analysis and the correction of any existing occlusal disharmony should precede the accepting of such a jaw relation record.* The limitations of such a method are obvious. Yet, such a jaw relation record is better than an inaccurate interocclusal record between the remaining natural teeth. Unless a record is made that does not influence the closing path by reason of its bulk and the consistency of the recording medium, direct apposition of opposing casts at least eliminates the possibility of the patient's giving a faulty jaw relationship.

Interocclusal records with posterior teeth remaining. A *second method*, which is a modification of the first, is used when sufficient teeth remain to support the partial denture (Kennedy Class III), but the relation of opposing teeth does not permit the occluding of casts by hand. In such cases, jaw relations must be established as for fixed restorations using some kind of interocclusal record.

The least accurate of these is the interocclusal wax record. The successful recording of centric relation with an interocclusal wax record will be influenced by the bulk and the consistency of the wax and the accuracy of the wax after chilling. Excess wax contacting mucosal surfaces may distort soft tissues, thereby preventing accurate seating of the wax record onto the stone casts. Distortion of wax during or after removal from the mouth may also interfere with accurate seating. Therefore a definite procedure for making interocclusal wax records is given as follows:

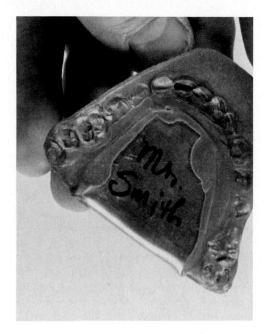

Fig. 16-1. An impression wax (Aluwax) wafer is reinforced with ash No. 7 metal. Reinforcement is folded over wafer and should be shaped to just clear lingual surfaces of teeth in lower arch. A water bath is used to uniformly soften impression wax.

A uniformly softened, reinforced wafer of impression wax is placed between the teeth, and the patient is guided to close in centric relation (Fig. 16-1). Correct closure should have been rehearsed prior to placement of the wax so that there will be no hesitancy or deviation on the part of the patient. The wax is then removed and immediately chilled thoroughly in room-temperature water. It should be replaced a second time to correct the distortion resulting from chilling and again chilled after removal.

All excess wax should now be removed with a sharp knife. It is most important at this time that all wax contacting mucosal surfaces be trimmed free of contact. The chilled wax record again should be replaced to make sure that no contact with soft tissue exists.

A wax record should be further corrected with an impression paste, which is used as the final recording medium. Some impression pastes are more suitable than others for this purpose. Generally a material that sets quite hard is preferred.

In the making of such a corrected wax record, the opposing teeth (and also the patient's lips and the dentist's fingers) should first be lightly coated with petroleum jelly or a silicone preparation. The impression paste is then mixed and applied to both sides of the metal-reinforced wax record. It is quickly placed, and the patient is assisted with closing in the rehearsed path, which will this time be guided by the previous wax record. After the paste has set, the corrected wax record is removed and inspected for accuracy. Then any excess projecting beyond the wax matrix should be removed with a sharp knife.

Such a record should seat on accurate casts without discrepancy or interference and will provide an accurate interocclusal record. When an intact opposing arch is present, use of an opposing cast may be dispensed with and a hard stone may be poured directly into the impression paste record to serve as an opposing cast. However, although this may be an acceptable procedure in the construction of a unilateral fixed partial denture, the advantages of having casts properly oriented on a suitable articulator contraindicates the practice. The only exception to this is if the maxillary cast on which the partial denture is to be fabricated has been mounted previously with the aid of a face-bow. In such an instance an intact lower arch may be reproduced in stone by pouring a cast directly into the interocclusal record.

An interocclusal record also may be made with an adjustable frame (Fig. 11-22). Reference to this method has previously been made in Chapter 11. The adjustable frame was devised for use with materials that offer no resistance to closure, such as zinc oxide and eugenol impression pastes.

Some of the advantages of using a metallic oxide paste over wax as a recording medium for occlusal records follow: (1) uniformity of consistency, (2) ease of displacement on closure, (3) accuracy of occlusal surface reproduction, and (4) dimensional stability; also (5) some modification in occlusal relationship is possible after closure, if made before the material sets, and (6) distortion is less likely during mounting procedures.

Three important details to be observed when you are using such a material are as follows:

1. Make sure that the occlusion is satisfactory before making the interocclusal record.

2. Be sure that the casts are accurate reproductions of the teeth being recorded.

3. Trim the record with a sharp knife whenever it engages undercuts, soft tissues, or deep grooves.

Occlusal relations using occlusion rims on record bases. A *third method* is used when one or more distal extension areas are present, when a tooth-bounded edentulous space is large, or when opposing teeth do not meet. In these instances, occlusion rims on accurate jaw relation record bases must be used. *It should not be necessary to add that simple wax records of edentulous areas are never acceptable, despite the unfortunate continuation of this practice. Any wax, however soft, will displace soft tissues. It is totally impossible to seat such a wax record on a stone cast of the arch with any degree of accuracy.*

In this method the recording proceeds much the same as in the second method, except that occlusion rims are substituted for remaining teeth. It is essential that accurate bases be used to help support the occlusal relationship. Shellac bases may be adapted to the casts and then corrected with some kind of impression paste. This is best done by first burnishing tinfoil onto the lubricated cast, mixing a suitable zinc oxide and eugenol impression paste and applying it to the shellac base, and then seating the shellac base onto the cast until the paste has set. The tinfoil adheres to the impression paste, giving a tinfoil-lined correction of the original base. Such a corrected base is entirely acceptable for jaw relation records. Shellac bases also may be lined with some self-curing resin to accomplish the same purpose. In either case, undercuts on the cast must first be blocked out, and tinfoil is required. When resin is employed, a tinfoil substitute is required.

Record bases also may be made entirely of self-curing resin. Those materials used in dough form lack sufficient accuracy for this purpose unless they are corrected by relining. A resin base may be formed by sprinkling monomer and polymer into a shallow matrix of wax or clay, after blocking out of any undercuts. If the matrix and blockout have been formed with care, interference to removal will not occur, and little trimming will be necessary. When the sprinkling method is used and sufficient time is allowed for progressive polymerization to occur, such bases are the most stable and accurate obtainable short of using cast metal, vulcanite, or compression molded and processed resin bases for jaw relation records. See Fig. 17-44.

Jaw relation records made by this method accomplish essentially the same purpose as the two previous methods. The fact that record bases are used to support edentulous areas does not alter the effect. Therefore in any of these three methods the skill and care used by the dentist in making occlusal adjustments on the finished prosthesis will govern the accuracy of the resulting occlusion.

Methods for recording centric relation on record bases. There are many ways by which centric relation may be recorded when record bases are used. The least accurate is the use of softened wax occlusion rims. Modeling plastic occlusion rims, on the other hand, may be uniformly softened by flaming and tempering, resulting in a generally acceptable occlusal record. This method is time proved, and when competently done, it is equal in accuracy to any other method.

When wax occlusion rims are used, they should be reduced in height until just out of occlusal contact. A single stop is then added to maintain its terminal position while a jaw relation record is made in some uniformly soft material, which sets to a hard state. Quick-setting impression plaster, impression paste, or self-curing resin may be used. With any of these materials, opposing teeth must be lubricated to facilitate easy separation. Whatever the recording medium, it must permit normal closure into centric relation without resistance and must be transferable with accuracy to the casts for mounting purposes.

Relative to the third method, some mention must be made of the ridge on which the record bases are formed. If the prosthesis is to be tooth supported or a distal extension base is to be made on the anatomic ridge form, the bases will be made to fit that form of the residual ridge. But, if a distal extension base is to be supported by the functional form of the residual ridge, it is necessary that the recording of jaw relations be deferred until the master cast has been corrected to that functional form. Record bases must be as identical as possible to those of the finished prosthesis. Jaw relation record bases are useless unless they are made on the same cast to which the denture will be processed, or a duplicate thereof, or are themselves the final denture bases. The latter may be either of cast alloy or a processed resin base. Therefore, for distal extension dentures that are to be made to conform to the functional form of the edentulous ridge, the recording of final jaw relation records must be deferred until the functional impression has been accomplished, the functional ridge form has been reproduced on the stone cast, and accurate record bases have been fabricated to fit that functional form.

Jaw relation records made entirely on occlusion rims. The *fourth method* is used when no occlusal contact exists between the remaining natural teeth, such as when an opposing maxillary complete denture is to be made concurrently with a lower partial denture. It may also be used in those rare situations in which the few remaining teeth do not occlude and will not influence eccentric jaw movements. Jaw relation records are made entirely on occlusion rims when either arch has only anterior teeth present (a fixed anterior restoration is considered the same).

In either case, jaw relation records are made entirely on occlusion rims. The occlusion rims must be supported by accurate jaw relation record bases. Here the choice of method for recording jaw relations is much the same as that for complete dentures. Either some direct interocclusal method or a stylus tracing may be used. As with complete denture construction the use of a facebow, the choice of articulator used, the choice of method for recording jaw relations, and the use of eccentric positional records are optional according to the training, ability, and desires of the individual dentist.

The same principles of occlusion apply to such a partial denture just as they do to a complete denture. If the dentist believes that he can adjust occlusion adequately in the mouth, a simple hinge mounting is all that is needed. On the other hand, if he believes in the use of a fully adjustable instrument with the casts mounted to the hinge axis, then he should do so with a partial denture. In between these two extremes we find the majority of dentists who are trained in prosthodontics using a simple face-bow mounting on a semiadjustable articulator (Hanau, Whip-Mix, and so forth) and recording jaw relations to correctly orient casts and adjust the articulator by means of either static records or a stylus tracing.

Establishing occlusion by the recording of occlusal pathways. The *fifth method* of establishing occlusion on the partial denture is the registration of occlusal pathways and the use of an occluding template rather than a cast of the opposing arch. When a static jaw relation record is used, with or without eccentric articulatory movements, the prosthetically supplied teeth are arranged to occlude according to a specific concept of occlusion. On the other hand, when a functional occlusal record is used, the teeth are modified to accept every possible eccentric jaw movement.

These movements are made more complicated by the influence of the remaining natural teeth. Occlusal harmony on complete dentures and in complete mouth rehabilitation may be obtained by the use of modern instruments and techniques. Schuyler has emphasized the importance of establishing first the anterior tooth relation and incisal guidance before proceeding with any complete oral rehabilitation. Others have shown the advantages of establishing canine guidance as a key to functional occlusion before proceeding with any functional registration against an opposing prosthetically restored arch. This is done on the theory that the canine teeth serve to guide the mandible during eccentric movements when the opposing teeth come into functional contact. It also has been pointed out that the canine teeth transmit periodontal proprioceptor impulses to the muscles of mastication and thus have an influence on mandibular movement even without actual contact guidance. However, as long as the occlusal surfaces of unrestored natural teeth remain in contact, as in many a partially dentulous mouth, these will always be the primary influence on mandibular movement, and the degree of occlusal harmony obtainable on a fixed or removable restoration will depend on the occlusal harmony existing between these teeth.

Regarding occlusion, Thompson has said: "Observing the occlusion with the teeth in static relations and then moving the mandible into various eccentric positions is not sufficient. A dynamic concept is necessary in order to produce an occlusion that is in functional harmony with the facial skeleton, the musculature, and the temporomandibular joints."* To this need only be added "and with the remaining natural teeth," and we have defined the requirements for partial denture occlusion.

*From Thompson, J. R.: In Sarnat, B. S., editor: Temporomandibular disorders: diagnosis and dental treatment in the temporomandibular joint, Springfield, Ill., 1951, Charles C Thomas, Publisher.

In the registration of occlusal pathways, an occlusion rim of a suitable hard wax, such as Peck's purple hard inlay wax, is attached to an accurate jaw relation record base. This base must be securely attached to the partial denture framework. It may be the final denture base of processed resin or metal. The occlusion rim is worn by the patient for a period of time, preferably for twenty-four hours or more and preferably during sleep. It is removed by the patient only while eating.

Whereas some of the methods described previously may be applied to the construction of partial dentures in both arches simultaneously, this method requires that an opposing arch be intact or restored to the extent of planned treatment. If partial dentures are planned for both arches, a choice is necessary as to which denture is to be made first and which is to bear a functional occlusal relation to the opposing arch. Generally the maxillary arch is restored first and the mandibular partial denture occluded to that restored arch. Similarly, if the maxillary arch is to be restored with a complete denture or a fixed partial denture or crowns, this is done before establishing the occlusion on the opposing partial denture.

Regardless of the method used for recording jaw relations, when one arch is completely restored first, that arch is treated as an intact arch even though it is wholly or partially restored by prosthetic means. It is well to consider at the time of treatment planning the possible advantages of establishing the final occlusion to an intact arch.

By wearing and biting into a wax occlusion rim, a record is made of all extremes of jaw movement. The wax occlusion rim must maintain positive contact with the opposing dentition in all excursions and must be left high enough to assure that a record of the functional path of each cusp will be carved in wax. This record should include not only voluntary excursive movements but also involuntary movements and changes in jaw movement caused by changes in posture. Extreme jaw positions and habitual movements during sleep should also be recorded.

The occlusal paths, thus recorded, will represent each tooth in its three-dimensional aspect. Although the cast poured against this will resemble the opposing teeth, it will be wider than the teeth that carved it because it represents those teeth in all extremes of movement. The recording of occlusal paths in this manner eliminates entirely the need for attempting to reproduce mandibular movement on an instrument.

Occlusion thus established on the partial denture will have more complete harmony with the opposing natural or artificial teeth than can be obtained by adjustments in the mouth alone, because occlusal adjustment to accommodate voluntary movement does not necessarily prevent occlusal disharmony in all postural positions or during periods of stress. Furthermore, occlusal adjustment in the mouth without occlusal analysis is limited by the dentist's ability to interpret correctly occlusal markings made intraorally, whether by articulating ribbon or by other means.

The registration of occlusal pathways has still further advantages. It makes possible the obtaining of jaw relations under actual working conditions, with the denture framework in its terminal position, the opposing teeth in function, and an opposing denture, if present, fully seated. In some instances it also makes possible the recovery of lost vertical dimension, either unilaterally or bilaterally, when overclosure or mandibular rotation has occurred, rather than perpetuating an abnormal mandibular relationship.

Step-by-step procedure for registering occlusal pathways. The technique for the registration of occlusal pathways is as follows:

1. Support the wax occlusion rim by a denture base having the same degree of accuracy and stability as the finished denture base. Ideally, this would be the final denture base, which is one of the advantages of making the denture with a metal base. Otherwise, make a temporary base of sprinkled self-curing acrylic resin, which is essentially identical to the final resin base. In any distal extension partial denture, make this base on a cast that has been corrected to the functional or supporting form of the edentulous ridge (Fig. 16-2).

Place a film of sticky wax upon the base before the wax occlusion rim is secured to it. The wax used for the occlusion rim should be hard enough to support biting stress and should be tough enough to resist fracture. Peck's purple hard inlay wax has proved to be suitable for the majority of patients. However, some individuals with weak musculature or tender mouths may have difficulty in reducing this wax. In such situations use a slightly less hard wax. Make the occlusion rim wide enough to record all extremes of mandibular movement.

2. Have the patient wear the occlusion rim for a period of twenty-four hours or longer. It should be worn constantly, including nighttime, except for removal during meals. Instruct the patient in the removal and placement of the partial denture supporting the occlusion rim and advise him that by chewing and gliding, the wax will be carved by the opposing teeth. Therefore the opposing teeth must be cleaned occasionally of ac-

Fig. 16-2. A, After correction of edentulous area to functional form, framework is reseated accurately on corrected master cast, any undercuts are blocked out with clay, and a tinfoil substitute is applied to surface of cast. **B,** A new resin base is made with self-curing acrylic resin by sprinkling to form a record base that is as nearly as possible identical to form of finished denture base. After curing, framework is lifted and any flash or excess is trimmed away. This base is then used to establish occlusal relations by whatever method is indicated, depending upon opposing dentition and dentist's preference.

Fig. 16-3. Example of a completed occlusal registration in a hard inlay wax supported by accurate record bases. Note that width of each cusp in all extremes of mandibular movement is recorded as a continuous glossy surface. Yet, anatomy of each opposing tooth is well defined. Completed registration must be placed back onto master cast without intervening debris or discrepancy and secured there with sticky wax so that accuracy of occlusal registration will be maintained.

cumulated wax particles. It is necessary that the patient comprehend what is being accomplished and understand that both voluntary and involuntary movements must be recorded.

Before dismissing the patient, add or remove wax where indicated to provide continuous contact throughout the chewing range. To accomplish this, repeatedly warm the wax with a hot spatula and have the patient carve the warmed wax rim with the opposing dentition, each time adding to any areas that are deficient. Support with additional wax any wax left unsupported by its flow under occlusal forces. It is important that the wax rim be absolutely dry and free of saliva before additional wax is applied. Each addition of wax must be made homogeneous with the larger mass to avoid separation or fracture of the occlusion rim during the time it is being worn. Leave the wax occlusion rim from 1 to 3 mm high, depending on whether or not vertical dimension is to be increased.

3. After twenty-four hours the occlusal surface of the wax rim should show a continuous gloss, indicating functional contact with the opposing teeth in all extremes of movement (Fig. 16-3). Any areas deficient in contact should be added to at this time. The reasons for maintaining positive occlusal contact throughout the time the occlusion rim is

being worn are that (a) all opposing teeth may be placed in function; (b) an opposing denture, if present, will become fully seated; and (c) vertical dimension in the molar region will be increased, thus repositioning the head of the mandibular condyle and allowing temporomandibular tissues to return to a normal relationship.

On the other hand, if during this period the wax occlusion rim has not been reduced to natural tooth contact, warm it by directing air from the air syringe through a flame onto the surface of the wax. By holding the wax rim with the fingers while warming it, a gradual softening process will result, rather than a melting of the surfaces already established. Repeatedly warm the occlusion rim and replace it in the mouth until the occlusal height has been reduced and lateral excursions have been recorded. At this time, support with additional wax those areas left unsupported by the flow of the wax to the buccal or lingual surfaces. At the same time, trim the areas obviously not involved, thus narrowing the occlusion rim as much as possible. Remove also those areas projecting above the occlusal surface, which by their presence might limit functional movement.

Having accomplished seating of the denture and changes in mandibular position by the previous period of wear, it is possible to

Fig. 16-4. Four views of an occlusal registration for a lower Class II partial denture. **A,** Occlusal registration in wax returned to master cast. Note extreme horizontal movement recorded. **B,** Same cast boxed with clay, leaving multiple occlusal surfaces exposed as vertical stops. **C,** Effect of occlusal stops, eliminating any possible changes in vertical dimension on articulator. **D,** Processed denture remounted for occlusal readjustment. Note modification in occlusal anatomy of stock artificial teeth and slight increase in height of occlusal plane. This is in harmony with natural tooth contact elsewhere in arch.

complete the occlusal registration at the chair. However, if all involuntary movements and those caused by changes in posture are to be recorded, the patient should again wear the occlusion rim for a period of time.

4. After a second twenty-four to forty-eight hour period of wear the registration should be complete and acceptable. The remaining teeth serving as vertical stops should be in contact, and the occlusion rim should show an intact glossy surface representing each cusp in all extremes of movement.

Not all natural teeth formerly in contact will necessarily be in contact on completion of the occlusal registration. Those teeth that have been depressed over a period of years and those that have been moved to accommodate overclosure or mandibular rotation may not be in contact when mandibular equilibrium has been reestablished. Such teeth may possibly return to occlusal contact in the

future or may have to be restored to occlusal contact after initial placement of the denture. Since the mandibular position may have been changed during the process of occlusal registration, the cuspal relation of some of the natural teeth may be different than before. This fact must be recognized in determining the correct restored vertical dimension.

The completed registration is now ready for conversion to an occluding template. This is usually done by boxing the occlusal registration with modeling clay after it has been reseated and secured onto the master or processing cast (Figs. 16-4 to 16-7). Only the wax registration and areas for vertical stops are left exposed. It is then filled with a hard stone to form an occluding template. (See Chapter 17.)

It is necessary that stone stops be used to maintain the vertical relation rather than relying on some adjustable part of the articulat-

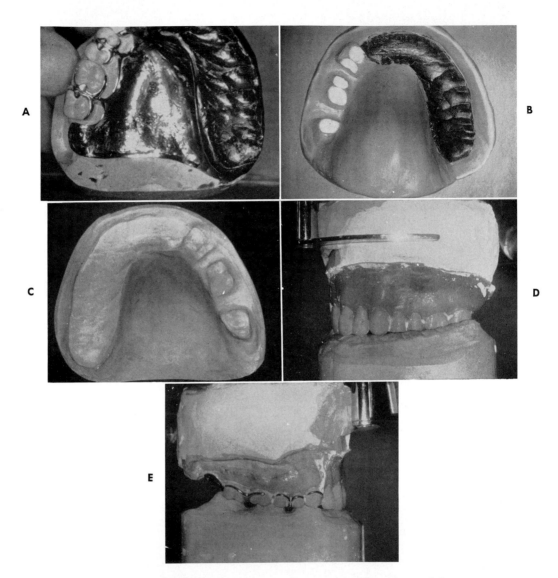

Fig. 16-5. Five views of an occlusal registration for an upper Class II partial denture. **A,** Partial view of occlusal registration returned to master cast. Again, note extreme horizontal movement recorded. **B,** Same cast boxed with clay, leaving multiple occlusal surfaces exposed as vertical stops. **C,** Occlusal view of occluding template. **D,** Processed denture remounted for occlusal readjustment. Note modification of teeth even to point of disregarding interdigitation, to effect good occlusion with template. Anterior teeth must be tried in mouth and positioned for esthetics before posterior teeth are arranged. **E,** Occlusal stops in full contact after processing and occlusal readjustment following remounting.

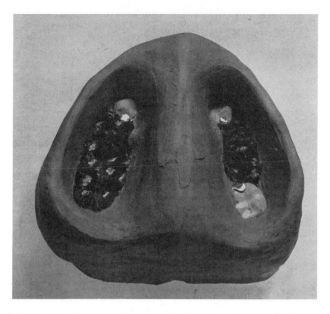

Fig. 16-6. Completed occlusal registration boxed with clay prior to pouring template in a hard die stone. Occlusal surfaces of adjacent abutment teeth are left exposed to serve as stone-to-stone vertical stops. Clay is trimmed just to margins of registration and raised in center to provide an arch for lingual access while arranging teeth to occlude with template.

Fig. 16-7. Rather than use clay sufficient to arch across from one side to another, the same may be done with wax with less time and material. It is better that the clay form a more acute angle with the occlusal wax registration and exposed occlusal surfaces than illustrated here.

ing instrument, which might be changed accidentally (Fig. 16-8). Also, by using stone stops and by mounting both the denture cast and the template before separating them, a simple hinge instrument may be used.

Because of its simplicity and the accessibility it affords in arranging teeth, the Hag-man Junior Balancer is preferred as an articulating instrument for use with an occluding template (Fig. 16-9). In this application the instrument is used as a hinge only, with all other moving elements securely locked in a fixed position. However, any hinged articulator may be similarly used.

Materials for artificial posterior teeth. Modern resin teeth are preferred by some over porcelain teeth because the former are more readily modified and thought to more nearly resemble enamel in their action against opposing teeth. Resin teeth with gold occlusal surfaces are preferably used in opposition to natural teeth, restored natural teeth, and gold occlusal surfaces, whereas porcelain teeth are generally used in opposition to other porcelain teeth.

Some changes in this concept have occurred in recent years. Sears and, later, Myerson have introduced the feasibility of using porcelain and resin teeth in opposition and the advantage of reduced frictional resistance by doing so. Myerson has compared the effect of porcelain teeth against resin teeth to that of a diamond stylus against a vinyl phonograph record, which results in less wear by friction than does the less hard sapphire stylus. For this to be truly compar-

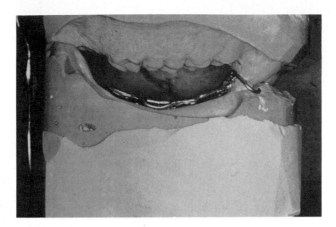

Fig. 16-8. Profile view of an occlusal template and one of its vertical stops. Despite the fact that this is a record of all extremes of mandibular movement for this patient, anatomy of occluding teeth can easily be identified.

Fig. 16-9. Completed upper partial denture with artificial teeth arranged and modified to occlude with a template made from a wax occlusal registration. Hagman Junior Balancer is used as a hinge alone, with all adjustable elements securely locked before the cast and template are mounted. Stone stops are used to preserve vertical relation. Note notch in upper cast for keying cast to articulator to facilitate accurate remounting after processing.

able, the porcelain tooth should possess a glazed surface, but experience has shown that even a polished vacuum-fired porcelain surface causes limited wear and reduced frictional resistance when in opposition to a modern resin artificial tooth.

A second fact also has been recognized, which is that resin tooth surfaces may in time become impregnated with abrasive particles, thereby becoming an abrasive substance themselves. This may explain why resin teeth are sometimes capable of wearing opposing gold surfaces. *An evaluation of occlusal contact or lack of contact, however, should be meticulously accomplished at each six-month recall appointment regardless of the choice of material for posterior tooth forms.*

Although some controversy still may exist in regard to the use of porcelain or resin artificial teeth, there is broad agreement that narrow occlusal surfaces are desirable. Posterior teeth that will satisfy this requirement should be selected, and the use of tooth forms having excessive buccolingual dimension should be avoided.

It has been our observation that artificial posterior resin teeth become excessively abraded in comparatively short periods of time regardless of the material by which they are opposed. The attendant ills of excessive abrasion of occlusal surfaces may often be avoided by using porcelain teeth to oppose porcelain teeth, gold occlusals to oppose other gold occlusal surfaces or natural teeth, and removal of the denture on retiring.

Acrylic resin teeth are easily modified and readily lend themselves to construction of cast gold surfaces on their occlusal portions. A simple procedure for fabricating gold occlusal surfaces and attaching them to acrylic resin teeth is described in Chapter 17 under posterior tooth forms.

Arranging teeth to an occluding template. The occlusal surface of the artificial teeth, porcelain or resin, must be modified to occlude with the template. In this method they are actually only raw materials from which an occlusal surface that is in harmony with an existing occlusal pattern is developed. Therefore the teeth must be occluded too high and then modified to fit the template at the established vertical dimension.

Teeth arranged to an occluding template ordinarily should be placed in the center of the functional range. Whenever possible, the teeth should be arranged buccolingually in the center of the template. When natural teeth have registered the functional occlusion, this may be considered the normal physiologic position of the artificial dentition regardless of its relation to the residual ridge. On the other hand, if some man-made occlusion in the opposing arch has been recorded, such as that of an opposing denture, the teeth should be arranged in a favorable relation to their foundation, even if this means arranging them slightly buccally or lingually from center of the template.

The teeth are usually arranged to interdigitate with the opposing teeth in a normal

Fig. 16-10. A, View of interdigitation sometimes possible when teeth are arranged to an occlusal template. This is possible only when gross migration of opposing teeth has not occurred. **B,** View of modification to occlusal surfaces necessary when customary interdigitation would create objectionable spaces. Note that original cusp-to-cusp relation of artificial teeth has been altered until marginal ridges have actually become interdigitation cusps. Such an occlusal relationship is entirely permissible and effective.

cuspal relationship. As is customary, whenever possible the mesiobuccal cusp of the maxillary first molar is located in relation to the buccal groove of the mandibular first molar and all other teeth arranged accordingly. With functional occlusion, however, it is not absolutely necessary that a normal anteroposterior relation be reestablished. (See Fig. 16-10.) In the first place the opposing teeth in a broken dental arch may not be in normal alignment, and interdigitation may be difficult to accomplish. In the second place the occlusal surfaces will be modified so that they will function favorably regardless of their anteroposterior position (Fig. 16-11). Since cusps modified to fit an occlusal template will be in harmony with the opposing dentition, it is not necessary that the teeth themselves be arranged to conform to the usual concept of what constitutes a normal anteroposterior relationship.

Making the occluding template of metal. Some indicator must be used to guide the alteration of occlusal surfaces to fit the template. Articulating paper has several disadvantages when used for this purpose. One is that it does not conform readily to irregular surfaces and quickly becomes perforated, giving irregular markings. Another is that the waxlike substance with which the paper is impregnated tends to accumulate on the surface of the template, changing the vertical relation somewhat and giving false marks on the teeth. An inked marking tape (silk ribbon, dental tape, or typewriter ribbon) is superior to articulating paper because it will not tear and yet will conform better to irregular surfaces (Fig. 16-12). In this regard it

Fig. 16-11. Occlusal surfaces after remounting and final occlusal readjustment to template. Note functional occlusal anatomy resulting. This is an entirely different occlusal surface from that which was present on the stock artificial teeth as manufactured.

Fig. 16-12. When you are arranging teeth to an occluding template, marking tape should be used in positioning and modifying each tooth to fit template. Note that at this early stage articulator has been opened approximately 0.5 mm, as evidenced by slight space at vertical stop.

also permits more accurate marking of proximal surfaces as they are being ground to fit the denture framework. An ink mark may be more reliably interpreted than may a crayon mark made with articulating paper.

The inked ribbon may be held with forceps, such as the Miller articulating paper forceps, or in a wire frame (Fig. 16-13). The latter is easily made of orthodontic wire and holds the ribbon taut at all times, whereas the forceps are designed primarily for use with articulating paper.

One of the hazards of arranging teeth to a stone template is that the template becomes abraded by continuous closure against the artificial teeth as they are being adjusted to occlude with the template. It is inevitable that during the process of alternately marking and grinding occlusal surfaces the stone template is subjected to considerable abuse and wear (Fig. 16-14). This abrasion can be minimized by using the hardest dental stone available for the template and by avoiding forceful contact of the template with the oc-

clusal surfaces of the teeth. It also can be avoided by electroplating the wax occlusal registration, thus forming a relatively indestructible occlusal template. (See Figs. 16-15 to 16-20.) The technique is as follows:

Low-fusing metal has been preferred to stone as an occluding cast material, but molten metal cannot be poured into a wax mold. Electroplating permits a metallic surface to be formed on the wax record with accuracy and with greater hardness than low-fusing metals. Electroforming with silver has proved to be the simplest and most satisfactory method.

Interest in electroplating has been revised since the advent of the Thiokol and Silicone impression materials. The change from time-honored copper dies to silver dies was made necessary by the introduction of these new impression materials when electroformed dies were preferred to stone dies.

The technique for electroplating the occlusal template is basically identical with electroplating of Thiokol and Silicone impressions. The main differences are that the vessel containing the electrolyte must be larger, the leads must be attached

Fig. 16-13. Drawing of a wire holder for marking tape or typewriter ribbon. Wire used is 0.036-inch orthodontic wire. Ribbon is held taut at either end after passing over inner arch (over, under, and then over).

Fig. 16-14. Stone occlusal template before and after use. **A,** Occlusal surfaces are unmarred by abrasion. **B,** Evidence of abrasion through articulating marks shows damage and therefore inaccuracy resulting from abrasion and crushing forces as template is tapped against opposing teeth. If occlusal surfaces during remounting are readjusted to fit this altered surface, some occlusal inaccuracies are inevitable, which must then be compensated for by occlusal adjustment of completed denture.

Fig. 16-15. Homemade equipment for electroplating wax occlusal registration. Milliamperage can be varied from 35 to 200 ma. Electrolyte in glass container is silver potassium cyanide; anode is pure silver. Commercial electroplating equipment may be purchased, or equipment may be assembled as shown by diagram in Fig. 16-16. Work is suspended in solution from an alligator clip superstructure attached to one side of electric circuit. Anode may be suspended or placed in a refrigerator dish as illustrated. The variable factor of the distance from anode to work may be eliminated by agitating the solution with an aquarium aerator pump, open end of plastic tubing being held in solution by passing it through an egg-shaped fishing sinker.

Fig. 16-16. Diagram and parts needed for making electroplating device for silver plating Thiokol and silicone impressions and wax occlusal registrations. S. W., Toggle switch; *T*, small filament transformer; *P.L.*, pilot light; *B.R.*, full-wave bridge rectifier; *V.R.*, variable rheostat; *M.A.*, milliammeter; *F.R.*, fixed resistor. Parts required include 6.3-volt filament transformer, milliammeter, 1.5 Å full-wave bridge rectifier, 50-ohm, 4-watt variable rheostat, pilot light, 2 SPST switches, 10-watt, 50-ohm wire-wound resistor, and utility cabinet. (Courtesy Dr. Paul E. Hammons.)

Fig. 16-17. Leads are attached below wax occlusal registration with sticky wax, and denture framework is coated with a protective lacquer (Kerr plate mask). Occlusal registration is then metalized with a silver lacquer, which is carried down lingual surface to join wire leads. (From McCracken, W. L.: J. Prosthet. Dent. **8:**955-963, 1958.)

Fig. 16-18. Wax occlusal registration after electroplating. Note wire staples added to wax to provide retention to stone that will be poured against silver surface. Leads and protective lacquer over metal framework are now removed prior to reseating occlusal registration onto master cast.

Fig. 16-19. After denture framework has been accurately reseated onto master cast and secured there with sticky wax, a clay matrix is formed, leaving one or more occlusal surfaces on each side exposed to serve as vertical stops. Clay is made to rise from borders of registration at a 45-degree angle and is arched across midline to provide lingual access when arranging teeth to template. Exposed occlusal surfaces are painted with a separator, and stone is vibrated into clay matrix to form remainder of occluding template.

Fig. 16-20. A, Electroformed silver occluding template with stone stops anteriorly to preserve vertical dimension. **B,** Another electroformed occluding template involving six opposing teeth (functional width of each cusp is readily discernible). (**A** from McCracken, W. L.: J. Prosthet. Dent. **8:**955-963, 1958.)

bilaterally in a manner that will allow the denture to be suspended in the solution, and the denture framework must be protected from the electrolytic current.

Ten milliamperes of current per tooth, plus 10 for the leads, is sufficient. Greater amperage would cause the electroplating to be too soft. The total area of the anode immersed in the solution should not be more than twice the area to be plated. The distance from the anode to the surface to be plated should be about 4 inches.

Since the number of teeth involved will vary, the plating machine must have a widely variable output. The machine being used is a self-made device with a variable output of from 35 to 200 ma, although suitable machines ready for use may be purchased.

The wax occlusal registration is metallized with Staco silver lacquer, and the leads are painted down the lingual side to joint with a T-shaped wire lead. This lead is attached to the wax rims with sticky wax. It is very important that all parts of the denture framework be painted with a protective lacquer, such as Kerr's Plate Mask, to prevent the casting itself from being plated.

At 10 ma per tooth, the occlusal registration to be plated should be left in the solution approximately five hours. A uniform plate of sufficient thickness will result. A heavier plate seems to cause some curling of the edges and pulling away from the wax surface. This leads to inaccuracies and must be avoided. Since the plated surface will be backed up with stone, a thin plate is all that is needed.

The attachment of the stone backing to the silver plate was a problem at first. In some cases, the metal separated from the stone backing due to the absence of mechanical attachment. The problem has been solved by imbedding two or more wire staples into the wax surface of the occlusal registration before plating. These staples become

part of the plated surface and aid in securing the metal to the stone. The small tip end of each staple projecting through the metal template can easily be ground away without marring the surfaces of the template.

The plated surface is boxed with clay, and stone is poured against it in the same manner as an unplated wax record. The articulator mounting and occluding the teeth to the template is the same, except for the advantages of the metal surface over a stone surface.

It is not expected that the silver plating of a wax occlusal record will receive wide acceptance because of the added step of electroplating. But just as there are those who prefer to work with electroformed dies, so there may be some who would prefer to arrange teeth to a metal template.*

Functional registration of occlusal surfaces for fixed partial dentures and single crowns. Many of the advantages to be found in the registration of occlusal pathways for removable partial dentures may be applied also to the construction of fixed restorations and individual crowns. A more harmonious occlusion results from establishing a functional relationship than when only a centric occlusal relation is recorded.

Since fixed restorations and individual crowns are often essential to adequate mouth preparations for partial dentures, it is necessary that methods for obtaining occlusal harmony on those restorations be considered in this chapter. It has been stated previously that analysis and adjustment of the natural occlusion is an essential part of mouth prepa-

*From McCracken, W. L.: Functional occlusion in removable partial denture construction, J. Prosthet. Dent. **8:**955-963, 1958.

rations. It is equally essential that any occlusion reconstruction be done in harmony with the accepted or corrected natural occlusion. It is doubtful that this is possible without having some record of the existing occlusal pattern.

Functional occlusion for fixed partial dentures and crowns must be established entirely at the chair, because the patient cannot be given a restoration that he can remove at mealtime. Although such a jaw relation record does not possess all the advantages of an occlusal registration made during a twenty-four-hour period, it does create an occlusion that is in harmony with the majority of jaw movements. Occlusal discrepancies on the finished restoration caused by changes in posture can be recorded and eliminated only by having the patient wear an unpolished gold restoration or one made dull by sandblasting for a period long enough to register any remaining interference. This limitation of a functional registration done at the chair should be recognized and then corrected on the finished restoration.

Establishing functional occlusion on a single crown. The method of registering functional occlusion on a single crown was mentioned previously in conjunction with the making of a crown pattern to fit a denture clasp (Chapter 13). In this technique a thin coping of self-curing resin is made to support the wax pattern. An occlusal pattern is then established directly in the mouth with little danger of fracture or distortion. Any hard inlay wax may be used for this purpose.

Either removable dies or individual dies in conjunction with a solid cast may be used to establish vertical surfaces on the wax pattern, which will satisfy requirements for marginal contact, guiding planes, and contours for clasp retention and reciprocation. This may be done prior to establishing occlusal relations, or the occlusal aspect of the pattern may be completed first and the pattern then returned to the cast for the shaping of vertical surfaces.

When individual dies are used, occlusion is usually established first and then the pattern is placed on a solid cast of the arch to contour the crown in relation to the path of placement. This is done with the aid of a surveyor. Finally the pattern is returned to the individual die to refine the margins. When removable dies are used, the contouring of vertical surfaces may be done first, then the occlusal relationship may be established in the mouth, and finally the pattern is returned to the die for the refinement of the margins.

When several such restorations are to be made for the same arch, it is best that as many wax patterns be made concurrently as possible. On the other hand, it may be necessary to restore only one or two teeth at a time to preserve vertical and horizontal relations. This may sometimes be facilitated by making plastic temporary crowns for all prepared teeth in harmony with the existing occlusion, and then using these temporary crowns alternately as guides while establishing a functional occlusion on the wax patterns.

As with an occlusal registration for a partial denture, the completed occlusal registration should have a glossy surface and should make contact with the opposing teeth throughout the functional range. Sufficient chewing time must be allowed for any excess wax to be eliminated, with the teeth elsewhere in the arch again in contact.

The occlusal surface thus established will be broader than will a natural tooth. In the registration for a removable partial denture or a fixed partial denture this is converted to a template and an occlusal surface of acceptable width formed to occlude with only a part of the template. The occlusal registration for a crown pattern, on the other hand, is the wax pattern that becomes the finished casting. This occlusal surface is much too wide and has too much occlusal contact to be within the toleration limits of periodontal support. The wax pattern must therefore be narrowed to reduce the width of the occlusal table. Spillways should be added to further reduce the occlusal area and to increase masticating efficiency. This is generally done to conform to concepts of normal occlusal anatomy, the objective being to further reduce the area of occlusal contact and to assure maximum efficiency. A crown restoration thus formed will possess maximum efficiency without interference, in harmony with all eccentric movements and with the other teeth in the arch.

Step-by-step procedure for recording occlusal pathways for a fixed partial denture. The objectives in establishing functional occlusion on a fixed partial denture are the

Fig. 16-21. Establishing functional occlusion for a fixed partial denture by means of an occlusal registration of opposing teeth. **A,** Acrylic resin frame with hard inlay wax occlusal surface. **B,** Occluding template poured against wax registration with stone stops anterior and posterior. **C,** Resulting template to which occlusal surfaces of restoration will be formed.

same as for a single crown. The method, however, is somewhat different.

Functional occlusion for a fixed partial denture is established by means of an occlusal registration on an acrylic resin or cast metal frame or platform. The technique of occlusal registration is much the same as for removable partial denture occlusion except that the frame is not removable by the patient, and therefore occlusal registration must be done entirely at the chair. (See Fig. 16-21.)

The technique for establishing functional occlusion for a fixed partial denture is as follows:

1. Although a cast metal frame may be used, one made of acrylic resin is adequate for the purpose. The frame may be made on a cast from a separate alginate hydrocolloid impression of the prepared teeth or from a second pour of a rubber-base impression. The cast containing trimmed dies is not used for making a frame, for fear of marring its surface.

Clay or utility wax is added to block out the gingival one fourth of the prepared teeth and the adjacent soft tissues and edentulous areas. This eliminates any interference to the seating of the frame onto the working cast. Any irregularities in the preparations are also blocked out. Then a wax or clay matrix is formed to confine the self-curing acrylic resin within the desired limits.

The cast is painted with tinfoil substitute, which is allowed to dry. Self-curing acrylic resin is then applied, using the sprinkling method, until a resin platform of the desired thickness has been obtained. The occlusal portion is left wide but thin.

After polymerizing at least an hour, but preferably overnight, the frame is lifted from the cast and trimmed of excess. It should be no bulkier than is necessary for strength. The only adjustment that should be necessary in the mouth is the reduction of the occlusal plane to provide space for the registration wax.

2. The resin frame must seat accurately on the abutment teeth, and there must be no contact with soft tissues. The occlusal surface should be reduced sufficiently to provide ample clearance for the registration wax. Apply a film of sticky wax to the dried frame and

than add a hard inlay wax to the occlusal surface.*

While the wax is still soft, place the resin frame in the mouth and ask the patient to make centric contact and excursive movements. Add wax where deficient and support the width bucally and lingually with additional wax. Reduce excess width as well as excess height at the limits of excursive movements. Do not add to glossy areas, but only those areas in which contact is deficient. This registration differs from the partial denture registration, in which the occlusion rim is left 1 to 3 mm high for the patient to reduce during a twenty-four-hour period. The fixed partial denture registration is done entirely at the chair and can only record voluntary movements at the vertical level determined by the other teeth in the arch. As mentioned repeatedly in preceding paragraphs, this should be an occlusion that is acceptable or made so by previous occlusal adjustments or reconstruction.

The completed registration should make contact with the opposing teeth throughout the functional range. The registration should have an intact glossy surface and will be much wider than will the occlusion on the finished restoration.

3. The completed occlusal registration is treated much the same as a registration for a removable partial denture. A hard die stone is poured against it, or it may be metallized and electroplated. In either case, seat it accurately on the working cast and secure it there with sticky wax.

Form a clay matrix at a 45-degree angle from the margins of the registration, leaving the cast exposed anteriorly and posteriorly to provide vertical stops. Pour stone directly against the wax registration or the electro-plated surface. After this has set, mount the cast and opposing template on some kind of hinge articulator before the two are separated. The resulting mounting will not be dependent on the articulator for maintaining the vertical relation because stone-to-stone stops will have been provided for this purpose.

Patterns are waxed to occlude with the opposing template. Generally, occlusal relations with the opposing teeth will not be jeopardized from an esthetic standpoint by carving restorations to a template alone. However, when interdigitation or the correct horizontal overlap might be difficult to ascertain when a template alone is used, another procedure may be followed. In this procedure a conventional mounting to an occluding cast is made first, using an occluding stone cast that has been poured directly into a wax or other interocclusal record (Fig. 16-22, *A*). This provides an anatomic opposing cast for the establishment of interdigitation and the desired amount of horizontal overlap. This is frequently desirable from an esthetic standpoint and to avoid a cusp-to-cusp occlusion on the completed restoration.

An occlusal registration made on an acrylic resin frame is then positioned on the working cast as described previously and a clay matrix formed around it, leaving stone exposed at either end for a vertical stop. The opposing anatomic cast is then lubricated or treated with some separating medium such as a solution of sodium silicate, the occlusal registration filled with stone, and the anatomic cast seated into the stone (Fig. 16-22, *B*). Sufficient thickness of stone must remain for strength.

After the occlusal template has set, it may be separated and trimmed. Two articulator mountings are thus obtained; one is an anatomic opposing cast, and the other is a removable stone template complete with vertical stops to which a functional occlusion may be perfected that will be free of eccentric interference. The same degree of occlusal harmony is possible by the method as with the functional occlusal record alone, with the added advantage of assuring an acceptable esthetic relationship with the opposing teeth. Occlusal surfaces may be made as narrow as desired, and occlusal anatomy should be added for masticating efficiency. Finished castings and the assembled fixed partial den-

---

*For an occlusal registration done entirely at the chair, any inlay wax may be used rather than the harder Peck's purple inlay wax that is used for recording occlusal pathways on a removable partial denture.

In recent years interest in the functionally generated path has led to the development of special waxes for this purpose, such as the Jelenko "Hi-Fi" wax. These waxes are suitable only for direct registration at the chair and cannot be worn by the patient away from the operatory; but then neither can a registration frame be worn outside the dental office because it must be removed by the patient during mealtime, which would leave prepared abutment teeth exposed. When this softer type of wax is used at the chair, it is best supported at its border by a harder inlay wax to prevent distortion at the limits of excursion.

A   **B**

Fig. 16-22. Articulated casts providing both anatomic and functional registrations of opposing teeth on same articulator. **A,** Conventional mounting to an occluding cast obtained on a wax interocclusal record. Correct vertical relationship is maintained by natural tooth contact anteriorly; otherwise a stone stop should be provided rather than depend on vertical stop of articulator alone. **B,** Occluding stone template formed from a functional occlusal registration is interposed between the two casts to establish functional occlusal surfaces on restorations. This removable template overlays opposing anatomic cast and is extended anteriorly and posteriorly to provide vertical stops when template is in use.

Fig. 16-23. Hanau twin-stage occluder. An anatomic occluding cast is attached to one upper arm and an occlusal template to the other. Better esthetic results are made possible by occluding wax patterns to both a functional and an anatomic cast. (Courtesy Hanau Engineering Co., Buffalo, N.Y.)

ture then should be reoccluded to the template to eliminate discrepancies caused by spruing and soldering.

Fig. 16-23 illustrates an articulator made by the Hanau Company, called the twin-stage occluder, which further facilitates the use of both a functional and an anatomic cast when occluding wax patterns to a functional record. Fig. 16-24 shows an improved version of the Verticulator made by the Jelenko

Company for use with either full arch or sectional casts, which also permits the use of dual opposing surfaces. Two upper arms are provided, both machined to fit a single lower arm. A static interocclusal record may be attached to one arm and a functional record to the other, and the two can be interchanged at will.

One disadvantage of using a simple hinge articulator as illustrated in Fig. 16-22 is the

Fig. 16-24. Two models of Jelenko Verticulator. Designed for use with Pankey-Mann technique, they are suitable for use with either an anatomic occluding cast or a functionally generated path. However, since only vertical movement is permitted, with positive metal-to-metal vertical limitation, instrument is best suited for use with functionally generated path. Dual model permits an interchange between a functional cast and an anatomic cast by substituting two matched and identical upper members. (Courtesy J. F. Jelenko & Co., Inc., New York, N.Y.)

small arc of closure dictated by the proximity of the hinge to the occlusal surface. An occluding template is most effectively used when vertical or nearly vertical closure is possible. When an instrument such as the Hagman Balancer is used, the arc of closure is sufficiently great that it may be considered nearly vertical at the plane of occlusion. Otherwise it is best that an instrument such as the Jelenko Verticulator (Fig. 16-24), which permits only vertical closure, be used in conjunction with an occluding template. The Verticulator has a further advantage of providing a spring-loaded metal-to-metal stop, which positively prevents possible abra-

sion of the occluding surfaces and loss of the established vertical dimension.

A fixed partial denture restoration made with functional occlusal surfaces should have a harmonious occlusion in centric and in all voluntary eccentric positions. As with a single crown, any remaining eccentric interference must be eliminated in the mouth. Since these are not caused by voluntary movements, it is best that the patient wear the restorations with dull occlusal surfaces (preferably sandblasted surfaces) for a period of twenty-four hours or more. Any remaining interference may then be identified by shiny areas in eccentric position, and these may be eliminated before final polishing. Indeed, it may be esthetically desirable at times to leave occlusal surfaces unpolished, with only a satin finish created by sandblasting.

Establishing jaw relations for a mandibular removable partial denture opposing a maxillary complete denture. It is not uncommon for a mandibular removable partial denture to be made to occlude with an opposing maxillary complete denture. The maxillary denture may already be present or it may be made concurrently with the opposing partial denture. In any event, the establishment of jaw relations in this situation may be accomplished by one of several methods previously outlined.

If an existing maxillary complete denture is satisfactory and is not to be replaced, that arch is treated as an intact arch as though natural teeth were present. A facebow transfer is made of that arch and the cast mounted on the articulator in the usual manner. Maxillomandibular relations may be recorded on accurate record bases attached to the mandibular partial denture framework, using one of the recording mediums previously outlined, such as wax, modeling plastic, quick-setting plaster, impression paste, or quick-curing acrylic resin. Centric relation is thus recorded and transferred to the articulator. Eccentric records can then be made to program the articulator.

In rare instances, when the mandibular partial denture replaces all posterior teeth and the anterior teeth are noninterfering, a central bearing point tracer may be mounted in the palate of the maxillary denture and centric relation recorded by means of an intraoral stylus tracing against a stable mandibular base.

If the relationship of the posterior teeth on the maxillary denture to the mandibular ridge is favorable and the complete denture is *stable*, jaw relations may be established by recording occlusal pathways in the mandibular arch the same as for any opposing intact arch. The success of this method depends upon the stability of the denture bases, the quality of tissue support, the relation of the opposing teeth to the mandibular ridge, and the interrelation of existing artificial and natural teeth.

More times than not, the existing maxillary complete denture will have been made to occlude with malpositioned mandibular teeth, which have since been lost, or the teeth

will have been arranged without consideration for the future occlusal relation with a mandibular partial denture. Too frequently one sees a maxillary denture with posterior teeth arranged close to the residual ridge without regard for interarch relationship and with an occlusal plane that is too low. In such instances the least that can be done is to reposition the posterior teeth on the maxillary denture before establishing maxillomandibular relations. This can only be justified when the maxillary denture is otherwise satisfactory as to fit, appearance, and occlusion elsewhere in the arch. Usually, however, a new maxillary denture must be made concurrently with the mandibular partial denture, and jaw relations may be established in one of two ways.

If the mandibular partial denture will be tooth supported (a Kennedy Class III arch accommodating a bilateral removable prosthesis), that arch is restored first. The same applies to a mandibular arch being restored with fixed partial dentures. In either situation the mandibular arch is completely restored first, and jaw relations are established as they would be to a full complement of opposing teeth. Thus the maxillary complete denture is made to occlude with an intact arch, and the procedure for doing so need not be included here.

On the other hand, as is more frequently the situation, the mandibular partial denture may have one or more distal extension bases. The situation then requires that either the occlusion be established on both dentures simultaneously or the maxillary denture be completed first.

After the making of final impressions, which includes the correction of the mandibular cast to establish optimal support for the bases of the partial denture (the denture framework must be made previously if a wax correction method is used), the maxillary occlusion rim is contoured, vertical relation with the remaining lower teeth is established, and a face-bow transfer of the maxillary arch is made. The maxillomandibular relations may be recorded by any one of the several methods previously outlined and the articulator mounting completed. Occlusion may be established as for complete dentures, taking care to establish a favorable tooth-to-ridge relationship in both arches, an optimal occlusal plane, and cuspal harmony between all occluding teeth.

After try-in, either of two methods may be used. Both dentures may be processed concurrently and remounted for occlusal correction, or the maxillary denture may be processed first, and after it is remounted, the teeth, still in wax on the partial denture, are adjusted to any discrepancies occurring.

Up to the point of establishing the final occlusion on the partial denture, jaw relations, articulator mounting, and try-in are accomplished as though both dentures were to be completed at the same time. The teeth on the mandibular partial denture are arranged in wax so that a favorable ridge relationship and occlusal plane will have been established. The maxillary denture alone is then remounted to adjust the occlusion to the remaining natural teeth and is placed in the mouth as a completed restoration.

The teeth in wax are removed from the partial denture base and replaced with hard inlay wax occlusion rims secured to acrylic resin bases, which are attached to the denture framework. A functional occlusal record by registering occlusal pathways is then accomplished, treating the opposing complete denture as an intact arch. The occlusal registration thus obtained is placed back on the master cast, boxed with clay, and an occluding template formed complete with stone-to-stone vertical stops. The same articulator may be used, replacing the original upper cast with the template, or the mandibular cast and the template may be mounted on a simple hinge-type articulator.

It is necessary that the acrylic resin record base be removed by softening it over a flame before the teeth are rearranged to occlude with the template. The teeth that were formerly arranged to occlude with the maxillary denture are then modified to fit the template, and the denture bases are waxed and processed. Investing must be done in such a manner that the cast may be recovered intact and remounted for occlusal refinement to the template.

Occlusion thus established on a mandibular partial denture opposing a maxillary complete denture provides occlusal harmony. Not only does stability of both dentures result, but trauma conducive to tissue changes beneath both dentures is held to a minimum. The harmony of occlusion thus established justifies the added steps necessary to accomplish such results.

Correction of occlusal discrepancies created during processing must be accomplished before the patient is permitted to use the denture(s). Methods by which these discrepancies may be corrected are discussed in Chapter 17.

SELF-ASSESSMENT AIDS

1. See if you will buy this statement: Occlusal harmony exists when the masticating mechanism can carry out its physiologic functions while the factors of occlusion remain in a healthy state; the factors of occlusion being the temporomandibular joints, the neuromuscular mechanism, and the teeth and their supporting structures.
2. Occlusal harmony between a removable partial denture and the remaining natural teeth is a major factor in preserving the health of the supporting structures of the natural teeth. True or false?
3. The establishment of a satisfactory occlusion for a partial denture patient should include five considerations or procedures by the dentist. Can you recall these five "musts"?
4. Define "centric relation" in your own words.
5. What is "centric occlusion"?
6. What is meant by the term "eccentric occlusion"?
7. Describe a "balanced occlusion."
8. Two methods are commonly used to develop an acceptable occlusion for a removable partial denture patient. Can you give a brief description of these two methods?
9. What records are necessary to correctly orient casts to an arcon type articulator and program the articulator?
10. A harmonious relationship of opposing occlusal and incisal surfaces, in itself, is not adequate to assure stability of distal extension removable partial dentures. What other factor must be recognized and dealt with to minimize unwanted leverages?
11. There are differences among dentists in developing contacts of opposing teeth in centric and eccentric positions for partially edentulous patients. When you answer the following queries correctly, honestly try to rationalize the recommendations contained in this text:
    a. Simultaneous contacts of opposing posterior teeth must occur in centric occlusion. True or false?
    b. Occlusion for tooth-borne removable partial dentures may be arranged to duplicate the occlusion seen in a harmonious natural dentition. True or false?
    c. Under what circumstances is a balanced occlusion desirable for the partially edentulous patient?
    d. Should working side contacts be developed when a mandibular distal extension

denture is opposed by natural teeth (assuming all mandibular posterior teeth are missing)?

e. You are treating a patient with a Class I maxillary arch. Is it beneficial to develop balancing and working contacts? Explain your answer. What about protrusive contacts?

f. Are balancing side contacts for a Class II maxillary arch desirable?

g. What are the desirable contact relationships of artificial-natural teeth when one arch is a Class IV arch?

h. What is the most distal extent that an artificial tooth should be arranged in in a Class I or II mandibular arch?

12. A patient requires a tooth-borne mandibular removable partial denture. The remaining teeth are maximally interdigitated; however, this position does not coincide with centric relation. There is no TMJ pathology, no neuromuscular disorders, and no periodontal conditions aggravated by occlusion. Would you insist that the patient be restored to have maximum interdigitation coincide with centric relation? Why or why not?

13. Under what circumstances would you develop an occlusion for a partially edentulous patient so that maximum intercuspation coincided with centric relation?

14. When must the dentist determine the horizontal jaw relation in which he will develop the occlusion for the partially edentulous patient? Why?

15. After the horizontal relationship of the jaws to which the occlusion will be developed has been determined, occlusal relationships may be established by five methods. The choice of method will be determined by the existing partially edentulous situation of the patient, location of remaining teeth in each arch, and the prior correction of any existing occlusal discrepancies. These five methods are (a) direct opposition of casts, (b) interocclusal records with posterior teeth remaining, (c) occlusal relations using occlusion rims, (d) jaw relation records made entirely on occlusion rims, and (e) recording functionally generated paths. You should be able to rationalize and briefly discuss each of the five methods.

16. What are the disadvantages of using wax for making interocclusal records?

17. When developing an occlusion for a partially edentulous patient using the functionally generated path technique, why may occluding frames be used rather than an articulator?

18. What are the disadvantages in developing an occlusion to a stone template or stone teeth on a cast?

19. Materials of which the occlusal surfaces of artificial posterior teeth are made deserve serious consideration by the dentist. These considerations should be based on minimizing attrition of occlusal surfaces, maintaining the established vertical dimension of occlusion, and maintaining positive contact of posterior teeth as planned. To best accomplish the preceding, please give the material of choice for opposing occlusal surfaces for (a) porcelain, (b) enamel, (c) restored natural teeth, and (d) fixed partial denture pontics with gold occlusal surfaces.

20. Acrylic resin posterior teeth lend themselves to easier modification than do porcelain teeth when the interresidual ridge distance is small or when an edentulous space to be restored with the denture is grossly restricted. However, acrylic resin teeth have one big drawback when occluded against any other occlusal surface, including acrylic resin. Know what this drawback is?

21. The occlusal surfaces of acrylic resin teeth attached to a denture may be duplicated in gold and attached to the same teeth. Did you consult Chapter 17 to see how this is accomplished?

22. Occlusal discrepancies created during processing procedures *must* be corrected before the patient is given possession of the dentures. True or false?

17 LABORATORY PROCEDURES

This chapter will cover only those phases of dental laboratory procedures that are directly related to partial denture construction. Familiarity with laboratory procedures relative to the making of fixed restorations and complete dentures is presumed. Such information is already available in the numerous excellent textbooks on those subjects and will not be duplicated here. For example, the principles and techniques involved in the waxing, casting, and finishing of single inlays, crowns, and fixed partial dentures are adequately covered in lecture material and textbooks and in manuals available to the dental student, the dental laboratory technician, and the practicing dentist. Similarly, knowledge of the principles and techniques for mounting casts, articulating teeth, and waxing, processing, and polishing complete dentures is presumed as a necessary background for the laboratory phases of partial denture construction. Therefore this chapter will be directed specifically toward the laboratory procedures involved in the making of a removable partial denture.

DUPLICATING A STONE CAST

A stone cast may be duplicated for one of three purposes. One is the duplication in stone of the original or corrected master cast to preserve the original. Upon this duplicate cast the denture framework may be fitted without danger of abrading or fracturing the surface of the original master cast. Most of the better commercial dental laboratories have adopted a policy of doing all work on a duplicate cast, including the fitting procedures. The finished casting is then returned to the dentist after all fitting has been completed on the duplicate cast.

The student or the dentist doing his own laboratory work should likewise follow the policy of making a duplicate cast for fitting the denture framework. Although some dental laboratories also may use the duplicate cast for blockout, it is preferable to do the blockout on the master cast just prior to a second duplication rather than to use the duplicate cast for this purpose. After blockout of the master cast a second duplication is done for making an investment cast. Upon this investment cast the wax or plastic pattern is formed, and the metal framework is ultimately cast against its surface.

A blocked out master cast should be duplicated in stone if wrought-wire retainers are planned as components of the framework for the removable partial denture. The contouring of wrought-wire retainers may be accomplished on this cast and transferred to the duplicate investment cast in the exact same relationship to which it was contoured on the duplicate stone cast. This use of a duplicate stone cast of the blocked out master cast avoids marring the master cast or investment cast. (See Fig. 17-12.)

Although both the fitting cast and the investment cast must be an accurate reproduction of the original, the fitting cast is made of a hard stone and is not directly involved in the making of the metal framework. The investment cast, on the other hand, must possess the properties of a casting investment, such as the ability to withstand burnout temperatures while providing the necessary mold expansion. Gold alloys and also Ticonium are cast to plaster-bound silica investments, whereas the higher melting stellite alloys are cast to investments containing quartz held together by a suitable binder so that they will withstand the higher casting temperatures necessary with these alloys. Although the latter are generally harder than are gypsum investments, any investment cast may be easily abraded and must be handled carefully to preserve the accuracy of its surface. The practice of treating the dried investment cast by dipping it in melted resin and beeswax reduces considerably the danger of its becoming abraded during subsequent handling.

The use of preformed plastic patterns eliminates some of the danger of altering the surface of the investment cast in the process of forming the pattern. With free-hand waxing, considerable care must be taken not to score or abrade the investment cast. The student, however, needs the experience of free-hand waxing to give him a better comprehension of the bulk and contours necessary to produce an acceptable denture framework. A continuation of this practice is recommended. For the same reasons it is also recommended that the laboratory technician be experienced in the use of wax shapes and free-hand waxing before he is allowed to use preformed patterns.

Duplicating materials and flasks. Duplicating materials are colloidal materials, which are made fluid by heating and return to a gel on being cooled.

The cast to be duplicated must be placed in the bottom of a suitable flask, called a duplicating flask. It is necessary that a duplicating flask contain the fluid material to facilitate cooling, to facilitate removal of the cast

from the mold without permanent deformation or damage to the mold, and to support the mold while it is being filled with the cast material. Numerous duplicating flasks are on the market (Fig. 17-1). One type is a metal bell with holes in the top for pouring. Another is a simple metal ring with removable bottom and top, the latter having a center hole for pouring. Still another has the top and bottom secured with thumb screws.

To Dr. Noble G. Wills is due much credit for his untiring efforts in furthering the development of accurate cast duplication equipment. Two of these duplicating flasks are illustrated in Fig. 17-1. They consist of a machined metal top and bottom fitting onto a formica ring 2 or 2¼ inches high. Formica rather than metal is used for the ring because Formica acts as an insulator to prevent too rapid cooling through the sides of the flask. The center hole in the top of each type is provided with a filling reservoir, or "feeder ring." Although not all duplicating flasks provide for a filling reservoir, it is most desirable that a ring superstructure be provided to serve as a reservoir for feeding the warm material into the mold. Thus as cooling and subsequent shrinkage occur, additional fluid

Fig. 17-1. Five types of duplicating flasks. Upper left, Wills flask, type E; upper right, Wills flask, type F. Both these flasks have a formica ring, 4-inch inside diameter and are 2 inches in height. Formica is used for its non-heat–conducting property and is machined with a 5-inch inside taper. In the center is a bell-shaped flask; lower left, Kerr duplicating flask; lower right, a lightweight brass flask in common usage.

material is fed into the mold from the reservoir above. This is similar to the cooling of dental gold after casting. Gold requires an additional bulk of metal so that on cooling, the piece being cast can draw on additional metal from the reservoir, which we call the *button*. Without the additional bulk of metal the casting would likely show porosity. In duplication, cooling from the bottom of the flask causes the duplicating material to shrink, which has a tendency to draw the chilling solution into closer adaptation to the cast.

The metal bottom of one of the types is provided with legs to hold it off the bottom of the cooling tank, thus allowing circulation of water beneath (Fig. 17-2). Although initially the flask should not be immersed completely in running water, any depth short

of the metal top is permissible because of the insulating properties of the formica ring.

The principal difference in the two types is in the disassembly of the flask to remove the cast from the mold (Fig. 17-3). One type has a lid that is machined to provide a definite undercut for securing the mold to the lid. The bottom and the formica ring may be removed to permit flexing the mold while the cast is being removed, but the mold remains securely attached to the lid at all times. Then the tapered ring may be placed back over the mold to support it while it is being filled. While this type provides support for the mold at all times, any accidental dislodgement from the undercut metal top would lead to permanent deformation of the mold. This hazard is eliminated in the second type, which permits complete disassembly of the

Fig. 17-2. Wills type D flask, made entirely of aluminum, with a ring 1¾ inches high. Upper portion of top lid has a depressed surface for holding surplus duplicating material, thus serving as a reservoir. This flask is competitively priced because costlier formica ring is not used.

Fig. 17-3. Underside of lids from two types of Wills duplicating flasks. Type E on left is undercut for locking duplicating material to lid, whereas type F (right) is keyed to permit complete removal of mold from flask and later repositioning.

mold from the flask to facilitate removal of the cast from the mold. The inside of the ring is tapered, and every part is keyed to facilitate the return of the mold to its original relationship with the flask. This type is preferred for school use.

The technique for duplicating is the same for any cast, whether or not blockout is present. However, if wax or clay blockout is present, the temperature of the duplicating material must not be any higher than recommended by the manufacturer to avoid melting and distorting the blockout material.

Any clay used for blockout prior to duplication must be of the insoluble type (Chapter 10). Therefore only an oily base clay may be safely used for this purpose.

Although ordinary baseplate wax may be used for paralleled blockout and ledges, care must be taken that the temperature of the duplicating material not be high enough to melt the wax. The use of prepared blockout material may be preferred, such as Ney blockout wax or Wills undercut material. A

formula has been given in Chapter 10 for those preferring to prepare their own blockout material.

Duplicating procedure. The equipment needed for duplication is as follows (Fig. 17-4):

Bunsen burner and tripod
Enamel or stainless steel double boiler (aluminum utensils should not be used, as aluminum seems to have a deleterious effect on the composition of the duplicating colloid)*
Duplicating flask
Plaster bowl (600 ml)
Stiff spatula (Kerr laboratory spatula or Buffalo dental No. 4 R)
Vibrator
Rubber suction cup
No. 7 spatula

Step-by-step procedure (Fig. 17-6). Although the procedure given describes the use of the Wills late-model flask, it applies as well to the use of any duplicating flask.

---

*Ready Duplicator may be used in lieu of an enamel or stainless steel double boiler (Fig. 17-5).

Fig. 17-4. Armamentarium for preparing material for duplicating: double boiler, ring stand, Bunsen burner, stiff laboratory spatula for stirring duplicating material and for mixing cast material in plaster bowl, No. 7 wax spatula for directing stream of fluid duplicating material over critical areas of cast, vibrator, duplicating flask with feeder ring, and rubber suction cup for extracting cast from chilled mold.

1. New hydrocolloid duplicating material is usually packaged in a semidried state. It may be in the form of a crumbled meal. In such case, further chopping is unnecessary. If in bulk form, it must be chopped into fine particles. This is greatly facilitated by running it through a kitchen food chopper. Any duplicating material being reused should similarly be reduced to small pieces before heating.

Heat the duplicating material in the top of the double boiler, stirring to dissipate lumps. New material must be diluted with water in the proportions recommended by the manufacturer; material being reused may be diluted if needed to replace water lost by evaporation. Remember that duplicating material may be further thinned with warm water during preparation as it becomes necessary, but the incorporation of dry material into a mix that is too thin is much more difficult to accomplish. Therefore it is best that any thinning be done by adding water slowly until the right consistency has been obtained.

When a smooth, creamy mix has been obtained, remove the upper pan of the double boiler from the burner and *continue stirring* until the temperature has dropped to 120° F. At this temperature, which is just low enough not to burn a finger immersed in it, the duplicating material is ready to pour.

2. For four minutes just prior to duplication, immerse the cast in water at about 85° F, preferably in water (slurry) that has lost its ability to etch the surface of the stone. Do this while the duplicating material is being cooled to a usable temperature. Immerse the cast upside down to allow the escape of any air trapped beneath sheets of wax placed on the master cast for relief. Another effective method is to immerse the blocked-out cast in clear slurry water in a rubber mixing bowl and place the bowl in an activated vacuum bell jar for two minutes just prior to duplication (Fig. 17-7).

Water that has been allowed to stand for some time with pieces of dental stone or plaster in it will have lost its ability to etch the surface of a stone cast. *Therefore any soaking of a stone cast should be done in water prepared for that purpose rather than in tap water.*

When pieces of plaster or stone have been previously placed in tap water, solution will occur until the water becomes saturated with calcium sulfate. Once the water has become saturated, an equilibrium occurs with no further dissolution taking place. A stone cast placed in such water will not become etched because the water already contains all the calcium sulfate it can hold. A container of such water should be available in the laboratory for use any time a cast needs to be soaked, such as prior to duplication or prior to repouring a portion of the original cast.

The broken pieces of plaster or stone should be small to medium in size but not fine enough to remain suspended in the water when it is agitated. These pieces should remain in the water at all times to maintain the equilibrium of the calcium sulfate. When used, the water should be clear.

Blow surface moisture off of the cast with compressed air, and center the cast in the bottom of the duplicating flask over a small

Fig. 17-5. Ready Duplicator maintains duplicating material at a controlled temperature and ready for immediate use. Duplicating hydrocolloid flows through a rubber hose at base of duplicator, and rate of flow is controlled by a manually operated shut-off valve. Its use is particularly suited when several duplications are accomplished daily. (Courtesy Ticonium Division, CMP Industries, Inc., Albany, N.Y.)

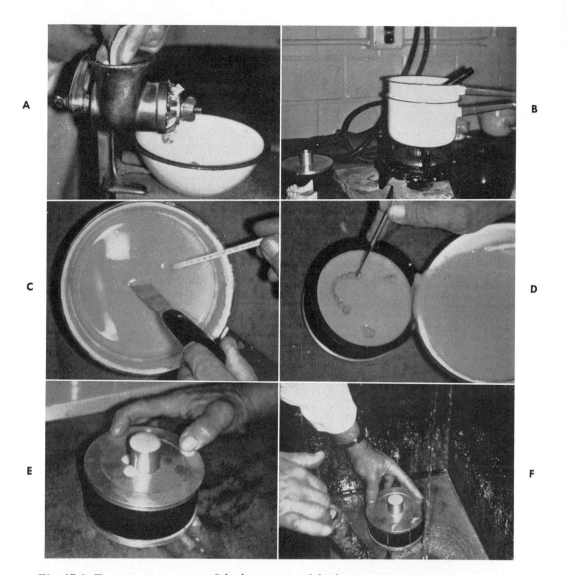

Fig. 17-6. Ten steps in process of duplication. **A,** If duplicating material is being reused, it should be ground into small pieces before being heated, to avoid lumps and uneven consistency. **B,** Material is then placed in top of a double boiler and stirred well with a spatula until it has reached a smooth, creamy consistency. Warm water may be added sparingly to dilute it if necessary, but avoid overdilution. **C,** Remove pan from double boiler and continue stirring until temperature has dropped to about 120° F. This is a temperature at which finger may be immersed without burning, but it is more accurately checked with a thermometer. **D,** Cast to be duplicated, which has been immersed in water just prior to duplication, is placed in bottom of duplicating flask, over a small pellet of clay. A small continuous stream of duplicating material is poured in at a posterior end of cast while material is guided over critical areas with a No. 7 spatula held in other hand. **E,** After filling flask, top and feeder ring are positioned, and duplicating material is added to fill completely the feeder ring. **F,** Flask is placed in running tap water about 2.5 cm (1 in) deep until material in feeder ring has completely gelled, with a depression in its center to show that shrinkage has occurred. Then flask may be completely immersed in running tap water for an additional thirty minutes.

Fig. 17-6, cont'd. G, Feeder ring is removed and projecting material cut off flush with top of flask. **H,** Flask is inverted and bottom of flask removed, exposing base of cast. In this position, open end now becomes top of mold and original top of flask becomes the bottom. Excess duplicating material is then removed around base of cast. **I,** Rubber suction cup is applied to base of cast *under water*. Mold is then removed from flask and flexed gently around sides as cast is removed with suction cup acting as a handle. **J,** *Mold* is inspected for defects. It is then returned to flask precisely in its original position, original lid placed on bottom for support, and stone or investment, properly proportioned and spatulated, is slowly vibrated around arch, tooth by tooth, to avoid trapping air or diluting material with moisture. Mold is then completely filled and either immersed in still water or covered with a wet towel or a bell jar to prevent dehydration of mold at expense of water of crystallization of cast material. Although a duplicating mold will not be poured a second time, its dimensional accuracy must be preserved until cast material has completely set.

Fig. 17-7. Entrapped air in blocked-out master stone cast may be eliminated prior to duplication by placing cast in a rubber mixing bowl, three-quarters filled with clear slurry water, and placing bowl under a bell jar and activating a vacuum for two minutes.

pellet of clay. Press the base of the cast firmly against the bottom of the flask.

3. With one hand, slowly pour the duplicating material into the flask just behind one posterior end of the cast. A stream of duplicating material about 3 mm (⅛ in) in diameter should be poured continuously at this point until the base of the cast has been completely covered. At this time, with the No. 7 spatula in the other hand, guide the material around the teeth, into interproximal spaces, and on critical tooth surfaces. This prevents trapping air bubbles in critical areas.

After the teeth have been completely covered, fill the flask within 3 mm (⅛ in) of the top. Then interrupt the pouring while positioning the metal top and feeder ring, after which completely fill the mold to the top of the feeder ring.

4. Now place the flask in about 2.5 cm (1 in) of cold (preferably running) water. The water should cover no more than the metal base and the lower 12 mm (½ in) of the formica ring so that initial cooling will occur only through the metal bottom.

Although cooling *must* be done slowly and from the bottom to control shrinkage and avoid distortion, it is not absolutely necessary that cooling be hastened by using cold water. Time permitting, a hydrocolloid mold may be bench cooled without affecting its accuracy, whereas too rapid cooling may cause distortion. With this in mind, allow the mold to set completely in a shallow water bath. However, to facilitate early separation of the mold, when the feeder ring has gelled, immerse the flask in cold running water, where it should be left for at least fifteen minutes to assure chilling throughout.

5. After thorough chilling, remove the flask from the water bath and remove the feeder ring. Cut off the hydrocolloid projecting above the lid flush with the top of the lid. Then invert the flask and remove the bottom, exposing the base of the cast. Remove any hydrocolloid covering the base of the cast and the flattened piece of clay, leaving the smooth base of the cast exposed.

The inside of the formica ring is tapered; therefore it may be removed by sliding it away from the top, leaving the mold attached only to the top. In the inverted position the top now has become the bottom and will remain so during the subsequent procedures.

The original bottom, now removed, will not be replaced on the mold, as this becomes the open end into which the cast material is poured.

If the top of the flask is undercut, the mold is not removed from it, and it becomes the base for supporting the mold. If the flask has a top that is keyed but not undercut, the mold is removed from it also to facilitate flexing as the cast is being removed from the mold. In either case, removal is best accomplished by applying a rubber suction cup to the base of the cast under running tap water and lightly flexing the mold while extracting the cast.

The suction cup is used as a convenient handle. Without it, the mold would have to be cut away to expose enough of the sides of the cast for a finger grip. After pouring and removing the duplicate cast, an excess would result where the mold has been cut away. Although this may be trimmed on the cast trimmer, it must be remembered that the base of the cast has been scored in three places to facilitate repositioning on the surveyor. If the scored areas are inadvertently trimmed away, there will be no record of the path of placement on the duplicate cast to aid in positioning it on the surveyor for locating contour lines. This necessity does not exist when clasp ledges (indices) were formed on the master cast. However, when waxing is to be done in relation to a survey line only, it is necessary that the original cast position be recorded on the duplicate cast. On the other hand, such a record always must be preserved on a duplicate stone cast to be used for fitting. This is particularly true when wrought-wire clasp arms must be accurately adapted in relation to the height of contour of the abutment teeth.

6. After removing the cast, replace the mold in the flask in exactly the same position as before. This is made possible by the keyed relationship of the parts of the flask. Reposition the hydrocolloid in the tapered formica ring so that the longer of the three grooves in the hydrocolloid mold points to the centering screw on the outside of the ring. Replace the keyed top, which is to become the bottom, and invert the ring so that the open end of the mold is up. If the reassembly is properly done, the mold is in exactly the same relation to the flask as before; otherwise distortion of the mold may result.

Remove any free moisture from the mold by inverting it and blowing it out with a gentle stream of compressed air. Care must be taken not to hold the stream of air on any area long enough to cause dehydration of that area.

With the correct amount of water in the plaster bowl, add a measured amount of stone or investment, following the manufacturer's recommendations. The correct water-powder ratio is given by the manufacturer for each 100 g of powder.

Mix thoroughly with a stiff spatula or a mechanical mixer. *Vacuum mixing is always preferable, to eliminate entrapped air.* If this equipment is not available, knead the mixture on the vibrator to remove as much air as will come to the surface. Many of the small air voids in a cast are due to air bubbles' being carried into the mold in the mix rather than to air trapped in the mold during pouring.

Fill the hydrocolloid mold in much the same manner as an impression of a dental arch. With the No. 7 spatula, add small amounts of material only at one posterior end while using the vibrator. The material is thus made to flow around the arch by the weight of the material behind it. Add material only at the original site until all critical areas of the mold have been filled. In this manner, excess moisture is pushed ahead of the material until it reaches the extreme opposite end of the mold, where it should be expelled and discarded. This avoids any dilution of the mix by the moisture remaining in the mold, minimizes the chances of trapping air, and results in a uniformly dense cast.

7. Immediately on filling the mold, partially immerse it in still water and allow it to set for about thirty minutes. Partial immersion supplies the cast material with needed water of crystallization, some of which may otherwise be taken up by the hydrocolloid, resulting in a chalky cast surface. On the other hand, partial immersion should not be for longer than approximately 45 minutes, and never overnight, or etching of the surface of the cast will result.

After the cast material has hardened, remove the flask from the mold and *break the mold away from the cast* rather than attempt to remove the cast from the intact mold. The mold should not be poured a second time anyway, and fresh surfaces of the cast may be rubbed off in withdrawing it from the mold. *Therefore the mold should always be broken away from the cast.*

Duplicating material may be washed and placed in water in a covered jar for reuse, especially when it will likely be reused in the near future. However, if any doubt exists as to its texture, it should be discarded. One should not attempt to revitalize old duplicating material by replenishing with new. Instead, any questionable material should be discarded and a new batch of material mixed as needed.

A freshly duplicated cast should not be handled unnecessarily, particularly one made of investment material, until it has been allowed to dry in air or in an oven. *An investment cast should not be trimmed on a cast trimmer, as this causes a slurry of investment to splash over the cast, which may not then be entirely removed by rinsing.* For that matter an investment cast should not be rinsed at all. Instead it should be hand-trimmed with a sharp knife, and any powdered residue should be carefully blown off.

After initial drying and trimming, an investment cast should be dried in an oven at 180° to 200° F for sixty to ninety minutes depending on the size of the cast. Then it should be removed and immediately lightly sprayed with a plastic model spray. A build-up of the plastic spray on the investment cast must be avoided.

Some of the advantages of spraying an investment cast are (1) it provides a smooth dense surface on the investment cast, (2) it facilitates the development of wax and plastic patterns in that these substances adhere better to the sprayed cast than they will to an untreated refractory cast, and (3) it helps prevent marring of the cast during handling.

WAXING THE PARTIAL DENTURE FRAMEWORK

Experience with free-hand waxing and the use of ready-made wax shapes is recommended as a prerequisite to the use of preformed plastic patterns (Fig. 17-8). Unless plastic patterns are selected and used with care, they are better not used at all. The fact that they facilitate rapid production of partial denture castings has led to their widespread use in commercial laboratories, but this alone does not justify their use. Even when plastic patterns are used, parts of the denture

Fig. 17-8. Preformed plastic patterns are available in many different shapes and sizes. Being a soft plastic material, they have a tendency to regain their original carded shape after being adapted to refractory cast unless a "tacky" liquid is first applied to cast. (Courtesy J. F. Jelenko & Co., Inc., New York, N.Y.)

framework must be waxed free-hand to avoid excessive bulk and to create the desired contours. (See Fig. 17-9.)

The use of ready-made wax shapes facilitates free-hand waxing to the point that an experienced dentist or dental laboratory technician can complete a wax pattern in little more time than is necessary when plastic patterns are used. Much of the speed with which a wax pattern may be produced depends on how well the step-by-step procedure is organized to take fullest advantage of the wax shapes.

The student in the preclinical laboratory should begin his waxing experience on a stone cast rather than on the softer investment cast, so that he may be free to modify and correct his errors as they are pointed out to him. Only after having a clear understanding of the location, bulk, and contours of the various parts of the wax pattern being done should he be allowed to wax on the investment cast. Since corrections on the investment cast may result in a rough casting, it is imperative that the waxing on the investment cast be done in a positive manner with a minimum of changes and corrections.

The same applies to the making of a removable partial denture framework in the undergraduate dental clinic. Although the typical dental student probably will not fabricate his own partial denture castings after graduation, it is essential that he have a background and experience in dental laboratory procedures that will enable him to design the denture framework and prescribe how it is to be fabricated (Fig. 17-10). Not only this, but he must also be capable of evaluating the finished product to the end that the quality of dental laboratory services is maintained (Fig. 17-11).

With this in mind, it is desirable that two or more partial denture frameworks be waxed to completion, if not cast and finished, by the clinical student himself. To avoid discrepancies occurring as a result of inept waxing and subsequent corrections on the investment cast, it is most desirable that the student first do a practice wax pattern on a duplicate stone cast. After all corrections have been approved by his instructor, waxing on the investment cast may be done with confidence and dispatch, resulting in a casting of high quality. Although this policy may be

Fig. 17-9. Three steps in making of a denture framework using blockout ledges and ready-made pattern forms. **A,** Master cast with shaped blockout ledges for location of retentive and nonretentive clasp arms. **B,** Completed pattern using an anatomic replica pattern, plastic clasp forms resting on investment ledges, and retention mesh anteriorly. Pattern is then waxed to completion. **C,** Finished casting returned to master cast. Blockout ledges may be seen below three lingual clasp arms.

Fig. 17-10. Technician should receive from dentist a master cast, **A,** that has been surveyed and had reference lines scratched on two sides and dorsal aspect of base of cast or has been marked for tripoding. Upon this cast, outline of denture framework should be drawn precisely, without marring cast, where component parts of framework are to be placed and their dimensions indicated. In addition, written instructions, including waxing specifications, which ideally should accompany the outlined master cast, must be included (see Fig. 18-2). From such a work authorization, the technician may be expected to return a polished casting that accurately conforms to penciled design, as in **B.**

Fig. 17-14. Outline for retentive wrought-wire arm is outlined on cast following ledge index. An 18-gauge round wax strip is adapted to penciled outline. Wax strip straightened out determines length of 18-gauge wrought wire (Type II) required to form direct retainer arm.

Fig. 17-15. Wrought-wire arm is closely and passively adapted to abutment tooth. Note taper of arm from distobuccal aspect of abutment to retentive end. "Foot" is just lingual to crest of residual ridge to provide space for cervical end of artificial molar.

so tapered that the terminal portion of the wire engaging the undercut is approximately one half the diameter of the 18-gauge wire. (See Chapter 11.)

d. With contouring pliers, contour the tapered portion of the wire to contact the the buccal surface of the premolar starting the contour near the tapered terminal end of the wire. The wire must accurately follow the ledge index on the cast. Continue contouring the wire to contact the tooth slightly lingual to one half the width of the distal surface of the tooth.

e. With the contoured portion of the wire held in position against the abutment tooth, mark the wire with a pencil at the exact spot where the wire must turn inferiorly toward the residual ridge. Also, carefully estimate the length of this upright portion of the wire according to the outline on the cast. Make a bend in the wire at the previously marked spot so that the vertical portion of the wire will contact the guiding plane area of the abutment tooth. The wire cannot be placed back on the cast at this time. Having estimated the length of the vertical portion of the wire, make a bend so that the remaining portion of the wire contacts the residual ridge region of the cast and is directed posteriorly. Two millimeters from the untapered end of the wire, make a bend so that the end of the wire projects almost vertically upward.

Fig. 17-16. Portion of wrought wire contacting distal of abutment is placed as far inferiorly as possible, since master cast was blocked out in this area. Such a position will have less of a tendency to "top-load" the tooth in resisting horizontal rotation of denture. Small angled piece of wire at distal of conformed arm facilitates handling of warm clasp arm with cotton forceps in later waxing procedures and provides mechanical attachment of retainer arm, which will be embedded in cast framework.

f. The formed wire should accurately and passively conform to the outline on the stone cast (Figs. 17-15 and 17-16). Wrought wire can be accurately and rather quickly adapted without nicks or having become strain-hardened. Practice first with paper clips. Place the formed wire and cast aside until the wax pattern has been developed on the other stone cast.

3. Adapt one thickness of 24-gauge casting sheet wax (green or pink) or adhesive wax

Fig. 17-17. Lingual bar pattern is made of half-pear–shaped, 6-gauge wax form, reinforced on tissue surface with 24-gauge sheet wax for rigidity. Bar is trimmed to conform to outline of denture base on one side and minor connector outlined on distal extension side.

Fig. 17-18. This minor connector (arrow) forms part of direct retainer assembly for abutment tooth. Its contact with guiding plane, in conjunction with guiding plane surfaces on opposite side of arch, will assure only one path of placement and removal of completed restoration.

on the lingual aspect of the alveolar ridge to cover the outline of the lingual bar major connector. Be careful not to stretch the wax, thereby altering its thickness.

4. Adapt a piece of 6-gauge half-pear–shaped wax over the sheet wax to conform to the pencil lines denoting the lingual bar and showing through the sheet wax. The greater bulk of the half-pear shape must be at the lower border, with the tapered edge near or along the top pencil line. The thickness of the wax shape and the sheet wax previously adapted, plus a small amount of wax added to maintain a half-pear shape, will be the thickness of the major connector before polishing.

5. Cut away the sheet wax extending above the outline of the lingual bar and also below the half-pear–shaped wax, which has now become the lingual bar, and cut off both the bar and sheet wax even with the distal aspects of the premolar abutments or according to the outline of these areas (Fig. 17-17). Use a fairly dull instrument (Roach carver) for this purpose to avoid scoring the cast.

6. Seal the inferior and superior borders of the bar to the cast. It is important that the wax be sealed to the cast throughout its course, yet that the original half-pear shape be preserved. Should any part of the wax pattern not be sealed to the cast, the pattern may become dislodged during the application of the outer investment, resulting in the investment's seeping under the pattern. This would result in a false undersurface on the casting.

7. Adapt a piece of 8-gauge half-round wax to the full extent of the guiding plane on the distal surface of the left premolar (flat side to the guiding plane surface). Cut the wax off slightly inferior to the marginal ridge and seal the wax to the cast. Taper the wax superiorly to a feather edge (Fig. 17-18).

8. Adapt a piece of 10-gauge round wax strip from the superior border of the lingual bar up the embrasure between the first and second premolars, then over the marginal ridges, and into the rest seats prepared in the premolars. This minor connector should pass perpendicularly from the lingual bar up the interdental embrasure. A rule previously stated is that any crossing of gingival tissues by components of the framework should be abrupt and definite. A second rule to be followed is that minor connectors should conform to interdental embrasures whenever possible and should be so shaped to present as little bulk to the tongue as possible. Seal the wax shape to the cast, converting it to an embrasure form, and wax the occlusal rests to conform to the outline of the rest seat preparations (Fig. 17-19). Strengthen the wax at the marginal ridges if necessary. The final form of the pattern for the occlusal rests should be representative of the occlusal anatomy before the rest seats were prepared.

9. Cut two pieces of 24-gauge casting sheet wax (green or pink), which, when joined at the crest of the tooth-bounded edentulous ridge, will cover the penciled outline of the cast base (Fig. 17-20). Adapt the lingual portion first, being careful not to

Fig. 17-19. Gingival margins were relieved and interproximal undercuts were blocked out on master cast parallel to path of placement. Therefore this minor connector does not engage an undercut. In fact, the only components of the framework engaging undercuts are the terminal ends of retentive direct retainer arms. See Fig. 4-28 for interproximal conformation of this component on a finished framework.

Fig. 17-20. Twenty-four–gauge sheet wax is adapted over outline of lingual portion of cast denture base area. Outline will show through pink sheet wax, thus permitting accurate trimming of wax. Use of 24-gauge sheet wax permits some adjustment of denture base to alleviate sore spots if such occur after patient uses restoration.

stretch the wax. Trim this wax just 0.5 mm inferior to the penciled outline of the lingual portion of the cast base area. Seal the wax along its edges and to the adjacent end of the major connector.

10. In a like manner, adapt and seal the other piece of 24-gauge sheet wax over the buccal portion of the cast base, joining both pieces over the crest of the ridge in a smooth junction (Fig. 17-21).

11. Adapt a length of 8-gauge half-round wax on the guiding plane, proximal surfaces of the right side abutments (flat side against the guiding plane), attaching one end to the cast base pattern gingivally and carrying the other end over the marginal ridge and into the rest seat preparations (Fig. 17-22). Seal the wax along its edges and to the cast base pattern after the wax has been trimmed to conform to the outline of the rests and guiding plane areas.

12. Being guided by the index ledge, adapt a piece of 12-gauge half-round wax on the lingual surface of the right premolar abutment, and connect the distal end of the strip of wax to the previously formed minor connector on the same tooth. On this particular abutment and also on the molar abutment, the retentive clasp arms will be on the buccal surfaces and the reciprocal arms on the lingual surfaces. Reciprocal arms are nonreten-

Fig. 17-21. Buccal portion of cast base pattern is added, and wax is trimmed to conform to outline of framework. Forming this portion of cast base pattern is best done in two steps as described to avoid thinning 24-gauge sheet wax. Two halves are then carefully joined and sealed at crest of residual ridge.

tive and therefore should not be tapered except to avoid abruptness and irritation to the tongue by the terminal end of the clasp arm. Reinforce the junction of the reciprocal arm pattern with the minor connector to which it is attached (Fig. 17-23).

13. Adapt a piece of 8-gauge half-round wax to the lingual surface of the molar abut-

Fig. 17-22. Occlusal rests may be carved to form before other components of direct retainer assemblies are formed in wax. Rests should conform to occlusal morphology present before rest seats were prepared.

Fig. 17-23. Reciprocal components must be rigid and since they do not engage undercuts need not be tapered for the sake of flexibility. Reciprocal arm on molar restores lingual anatomy of abutment crown.

ment, being guided by the lingual ledge of the abutment crown. Connect the strip of wax to the previously formed minor connector. Add sufficient wax to have the lower portion of this reciprocal arm as thick as the lingual extent of the ledge on the crown. Superiorly, wax must be added to restore the normal contour of the lingual surface of the crown and feathered to the lingual height of the crown (Fig. 17-23). The terminal end of the reciprocal arm should have a taper corresponding to the taper of the lingual ledge in this area as viewed from above.

14. Beginning at the inferior border of the reciprocal arm of the right premolar at its junction with the minor connector, adapt a piece of 14-gauge round wax over the outline of the lingual portion of the border of the cast base. Carry the wax form up to the inferior border of the reciprocal arm on the molar abutment. Seal this piece of wax on the outside border without appreciably altering its form. This piece of wax will provide an adequate thickness for the border of the cast base and at the same time will form an undercut finishing line on the cast base (Fig. 17-24).

15. Up to this point the forming of the wax pattern has been done primarily on the lingual surfaces of the cast. The rationale of this procedure is to avoid distortion of any buccal components of the pattern by handling of the cast while accomplishing the heavier lingual waxing.

16. Perfect the waxing done thus far by smoothing and adding to the weak points. Smoothing does not mean polishing or flam-

Fig. 17-24. Fourteen-gauge round wax added as described forms a trough to support and retain acrylic resin supporting artificial teeth. Therefore a smooth junction between framework and acrylic resin is made without danger of cracks in resin appearing after denture has been in use. Since border of cast base pattern is thickened by addition of 14-gauge round wax, resultant casting can be gently rounded at borders, making it more comfortable for patient than having borders finished as sharp edges.

ing the wax pattern, either of which affects only the highest part of the convex surfaces and serves only to flatten and alter the shape of the wax. Rather smoothing should be done by gentle carving, which preserves the original form of the wax pattern. Therefore, as weak areas become evident, reinforce them by flowing on additional wax and blending it into the original waxing with a hot spatula and by carving. In the process of smoothing,

Fig. 17-25. Twelve-gauge half-round wax form is attached to minor connector on guiding plane and runs posteriorly just lingual to crest of residual ridge. Placed in this position, interference to arranging artificial posterior teeth will be minimized. Lower portion of ladderlike structure should be superior to inferior portion of major connector. Otherwise, a butt-type junction of major and minor connector would be difficult to construct.

Fig. 17-26. Longitudinal pieces forming a portion of minor connector are joined with 12-gauge half-round wax forms (arrow). Two buccal loops of 18-gauge round wax form are attached to longitudinal piece of wax near crest of residual ridge. A minor connector extending on both buccal and lingual slopes of residual ridge will, in all probability, strengthen acrylic resin denture base and minimize warping.

gently trim away all excess wax around the borders of the pattern with a Roach carver. Exercise caution to avoid any alteration of the surface of the cast.

17. Retention for the attachment of resin base on the distal extension side is added next. This consists of two parallel pieces of 12-gauge half-round wax connected with cross rungs to form a ladderlike framework. Beginning at the base of the vertical minor connector on the left second premolar, adapt a piece of 12-gauge half-round wax along the lingual surface of the residual ridge at the ridge crest (convex side up). Extend this piece of wax approximately two thirds the length of the edentulous area. Seal and blend the proximal end of the wax into the minor connector at its point of origin and just tack the distal end to the cast. The retentive frame need not be sealed to the cast throughout its course (Fig. 17-25).

About 5 to 7 mm inferior to the longitudinal piece of wax, adapt another piece of 12-gauge half-round wax parallel to the first piece and of the same length. The anterior end of the lower wax strip will be attached to the distal end of the major connector. At its point of origin, add wax to reinforce and blend it into the major connector (Fig. 17-25).

At equally spaced intervals of about 4 to 5 mm join the two longitudinal pieces with connecting bars of 12-gauge half-round wax strips. This forms the rungs of the ladderlike construction (Fig. 17-26). Each end of the rung must be attached securely to the longitudinal pieces with additional wax so that reinforcement rather than weakness will exist at each junction point. None of these crossbars need be sealed to the cast except at their ends.

From one rung of the ladder, usually the third from the end, curve a piece of 18-gauge round wax over the buccal side of the ridge to join the most distal rung at the end of the framework. This will provide additional support to the buccal flange of the resin denture base. To facilitate casting from lingually placed sprues, this buccal loop should be continuous with any two cross rungs. Attach the buccal loop securely with additional wax but do not seal it to the cast in its entire length. In a long span, such as a distal extension situation from a canine or first premolar abutment, two such buccal loops should be used; otherwise one will usually suffice (Fig. 17-26).

A butt-type joint finishing line of the major connector and the resin base retention ladder (minor connector) is made. The purpose of

Fig. 17-27. Round 14-gauge wax is used to form a direct connection of major connector to minor connector contacting guiding plane surface (arrow). Round form is modified to present a flat surface facing posteriorly and an angled surface anteriorly, thus forming a desired butt joint between major and minor connector.

Fig. 17-28. Eighteen-gauge round wax form is used to strengthen connection between major and minor connector (arrow). This could be accomplished with half-round 12-gauge wax form also. It is absolutely necessary that a strong, rigid union exist between major connector and minor connector to which acrylic resin denture base will be attached.

this type joint and finishing line is twofold. First a smooth, flat, continuous surface between the major connector and the acrylic resin denture base will result, which is less noticeable to the tongue than is a "hump" surface. Second a butt-type joint is stronger and more resistant to "working" the resin and producing strain fissures than other type joints. Place a strip of 14-gauge round wax about half-way up the lingual surface of the guiding plane minor connector and continue the wax strip inferiorly and on top of the previously formed joint between the ladder and the major connector. Seal this wax to the cast and to the superior border of the major connector. In the process of sealing the 14-gauge round wax, a half-round shape should result. Then additional wax may be added to provide the greatest bulk toward the lingual surface. The minor connector contacting the guiding plane surface is thickest at its gingival portion and tapers to a very thin form as it approaches the marginal ridge of the abutment. A minor connector thus established (a rectangular, wedge shape) provides the least interference with the placement of the adjacent artificial tooth. Blend the anterior side into the major connector with a hot wax spatula. Flatten the posterior portion with a warm spatula and carve it to form (Fig. 17-27).

All junctions with the major connector

should be reinforced and blended smoothly into its contour (Fig. 17-28). After the butt-type joint is formed, in most instances and especially in those instances where the longitudinal sections of the ladder are separated by more than 4 to 5 mm, an 18-gauge round wax reinforcing element should be provided between the butt joint and the most anterior rung of the ladder (Fig. 17-28).

18. Accomplish the procedure described in 14 on the buccal portion of the cast base pattern.

19. Small "nailheads," as additional acrylic resin retentive elements, are now placed on both the cast base and the minor connector (ladder) for attachment of the resin base on the distal extension side (Fig. 17-29). For the latter the nailheads serve to attach a resin tray for making a secondary impression and are removed before the denture base is processed.

A nailhead is quickly and easily made by holding one end of a 5 to 7.5 cm (2 to 3 in) piece of 18-gauge round wax to the area the nailhead is to occupy, sealing the end to the pattern with a hot waxing instrument, holding the strip until the junction has hardened, and then cutting the 18-gauge wax strip about 2 mm above the junction. With a warm wax spatula the protruding end of the wax can be "mushroomed" by simply applying a little pressure.

Fig. 17-29. Small mushroom "nailhead" configurations are attached to cast base portion of wax pattern (arrows). These nailheads serve as additional retentive elements for the acrylic resin supporting artificial teeth. They should be so positioned that no interference to arranging artificial teeth will be encountered. Six to eight nailheads are quite sufficient on short-span bases (not more than two missing posterior teeth).

Nailheads on the cast denture base are confined within the undercut finishing lines and must be placed so that they will neither interfere with the arrangement of the artificial teeth nor protrude through the resin supporting the artificial teeth. Two rows of three or four nailheads are ample. One row should be placed lingually and about halfway between the border of the cast base pattern and the crest of the residual ridge. The other row is similarly located but placed on the buccal side of the cast base pattern.

20. Form the cast retentive direct retainer arms. The creation of the wax pattern has now progressed up to the point of adding the planned retentive clasp arms. These have been classified in Chapter 6. When a cast retentive clasp of any type (other than an I bar type) is to be used, it must be waxed in relation to the height of contour with the terminal one fourth of the tapered clasp arm progressively engaging a retentive undercut.

The location and extent of the undercut to be utilized as well as the remaining portion of the retentive arm are established first on the master cast, and the clasp arm is outlined from its origin to its terminus. A wax ledge is carved to establish the location of the inferior border of the clasp arm. In fact, this ledge should be carved the width of a pencil line cervically to the planned inferior border and terminus of the arm to allow for smoothing and polishing the completed casting. Otherwise the inferior border of the cast arm would occupy a position occlusal to its planned position. This ledge is duplicated on the refractory cast, and the clasp arm is waxed or the plastic pattern is placed with its inferior border along the ledge.

Cast retentive clasp arms are most satisfactorily made utilizing preformed plastic patterns that are uniform in dimensions and taper (Fig. 17-8). Students and technicians alike, however, should have had experience in free-hand waxing and in the use of wax shapes. Twelve-gauge half-round wax is used to form the outline of the clasp, which is then sealed to the cast. Some reinforcement at the point of origin and addition of wax along the length of the arm is necessary to create a tapered arm by carving. Of course, some trimming along the sealed edges will also be necessary. The finished pattern should have a uniform taper throughout its course, terminating in a predetermined infrabulge area. With a circumferential clasp the height of contour is crossed at about three fourths the length of the retentive arm (never less) as the diameter of the clasp arm decreases and the terminal one fourth progressively engages the tooth undercut.

With a bar-type clasp arm the height of contour is not always crossed by the clasp arm, but the clasp must have a uniform taper from its point of origin to its termination in the undercut area. The point of origin of a bar clasp arm is at the cast denture base or where it emerges from an acrylic resin denture base. Its taper therefore should begin at this point rather than at its attachment to minor connectors of the denture framework. Any portion thereof that will be embedded in a resin base must be considered a rigid connector and not part of the retentive clasp; therefore only the exposed part is tapered to form the bartype clasp arm.

A cast clasp arm should not be indiscriminately polished and then "pliered" to place. Rather, waxing should be done in such a manner that a minimum of finishing is necessary and its intended relationship to the abutment tooth is maintained.

With the preceding information and suggestions the patterns for the cast retentive arms may be accomplished. Being guided by

Fig. 17-30. Wax pattern for cast circumferential retainer arm on buccal surface of molar abutment. Since this is a retentive arm, it is tapered from its attachment area to its terminus. Bar-type direct retainer arm (arrow) joins cast base pattern. From its retentive tip to its junction with cast base pattern, clasp is carved to a tapering, half-round form. Note that inferior portion of assembly is 6 to 7 mm inferior to gingival sulcus to avoid impingement of tissue and possible strangulation. The only portion of bar-type retainer arm occupying an undercut is terminal one third to one fourth of horizontal portion in contact with tooth.

Fig. 17-31. Previously formed wrought-wire retainer arm is attached to wax pattern and is in a passive relation to both abutment tooth and pattern.

the index ledge on the buccal surface of the molar abutment tooth, adapt a piece of 12-gauge half-round wax (flat side to abutment) and attach it to the minor connector (body of the direct retainer). Add a small amount of wax to the clasp arm so that it can be carved to a taper that conforms to the relative dimensions of a cast retentive arm as illustrated in Fig. 6-5. Reinforce the junction of the clasp arm with the body of the clasp by adding sufficient wax to provide a uniform taper from the body to the terminal end of the arm (Fig. 17-30). The student is reminded that in the formation of *all* wax pattern junctions, the end result must be a solid, homogeneous pattern without pits, voids, cracks, or fissures.

The bar-type retainer is formed next by first adapting a piece of 12-gauge half-round wax (flat side to abutment) on the buccal aspect of the right premolar abutment, being guided by the ledge index on the simulated refractory cast. Carefully cut (vertically) this piece of wax at the designated anterior portion of the retainer. Join another piece of 12-gauge half-round wax (flat side to cast) to the anterior end of the crosspiece on its underneath side. Adapt the wax to follow the

inferior border of the outline of the retainer assembly and seal the end of the cast base pattern. Add sufficient wax with a hot spatula to provide a continuous taper from the retentive tip of the bar-type arm to its junction with the pattern for the denture base. The bar retainer is sealed to the cast in its entire length. Carve the wax to the outline form on the cast (Fig. 17-30). The thickest and broadest portion of the bar retainer will be at its junction with the denture base.

21. Perfect the waxing done thus far by carving, smoothing, and adding to weak points. The use of binocular loops (or any magnifying systems) to carefully inspect the pattern at this stage will probably disclose discrepancies heretofore unobserved.

22. Attach the wrought-wire retentive arm. Hold the previously formed wrought-wire retainer in a pair of cotton forceps by the small upright portion of the "foot" and warm it *over* a flame. Place the wire on the cast in its intended position in the wax pattern. It is usually necessary to hold a hot instrument against the retentive arm to dissipate enough heat so that the foot and upright portions of the retainer will be passively and completely embedded in the wax pattern (Fig. 17-31). However, the wrought wire need not be hot enough to excessively pool the wax pattern and change its desired form. Carefully inspect the area where the retentive arm emerges from its embedded position in the minor connector to ascertain that the wire arm is postively surrounded by wax without evidence of wax fissures or cracks.

Fig. 17-32. Completed wax pattern for a mandibular Class II partial denture framework.

Fig. 17-33. Meticulous attention to detail and neatness in forming wax patterns not only assures the quality of the framework but also saves time in finishing the resultant casting. **A,** Right side view. Note retentive "nailheads" on both cast base pattern and minor connector for denture base. The three nailheads on minor connector serve to retain "impression tray" for making a secondary impression and are of no further use after this procedure has been accomplished. **B,** Left side view. Buccal loops have been so placed that they will not interfere with arranging artificial posterior teeth. In some instances, because of lack of interresidual ridge space, acrylic resin teeth must be used but almost always having their occlusal surfaces duplicated in gold.

The wax pattern is now completed and ready for spruing and investing (Figs. 17-32 and 17-33). An alternate method for forming the wrought-wire retentive clasp arm is illustrated in Fig. 17-34. The method illustrated is particularly applicable to short abutment teeth and will avoid two right-angle bends in the wrought wire.

Waxing metal bases. A technique for forming the retentive framework for the attachment of resin bases has been given. Two basic types of metal bases may be used instead of the resin base. The advantages of using cast metal bases is preference to resin bases have been discussed in Chapter 8.

The type of base to be used must be determined prior to blockout and duplication so that the relief over each edentulous ridge may be provided or eliminated as required. For a resin base full relief for the retentive frame must be provided. For a full metal base no relief over the ridge is used. For a partial metal base the junction between metal and resin must be clearly defined by trimming the relief along a definite, previously determined line.

One type of metal base is the full base with a metal border to which tube teeth, cast copings, or a resin superstructure may be attached. If porcelain or plastic tube or grooved teeth are used, they must be positioned first and the pattern waxed around them to form a coping (Fig. 17-35). The teeth are then attached to the metal base by cementation or, with the use of resin teeth, attached with additional acrylic resin under

Fig. 17-34. A, Blocked-out master cast is duplicated in refractory investment and also in dental stone. **B,** An 18-gauge, round wrought-wire clasp is carefully adapted to duplicate stone cast being guided by ledge index created in wax on master cast for its placement. Required length of wire for making clasp is easily determined by laying an 18-gauge, round wax strip to planned outline and then measuring the wax strip. **C,** Lingually, wrought wire is contoured to conform to thickest portion of finishing line at junction of lingual bar and minor connector used to retain denture base. **D,** Contoured clasp is transferred to duplicate refractory cast and will occupy exact position that it occupied on duplicate stone cast. Waxing the pattern for the framework is completed in the usual manner.

Fig. 17-35. Stock porcelain or resin tube tooth, or an artificial tooth used as a tube tooth, should be ground to accommodate a cast coping as illustrated. A hole is drilled from underside of tooth, or if one is already present, it is made larger. Then tooth is ground to fit ridge with enough clearance for a minimum thickness of metal. A 45-degree bevel is then formed around base of tooth, and finally a collar is created on lingual side, extending to interproximal area. Tooth is then lubricated and wax pattern for denture base formed around it.

pressure, a so-called "pressed-on" method of attaching resin teeth to a metal base. Another method of attaching teeth is to wax the base to form a coping for each tooth, either by carving recesses in the wax or by waxing around dummy teeth. Rather than attaching a stock tooth, the full tooth may be waxed into occlusion, the base invested, and the wax patterns replaced with a processed acrylic resin tooth. This method permits some variation in the dimension and form of the supplied teeth not possible with stock teeth. It is particularly applicable to abnormally long or short spaces or when a stock tooth of desired width is not available. With modern cross-linked acrylic resins, such processed teeth are fairly durable; however, the addition of gold occlusal surfaces is indicated.

Wax patterns of the teeth to be supplied may be waxed directly onto a metal base and then cast in gold and attached to the base by soldering. In this method the prosthetically supplied teeth are carved as for resin veneer fixed partial denture pontics. After attachment to the metal base, resin veneers are then processed to match any adjacent veneered abutment crowns. Teeth visible are generally abutted to the ridge, and cast flanges are used only in the posterior part of the mouth. This method is generally used only in conjunction with full mouth reconstruction. Both the denture framework and the cast pontics are usually made of gold to facilitate assembly by soldering.

When artificial teeth are to be arranged to occlude with an opposing cast or an opposing template, the metal base must be formed with a boxing for the attachment of the tissue-colored denture resin supporting the teeth. This is the most common method of attaching teeth to a metal base. The wax pattern for the base is formed from one thickness of 24-gauge casting wax, which is then reinforced at the border, and a boxing is formed for the retention of the resin superstructure. Since metal borders are more difficult to adjust than resin, they are usually made somewhat short of the area normally covered with a resin base. Also, since border thickness adds objectionable weight to the denture, it is made with only a slight border roll. This is one disadvantage of the full metal base, in that the border accuracy of the impression registration cannot be used to fullest advantage, and the contouring of facial and lingual surfaces cannot be as effective as with a resin base in which added bulk can sometimes be used to advantage.

The border is first penciled lightly on the investment cast, and then the 24-gauge sheet casting wax is smoothly adapted. Considerable care must be taken not to stretch and thin the sheet wax in adapting it to the cast. To avoid wrinkling, the wax should be adapted in at least two longitudinal pieces and joined and sealed together at the ridge crest. The wax is then trimmed along the penciled outline with a dull instrument to avoid scoring the investment cast.

A single piece of *14-gauge round* wax is now adapted around the border *over* the sheet wax. With a hot spatula this must be sealed to the cast along its outer border. The inner half of the round wax form remains untouched. Then, sufficient wax is flowed onto the round wax to blend it smoothly into the sheet wax, thus completing a border roll. Wax is added when needed to facilitate carving without trimming the original 24-gauge thickness. The result should be a rounded border blending smoothly into the sheet wax.

The boxing for the resin, which will in turn support the artificial teeth, is now added, again using *14-gauge round* wax. The proposed outline for the boxing is identified by lightly scoring the sheet wax. On this scored line the 14-gauge round wax is adapted, thus forming the outline of the boxing.

With additional wax the ditch between the sheet wax and the outer border of the round wax is filled in and blended smoothly onto the sheet wax. This is done in the same manner as the border, adding sufficient wax to allow for smoothing and carving. As mentioned previously, the pattern should not be flamed or polished with a cloth. Instead the pattern must be smoothed by carving.

The result thus far should be a pattern reinforced at the border and at the boxing and slightly concave in between, with some of the original sheet wax exposed. The inside of the boxing is not sealed to the sheet wax, thus leaving a slight undercut for the attachment of the resin. With a sharp blade the margins of the boxing are then carved to a knife-edge finishing line. With the back side of the large end of the No. 7 wax spatula this margin may be lifted slightly, further deepening the undercut beneath the finishing line.

In addition to the undercut finishing line, retention spurs, loops, or nailheads are added for retention of the resin to be added later. Spurs are usually made of 18-gauge or smaller round wax attached at one end only at random acute angles to the sheet wax. Loops are small-gauge round (wax, resin, or metal) circles attached either vertically or horizontally with space beneath for the resin attachment. Nailheads are made of short pieces of 18-gauge round wax attached vertically to the sheet wax, with the head flattened with a slightly warmed spatula. Any method of providing retention is acceptable if it permits positive attachment of the resin and will not interfere with the placement of artificial teeth.

A metal base waxed as described will provide optimal contours with a minimum of bulk and weight and with adequate provision for the attachment of artificial teeth to the metal base. Properly designed, the more visible portions of the metal base will be covered with the acrylic resin supporting the supplied teeth.

ANATOMIC REPLICA PATTERNS

A technique for obtaining a duplication of the palatal portion of a maxillary cast was developed originally by William Thompson as an aid to phonetics. This was called the *Thompson Tru-Rugae technique*. It was soon discovered that many other advantages also resulted from anatomic replica patterns. It was found that patients became accustomed to an anatomic replica palate much more readily than to a smooth highly polished surface or to the concentrated bulk of palatal bars. It has been claimed that an irregular palatal surface seems to improve mastication by giving the tongue a "washboard" surface against which to press out the softer food particles and thereby separate them for mastication by the teeth.

The appearance of the denture to the patient is seemingly improved by its anatomic form and by the fact that the surface is never highly polished. This fact is readily recognized and makes the patient aware of the fact that it is a personalized reproduction of his own palate rather than a foreign body to be tolerated.

The irregular contour of the anatomic replica palate adds rigidity to the casting by its corrugated shape, thus permitting the use of thinner castings than would be permissible with a smooth, uncorrugated surface. This adds to patient acceptance and comfort by decreasing both weight and bulk.

To the laboratory the anatomic replica palate means a saving in polishing time and in finishing and polishing materials.

The original Thompson technique was cumbersome but worthy of note because it led to later developments in anatomic replica techniques. Walker and Orsinger are credited with originating the present technique for palate reproduction, a description of which appeared in 1954. It is now almost a universally accepted technique for making full and partial palate reproductions.

The material is available as a Tru-Rugae kit and contains all the materials needed to make anatomic replica palates for complete and partial dentures. Whether used as a pattern to be burned out and cast or, in slightly thicker form, as an anatomic pattern of the palate to be discarded when boiling out a flasked denture, the technique is essentially the same. Walker and Orsinger listed the equipment and material required as follows:

> Cardboard box approximately 6 by 6 by 2 inches deep [to permit reuse of the polymer]
> Camel's-hair brush, large water coloring size, or larger
> Small nasal atomizer (DeVilbiss Economy Atomizer No. 182 is satisfactory)*
> Wax spatula
> Iris or cuticle scissors
> Powder: Ethyl methacrylate powder, Dupont Lucite HG-24 or equal

----

*Compressed air–operated spray guns give a much finer and more uniform spray than the hand-operated atomizer and are not subject to clogging. Tow of these are the Thayer-Chandler air brush and the Dupli-Color touch-up spray gun, model A, both of which require compressed air for operation.

> Liquid: Methyl methacrylate monomer, or any denture base liquid acrylic resin
> Coloring material for liquid: Prussian blue, artist's color ground in oil
> Pattern cement: Pre-formed plastic pattern scraps dissolved in acetone
> Plasticizers: Methyl salicylate, camphor, rosin, or suitable commercial plasticizers such as Dow Resin 276. . . . [The plasticizer is added to the liquid in the atomizer or spray gun only, about six drops to the small atomizer, correspondingly more to the larger spray gun.]*

The following formula for a liquid is used at Lackland Air Force Base and contains a plasticizer:

Camphor	75 ml
Oil of wintergreen	75 ml
Acrylic resin monomer	350 ml
Sudan red	Pinch

Procedure for making an anatomic replica pattern. The procedure for making the anatomic replica pattern (or wafer) is as follows:

1. Make an alginate impression of the master cast. The buccal and labial borders of the impression extending beyond the impression tray should be shortened to provide better access to the palatal area. Rinse the impression to remove any loose particles, and remove excess moisture with compressed air. Leave the surface damp but free of surface moisture.

2. Fill the impression with powder from the cardboard box. (It is suggested that only enough powder be kept in the box to completely fill a hydrocolloid impression rather than to reuse larger quantities. Since this material becomes contaminated, it can be screened to remove foreign particles and replenished with fresh powder from the original container.)

3. Invert the impression over the cardboard box and dump out the surplus powder. Give the back of the hand holding the impression three or four slaps to remove more excess powder. This leaves powder layer No. 1 in the impression, which now has a fine sugar-coated appearance.

4. Using the atomizer, or preferably an air gun giving a fine misty spray, spray the face of the impression, as it is held in the other

----

*From Walker, T. J., and Orsinger, W. O.: Palate reproduction by the hydrocolloid-resin method, J. Prosthet. Dent. 4:54-66, 1954.

hand, with monomer. In this manner the liqud is prevented from building up in deeper areas of the impression. The monomer should contain several drops of plasticizer, depending on the size of the container.

5. Immediately fill the impression again, and dump and tap out the excess powder. This is powder layer No. 2, which is then sprayed with monomer as before. Use sufficient liquid to saturate the powder particles.

Ordinarily three layers of powder are sufficient to make a pattern thick enough for casting. (For palate reproductions on complete dentures, five or six layers may be necessary.) The thickness will be determined by how hard the operator shakes or taps out the excess powder from the impression and also by the length of time the second and third applications of powder are left on the impression before they are tapped off. The longer they remain on the impression, the thicker the wafer will be, because the powder picks up more liquid as it stands.

6. Set the impression under an inverted container or in a bell jar to prevent evaporation of the monomer and to allow the liquid to penetrate more thoroughly the grains of powder. This results in a finer surface and a more uniform thickness after cementation on the refractory cast. (This precaution applies equally well to any procedure in which denture bases are made by a sprinkling method.) An inverted bowl or glass refrigerator jar prevents evaporation and allows more thorough penetration of the monomer during polymerization.

7. When the plastic wafer has reached a flexible polymerized state (in about thirty minutes), strip it out of the impression completely. With fine iris scissors, trim the wafer to correspond to the outline of the palatal coverage previously penciled lightly on the refractory cast. Discard the cuttings, leaving only the wafer to be cemented to the refractory cast. If a definite ledge for a finishing line was established on the master cast with relief wax, the plastic wafer should extend about 2 mm beyond the platform that has been reproduced on the investment cast. This establishes the finishing line on the tissue side of the casting. (The undercut finishing line on the exposed side will be waxed on the plastic wafer about 2 mm in front of its trimmed edge.)

8. With a fine camel's-hair brush, paint a uniform layer of pattern cement on the investment cast inside the penciled outline. If preferred, this cement can be made up by dissolving plastic pattern forms in acetone. If it becomes too thick, it may be thinned with monomer. Excess cement should be avoided because it will cause irregular borders to be reproduced in the casting. Press the plastic wafer to place on the cast, making sure it conforms to the penciled outline. The remainder of the pattern then may be completed in the usual manner. If it is necessary to store the wafer overnight before completing the pattern, it should be covered with an inverted glass container or placed under a bell jar to maintain its plasticity. Refrigeration will also maintain the plasticity of anatomic replica patterns for extended periods.

In making cast palate reproductions for a complete upper denture the method is essentially the same as that used for a partial denture. For resin palate reproductions an alignate hydrocolloid impression of the master cast is also used. The wafer is sprayed into the impression somewhat thicker than for a metal casting, then it is removed after polymerizing and trimmed as above. The wafer is not cemented to the master cast but merely waxed to place to form the palate of the denture. This is done before the denture is invested for processing. The palate of the original base is then cut out and replaced with the anatomic palate wafer. This is discarded during boilout, leaving a mold that results in an anatomic replica palate on the completed denture.

SPRUING, INVESTING, BURNOUT, CASTING, AND FINISHING THE PARTIAL DENTURE FRAMEWORK

Brumfield has listed some of the factors that influence the excellence of a dental casting:

1. Care and accuracy with which the model [cast] is reproduced.
2. Intelligence with which the case [framework] is designed and proportioned.
3. Care and cleanliness in waxing up the model [cast].
4. Consideration of the expansion of the wax due to temperature.
5. The size of the sprues.
6. The length of the sprues.

7. The configuration of the sprues.
8. Points of attachment and manner of attachment of the sprues to the cast.
9. Choice of investment.
10. The location of the pattern in the mold.
11. The mixing water: amount, temperature, and impurities.
12. The spatulation of the investment during mixing.
13. The restraint offered to the expansion of the investment, due to the investment ring.
14. Setting time.
15. Burn-out temperature.
16. Burn-out time.
17. Method of casting.
18. Gases: adhered, entrapped, and absorbed.
19. Force used in throwing the metal into the mold.
20. Shrinkage on cooling.
21. Removal from the investment after casting.
22. Scrubbing, pickling, etc.
23. Polishing and finishing.
24. Heat handling.*

Spruing. Brumfield describes the function of the sprues as follows:

The sprue channel is the opening leading from the crucible to the cavity in which the appliance [framework] is to be cast. Sprues have the purpose of leading the molten gold from the crucible into the mold cavity. For this purpose, they should be large enough to accommodate the entering stream, and of the proper shape to lead it into the mold cavity as quickly as possible, but with the least amount of turbulence. The sprues have the further purpose of providing a reservoir of molten metal from which the casting may draw during solidification, thus avoiding porosity due to shrinkage. The spruing of the cast may be roughly summarized in three general rules.

1. The sprues should be large enough that the molten metal in them will not solidify until after the metal in the casting proper has frozen. (8- to 12-gauge round wax is usually used for multiple spruing of partial denture castings.)

2. The sprues should lead into the mold cavity as directly as possible and still permit a configuration which will induce a minimum amount of turbulence in the stream of molten metal.

3. Sprues should leave the crucible from a common point and be attached to the case [pattern] at its bulkier sections. That is, no thin sections of casting should intervene between two bulky, unsprued portions.

The configuration of the sprues, from their point of attachment at the crucible, until they reach the mold cavity may be influential in reducing turbulence. One of the more important sources of difficulty in casting is the entrapment of gases in the mold cavity, before they have a chance to escape. If the sprue channels contain sharp right angle turns, great turbulence is induced which is calculated to entrap such gases and so lead to faulty castings. Sprue channels should make long radii, easy turns and also enter the mold cavity from a direction designed to avoid splashing at this point.

As pointed out, the sprues should be attached to the bulky points of the mold [pattern]. If two bulky points exist with a thin section between them, each of the bulky spots should be sprued. The points of attachment should be flared out and local constrictions avoided. If this practice is followed, the sprue, being bulky enough to freeze after the case [framework] has frozen, will continue to feed molten metal to the case [framework] until it has entirely solidified, thus providing sound metal in the casting proper with all shrinkage porosity forced into the sprue rod, which is later discarded.*

There are two basic types of sprues: multiple and single (Figs. 17-36 and 17-37). The majority of partial denture castings require multiple spruing, using 8- to 12-gauge round wax shapes for the main sprues and 12- to 18-gauge round wax shapes for auxiliary sprues. Occasionally, however, a single sprue is preferred for full cast palates and cast metal bases for the mandibular arch when these are used as complete denture bases. With partial dentures the use of a single sprue is limited to those maxillary frameworks in which, because of the presence of a palatal plate, it is impossible to locate multiple sprues centrally. In such situations the single sprue may be used advantageously. A single sprue must be attached to the wax pattern so that the direction of flow of the molten metal will be parallel to the long axis of the single sprue. In some instances the investment cast may have to be cut away anteriorly to make room for the attachment of the sprue; in others the sprue may be attached posteriorly. One disadvantage of using a single sprue for large

---

*From Brumfield, R. C.: Dental gold structures, analysis and practicalities, New York, 1949, J. F. Jelenko & Co., Inc.

*From Brumfield, R. C.: Dental gold structures, analysis and practicalities, New York, 1949, J. F. Jelenko & Co., Inc.

Fig. 17-36. View of a sprued wax pattern. Three 8-gauge sprues attached to lingual bar and three 12-gauge sprues attached to denture base minor connector and direct retainer assemblies are joined at central sprue hole in investment cast.

Fig. 17-37. Full cast denture bases and broad palatal coverage patterns are best sprued with a single main sprue located posteriorly. Where a cast denture base for a completely edentulous arch is being sprued, single sprue may be located anteriorly.

castings is that an extra long investment ring must be used.

Some important points to remember in multiple spruing are as follows:

1. Use a few sprues of large diameter rather than several smaller sprues.
2. Keep all sprues as short and direct as possible.
3. Avoid abrupt changes in direction; avoid T-shaped junctions as much as possible.
4. Reinforce in all junctions with additional wax to avoid constrictions in the sprue channel and to avoid V-shaped sections of investment that might break away and be carried into the casting.

Step-by-step procedure. The laboratory procedure for multiple spruing is essentially the same for all mandibular castings and maxillary castings except those with a palatal plate. The following technique is given for a typical mandibular Class II partial denture casting:

1. Reduce the base of the cast to about 12 mm (½-in) thickness. Trim all edges of the cast until it is slightly larger than the wax pattern and tapers from the occlusal aspect toward the base.
2. Cut a 9 mm (³⁄₈-in) hole through the cast centered on a line joining the distal ends of the major connector on each side. The hole must be large enough to accommodate the main sprue from which other sprues will lead to the framework. (Stainless steel sprue cones may be purchased for forming the main sprue hole. These are available in sev-

eral sizes and shapes and are used to form the hole in the investment cast at the time the cast is poured into the duplication mold.)

3. Roll one half sheet of softened pink baseplate wax into a rod of such diameter that it will just pass through the hole cut in the base of the cast when it is inserted from the bottom. Allow the wax rod to protrude slightly on the wax pattern side of the cast. Seal this portion to the cast all around its border. The long portion protruding from the underside of the cast will serve as a handle during investment. The slight projection on the wax pattern side serves as an extrusion, with the sprue leads attached approximately 4.5 mm (³/₁₆ in) below the tip of the main sprue. By using this overjet principle of spruing, the initial thrust of molten metal is directed against the tip of the main sprue reservoir, and the turbulence that is created is confined to this area rather than at the entrance to the pattern mold cavity.

4. From this main sprue, attach three pieces of 8-gauge round wax extending radially to the lower border of the lingual bar major connector. Direct one piece to the central portion of the connector and the other two to just anterior to the finishing lines where the major connector joins the base retention on one side and the cast base on the other side. Thus the molten metal is fed to portions of the clasp assembly as well as to the bar itself. Attach these spures to the bulkiest part of the major connector, being careful not to involve any critical margins. In spruing a tooth-borne partial denture framework consisting of four clasp assemblies, four such sprues should be used, each attached to the major connector just below the clasp assembly.

5. In a similar manner, using pieces of 12-gauge round wax, connect the main sprue to the retentive framework or to any metal bases. In attaching to a retentive framework, make sure this is at the junction of a crossbar, thus assuring a free flow of metal with a minimum of changes in direction. A 12-gauge, round wax sprue is attached to the body of each direct retainer assembly on the cast denture base side. These sprues so placed will ensure the casting of the bar-type retainer, the circumferential retainer, and the buccal portion of the cast base pattern.

6. Reinforce all points of junction between the sprues and the denture framework with

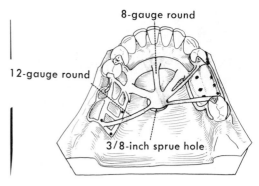

Fig. 17-38. Wax pattern is sprued as illustrated.

Fig. 17-39. Trimmed investment cast and sprued pattern are secured to sprue former.

additional wax. The spruing is now completed (Fig. 17-38).

Investing the sprued pattern (Fig. 17-39). The investment for a partial denture casting consists of two parts: the investment cast upon which the pattern is formed and the outer investment surrounding the cast and pattern. The latter is confined within a metal ring, which may or may not be removed after the outer investment has set. If the metal ring is not removed, it must be lined with a layer of asbestos to allow for both setting and thermal expansion of the mold in all directions.

The investment must conform accurately to the shape of the pattern and must preserve the configuration of the pattern as a cavity after the pattern itself has been eliminated through vaporization and oxidation. Brumfield has listed the purposes of the investment as follows:

1. Investment provides the strength necessary to hold the forces exerted by [the] entering stream of molten metal until this metal has solidified into the form of the pattern.
2. It provides a smooth surface for the mold cavity so that the final casting will require as little finishing as possible and in some cases a de-oxidizing agent to keep surfaces bright.
3. It provides an avenue of escape for most of the gases entrapped in the mold cavity by the entering stream of molten metal.
4. It, together with other factors, provides necessary compensation for the dimensional changes of the gold [alloy]* from the molten to the solid, cold state.†

The investment for casting gold alloys is a plaster-bound silica material, so compounded that the total mold expansion will offset the casting shrinkage of the gold, which varies from 1% to 1.74% (the highest figure being the shrinkage of pure gold). Generally, the higher the percentage of gold in the alloy, the greater the contraction of the casting upon solidifying.

Only one chromium-cobalt alloy has a sufficiently low melting temperature to be cast into a plaster-silica investment mold. According to Peyton, for the others having a higher melting temperature, an investment containing quartz powder held together by an ethyl silicate or sodium silicate binder is generally used. Expansion to offset casting shrinkage for the chromium-cobalt alloys is accomplished primarily through thermal expansion of the mold and must be sufficient to offset their greater casting shrinkage, which is in the order of 2.3%. For this reason the metal ring is usually removed after the mold has hardened, to allow for the greater mold expansion necessary with these alloys. Since the investments for chromium-cobalt alloys are generally less porous, there is greater danger of entrapping gases in the mold cav-

ity by the molten metal. Spruing must be done with greater care, and in some instances, provision for venting the mold is necessary to avoid defective castings.

Step-by-step procedure. The technique for applying the outer investment is usually referred to as "investing the pattern." Actually, the cast upon which the pattern is formed is part of the investment also. The following technique is given as being representative of, and applicable to, all partial denture castings:

1. Just before mixing the investment, line the ring with one layer of sheet asbestos. The asbestos should be 6 mm (¼ in) shorter than the ring at the crucible end. The asbestos permits hot gases to escape at the back through the asbestos; yet some investment in contact with the ring at the crucible end prevents the investment from falling out during handling of the ring after heating. Wet the asbestos after it is in place, but do not pack it tightly against the walls of the ring. (Step 1 is omitted if a split type forming flask is used that will be opened and removed as soon as the investment has set.)

2. Unless the investment cast has been dipped in beeswax, which prevents it from absorbing water from the painting investment, it must be soaked in room-temperature water before painting. In such case, immerse the cast with the sprued pattern in a pan of water at about 85° F no longer than four minutes. Water saturation of an untreated investment cast assures a good bond between the old investment and the new, but cold water must not be used for fear the pattern will shrink and be loosened from the cast.

3. Mix 100 g of investment, using 2 ml more water than was used to make the investment cast. (If the investment for the cast required 28 ml of water per 100 g of powder, the painting mix should be 30 ml of water per 100 g.) Spatulation must be thorough and should continue for about sixty seconds to distribute water throughout the mix when mixed by hand. Remember that a well-spatulated mix gives greater expansion and that mechanical spatulation, under vacuum conditions, usually results in the best mix possible.

Paint the pattern with a wetting agent (de-bubblizer) just prior to applying the investment to reduce the surface tension of the wax so that the outer investment readily cov-

---

*Note the substitution of the word *alloy*, as the same principles apply whether the metal be a precious metal alloy or a chromium-cobalt alloy. In some of the latter alloys the cobalt is partially replaced by nickel; such alloys are sometimes described as "stellite" alloys.
†From Brumfield, R. C.: Dental gold structures, analysis and practicalities, New York, 1949, J. F. Jelenko & Co., Inc.

ers and adheres to the pattern. With a brush carrying the mixed investment, start at one end of the cast and work the investment under the sprues. Use only indirect vibration, the hand supporting the cast being between it and the vibrator. Keep working the investment under the wax sprues, working from one side of the cast around to the other. Proceed to invest the remainder of the pattern in the same manner. Wrought-wire retentive clasp arms also must be covered with investment. The entire pattern should be covered with about 6 mm (¼ in) of investment. An even layer of investment is necessary to assure uniform expansion of the mold. Set the invested pattern aside until the outer investment has set (unless the vibrator will remain off, do not place the pattern on the same bench or vibration transferred through the bench will cause the investment to pull away from the pattern).

4. After the painting investment has reached its initial set (in about ten minutes), it may be invested in the casting ring or flask former. Just before investing the assembly in the casting ring, dip the assembly in water to again wet the outer investment, shaking off any excess water. Four hundred grams of powder will be ample, mixed with the same proportion of water as before. *Only hand spatulation for about sixty seconds should be used, since some air in the outer investment is necessary to aid in venting the mold.*

One type of casting ring (Ney partial denture casting ring) has no crucible former and consists of a large heavy metal ring with an opening at one end about the diameter of an inlay casting ring. The other end is open to accommodate the invested pattern. To use this ring the invested pattern is inserted with its main sprue protruding through the center of the smaller opening. The invested cast in this position should have sufficient space above for an adequate bulk of investment to cover it. In this position, connect the main wax sprue with the sides of the ring at its mouth, thus closing the opening. The main sprue protruding through the wax seal may be held between two fingers while the ring is held inverted in the palm of the hand. The invested cast is now completely covered with investment, filling the ring to the top. A glass slab may be slid over the top of the filled ring to permit inverting the ring on the bench while the investment sets. The crucible is then cut into the hardened investment at the main sprue.

A second type of ring has a crucible former. Representative of this type are the Kerr and Jelenko partial denture casting rings. This type is perhaps the most frequently used. The invested cast is attached to the crucible former by placing the main sprue into the hole and sealing it to the crucible former. Care must be taken that the invested cast is centered in the ring, with sufficient space all around and at the top for adequate thickness of outer investment. The casting ring is seated onto the crucible former and filled with investment, thus embedding the cast in investment as previously outlined.

Dr. Noble G. Wills has developed an innovation to the spruing and investing of a partial denture, which is a valuable aid in securing the investment cast to the sprue former and in regulating the height of the cast in the ring.

For a long time a tapered sprue cone of metal has been used to form the sprue hole in the investment cast, thus eliminating the need for cutting a 9 mm (⅜-in) sprue hole in the base of the cast later. The sprue is then reinserted into the cast just prior to investment, where it is retained by friction.

The Wills sprue pin is a machined brass untapered screw ⅜ inch in diameter and threaded with a No. 16 thread. This fits into a threaded hole in a metal sprue former made to accommodate the Kerr or the Jelenko partial denture casting ring (Fig. 17-40). Projecting from the screw is a pin that is used to retain the threaded sprue in the hydrocolloid mold as the investment cast is being poured into it (Fig. 17-41). The threaded sprue must be lubricated with petrolatum or silicone jelly so that it may be removed from the cast with ease. A screwdriver is then used to remove the sprue from the cast, leaving a threaded sprue hole comparable to that in the sprue former.

After the wax pattern is completed and ready to invest, the brass sprue pin is screwed halfway into the base of the cast, and the other half is screwed into the sprue former. Thus the investment cast is held securely to the sprue former, and by inserting a screwdriver through the hole in the sprue former and engaging the slot in the threaded sprue, its height in relation to the ring can be adjusted.

Fig. 17-40. Wills threaded sprue former and matching casting ring. Base and ring may be either the Kerr or the Jelenko size, but both must match. Projection on ⅜-inch rod threaded with a No. 16 thread is for positioning lubricated sprue into duplication mold prior to pouring investment cast.

Fig. 17-41. Threaded sprue being held in duplication mold by pointed projection. Sprue is first lubricated with petrolatum or silicone jelly. Note slotted end to facilitate withdrawal from cast and, later, to adjust with a small screwdriver the height of wax pattern in casting ring.

Since there is some probability that the sharp edges of investment making up the threaded sprue channel may become broken off by the force of the molten metal and thus be carried into the mold proper, the threaded sprue hold should be reamed slightly and the particles eliminated just prior to placing the investment in the furnace.

A third type of casting ring is the split-type forming flask, which is opened and removed as soon as the investment has set. This flask is available in various diameters and heights, but the medium size will accommodate about 90% of all wax patterns. This type of casting ring does not use a crucible former. Instead the flask is placed on a glass slab and nearly filled. Then the invested cast (sprue up) is embedded into it, using the sprue as a handle until the investment reaches a consistency sufficient to support the weight of the cast. Sometimes a copper screen is used inside the split-type flask to support the investment during heating and casting. This is not necessary if care is taken to avoid too rapid burnout or careless handling of the heated mold.

5. Allow the investment to set for at least an hour. At the end of this time, if the first type of ring was used, cut away the wax and

protruding main sprue in such a manner as to form a concavity in the investment with the deepest part at the sprue. If the second type was used, merely remove the crucible former, which will leave the investment concaved or funnel shaped. The concavity may be deepened if desired by trimming the walls uniformly smooth, maintaining the funnel shape. If a split-type flask is used, a crucible may be formed by carving a funnel in the mold at the main sprue. Finally, trim the two faces of the mold to be parallel, using the edges of the ring as a guide. This is done by rubbing the mold over a piece of wire mesh screening (Fig. 17-42). If the split-type ring was used, it is now removed by sliding off the retaining clip, which allows the ring to be opened.

Burnout. The burnout operation serves three purposes: it drives off moisture in the mold, it vaporizes and thus eliminates the pattern, leaving a cavity in the mold, and it expands the mold to compensate for contraction of the metal on cooling.

Brumfield has this to say about burnout:

The time required to drive off the water is mainly a function of the amount of heat available and of the closeness of the heating element to the

Fig. 17-42. Excess investment may be trimmed flush with rim of casting ring or flask by rubbing it over a piece of wire mesh or screening material. (Courtesy Ticonium Division, CMP Industries, Inc., Albany, N.Y.)

investment when placed in the furnace. If the furnace is large and a number of molds are burned out at the same time, the burn-out will require more time than would be the case with a single mold in the same furnace. . . .

The temperature of the mold is held down during early stages of burn-out by the vaporization of the water. Water will not rise appreciably above its boiling point until it is all vaporized. At the end of 60 minutes, the water is practically all driven off and the temperature at the inside of the mold will rise fairly rapidly to near the temperature of the furnace. Complete equalization, however, requires another 70 minutes, giving a total burn-out time of about two and one-quarter hours for eliminating the water and raising the temperature of the mold approximately 1300° F. The so-called soaking period often recommended to be given the mold, after furnace pyrometer shows the full burn-out temperature, is designed to allow time for the water to be eliminated from the mold and the mold temperature to rise to that of the furnace.

During the time the water is being eliminated, the wax is being eliminated through vaporization and oxidation of carbon. Vaporization of wax ordinarily does not require as much time as that for vaporization of the water and will often have been completed when the temperature on the inside of the furnace has risen to about 1000° F. The carbon residue may require more time for elimination. The more oxidizing the atmosphere of the eliminating furnace the better from the standpoint of eliminating wax. . . .

It is essential that the time of burn-out be sufficient to entirely eliminate the moisture. If the moisture is not eliminated, its presence has two bad effects on the casting. The casting made from an incompletely eliminated ring is apt to be porous due to the continued emission of steam by the investment. Second, the venting of the mold cavity is largely accomplished through the interstices of the investment itself. Although the investment is finely ground and these interstices are invisible to the eye, they nevertheless exist in very considerable amounts. Most investments contain voids (that is, spaces not occupied by investment particles), which amount to as much as 50 per cent of the total volume occupied. It is through these void spaces that the gases entrapped in the mold cavity by the entering stream of molten metal are able to depart with sufficient rapidity to avoid porosity in the casting. If these spaces are already occupied by steam from the incompletely eliminated mold or by finely divided particles of carbon residue from the wax, the entrapped gases cannot escape and porosity results from their inclusion in the casting. It is better to err on the side of too long a burn-out than in the opposite direction.*

For the investment to heat uniformly it should be moist at the start of the burnout cycle. Steam will then carry the heat into the investment during the early stages of the burnout. Therefore if the investment is not burned out on the same day it is poured, it should be soaked in water for a few minutes before being placed in the burnout furnace.

Just prior to being placed in the furnace, the mold should be placed in the casting machine to balance the weight against the

---

*From Brumfield, R. C.: Dental gold structures, analysis and practicalities, New York, 1949, J. F. Jelenko & Co., Inc.

weight of the mold. At this time the mold should be properly oriented to the machine and its crucible and a scratch line made at the top for later repositioning of the hot mold.

The mold should be placed in the oven with the sprue hole down and the orientation mark forward. Burnout should be started with a cold oven, or nearly so. Then the temperature of the oven should be increased slowly to a temperature of 1250° F over a period of two hours. This temperature then should be maintained for at least a thirty-minute "heat-soaking" period to ensure uniform heat penetration. More time must be allowed for plastic patterns, particularly palatal anatomic replica patterns.

It is important that this temperature not be exceeded during the burnout period. (When a high heat investment is used, the manufacturer's instructions as to burnout temperature should be followed.) For all plaster-bound investments, contraction of the mold occurs beyond 1350° F, and breakdown of the binder begins at about 1450° F. To avoid loss of expansion and possible cracking, the soaking temperature should not exceed 1250° F.

Casting. The method of casting will vary widely with the alloy and equipment being used. All methods use force to inject quickly the molten metal into the mold cavity. This force may be either centrifugal or air pressure; the former is more commonly used. In any case, either too much or too little force is undesirable. If too little force is used, the mold is not completely filled before the metal begins to freeze. If too much force is used, excessive turbulence may result in the entrapment of gases in the casting. With centrifugal casting machines this is regulated by the number of turns put on the actuating spring. For the Thermotrol casting machine, for example, this is two to three turns.

The metal may be melted with a gas-oxygen blowtorch or by an electric muffle surrounding the metal. In some commercial casting procedures and in some dental laboratories the induction method may be used, which provides a rapid and accurate method of melting the metal. The cost of induction equipment prohibits its wide-spread use.

The blowtorch method may produce consistently excellent results, but the lack of temperature control leaves much responsibility on the skill and judgment of the dentist or technician. Since the temperature at which the metal is thrown into the mold has an important bearing on the excellence of the casting, the use of controlled melting with an electric muffle, such as the Thermotrol, eliminates many of the variables common to the blowtorch method. Properly adjusted, this machine indicates the temperature of the molten metal at the instant it is thrown into the mold.

Removing the casting from the investment. Chromium-cobalt alloys are usually allowed to cool in the mold and are not cleaned by pickling. Finishing and polishing, which are done with special high-speed equipment, require a technical skill in the use of bench lathes not ordinarily acquired by the dental student. The average dentist is more adept in the use of the dental handpiece, whereas the average technician is, by reason of his training, more proficient in the use of bench lathes for finishing and polishing larger castings. Just before being polished (high-shine), chromium–cobalt castings are electropolished, which is a controlled deplating process. The following therefore applies specifically to gold alloy castings being completed by the dental student or dentist.

After the casting is completed, allow the mold to cool until the sprue button has changed in color from red to black when viewed in shaded light. This will be about eight to twelve minutes after completion of a large casting. At this time, quench the hot ring in water. With most gold castings this will produce a fairly soft and ductile condition in the metal. However, the larger the flask and the greater the amount of investment surrounding the casting, the longer the period required for bench cooling prior to quenching. It has been pointed out that when the Ney partial denture flask is used, a cooling period of eight to twelve minutes is sufficient, but that if a flask with straight sides is used, it will hold approximately 60% more investment and therefore will require considerably more time for cooling. For the latter type of flask (such as the Kerr or Jelenko flask) it is suggested that twenty minutes be allowed for bench cooling to avoid the possibility that the casting will be too soft.

The practice of allowing the casting to completely cool in the investment is not recommended for gold alloys. Although it is true that all gold alloys capable of being hardened by slow cooling will harden if allowed to cool slowly in the investment, the difference between the outside and the center at any given instant may vary 200° F or more. Not only is heat hardening by this method uneven but shrinkage also is nonuniform, resulting in an inaccurate casting.

After removal of the investment from the casting by brushing under water with a stiff bristle brush, the casting should be further cleaned by *pickling*. Prior to pickling, detergent powder may be used to aid in removing investment particles.

When the casting is clean, it should be pickled in an acid pickling solution. Prevox, Jel-Pac, dilute sulfuric acid, or 30% to 50% hydrochloric acid may be used for pickling. The latter is objectionable because of the fumes and the fact that these fumes corrode laboratory instruments. It is essential that the pickling acid be clean and relatively colorless rather than have the typical greenish blue color of contaminated acid. Contamination results not only from repeated reuse of the solution but also from handling the casting with metal tongs during pickling. A contaminated acid contains excessive copper and other salts that will contaminate the surface of the casting, leading to tarnish and discoloration in the mouth.

When surface pits and irregularities on the casting become contaminated with foreign salts, later finishing and polishing may fail to remove them completely. When such a restoration comes in contact with sulfur-bearing foods, metallic sulfides are formed that exude from the pits and irregularities. Dark rings of stain and discoloration subsequently spread over a larger area, giving a tarnished appearance to the polished metal. This is the result of using an unclean pickling bath.

Under no conditions should the casting be heated and plunged into the pickling solution. Pickling is properly done by placing the casting in a clean porcelain dish and pouring the clean pickling solution over it to a depth sufficient to cover it. The dish then should be heated over a flame until the surface of the casting brightens. The pickling solution is poured off (flushing generously with water or base solution) and the casting washed with an abundance of water. If the acid solution is fresh and clean, no base metal deposits will occur to cause later discoloration of the polished casting in the mouth.

Finishing and polishing. Some authorities hold that the sprues should not be removed from the casting until most of the polishing is completed. Although it is true that this policy may prevent accidental distortion, it is difficult to adhere to and is therefore somewhat impractical. Instead, reasonable care should be exercised to avoid any distortion resulting from careless handling.

Actual polishing procedures may vary widely according to personal preference for certain abrasive shapes and sizes. However, several rules in finishing the casting are important. These are as follows:

1. High speeds are preferable to low speeds. Not only are they effective but in experienced hands there also is less danger of the casting's being caught and thrown out of the hands by the rotating instrument.

2. The wheels or points and the speed of their rotation should do the cutting. Excessive pressure heats the work, crushes the abrasive particles, causes the wheels to clog and glaze, and slows up the cutting.

3. A definite sequence for finishing should be adopted and followed in every case. Such a sequence for finishing a gold casting is given by Berger:

(a) Remove sprues with a jeweler's saw rather than separating discs. This saves gold and prevents accidentally cutting into essential parts of the case [framework].

(b) Grind off sprue stubs with ¾″ or ⅞″ heatless stones, 1/16″ thick. Rough grind entire case [framework] and shape bars, clasps, and saddles [metal denture bases]. Always grind bars and clasps lengthwise. Cross-grinding can weaken a bar or clasp by grinding it too thin in spots. [If the location of clasps has been properly surveyed, it should not be necessary to grind the insides of the clasps. Smoothing the inner surface and polishing should be all that is needed.]

(c) Finish grinding with barrel-shaped mounted stones of medium grit. Use above precaution in grinding bars and clasps.

(d) Sandpaper the entire appliance [framework] using fine arbor bands, following the above precautions as to bars and clasps.

(e) . . . rubber wheel the entire case [framework] carefully to remove all scratches. The better the case [framework] is rubber-wheeled, the easier the subsequent polishing steps become.

(f) The insides of the clasps and other inaccessible points may be polished readily and rapidly with a pointed rubber cylinder. Retentive clasps should be shaped with a uniform taper in both width and thickness throughout their entire length.

(g) The case [framework] is now ready for final polish. Use a B-20, 2-row brush wheel, with pumice or tripoli, or both, to remove all traces of rubber wheel marks.

(h) Finish this step with a tripoli-charged cloth buff or felt wheel and cones to get a velvety smooth finish.

(i) High gloss is imparted with a rouge-charged cloth or chamois buff.

(j) Boil case [framework] in a solution of [detergent] for several minutes and then with a hard brush remove all traces of polishing media. [This may also be accomplished by brushing with a solution of soap and household ammonia, or with commercial cleaning solutions.]*

4. Clean polishing wheels should be used. If contaminated wheels are used, foreign particles may become embedded in the surface, which will lead to later discoloration.

5. Be sure each finishing operation completely removes all scratches left by the preceding one. Remember that each successive finishing step uses a finer abrasive and therefore cuts more slowly and requires more time to accomplish.

Heat hardening. If the gold casting has been quenched in the investment, it is removed from the investment in its softest and most ductile condition. All grinding and finishing operations are performed while it is in this condition. *After finishing, and just before final polishing, precious metal alloys should be heat hardened.* Although chrome-cobalt alloys cannot be heat hardened, they have satisfactory physical properties in their original state as cast, plus whatever work-hardening occurs from manipulation and use.

Hardening gold castings by heat soaking.† Dental gold castings, which are subject to heat hardening, may be effectively hardened as follows when the casting is finished and ready for the final high polish:

1. Stabilize the furnace at the desired temperature by proper adjustment of the dial. See manufacturer's instructions for correct temperature for each alloy. (Yellow casting golds heat harden at temperatures between 600° and 700° F. White gold alloys heat

harden more effectively at temperatures as high as 800° F, except Jelenko Palloro and alloys of its type, which require somewhat different treatment. These should be quenched in the investment as soon as the casting machine stops, while the button is still red, and heat hardened by soaking for five minutes in a furnace stabilized at 600° F.)

2. Place the casting on a metal tray in the furnace, close the door, and allow to heat soak for fifteen minutes.

3. Remove the tray at the end of this period with the casting on it (do not touch the casting with cold tongs) and allow it to bench cool.

This treatment will produce from 85% to 100% of the strength given by the variable cooling–heat hardening process and will avoid any possibility of warpage because of heat treatment.

MAKING OF IMPRESSION TRAYS AND RECORD BASES

An individual impression tray may be made of self-curing acrylic resin, modeling plastic, or double-thickness baseplate material. Impression trays made from self-curing acrylic resin are preferred in most instances because of their accuracy and lack of dimensional change after being fabricated. Such trays may be made by either the "sprinkle-on" or the "adapting" technique on properly relieved casts. The adapting technique has been illustrated in Fig. 14-8. A sprinkle-on procedure for individual impression trays will be described in this section. However, adapting acrylic resin dough to a properly relieved cast is sufficiently accurate to make individual impression trays. Record or trial denture bases should be made by the sprinkle-on technique because of the requirement for close tissue adaptation of these bases.

The resin tray materials are packaged as a powder and liquid with activating chemicals added to induce polymerization when the two are mixed. They are mixed together in a jar in measured proportions and then adapted while in a doughy state to a moistened or lubricated cast. Polymerization is usually rapid with considerable exothermic reaction. They may be trimmed with scissors while soft and further trimmed after polymerizing. Although considered "dead" materials (that is, without elastic memory), they are not accurate enough to use as denture

---

*From Berger, H. R.: Finishing and polishing requires a careful technic, Jelenko Thermotrol Technician 1:7, Oct., 1947.
†From information taken from the physical properties chart of J. F. Jelenko & Co., Inc., New York, N.Y.

bases for jaw relation records or as trial bases when accuracy is essential.

Trial bases and bases for jaw relation records should either be made of materials possessing accuracy or be relined to provide such accuracy. Relining may be accomplished by seating the previously adapted base onto the tinfoiled or lubricated cast with an intervening mix of some zinc oxide–eugenol paste or with self-curing resin. Some use has been made of the mercaptan and silicone impression materials for this purpose, but the wisdom of using an elastic lining for jaw relation record bases is questionable. However, when rigid setting materials are used for this purpose, any undercuts on the cast must be blocked out with wax or clay to facilitate their removal without damage to the cast.

The ideal jaw relation record base and trial base is one that is processed (or cast) to the form of the master cast, becoming the permanent base of the completed prosthesis. Cast metal bases for either complete or partial dentures offer this advantage over resin-based dentures. Resin bases (either methyl methacrylate, vinyl combinations, or styrene) likewise may be processed directly to the master cast, thus becoming the permanent denture base. In either case, when undercuts are present, the master cast must be destroyed during removal of the base. Then existing undercuts must be blocked out inside the denture base before a cast is poured into it to make an articulator mounting. A second cast, which includes the undercuts, must be poured against the entire base to support it during the processing of the resin superstructure. When both the base and the superstructure are of resin, some care must be taken to avoid visible junction lines between the original resin base and the resin that supports the teeth and establishes facial contours.

Some self-curing acrylic resin materials are sufficiently accurate for use as trial and jaw relation bases. These are used with a sprinkling technique, which when properly done permits a base to be made that compares favorably with a processed base. A material must be selected that will polymerize in a reasonable time (usually a twelve-minute monomer) and will retain its form during the sprinkling process. Since polymerization with typical shrinkage toward the cast begins immediately, alternate addition of monomer and polymer in small increments results in reduced overall shrinkage and greater accuracy.

Technique for making a sprinkled acrylic resin record base or impression tray. The technique for sprinkling a record base will be given here. Some blockout of the cast is necessary in most instances, depending on the purpose for which the base is to be used. An individual impression tray requiring space for the impression material may be further relieved with sheet wax or wet asbestos. Sheet asbestos, such as is used to line inlay rings, may be dipped in water and adapted to the cast for this purpose. More than one thickness may be used, or wet asbestos may be added, using the wet asbestos as one would modeling clay. By painting the asbestos relief with a tinfoil substitute, it may be easily stripped out of the impression tray, leaving no trace of the relief material on either the cast or the tray.

Relief of undercut areas on the cast is best accomplished with a water-soluble modeling clay or baseplate wax. Modeling clay is easily formed and shaped on the cast and is easily removed from either the cast or the base with a natural bristle toothbrush under warm running water. Wax, on the other hand, must be flushed off the cast with hot water. It must be removed from the inside of the base by scraping and with a wax solvent, followed by flushing with water only hot enough to eliminate any residual wax.

Impression trays to be used with an alginate hydrocolloid impression material must be perforated to assure retention of the impression material within the tray. Areas over displaceable soft tissue also require perforation to avoid displacement of those tissues by hydraulic pressure. Perforation is best accomplished by using a bi-beveled surgical drill, which fits the dental handpiece but will not become clogged when drilling holes in resin materials.

The amount of relief used for an impression tray will depend on the type of impression material being used and the quality of the tissues being recorded. Trial bases and bases for jaw relation records, on the other hand, must have maximum contact with the supporting tissues. The accuracy of the base will be in proportion to the total area of intimate tissue contact provided. Those areas most frequently undercut and requiring blockout are the distolingual and retromylohyoid areas areas of the mandibular cast, the distobuccal and labial aspects of the maxillary cast, and, frequently, small multiple undercuts in the palatal rugae. These areas and any others are blocked out with a minimum of clay, to obliterate as little of the surface of the cast as possible. A close-fitting base may then be made that will have the necessary accuracy and stability and yet may be lifted from and returned to the master cast without abrading it.

Except for the presence of relief, the technique for sprinkling an impression tray is the same as that for a trial or jaw relation record base. The purpose for which it is to be used will influence the relief as follows: (1) an individual impression tray will have relief sufficient to accommodate the impression material; (2) an impression tray for making a fluid-wax functional impression prior to the making of the cast framework will have relief over the ridge areas to be recorded, with three or more tooth-bearing areas exposed and a clay matrix over the remainder of the cast; (3) an impression tray attached to the partial denture framework for making a functional impression will have sufficient relief to accommodate the impression material and permit its flow in the mouth; (4) a trial or jaw

relation record base will have undercuts blocked out but no relief over the supporting areas of the ridge.

If the impression tray or base is to be attached to a partial denture framework, the framework is first seated on the cast in its terminal position. This is done after the necessary blockout or relief or both have been placed. The cast and the blockout or relief is then painted with a tinfoil substitute of a type that may be painted onto a cold surface without leaving a heavy or uneven film, such as Al-Cote. This is essential to the accuracy of a denture base, but not all tinfoil substitutes are suitable for this purpose.

As soon as the tinfoil substitute has dried, the cast is wet with the monomer from a dropper bottle. The ordinary medicine dropper is not suitable for this purpose because the lumen is too large, resulting in an uncontrollable excess of monomer. The glass may be drawn to a fine tip over a flame but is easily broken. Instead the simple addition of a hypodermic needle of about 23 gauge to the glass lumen by flaming the glass tip around the needle provides a suitable syringe tip for the application of monomer in small quantities as needed (Fig. 17-43).

After the surface is wetted with the mono-

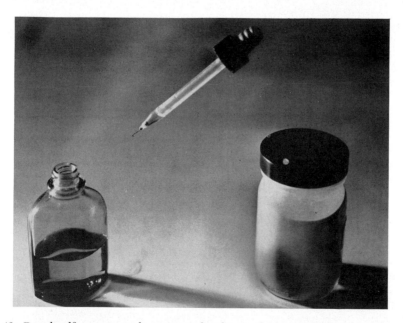

Fig. 17-43. Rapid self-curing acrylic resin in bottles used for sprinkling resin bases and so forth. A 23-gauge hypodermic needle has been sealed into tip of dropper barrel to limit size of drop and facilitate wetting the monomer without flooding. Large-mouthed bottle is of a size that can easily be held in hand, and it has a hole in rim the size of a No. 8 or 10 round bur to allow powder to be applied selectively to area involved.

mer, the polymer is sprinkled or dusted onto the wet surface until all the monomer has been absorbed. Sprinklng is best accomplished with a large-mouthed bottle with a single hole in the lid near the rim. The hole should be about the size of a No. 8 round bur. This facilitates the placement of the polymer without excess in any one area. A flexible bottle with suitable applicator tip also may be used. However, it seems that better control over the application of the polymer is possible when a bottle with a hole in the cap is used. The objective should be the uniform application of polymer over the entire ridge rather than the allowing of excess to accumulate at the border to be trimmed later. A self-curing acrylic resin material must be used that will retain its form during the sprin-

kling procedure without objectionable flow into low areas.

Once the polymer has been sprinkled in slight excess, the monomer is again added. Flooding must be avoided; therefore the monomer must be directed over the entire surface gradually until the polymer has just absorbed the monomer. *A few seconds' delay prior to the addition of excess monomer will allow the mass to reach a tacky consistency and prevent it from flowing when more monomer is added.* Then the monomer may be added in excess, which is immediately absorbed by the application of more polymer as before. This process is repeated selectively until a uniform layer has been built up, just thick enough so that none of the underlying cast or relief may be seen. Some areas will

Fig. 17-44. Stable record bases are required to correctly orient diagnostic casts representative of distal extension removable partial denture situations. Such bases are made with an autopolymerizing acrylic resin. **A,** Extent of record bases is outlined in pencil. Note that outline includes cingula of anterior teeth and distal surface of prospective terminal abutments. **B,** Interproximal undercuts are blocked out with wax. Other undercut areas involved in denture base design are also eliminated by blockout. Prominent or undercut rugae must be blocked out or covered with a soft quick-curing acrylic resin, which then becomes a part of record base. **C,** Utility wax is adapted to outline of cast in edentulous regions to confine acrylic resin when it is being applied. Wax should be adapted approximately 2 mm from penciled outline to provide adequate thickness of record base borders. **D,** A stiff 16-gauge wire is bent to conform to lingual alveolar ridge of lower cast and becomes a part of record base. This wire will strengthen final record base and will eliminate some flexibility of base.

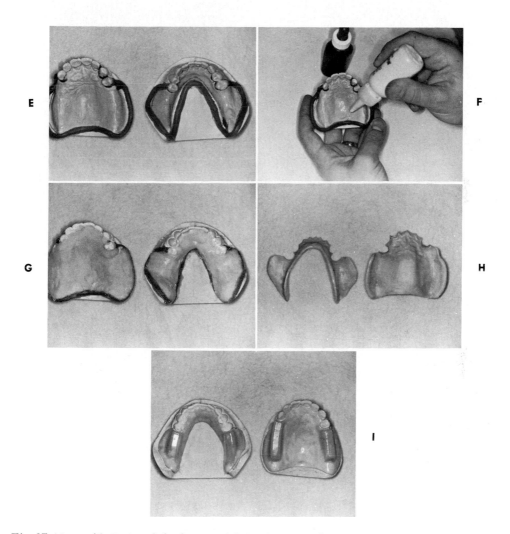

Fig. 17-44, cont'd. E, A tinfoil substitute (Al-Cote) is painted on cast to act as a separator. Two thin coats are applied, allowing first coat to dry before application of second coat. **F,** Acrylic resin is sprinkled on cast, alternating application of monomer and polymer. **G,** A uniform thickness (2 mm) of acrylic resin is sprinkled within record base outline. **H,** Record bases have been removed (after curing) and trimmed to established outlines. Note tissue detail and border thickness. **I,** Occlusion rims have been added to polished record bases. "Occlusal" surfaces of occlusion rims should be only as wide as occlusal surfaces of natural teeth they are representing. Attention must be given the fabrication of occlusion rims so that a natural arch form is maintained. In fact, occlusion rims should be thought of as replacements for lost natural teeth and their supporting structures for record-making purposes.

Fig. 17-45. Technique for making a record base attached to framework for a distal extension removable partial denture. **A,** Tissue undercuts are blocked out only enough to eliminate undercuts, and edentulous ridges are painted with a tinfoil substitute (Al-Cote). **B,** Framework is positioned on cast after tinfoil substitute has dried. A small amount of wax is added on either side of minor connector extension touching distal surface of premolars to avoid having acrylic resin "run under" connector at gingival of abutment tooth. **C,** Utility wax strips are used to confine "sprinkled-on" acrylic resin, and they outline extent of record base. Wax strips do not cover finishing lines of direct retainers and lingual bar. **D,** Cast is wet with monomer in a small area, and just enough polymer is added to take up monomer. This procedure is repeated until an overall thickness of 2 mm is obtained. **E,** All areas within wax boxing have been covered by acrylic resin. **F,** Record base has been removed from cast and trimmed. Only borders of record base are polished. **G,** A view of tissue surfaces. **H,** Occlusion rims are added to record base.

require further addition, particularly ridge crests and other prominent areas.

The final step in sprinkling is the addition of monomer sufficient to leave a wet surface. *Immediately*, the cast should be placed in a covered glass dish or covered with an inverted bowl. This permits final polymerization in a saturated atmosphere of monomer and prevents evaporation of surface monomer. The cast should not be placed in water nor any attempt made to accelerate polymerization. Slow polymerization is necessary so that shrinkage *toward* the cast will occur, earlier layers polymerizing first. Only thus will overall shrinkage be negligible and accuracy of fit be assured. Whereas this is of little consequence in the making of an impression tray, it is most essential in the making of a sprinkled resin base.

Although polymerization will be about 90% complete within an hour, and an impression tray may even be lifted within a half hour, a sprinkled denture base should be left *overnight* before being separated from the cast. It should then be lifted either dry or under lukewarm tap water. It should not be immersed in hot water, or some warpage may occur.

A sprinkled acrylic resin base made with the precautions outlined above will retain its accuracy for days, or even for an indefinite period, comparable to that of a heat-cured resin base (Figs. 17-44 and 17-45). Failure to do so can be attributed to faulty technique rather than to any inherent inaccuracy in the material itself, provided the proper material has been used. As with any resin base, storing in air results in some distortion because of dehydration. However, since the stone cast itself may not be stored in water, possible distortion of the resin from being immersed off the cast must be weighed against that occurring due to dehydration. Generally the latter is not sufficient to warrant keeping the resin base in water.

Technique for making an impression tray attached to a framework. Individual impression trays can be conveniently made by adapting a quick-curing acrylic resin dough to the relieved master cast and framework. Less time is required to make the trays by this method than with the sprinkle-on technique, and the required accuracy is not compromised when care is used in fabricating the trays (Fig. 17-46).

OCCLUSION RIMS

It has been explained that jaw relation records for partial dentures always should be made upon accurate bases that are either part of the denture casting itself or attached to it in exactly the same relation as the final denture base will be. Further, it has been stated that although the use of the final denture base is best for jaw relation records, a sprinkled or corrected acrylic resin base may be used satisfactorily. In any case, accuracy of the base supporting a maxillomandibular record must be assured before the function of occlusion rims can be considered.

Occlusion rims may be made of several materials. The material that is most commonly used to establish static occlusal relationships is the hard baseplate wax rim. However, use of a wax occlusion rim is likely to be inaccurate when the occlusal portion of the rim is pooled with a hot instrument or flamed, because of the fact that uniform softening cannot be assured. Also, some errors in repositioning apposing casts against wax occlusion rims for mounting on the articulator are likely to occur. When some soft material that sets to a rigid state, such as impression plaster or impression paste, is used in conjunction with wax rims to record static occlusal relations, many of the errors common to wax rims are eliminated provided some space exists between the occlusion rims or the opposing teeth or both at the desired vertical dimension to be recorded. Occlusion rims for static jaw relation records should be so shaped that they represent the lost teeth and their supporting structures. An occlusion rim that is too broad and extended beyond where prosthetically supplied teeth will be located is inexcusable. Such rims will substantially alter the shape of the palatal vault and arch form of the mandibular arch, crowd the patient's tongue, have a nonwelcomed effect on the patient, and will offer more resistance to jaw relation recording media than will a correctly shaped occlusion rim.

Modeling plastic may be used rather than wax for occlusion rims, with several advantages over the latter. It may be softened uniformly by flaming, yet becomes rigid and sufficiently accurate when chilled. It may be trimmed with a sharp knife to expose the tips of the opposing cusps to recheck or position an opposing cast into the record rim. Opposing occlusion rims of modeling plastic may be

Fig. 17-46. For legend see opposite page.

keyed with greater accuracy than opposing wax rims. Preferably, however, even those should be trimmed short of contact at the vertical dimension of occlusion, and plaster or impression paste should be interposed for the final record. As with wax rims, an adjustable frame to support the final record also may be used.

Occlusion rims of either extra hard baseplate wax or modeling plastic may be used to support intraoral central bearing devices or intraoral tracing devices or both. However, because of its greater stability, modeling plastic is preferable for this purpose also when the edentulous situation permits the use of flat plane tracings. An example of such a situation is when an opposing denture is being made concurrently with the partial denture. In such a case, modeling plastic occlusion rims provide greater stability than wax rims, with corresponding improvement in the predictable accuracy of such a jaw relation record. Although the sealing of opposing occlusion rims or the use of clips for complete denture jaw relation records, particularly for an initial articulator mounting, may be acceptable, the existence of a partial denture framework makes this practice hazardous. Since it is necessary that the dentist be able to see that the partial denture framework is in its original relation to the supporting teeth before the casts are articulated, the framework and attached base should be seated accurately on its cast before the opposing cast is repositioned in occlusion to it.

Occlusion rims for recording functional, or dynamic, occlusion must be made of a hard wax that can be carved by the opposing dentition. This method, outlined in Chapter 16, presumes that the opposing arch is intact or has been restored. Functional occlusion records by this method cannot be made when both arches are being restored simultaneously.

Rather an opposing arch must be as intact as the treatment plan calls for or must be restored by whatever prosthetic means the situation dictates. Opposing partial dentures or an opposing complete denture may be carried concurrently up to the final occlusal record. One denture is then completed and placed and the functional record made in opposition to it. Frequently this requires that all opposing teeth be articulated first in wax to establish optimal ridge relations and the correct occlusal plane. One denture is then carried to completion, and the teeth remaining in wax on the opposing denture are removed while the functional occlusal record is being made.

No single wax has been manufactured specifically for establishing functional occlusal records. Some inlay waxes are used for this purpose because they can be carved by the opposing dentition and because most of them are hard enough to support occlusion over a period of hours or days. A wax for recording functional crown and bridge occlusion, since it is established entirely in the dental office, is selected on the basis of how well it may

---

Fig. 17-46. Secondary impressions for distal extension mandibular removable partial dentures are made in an individual tray attached to the denture framework. **A,** The framework has been tried in the mouth and fits the mouth and master cast as planned. **B,** An outline of the resin tray is penciled on the cast. **C,** One thickness of baseplate wax is adapted to the outline to act as a spacer so that room for the impression material exists in the finished tray. Windows are cut in the wax spacer corresponding to the regions on the cast contacted by the minor connectors for the denture bases. **D,** The framework is warmed and pressed to position on the relieved master cast. All regions of the cast that will be contacted by the autopolymerizing acrylic resin dough are painted with a tinfoil substitute (Al-Cote). **E,** Quick-curing acrylic resin is mixed, and wafers of the material are made as described in Chapter 14. The resin material is adapted to the cast and over the framework with finger pressure. Excess material over the borders of the cast is removed with a sharp knife while the material is still soft. **F,** The cured resin trays and framework are removed from the cast, and the trays are trimmed to the outline of the wax spacer. **G,** Borders of the trays will be adjusted to extend within 2 mm of the tissue reflections. Holes then will be placed in the trays corresponding to the crest of the residual ridge and retromolar pads to allow the escape of excess impression material when the impression is made.

be carved by the opposing dentition in a relatively short period of time. Therefore a softer wax may be used than is required for the recording of occlusal paths over a period of twenty-four hours or more. For this latter purpose, Peck's purple hard inlay wax seems to satisfy best the requirements for a wax that is durable yet capable of recording a functional occlusal pattern. This wax is packaged in the form of sticks. A layer of sticky wax is first flowed onto the surface of the denture base. Two sticks of the inlay wax are then laid parallel along the longitudinal center of the denture base and secured to it with a hot spatula. This is the only preparation prior to the dental appointment. Since neither the height nor the width of the occlusion rim can be known in advance and since deep warming of a chilled wax rim is difficult, the rim is not completed prior to the appointment.

With the patient in the chair a hot spatula is inserted into the crevice between the two sticks of wax, making the center portion fluid between two supporting walls. Some transfer of heat to the supporting walls occurs, resulting in the occlusion rim's becoming uniformly softened. The patient is asked to close into this wax rim until the natural teeth are in contact, which establishes both the height and the width of the occlusion rim. Wax is then added or carved away as indicated and the patient asked to go into lateral excursions. Any excess wax is then removed, and any unsupported wax is supported by addition. Finally, wax is added to increase the vertical dimension sufficient to allow (1) for denture settling, (2) for changes in jaw relation brought about by the reestablishment of posterior support, and (3) for carving in all mandibular excursions. When sufficient height has been established, as well as sufficient width to accommodate all excursive movements, the patient is instructed and dismissed.

Although this discussion has been included in this chapter on laboratory procedures, the entire procedure of establishing occlusion rims for recording functional occlusion should be considered a chairside procedure rather than a laboratory procedure. It is necessary, however, that the purpose of a functional occlusal record be clearly understood so that subsequent laboratory steps may be accomplished in a manner that the effect of such an occlusal record may be reproduced on the finished denture.

MAKING A STONE OCCLUSAL TEMPLATE FROM A FUNCTIONAL OCCLUSAL RECORD

After final acceptance of the occlusal record as registered by the patient, the effectiveness of this method for establishing functional occlusion on the partial denture will depend on how accurately the following procedures are carried out. For this reason it will be given as a step-by-step procedure.

Step-by-step procedure

1. If the base of the master cast (or processing cast) has not been keyed previously, do this before proceeding. First reduce the thickness of the base if it is so thick that difficulty will be encountered in flasking. The base may not be reduced on this account after removal from the articulator, since the mounting record would be lost.

Keying may be done in several ways, but a method whereby the keyed portions are visible on the articulator mounting eliminates some possibility of remounting error. According to the preferred method, form a 45-degree bevel on the base of the cast by hand or with the model trimmer and then add three V-shaped grooves on the anterior and the posterior aspects of the base of the cast at the bevel (Fig. 17-47). The bevel serves to facilitate reseating the cast on the articulator mounting, and the mounting surfaces are made still more definite by the triangular grooves. Being placed at the beveled margin, the triangular grooves are visible at all times, and any discrepancy may be clearly seen.

2. Inspect the underside of the cast framework and denture bases, removing any particles of wax or other debris. Similarly, inspect and clean the master cast of any particles of stone, wax, blockout material, or any other debris that might prevent the casting from being seated accurately upon it.

Now seat the denture framework on the cast in its original terminal position. This is the position that was maintained by securing it with sticky wax while the trial denture base was being made, with all the occlusal rests seated. It is also the position that the casting assumed in the mouth while the occlusal record was being made and that must

Fig. 17-47. Base of any cast should be beveled and keyed as shown before mounting on articulator. Petroleum jelly is used as a separating medium to facilitate removal and remounting subsequent to processing. Keying should always be done prior to boxing and pouring an occlusal registration because cast and template must be mounted on articulator before they are separated.

be duplicated on returning the denture framework to the master cast. Holding the framework in this terminal position, secure it again with sticky wax. (If a processing cast is being used in place of the master cast, the denture base will have been made on that cast and the same precautions in returning the framework to its original position apply.)

3. With the denture framework and the occlusal record in position, form a matrix of clay around the occlusal record to confine the hard stone, which will form the stone occlusal template. (If electroforming has been done as mentioned in Chapter 16, the electroforming precedes Step 1. The clay matrix is the same for a metallized surface as for the wax record.)

The clay matrix should rise at a 45-degree angle from the buccal and lingual limits of the occlusal registration. Then arch either clay or a sheet of wax across from one side to the other, forming a vault that will permit lingual access when articulating the teeth.

Leave the occlusal surfaces of the adjacent abutment teeth or the corresponding surfaces of a processing cast exposed so that they may act as vertical stops. This will serve to maintain the vertical relation on the articulator. Unless such stone-to-stone stops are used, the vertical relation on the articulator may be

altered by the technician, either accidentally or otherwise. Any change in vertical relations is incompatible with a concept of dynamic occlusion, since the occlusal pattern is directly related to the degree of jaw separation. Although it may be true that vertical dimension may be changed when casts are mounted in relation to the opening axis of the mandible, *as long as natural cusps remain to influence mandibular movement, the vertical relation established with a functional occlusal record must not be changed on the articulator.*

Treat the surfaces of the adjacent abutment teeth left exposed with sodium silicate, Microfilm, or some other separating medium to ensure separation of the stone vertical stops.

4. If the wax record has not been metallized, use a hard dental stone to form the opposing template. This may be an improved stone such as Duroc, but the use of a stone die material such as Vel-Mix is preferred. Only the occluding surface need be poured in the harder stone, a less costly laboratory stone being used to back it up. If this is done, add the second layer to the first before the former takes its initial set, to avoid any possibility of accidental separation between the two materials.

Vibrate the stone only into the wax registration and against the stone stops. Pile on the rest of the stone and leave it uneven to facilitate firm attachment to the mounting stone. Attach the occlusal template to the articulator without provision for remounting, since only the working cast need be keyed for remounting.

5. After the stone template has set, attach the occluded casts to both arms of the articulator before separating the casts. The type of articulating instrument used is of little importance, since all eccentric positions are recorded on the template, and whatever instrument is used acts purely as a simple hinge or a tripod. Therefore any laboratory articulator or tripod may be used. Because of the easy access afforded in arranging artificial teeth and adjusting occlusion, the Hagman Junior Balancer is preferred over most other instruments for this purpose.

Casts should be attached to the articulating instrument selected with stone rather than with plaster. Mounting stones are available that have been especially formulated and prepared to minimize the setting expansion inherent in most gypsum products. The least amount of setting expansion of the mounting medium is most desirable to maintain the intended relationship of the opposing casts.

It must be remembered which arch is represented by the working cast, and the articulator mounting should be made accordingly. For example, for a mandibular denture the template is attached to the upper arm of the articulator, whereas for a maxillary denture the template is mounted upside down on the lower arm. The keyed base of the working cast attached to the opposing arm must be coated with a light coat of mineral oil or petroleum jelly to facilitate its separation from the mounting stone.

6. After the mounting has been completed, separate the casts and remove the clay. The template with its mounting may be removed from the articulator if a mounting ring or mounting stud permits; otherwise trimming must be done on the articulator. With pencil, outline the limits of the occlusal registration and carefully knife-trim any excess stone around its borders. Trim the vertical stops to a sharp edge on the buccal surface where they contact the working cast. Also remove any overhanging stone, leaving the occluding template and vertical stops clearly visible and accessible.

Remove the wax registration preparatory to arranging artificial teeth to the occluding template.

ARRANGING POSTERIOR TEETH TO AN OPPOSING CAST OR TEMPLATE

Whether posterior teeth are to be arranged to occlude with an opposing cast or an occlusal template, unless metal bases are part of the denture framework, the denture base upon which the jaw relation record has been made must first be removed and discarded. This statement is based on the assumption that where an adjustable articulator has been used to develop the occlusion, the trial dentures have been evaluated, the articulator mounting has been proved, and the articulator has been programmed for eccentric positions. Since record bases that are entirely tissue supported have no place in recording occlusal relations for partial dentures, the bases must be attached to the

denture framework. Metal bases being part of the prosthesis present no problem. The teeth may be arranged in wax or replaced on the metal base, depending on the type of posterior tooth being used, and these occluded directly to the opposing cast or template.

Unless occlusal relations are recorded on final resin bases, self-curing acrylic resin bases by the sprinkling method are the most accurate and stable of bases that may be used for this purpose. (An alternate method is the relining of the original impression bases, thus accomplishing the same purpose.) While static relations may be recorded successfully on corrected bases, functional registrations are best accomplished on new resin bases made for that purpose. In either case the denture cannot be completed on these bases, nor can the bases be removed conveniently from the retentive framework during the boilout after flasking. Therefore the metal framework must be lifted from the cast, and the original record base removed by flaming its underside: *Care must be taken not to allow the resin to catch on fire, or the cast framework will become discolored with carbon.* The framework is repolished and is then returned to its original position on the master cast and secured there with sticky wax before arrangement of the artificial teeth is begun.

Posterior tooth forms. Posterior tooth forms for partial dentures should not be selected arbitrarily. One should bear in mind at all times that the objective in partial denture occlusion is harmony between natural and artificial dentition. Whether the teeth are arranged to occlude with an opposing cast or to an occlusal template, they should be modified to harmonize with the existing dentition. In this respect, partial denture occlusion may differ from complete denture occlusion. In the latter, posterior teeth may be selected and articulated according to the dentist's own concept of what constitutes the most favorable complete denture occlusion, whereas partial denture occlusion must be made to harmonize with an existing occlusal pattern. Thus the occlusal surfaces on the finished partial denture may bear little resemblance to the original occlusal surfaces of the teeth as manufactured.

Posterior teeth for partial dentures should be considered *material from which a suitable occlusal surface may be formed rather than teeth to be articulated as well as possible with opposing surfaces.* The original occlusal form therefore is of little importance in forming the posterior occlusion for the partial denture.

Whereas the posterior teeth may be made of porcelain or resin, resin teeth are more easily modified and subsequently reshaped for masticating efficiency by adding grooves and spillways. Resin teeth are also more easily narrowed buccolingually to reduce the size of the occlusal table without sacrificing strength or esthetics. They also may be more easily ground to fit minor connectors and irregular spaces and to avoid retentive elements of the denture framework. *However, it is reemphasized that when acrylic resin teeth are used without gold occlusal surfaces, the occlusion must be evaluated quite frequently to make sure that the occlusal surfaces of the resin teeth have not worn out of contact in centric occlusion.* Aside from economics, the occlusal surfaces of acrylic resin teeth should be duplicated in gold to prevent excessive wear of the occlusal surfaces, thereby maintaining the planned occlusion for artificial posterior teeth (Fig. 17-48). It seems that the best combinations of opposing occlusal surfaces to maintain the established occlusion and avoid deleterious abrasion are porcelain to porcelain surfaces, gold surfaces to natural or restored natural teeth, and gold surfaces to gold surfaces.

Arranging teeth to an occluding surface. The procedure for arranging teeth to a static relationship with an opposing cast is essentially the same as for arranging teeth to an occluding template. On the other hand, articulation of artificial teeth on an adjustable instrument, which reproduces to some extent mandibular movement, will follow more closely the customary pattern for complete denture occlusion.

Step-by-step procedure. The procedure for arranging posterior teeth to an occluding template is as follows:

1. First raise the vertical adjustment of the articulator approximately 1 mm. If vertical stops are used, this will separate the stone stops by that amount.

2. With the aid of marking tape or articulating ribbon, mark the mesial and the ridge lap surfaces of the tooth to be placed against the most anterior minor connector on either side. Continue to mark and relieve this tooth until it conforms to and fits around the minor connector, occluding with the opposing surface at the existing vertical dimension. Modify the cusps of this tooth as required to occlude with the opposing surface.

3. Arrange the remaining teeth on that side in order, progressing posteriorly. Relieve the ridge lap and modify the occlusal surfaces as required to occlude optimally with the opposing surfaces. One or more teeth may have to be narrowed mesiodistally to establish a satisfactory mesiodistal relation with the opposing teeth. In other instances it may be necessary to leave a space between the first two teeth to accomplish this effect. Although intercuspation is desirable in most instances, it is not absolutely necessary when arranging to an occlusal template, since modified occlusal surfaces will function satisfactorily in any mesiodistal relation.

4. If a posterior abutment is present, the last tooth may have to be narrowed mesiodistally to fit the remaining space. This tooth also should be ground to conform to the contour of the minor connector, thereby effecting a more natural marginal contact relation with the abutment tooth.

5. Proceed to the opposite side of the arch and arrange the tooth or teeth in the same sequence, with each tooth lying adjacent to a minor connector being ground to fit that minor connector.

6. When all teeth have been arranged to the opposing surfaces, having been modified to occlude optimally at the existing vertical dimension, release the vertical element (pin or screw), leaving the occlusion uniformly high. When vertical stops of stone are used, the vertical element on the articulator may be removed entirely, since the absolute vertical dimension will be ultimately maintained by the stone stops. Otherwise the pin or screw should be returned to its original position. (This is, of course, difficult to reestablish without a calibrated pin; hence the value of having definite stone stops.)

Using marking tape or articulating ribbon as an indicator, the occlusal surfaces are now further modified until an optimal occlusal relationship at the selected vertical dimension of occlusion has been established. At least three factors must be considered:

a. The template surface may be easily abraded or otherwise damaged by re-

Fig. 17-48. For legend see opposite page.

peated closure against the teeth being arranged. This does not apply when opposing artificial teeth are being arranged and modified concurrently. When arranging teeth on a single denture, however, an opposing surface made of hard metal is the only way of eliminating this possibility; otherwise, violent tapping must be avoided.

b. Unreliable markings usually result when articulating paper is used. Areas of heavy contact become perforated, leaving only a small mark, whereas areas of lesser contact may make a heavier mark. This may be avoided by using a marking tape or an inked ribbon, which better conforms to irregular occluding surfaces, does not tear or become perforated, and remains constant with repeated use. Markings are thus more reliably interpreted. A ribbon holder has been described in Chapter 16 under the discussion on arranging teeth to an occluding template.

c. Wax from articulating paper eventually is deposited on opposing surfaces, having the effect of increasing the vertical dimension of occlusion and leading to false interpretation of occlusal interference. This too is avoided by using a marking tape or an inked ribbon, since the ink or dye does not create a false surface.

Regardless of the type of indicator used, stone stops are best left unmarked for better interpretation of absolute contact. Wax from articulating paper may create a false surface here also, changing the vertical relation. Although marking ink does not do this, it does make visualization of the vertical relation at the stops more difficult to interpret.

7. Except for the addition of spillways, perfect the occlusion while the teeth are still in wax. Only those errors occurring as a result of processing will then need to be corrected by remounting. Final waxing may be done off of the articulator, but the cast should be returned to it to correct for any tooth displacement resulting from waxing and carving.

TYPES OF ANTERIOR TEETH

Anterior teeth on partial dentures are concerned primarily with esthetics and the function of incising. These are best arranged in the mouth, since an added appointment for try-in would be necessary anyway. They may be arranged arbitrarily on the cast and then tried in, but a stone index of their labial surfaces should be made on the master cast after the final arrangement has been established.

From a purely mechanical standpoint, all missing anterior teeth are best replaced with fixed restorations rather than with the partial

---

Fig. 17-48. Gold occlusal surfaces, duplicating occlusal morphology of adjusted acrylic resin posterior teeth, are readily fabricated. **A,** Denture has been used by patient and all necessary occlusal adjustments have been accomplished on resin teeth in first two weeks of use. **B,** Stone matrix is poured over occlusal surfaces and extended over top one fourth of buccal surfaces. **C,** Stone matrix is extended to cover depth of lingual flange so that it can be positively relocated in same position after artificial teeth have been prepared for reception of gold occlusal surfaces. Buccal portion of matrix is trimmed so that wax patterns for gold surfaces will be about 1.5 mm thick. **D,** Stone matrices are painted with a separating medium, and wax patterns of occlusal surfaces are formed by flowing inlay wax into occlusal portions of matrix. Small retention loops are placed—one in each individual occlusal pattern. Patterns are sprued and cast in Type III gold. **E,** Wax patterns have been cast and polished. **F,** Acrylic resin artificial teeth are prepared for reception of gold occlusal surfaces by reducing their occlusal portion about 2 mm and making an undercut groove through central fossa of resin teeth. Groove should only be deep enough to accommodate retention loops on gold occlusal surfaces. **G,** Gold occlusals, stone matrix, and denture are assembled. Matrix is held in position with sticky wax. Tooth shade acrylic resin (autopolymerizing) is used to attach gold occlusal surfaces to denture by using the "sprinkle in" method of application. **H,** Procedure is completed by finishing and polishing tooth shade resin. Although original occlusal surfaces have been duplicated in gold and now occupy same position as original resin surfaces, a remounting cast should be made so that any possible resulting occlusal discrepancies can be corrected on an articulator, using new interocclusal records to mount lower cast and denture. (From Morris, A. L., and Bohannon, H. M., editors: Dental specialties in general practice, Philadelphia, 1969, W. B. Saunders Co.)

denture. However, for economic or cosmetic reasons or in situations in which several missing anterior teeth are involved, such as in a Class IV partially edentulous arch, their replacement with the partial denture may be unavoidable.

Some types of anterior teeth used on partial dentures are as follows:

1. Porcelain or resin teeth, attached to the framework with acrylic resin.

2. Ready-made resin teeth processed directly to retentive elements on the metal framework with a matching resin. This is called a *pressed-on* method and has the advantage of permitting prior selection and try-in of the anterior teeth, plus the advantage of using ready-made resin teeth for labial surfaces. These are then hollowed out on the lingual surface to facilitate their permanent attachment to the denture framework with resin of the same shade.

3. Resin teeth processed to a metal framework in the laboratory. Tooth forms of wax may be carved on the denture framework and tried in the mouth, adjusted for esthetics and occlusion, and then processed in a resin of a suitable shade. There is some question as to whether the shade and durability of such teeth are comparable to those of manufactured plastic teeth, but improvements in materials have led to improved quality and appearance of laboratory-made teeth. Moreover, such teeth may frequently be shaped and characterized to better blend with the adjacent natural teeth.

4. Porcelain or resin facings cemented to the denture framework. These may be tried in the mouth on a baseplate wax base and adjusted for esthetics. Ready-made plastic backings may be used, which become part of the pattern for the partial denture framework, and the teeth are then ultimately cemented to the denture framework. Esthetically these are less satisfactory than other types of anterior teeth, but they have the advantage of greater strength and are easily replaced. A record of the mold and shade of each tooth should be kept, and only the ridge lap of the replacement teeth need to be ground to fit. When replaceability is the main reason for its use, the stock facing should not be beveled, or difficulty will be encountered in replacing it. Replacement also may be accomplished by waxing and pro-

cessing a resin facing directly to the metal backing. Stock tube or side-groove teeth are not ordinarily used for anterior teeth on partial dentures because of the horizontal forces that tend to dislodge them.

5. The denture pattern may include anterior teeth hollowed out to receive resin veneers, the same as for veneer crowns and veneer pontics on fixed partial dentures. This is most applicable when the denture framework is to be cast in gold. Then labial surfaces may be waxed and the final carving for esthetics done in the mouth. A modification of this method is the waxing of the veneer coping on a previously cast gold base. These are then cast separately and attached to the framework by soldering. Esthetically the result is comparable to that obtained with resin veneer crowns. This method is particularly applicable when there is a desire to make the replaced teeth match adjacent veneered abutment crowns.

WAXING AND INVESTING THE PARTIAL DENTURE PRIOR TO PROCESSING RESIN BASES OR ATTACHMENTS

Waxing the partial denture base. Waxing the partial denture base prior to investing differs little from the waxing of a complete denture; the only difference is the waxing to and around exposed parts of the metal framework. Here, undercut finishing lines should be provided whenever possible. Then the waxing is merely butted to the finishing line with a little excess to allow for finishing. Otherwise, small voids in the wax may become filled with investing plaster, or fine edges of the investment may break off during boilout and packing. In either case, small pieces of investment may become embedded in the resin at the finishing lines. This is avoided by slightly overwaxing and then finishing the resin back to the metal finishing line with finishing burs. Abrasive wheels and discs should not be used for this purpose, as they will cut into the metal and may burn the resin. Pumice and a rag wheel should be used sparingly for polishing because it will cut the resin more rapidly than the metal and leave the finishing line elevated above the adjacent resin.

When waxing to polished metal parts not possessing a finishing line, it must be remem-

bered that no attachment will exist and that over a period of time there inevitably will be some seepage, separation, and discoloration of the resin in this area. This may be avoided to some extent by roughening the metal whenever possible to effect some mechanical attachment. The wax should be left thick enough so that the resin will have some bulk at its junction with the polished metal. Thin films of resin over metal should be avoided, and, in finishing, these should be cut back to an area of bulk with finishing burs. Otherwise any thin film of resin will eventually separate and become discolored and unclean due to marginal seepage.

Gingival form should be waxed in accordance with modern concepts of cosmetics and should be made as self-cleansing as possible. The dental student should familiarize himself with normal gingival architecture as found on diagnostic casts of natural dentition, beginning with the casts of each other's mouths usually made in basic technique exercises. In this manner he may have a better concept of gingival contours to be reproduced on prosthetic restorations.

In general, students and technicians alike seem to lack a clear concept of natural gingival architecture and are prone to leave too much tooth embedded in wax. Artificial teeth ordinarily should be uncovered fully to expose all the anatomic crown and even beyond when gingival recession is to be simulated. Relatively few prosthodontic patients are in an age bracket in which some gingival recession and exposed cementum would not normally be present, and this should be simulated on prosthodontic restorations in proportion to the patient's age. With partial dentures, gingival contours around the remaining natural teeth should be used as a guide to the gingival contours to be reproduced on the prosthesis. However, interproximal spaces are most always filled, particularly between posterior artificial teeth.

Frush has listed the following rules for varying the height of the gingival tissue at the cervical portion of the teeth:

(a) Slightly below the high lip line at the central incisors.
(b) Lower than the central incisor gum line [gingival margin] at the lateral incisors.
(c) Higher than the central or lateral incisor gum line [gingival margin] at the canine.

(d) Slightly lower than the canine at the premolar and variable for both premolars and molars.*

The correctly formed interdental papilla should be formed so that it will be self-cleansing. It should be carved so that it is in harmony with the interpretation of age and will be the deciding factor in the visible outline form of the tooth. As Frush has pointed out, even a drop of wax properly placed can change the appearance of a square tooth to one of tapering or ovoid appearance. A properly formed interdental papilla further enhances the natural appearance by increasing the color in this area.

The rules for forming the interdental papilla are given by Frush as follows:

(a) The papilla must extend to the point of tooth contact for cleanliness.
(b) The papillae must be of various lengths.
(c) The interdental papilla must be convex in all directions.
(d) The papillae must be shaped according to the age of the patient.
(e) The papilla must end near the labial face of the tooth and never slope inward to terminate toward the lingual portion of the interproximal surface.*

The denture should be waxed and carved as for a cast restoration, which it actually is, regardless of the material to be used or the method of processing. The fact that a split-mold technique is used for processing does not alter the fact that the form of the denture base is to be reproduced by a casting procedure. Therefore the denture pattern should be waxed with care in the same form as that desired for the finished restoration rather than attempting to shape facial contours on the prosthesis during the polishing phase (Fig. 17-49). Polishing should consist primarily of trimming away the flash, stippling polished surfaces when desired, and polishing lightly with brush wheels and pumice, followed by final polishing with a soft brush wheel and a nonabrasive shining agent such as "whiting." Gross trimming and polishing with pumice should not be necessary if the denture has been properly waxed prior to investing.

Since the polished surfaces of any denture

---

*From Frush, J. P.: Dentogenic restorations and dynesthetics, Los Angeles, 1957, Swissdent Foundation.

Fig. 17-49. A, Interdental papillae are convex and extend to contact points of adjacent teeth on a complete maxillary denture to simulate naturalness. Root indices were carved in wax before denture was processed. Stippling was accomplished with an eccentric No. 6 round bur. **B,** Buccal flange of a removable partial denture base is similarly treated as in **A.** Finishing of acrylic resin bases is simplified by careful waxing, carving, and investing prior to processing.

play an important part in both retention and the control of the food bolus, buccal and lingual contours generally should be made concave. Border thickness of the denture should be left as recorded in the impression. The only exceptions are the distolingual aspect of the lower denture base to avoid interference with the tongue, and the distobuccal aspect of the upper denture base to avoid interference with the coronoid process of the mandible. These are the only areas that cannot ordinarily be waxed to final contour before investing and may need to be thinned *by the dentist* at the time of final polishing.

Investing the partial denture. In investing a partial denture for processing a resin base, it must be remembered that the denture cast must be recovered from the flask intact for remounting. The practice of cutting the teeth off the cast to expose the connectors and retainers, which are then embedded in the upper half of the flask, is permissible only when an existing denture base is being relined and no provision has been made for remounting. (In such case, it seems that this practice has no advantage over investing the denture being so relined upside-down in the lower half of the flask.) Since some increase in vertical dimension has, in the past, been inevitable in any split-mold processing technique, this method results in the denture framework's being raised from the supporting teeth by the amount of increase. Whereas occlusal adjustment in the mouth may temporarily reestablish a harmonious occlusal relation with the opposing teeth, the denture framework must then settle into sup-

porting contact with the abutment teeth at the expense of the underlying ridge.

Changes in vertical dimension may be held to a minimum by using denture resins that can be placed in the mold in a fluid rather than a doughy state or those that may be injected in a fluid state into a closed mold. Dimensional changes occurring during relining may also be held to a minimum by using cold-curing resins for this purpose, thus avoiding the thermal expansion of a mold subjected to elevated temperatures.

When two opposing partial dentures are being made concurrently, one is sometimes processed and placed first and then the final occlusion established on the second denture to a fully restored arch. In such case, when there are no natural teeth in opposition, it is not necessary that the first denture be remounted after processing. In all other cases, remounting to correct for errors in occlusion is absolutely necessary. Flasking must be accomplished so that the cast may be recovered from the flask undamaged.

Since the partial denture impression (fluid-wax) may not be boxed prior to pouring the cast, metal mounting plates cannot be used as with complete denture impressions. Adding a mounting plate later with additional stone is not dependable, because if the cast separates between the two layers of stone, the mounting record is lost. The base of the stone cast must therefore be keyed by beveling and notching on at least three sides.

Minute voids in the base of the cast will have been reproduced in the stone-mounting, and although the obvious larger blebs

Fig. 17-50. Base of cast has been covered with 0.001 inch tin-foil prior to investing cast and denture for processing. Base of cast will be free of investing stone when recovered from processing flask and may be conveniently returned to original stone mounting on articulator for occlusal corrections or to preserve original face-bow mounting of a maxillary cast.

Fig. 17-51. **A,** Class I mandibular denture invested in lower half of flask. Master cast upon which denture will be processed is completely covered with investing stone, exposing only artificial teeth and waxed denture bases. There are *no* undercuts in invested lower half of flask, thus assuring separation of flask halves after investment procedure is completed. **B,** Maxillary Class I denture invested in lower half of an investing flask.

may be trimmed away, smaller blebs will remain. If the voids in the cast become filled with investing material, the effect is two particles trying to occupy the same space. This may be prevented by covering the base with tinfoil prior to investing (Fig. 17-50). By coating the base and sides of the cast with petroleum jelly, tinfoil may be easily adapted by burnishing it on with a towel. Not only does this keep the base of the cast isolated from investing material, but the cast also may be more easily recovered from the surrounding investment.

After tinfoiling has been done, the remainder of the cast should be coated with some reliable separator, such as mineral oil, petroleum jelly, sodium silicate, or tinfoil substitute. The entire cast, except for the wax and teeth, may then be invested in the lower half of the flask (Fig. 17-51). As with a complete denture only the supplied teeth and wax are left exposed to be invested in the upper half. Also, as with a complete denture, the investment in the lower half must be smooth and free of undercuts and must be coated with a separator to facilitate separation of the two halves of the flask.

An alternate and preferred procedure is to invest the cast only to the top of the tinfoiled base, smoothing the investment and applying a reliable separator. Then, a second layer of investment is placed around the anatomic portion of the cast, covering the natural teeth and the exposed parts of the denture framework. This is likewise smoothed and made free of undercuts and coated with a separator prior to pouring the top half of the flask. Recovery of the cast is thus made easier by having a shell of investment over the anatomic portion of the cast, which may be removed separately.

When the denture base is to be characterized by applying tinted resins to the mold, care should be taken not to embed the wax border in the lower half of the flask. Bennett has pointed out the need for investing only to the border of the wax, leaving the entire surface to be tinted reproduced in the upper half of the flask. With this precaution, tinting may be carried all the way to the border, and later removal of the flask will not mar the tinted surface. If tinting is not to be done or is to be done only at the cervical margins of the teeth and the interdental papillae, the wax border should be embedded in the lower half where it may be faithfully reproduced and preserved during polishing.

The use of resin materials that require trial packing is complicated by the presence of the retentive framework of the partial denture. With their use, trial packing must be done with a sheet of cellophane between two layers of the resin dough; otherwise the flask could not be opened without pulling the resin away from either the teeth in one half of the flask or the metal framework in the other. Resin dough is placed in each half of the flask, the sheet of cellophane placed between them, and the flask closed for trial packing. The flask is then opened, the cellophane removed, and the excess flash trimmed away. Final closure is then effected without the intervening sheet of cellophane.

Resin materials that require no trial packing have been developed. These are mixed as usual but are either poured into the mold or placed in the mold in a soft state. They offer little or no resistance to closure of the flask, yet the finished product is comparable to resin materials packed in a doughy state. They must be used in some excess, with the excess escaping between the halves of the flask. Although they are soft enough to allow the escape of gross excess, the use of a land space is advisable to avoid a thin film on the land area. Any film existing on the land area after deflasking may be interpreted as an opening of the flask by that amount, hence the need for some provision for an intervening space to accommodate the excess and to facilitate its escape as the flask is closed.

To provide such a land space the land area on the lower half of the flask may be painted with melted baseplate wax before the top half is poured. After wax elimination a space then remains to accommodate any excess resin remaining after the flask is completely closed. It is necessary that no plaster or wax be allowed to remain on the rim of the flask and that the flask make metal-to-metal contact before the second half is poured. Only in this way is it possible to see that the flask is completely closed prior to its being placed in the curing unit.

The pouring of the top half of the flask follows the same procedure as with a complete denture. Whereas it is not absolutely necessary that the entire top half be poured in

stone, it is necessary that a stone cap of some type be used to prevent tooth movement in an occlusal direction. This is due to the inability of plaster to withstand closing pressures. All plaster remaining on the occlusal surfaces of the teeth should be removed and a separator added before the stone cap is poured to facilitate its removal during deflasking. If the use of stone investment is preferred, a shell of improved stone or die stone may be painted or applied with the fingers onto the wax and teeth and this allowed to harden before the remainder of the flask is filled with plaster. If a full stone investment is preferred, some provision should be made for easy separation during deflasking. Not only should a separator stone cap be used, but metal separators or knife cuts radiating out to the walls of the flask should also be placed in the partially set stone. Deflasking is then easily accomplished by removing the stone cap and inserting a knife blade between the sections of stone.

Boilout should be deferred until the investing material has set for several hours or, preferably, overnight. Boilout must effectively eliminate all wax residue; therefore an adequate source of clean hot water must be available. Immersion of a flask containing the invested denture in boiling water for five minutes will adequately soften the wax supporting the artificial teeth so that flask halves may be separated and the remaining wax flushed out. After wax elimination with boiling water, the invested denture should be flushed with a solution of grease-dissolving detergent and again with clean boiling water.

Immediately after boilout the warm mold should be painted with a thin film of tinfoil substitute, being careful not to allow it to collect around the cervical portions of the teeth. A second coat should be applied after the first coat has reasonably dried, and packing of the mold should proceed immediately after this film has dried to the touch.

When the master cast for a distal extension partial denture has been repoured from a secondary impression, the supporting "foot" on the retention frame may not necessarily be in contact with the cast. Closing pressure within the flask may distort the unsupported extension of the metal framework, with subsequent rebound on deflasking. The finished denture base will then lack contact with the supporting tissues, resulting in denture rotation about the fulcrum line similar to that occurring after tissue resorption. *To provide support for the distal extension of the metal framework during flask closure, a self-curing resin should be sprinkled or painted around the distal end of the framework and allowed to harden before you proceed with packing the denture resin.*

PROCESSING THE DENTURE

Processing follows the same procedure as that for a complete denture. Denture base characterization may be added just prior to packing. This is most desirable when denture base material will be visible. Posterior resin bases alone ordinarily do not require characterization, but the dentist should select a denture base material that closely resembles the color of the surrounding tissues. The ideal resin base material for partial dentures is therefore one that (1) may be used without trial packing, (2) possesses a shade that is compatible with surrounding tissues, (3) is dimensionally stable and accurate, and (4) is dense and lends itself to polishing.

Layered silicone rubber flasking. There has never been any question concerning the merits of tinfoiling the denture before investing, which results in a tinfoil-lined matrix and eliminates the need for a separating film. The fact remains, however, that the use of a tinfoil substitute has become almost universal.

At best, any tinfoil substitute creates an undesirable film at the gingival margins of the teeth, resulting in microscopic separation between the teeth and the surrounding resin. This may be shown by sectioning a finished denture and by observing the marginal discoloration around the cervical portions of the teeth after several months in the mouth. To some extent, injection molding obviates this objection to the use of a tinfoil substitute—which is one of the principal advantages of injection molding over compression molding.

Since the use of compression molding is widespread and is likely to continue, some method that eliminates the use of a tinfoil substitute is needed. The layered silicone rubber method results in more complete adaptation of the resin around the cervical portions of porcelain teeth and more complete bonding to resin teeth. In addition, denture base tints may be applied directly to the mold without first applying a separating film.

A room-temperature–curing silicone rubber, which has sufficient body and toughness for the purpose, is applied to the wax surface of the denture and over the teeth just before the upper half of the flask is poured. The manufacturer's instructions must be followed as to mixing and time elapsed before the outer stone investment is added to ensure curing and bonding to the overlying investment. Boilout is then completed in the usual way.

A further advantage of the layered silicone rubber method is the ease with which deflasking is accomplished. If the wax carving of the denture has been completed with care prior to flasking, denture tints remain unaltered by unnecessary trimming and polishing of the processed denture.

All resin base materials available up to the present time exhibit some dimensional change, both during processing and in the mouth. The fit of the denture is therefore dependent, to a large extent, on the accuracy, or lack of accuracy, of the denture base material, since impression and cast materials in use today are themselves reasonably accurate. In an attempt to minimize dimensional changes in the denture base, materials and techniques are constantly being improved. Some of these use injection molding to provide a continuous source of material to the mold as curing shrinkage occurs. One technique utilizes hydraulic pressure within the top half of the flask to limit the shrinkage toward the cast only. It is claimed, by the originator of this technique, that processing by any other means results in both a distorted mold and a distorted cast, because of collapse of the stone or plaster around the myriad of small air voids inevitably present.

Denture base materials that may be poured into the mold or placed into the mold in a soft state are being used. This technique eliminates trial packing and excessive pressures, which leads to open flasks and altered vertical dimension, as is sometimes experienced with compression molding of resin base materials. Activated, or cold-curing, resins are frequently used to avoid mold expansion's occurring at higher temperatures. Materials other than acrylic resins are used with various techniques, some of these being styrene, vinyl, and, experimentally, epoxy resins. The main objective behind the development of newer techniques and materials is greater dimensional accuracy and stability, combined with strength and better appearance.

The study of the history of denture base materials is a most interesting one that has been covered elsewhere in dental literature. The future of denture base materials promises to be just as fascinating a study, but such a discussion cannot be included within the scope of this book. With newer materials the future of methyl methacrylate as a denture base material is uncertain despite its acceptance as the best material available for this purpose since its introduction in 1937. Although it has made possible the stimulation of natural tissue color and contours combined with ease of manipulation, the fact remains that it leaves much to be desired as far as accuracy and dimensional stability are concerned. Whether other and newer materials will eventually supplant methyl methacrylate as a denture base material remains to be seen. The fact is that the denture base of the future (1) must be capable of accurately reproducing natural tissue tones faithfully through the use of characterizing stains and customizing procedures and (2) must not require elaborate processing procedures and equipment, which would make the cost prohibitive for general usage.

REMOUNTING AND OCCLUSAL CORRECTION TO AN OCCLUSAL TEMPLATE

As long as dimensional changes continue to occur during the processing of resin denture bases or the resin attachment of teeth to metal bases, the processed denture will need to be remounted on the articulating instrument for correction of the altered occlusion. Even with improved denture base materials and processing techniques, some movement of artificial teeth will still occur due to the dimensional instability of the wax in which the artificial teeth were arranged. Until both sources of error can be eliminated, remounting will continue to be necessary.

The only alternate to remounting is the correction of the occlusion in the mouth. As has been discussed previously, the limitations to doing so successfully depend on the number of teeth involved, the stability of the denture bases, the accessibility of the occlusion, and the ability of the dentist to interpret and correct occlusal discrepancies.

How well the occlusion may be perfected by remounting will depend on the manner in which jaw relations were transferred to an instrument and how closely the instrument is capable of reproducing functional occlusion. But even though the articulator is capable of reproducing only a static centric relation, that relation at least should be reestablished prior to placement of the denture.

Whereas it is admitted that there are limitations to the perfection of eccentric occlusion in the mouth, some believe that it can be done with more accuracy than on an instrument that is incapable of reproducing eccentric positions. Correction for errors in centric occlusion, however, should not be included in this philosophy, for such is based on a premise that centric occlusion may be established satisfactorily by intraoral adjustment, followed then by a perfecting of eccentric occlusion. Because of denture instability and the inaccessibility of the occlusion for analysis, this is presuming more than anyone can justify. Even occlusal adjustment of natural dentition, in which each tooth has its own support, can best be done when preceded by an analysis of articulated diagnostic casts.

One cardinal premise must be accepted if prosthetic dentistry is to be anything more than a haphazard procedure. This is *that it is possible to transfer centric jaw relation to an instrument with accuracy and to maintain this relation throughout the fabrication of the prosthesis.* If this is true, then centric occlusion—coinciding either with centric jaw relation or with centric occlusion of the remaining natural teeth, or both—must have been established prior to initial placement of the prosthesis. This means that occlusal correction by remounting after final processing is an absolute necessity to the success of the restoration.

Remounting after processing is accomplished by returning the cast to a keyed relationship with the articulator mounting. Whereas the use of metal mounting plates attached to both surfaces may be desirable, it is not practical to do so with a partial denture cast. Stone to stone, properly keyed and free of debris, provides a sufficiently accurate surface for remounting.

A simple procedure, which greatly enhances the accuracy of the remounting surfaces, is the making of a stone split cast. After beveling and keying the base of the master cast, a separating film is applied and the inverted cast is encircled with a strip of lead boxing material. A thin layer of hard stone of a different color is then vibrated onto the base of the cast, and the exposed surface is left purposely uneven. Paper clips or washers may be partially embedded for added retention. After this thin layer of stone has hardened, it is attached to the articulator with mounting stone. Separation of the cast from the articulator and any subsequent remounting are then accomplished with opposing stone surfaces, resulting in greater accuracy.

It is most important that the mounting surfaces be free of particles that would prevent reestablishment of their original relationship. Therefore, tin foil of 0.001 inch thickness should be applied to the base of the cast prior to investing. This is easily accomplished by coating the surface of the cast with petrolatum and then applying the tin foil smoothly with the aid of a cloth towel. The original mounting surface of the cast is thus protected from contamination, and when the tin foil is stripped away after deflasking, the original surface may be returned to its original position. The opposing mounting surface on the articulator should be brushed and blown free of particles and then the base of the cast secured to it with sticky wax or modeling plastic. Stone may then be used for additional security, but only after the cast has first been secured with some reliable thermoplastic material. *A layer of cement, such as Duco cement, should never be used, since it introduces an intervening film that interferes with the accuracy of the remounting.*

Precautions to be taken in remounting. The following precautions should be taken to assure the accuracy of remounting to make final occlusal adjustment prior to the polishing and initial placement of the denture. These apply to all types of occlusal relationship records but are directed particularly to remounting to an occlusal template, when stone vertical stops are used.

1. Make sure that the base of the cast has been reduced before keying and mounting are done, so that it will not have to be altered later to get it into the flask.

2. Bevel the margins of the base of the cast so that it will seat in a definite boxlike manner in the articulator mounting.

3. Notch the posterior and the anterior aspects of the base to assure further its return to its original position. Notches at the margins are preferable to depressions within the base, as the former permit a visual check of the accuracy of the remounting.

4. Lubricate lightly the base and sides of the cast before it is mounted to facilitate its easy removal from the mounting stone.

5. Tinfoil the base and sides of the cast prior to flasking it so that traces of investment will not be present to interfere with remounting.

6. When remounting the cast secure it to the articulator with sticky wax or modeling plastic, followed by stone over both the mounting and the sides of the cast.

7. Before adjusting the occlusion, make certain that no traces of investment remain on the vertical stops.

8. Take care not to abrade the opposing occlusal surface during occlusal adjustment. The use of marking tape or inked ribbon is preferable to articulating paper. The artificial tooth is less likely to cut through and mar the opposing surface, and ink or dye will not build up a false opposing surface, as will the wax from articulating paper.

9. Occlusal readjustment to an occlusal template is complete when the stone vertical stops are again in contact. With other types of articulator mountings, readjustment is complete when the vertical pin is again in contact and any valid horizontal excursions are freed of interference.

Occlusal readjustment, as was the original articulation, is at the expense of the original tooth anatomy. Occlusal surfaces should be reshaped by adding grooves and spillways and by reducing the area of the occlusal table, thus improving the masticating efficiency of the artificial tooth. Although this may be done immediately after occlusal readjustment and prior to initial placement of the denture, it may be deferred until final adjustment has been completed. In any event, it is a necessary step in the completion of any removable prosthesis.

Porcelain teeth may be reshaped with abrasive or diamond mounted points. Plastic teeth lend themselves better to reshaping with small burs to restore functional anat-

Fig. 17-52. **A**, Stock, perforated tray is used to make an irreversible hydrocolloid (alginate) impression of denture and dental arch. Blockout of undercuts in denture base and of tips of direct retainers is necessary so that denture can be readily removed and replaced on a resultant remounting cast, as illustrated in **B**. **B**, Remounting cast poured in stone. Denture can be readily removed and replaced on cast for occlusal correction procedures using an articulator.

omy. Either type should be repolished judiciously to avoid reduction of cuspal contacts. Although cusps may be narrowed, spillways added, and the total area of contact reduced to improve masticating efficiency, critical areas of contact, both vertical and horizontal, must always be preserved.

The term *remounting* is also applied to the mounting of a completed prosthetic restoration back onto an instrument using some kind of interocclusal records. Discrepancies in occlusion resulting from processing of tooth-borne dentures may be corrected by reattaching the indexed processing cast and denture to the same instrument on which the occlusion was formulated. *However, because of some instability inherent in distal extension*

removable partial dentures, such dentures should be recovered from processing investment, finished, and polished for performing occlusal corrections by the use of new intraoral records. A remounting cast must be made by the dentist before occlusal corrections can be accomplished. This is simply done by first placing the denture in the mouth and making an irreversible hydrocolloid (alginate) impression of the denture and remaining teeth in the arch (Fig. 17-52). When the impression is removed, the denture usually will remain in the impression or can be accurately replaced. Undercuts in the denture bases are blocked out, the retentive elements of the framework are covered with a thin layer of molten wax, and a remounting cast is poured in the impression. The remounting casts are then oriented to the articulator by the same type interocclusal records that were used to orient the casts to formulate the occlusion. These procedures will be covered in Chapter 19 as an integral part of the initial placement appointment.

Occlusal harmony must exist before the patient is given possession of the dentures. Delaying the correction of occlusal discrepancies until the dentures have had a chance to settle is not justifiable.

POLISHING THE DENTURE

The areas to be considered in the polishing of a partial denture are (1) the borders of the denture bases, (2) the facial surfaces, and (3) the teeth and adjacent areas.

The borders on full metal bases will have been established previously. On partial metal bases and full resin bases the accuracy with which the border may be finished will depend on the accuracy of the impression record and how well this was preserved on the stone cast. Edentulous areas recorded from impressions in stock trays generally lack the accuracy at the borders that is found on casts made from impressions in individualized trays and by secondary impression methods. Border accuracy is determined also by whether or not the impression recorded a functional or a static relationship of the bordering tissue attachments.

Denture borders. The principal objectives to be considered in making an impression of edentulous areas of a partially edentulous arch are (1) maximum support for the partial denture base and (2) extension of the borders to obtain maximum coverage compatible with moving tissues. Although this second objective may be obtained with an adequate individualized impression tray, it is best accomplished with a secondary impression method. Not only should the *extent* of the border be recorded accurately but also its *width*. Both extent and width as recorded should be preserved on the stone cast. With the exception of certain areas that are arbitrarily thinned in polishing (mentioned previously in this chapter), finishing and polishing the denture borders should consist only of removing any flash and artifactual blebs. Otherwise borders should be left as recorded in the impression.

When the impression is made in a stock tray, both the extent and the width of the border will have been influenced by the tray itself. Some areas will be left short of the total area available for denture support, while others will be extended beyond functional limits by the overextension of the tray. In such areas the technician must interpret the anatomy of the mouth as best he can and arbitrarily trim the denture borders just short of obvious overextension. *This presumes an intimate knowledge of the anatomy of the mouth of the patient for whom the restoration is being made, which the technician does not possess.* Any overextension remaining after arbitrarily trimming the border has to be corrected in the mouth. We prefer to finish the borders of dentures ourselves, having painstakingly developed them during impression procedures.

Facial surfaces. The facial surfaces of the denture base are those polished surfaces lying between the borders and the supplied teeth. Methods have been proposed for making sectional impression records of buccal contours, thereby permitting the denture base to be made to conform to facial musculature. These have never received wide acceptance and may be considered impractical in removable partial prosthodontics.

Facial surfaces may be established in wax or may be carved into the denture base after processing. Generally it is desirable that it be done in wax as part of the wax pattern, both because it is easier to do so and because contours can best be established at a time when additions can be made if desired. Buccal surfaces should be made concave to aid in the retention of the denture by border molding, to preserve the border roll and thereby prevent food impaction, and to facilitate return of the food bolus back onto the masticating table. Lingual surfaces should be made concave to provide tongue room and to aid in the retention of the denture. If such contours are established previously in wax, finishing is not only more easily accomplished but border and gingival areas are also less likely to be inadvertently altered. Polishing of concave surfaces is always more difficult than polishing flat and convex surfaces, and this can largely be avoided by taking care to contour and polish the wax pattern prior to investing.

Finishing gingival and interproximal areas. The contouring of gingival and interproximal areas in the cured resin is difficult and generally unsatisfactory. The practice of doing so dates back to the days when vulcanite rubber was trimmed and shaped with Pearson-type chisels, and a trimming block was a necessary piece of equipment in any dental laboratory. Finishing was done with vulcanite burs and with brush wheels and pumice, creating the vertical interproximal grooves that for many years were typical of the "denture look." Not only is this contrary to modern concepts of denture esthetics but also gingival and interproximal carving of the denture resin around plastic teeth may not be done without some damage to the teeth themselves.

Modern cosmetic considerations demand that gingival carving be done around each tooth individually, with variations in the height of the gingival curve and in the length of the interdental papillae. Interproximally the papillae should be convex rather than concave. The gingival attachment should be free of grooves and ditches that would accumulate debris and stain and should be as free-cleansing as possible. All this precludes gross shaping and trimming of gingival areas *after* processing. Gingival carving should be done in wax, and investing should be done with care to avoid blebs and artifacts. Finishing should consist only of trimming around the teeth and the interdental papillae with small round burs to create a more natural simulation of living tissue, plus light stippling with an off-center round bur for the same reason. Polishing should consist only of light buffing with brush wheels and pumice and finally with a soft brush wheel and a nonabrasive polishing agent such as tin oxide.

Pumicing of gingival areas can only serve to polish the high spots, and although it may be done lightly, its use should be limited to light buffing of areas already made as smooth as possible by other means. Not only does heavy pumicing of the denture resin create a typical "denture look" but it also alters the surface of any plastic teeth present. If pumicing must be done, protect plastic teeth with adhesive tape during the process.

Any polishing operation on a partial denture done on a lathe is made hazardous by the presence of direct retainers, which can easily become caught in the polishing wheel. Although the least damage that might occur is the distortion of a clasp arm, there is a greater possibility that the denture may be thrown forceably into the lathe pan, with serious damage to the framework or other parts of the denture. The technician must be ever conscious of this possibility and must always cover any projecting clasp with the finger while it is near the polishing wheel. In addition, it is wise to keep a pumice pan well filled with wet pumice to cushion the shock should an accident occur. Any other lathe pan used in polishing should be lined with a towel or with a resilient material such as automobile undercoating material for the same reason.

SELF-ASSESSMENT AIDS

1. The dentist not only must be familiar with laboratory procedures but also must be proficient in executing them. True or false?
2. Although certain laboratory procedures may be delegated to a dental laboratory technician, the dentist will not be able to guide, direct, and "trouble shoot" such procedures unless he can perform them himself. True or false?
3. An intimate knowledge of dental materials employed in the construction of removable partial dentures is a must for the dentist. True or false?
4. Duplicate casts are required in many instances in treating partially edentulous patients. Can you name at least three of these instances?
5. What armamentarium and materials are required to duplicate a cast?
6. What is the difference between a reversible and an irreversible hydrocolloid? Which one is most commonly used in duplicating a cast?
7. Is it critical that the duplicating material chosen be compatible with the material from which the duplicate cast will be made?

8. Can you describe a "duplicating flask"?
9. How is reversible hydrocolloid prepared for duplicating purposes? What temperature of the hydrocolloid is sufficient to duplicate a cast?
10. If a blocked-out master cast is being duplicated, what precautions must be exercised to avoid distortion of the blockout material?
11. Can you give a step-by-step procedure for duplicating a stone cast with reversible hydrocolloid?
12. What is the danger of soaking a stone cast in tap water? A cast must be wet prior to duplicating it with hydrocolloid. How is this wetting accomplished?
13. Describe the procedure for recovering an investment cast from a duplicating mold and defend your answer.
14. For what reasons should an investment cast not be trimmed on a cast trimmer?
15. An investment cast on which the pattern for the framework will be developed should be oven dried after it is removed from the duplicating material. At what temperature and for how long?
16. An investment cast should be lightly sprayed with a plastic model spray immediately after drying. Can you give three valid reasons for spraying the cast?
17. You should already know the specifications for all components of a removable partial denture framework. Can you describe a logical order of creating the wax or plastic pattern for a mandibular removable partial denture framework to which a wrought-wire retainer arm will be attached?
18. What is meant by an anatomic replica pattern and where is it used?
19. How would you go about making an anatomic replica pattern? Does it have advantages over a free-hand pattern?
20. What is the purpose of "spruing" a wax pattern for a removable partial denture framework?
21. There are three general rules that should be followed in spruing any wax or plastic pattern for casting. Do you remember what they are?
22. After the pattern has been sprued, it must be covered with an investment (refractory) material to make a mold for casting. The outer investment must be the same material from which the cast was made. What are the purposes of the outer investment?
23. The casting shrinkage of gold alloys from the molten to the cold state is from _____% to _____%. The casting shrinkage of chromium-cobalt alloys is about _____%.
24. A casting ring, lined with asbestos, is used to confine the outer layer of investment around the pattern. The ring is not removed during

burnout or casting procedures for gold alloys. What is the purpose of the layer of asbestos in the ring?

25. After the investment material for a chromium-cobalt alloy casting has set, the ring is removed before burn out. Why?

26. What are the differences in composition of a refractory material for casting gold alloys and one for casting the high-heat type of chromium-cobalt alloys?

27. Give a step-by-step procedure for investing a sprued pattern that will be cast in gold. In chromium-cobalt alloy.

28. The casting mold is prepared to receive the molten alloy by a process known as "burn-out." Burnout serves three purposes. Can you state the three purposes?

29. Describe a burnout procedure for casting a removable partial denture framework in Type IV gold alloy.

30. Contracture of the mold for plaster-bound refractory investments occurs beyond _____°F.

31. Most refractory investments contain calcium sulfate that begins to break down at _____°F, resulting in a weak and brittle casting.

32. What different methods are used to melt gold alloys for casting? Chromium-cobalt alloys for casting?

33. After the casting is completed, how long should the mold be allowed to bench cool before the mold and casting are plunged in water?

34. What is the purpose of "pickling" a casting? Can you describe a pickling procedure?

35. If the wax pattern for a casting was neatly and properly developed and investing and casting procedures were correctly accomplished, finishing the casting should not be a time-consuming procedure. How would you finish a gold alloy removable partial denture framework. A chromium-cobalt alloy framework?

36. Describe a hardening heat treatment for a Type IV gold alloy framework.

37. Record bases, trial denture bases, and individual impression trays are conveniently made of autopolymerizing acrylic resin. What is an autopolymerizing acrylic resin and how does it differ from a heat-cured acrylic resin?

38. Record bases or trial denture bases should be fabricated by a "sprinkle on" technique using autopolymerizing acrylic resin, whereas individual or customized impression trays may be fabricated by "adapted" autopolymerizing acrylic resin. For what reason or reasons are the processes different?

39. Do you recall the procedures for making individualized acrylic resin impression trays as given in Chapter 14?

40. If you use a secondary or altered cast impression tray for a mandibular distal extension denture, you will attach an individualized tray to the framework. Can you give a step-by-step procedure for making such a tray?

41. Record bases and occlusion rims are necessary to record maxillomandibular relations for Class I and II arches and in Class III arches with long edentulous spans. Can you describe a step-by-step procedure for making record bases by the "sprinkle on" method to mount diagnostic casts?

42. A record base is attached to the framework for a distal extension mandibular denture and is made after the secondary impression has been made and recovery of the master cast. Could you make such a record base?

43. What purpose does an occlusion rim serve?

44. If an occlusion rim represents the missing teeth and supporting structures in a partially edentulous arch, should the occlusion rims be wider than the occlusal surfaces of the teeth they are replacing? Should occlusion rims not occupy the same position (bucco-lingually) the missing teeth occupied? There are several advantages to correctly proportioned occlusion rims as opposed to badly proportioned occlusion rims. Know what these advantages are?

45. Artificial posterior teeth were arranged on mandibular and maxillary trial bases (record) of acrylic resin attached to the respective frameworks. The arrangement was acceptable and approved. What procedures must now take place prior to the final arrangement of teeth and development of the external forms of the bases for processing?

46. Except around metal portions of the framework, should there be any difference in developing gingival contours, root indices, interdental papillae, lingual contours of individual teeth, and so on for removable partial denture bases and complete denture bases?

47. A partial denture must be so invested for processing acrylic resin bases that the processed denture and its cast can be recovered from the flask intact and unmarred. This procedure will facilitate and simplify correction of occlusal discrepancies due to processing. True or false?

48. Prior to investing the master cast and waxed denture in the lower half of a flask, what should be done to the base of the cast to facilitate recovery of the cast and remounting procedures?

49. After the processing flask containing the invested denture has been separated and residual wax flushed out, and a tinfoil substitute correctly applied, there is one observation that must be made and dealt with in regard to

the minor connector for attaching the resin base and its relation to the residual ridge. What is this observation and how is it dealt with before acrylic resin is packed in the mold?

50. Discrepancies in occlusion as a result of processing may be corrected by returning the processed denture and cast (intact) to the instrument on which the occlusion was developed—provided the dentures are tooth borne or the occlusion was developed using an occlusal template. Can you describe this type of process for correcting occlusal discrepancies?

51. Correction of occlusal discrepancies for distal extension dentures should be accomplished by an entirely different procedure than the above procedure. This procedure is described in Chapter 19.

52. Finishing and polishing the removable partial denture may be accomplished in the same manner as for a complete denture. However, polishing the removable partial denture on a lathe is made more hazardous because of the presence of _____.

18 WORK AUTHORIZATIONS FOR REMOVABLE PARTIAL DENTURES

A work authorization is a written direction for laboratory procedures to be performed in the fabrication of dental restorations. The responsibility of a dentist to the public and his profession in safeguarding the quality of prosthodontic services is discharged, in part, through meaningful work authorizations. Properly executed, they provide the means for increased professional satisfaction in a removable partial denture service.

A work authorization by a dentist is the same as granting "power of attorney"; it grants authority for others to act in his behalf. It bears the same relationship to a dental laboratory technician as the sextant does to a navigator—it plots his course.

Work authorizations are effective channels of communication when properly executed. They enhance the quality of the completed restorations by eliminating stereotyped production, and in its place provide for individually, scientifically considered prostheses.

WORK AUTHORIZATION

Content. The information contained in a work authorization should include (1) name and address of the dental laboratory, (2) name and address of the dentist originating the work authorization, (3) date of the work authorization, (4) identification of the patient, (5) desired completion date of the request, (6) specific instructions, (7) signature of the dentist, and (8) registered license number of the dentist. All these requirements can be accommodated in a simply designed form (Fig. 18-1).

Function. The following four important functions are performed by a work authorization: (1) It furnishes definite instructions for the laboratory procedures to be accomplished and establishes the acceptable minimum of quality for the services rendered. (2) It provides a means of protecting the public from the illegal practice of dentistry. (3) It is a protective document for both the dentist and dental laboratory technician if they become participants in a lawsuit to resolve matters between them. (4) It completely delineates the responsibilities of the dentist and the dental laboratory technician.

Characteristics. A work authorization must be legible, clear, concise, and readily understood. It is unreasonable to assume that laboratory technicians are decoding experts. Sufficient information must be included in a work authorization to enable the technician to study and execute the request. Many dentists are overly presumptive in assuming that a request can be acceptably fulfilled without proper directions.

It is sound practice to provide the dental laboratory technician with adequate written instructions for each required laboratory service in the construction of a restoration. Therefore a new work authorization should accompany the material returned to the laboratory for continuing progress in completing the restoration. In a modern dental practice it is highly improbable that a "one trip" laboratory service is adequate to provide a truly professional removable restoration.

No single work authorization form is adequate to furnish detailed instructions for accomplishing the laboratory phases in the construction of removable partial dentures, crowns and fixed partial dentures, and complete dentures or for accomplishing orthodontic laboratory procedures. Inherent differences in the many types of restorations themselves and differences in the laboratory phases necessary for their construction establish a requirement for individual work authorization forms.

DENTISTRY 16

WORK AUTHORIZATION – REMOVABLE PARTIAL DENTURES
University of Florida College of Dentistry

To: _____ Date: _____

From: _____

Patient Identification: _____

General Request: _____

_____

Date and Time Required: _____

Alloy for Framework: (specific by trade name) _____

Denture Base: (   ) Acrylic Resin   (   ) Metal   (   ) Combination

　　Specific by Trade Name: _____

Tooth Selection:

　　Anterior:　Make _____ Mold _____ Shade _____

　　Posterior:　Make _____ Mold _____ Shade _____

Specific Instructions: _____

_____

_____

_____

_____

_____

_____

_____

_____

_____

COLOR CODE ON CAST: Design – Green; Survey Lines – Black; Finishing Lines – Red
PLEASE WAX TO FOLLOWING SPECIFICATIONS – TYPE "D" GOLD: COBALT-CHROME IN PARENTHESIS

1. Lingual Bar – 6 GA. ½ Pear ι 24 GA. Sheet
2. Anterior, Posterior, and Single Palatal Bars – Two 26(28) GA. Sheet
3. Linguoplate Aprons ⎫
　 Cast Bases 　　　　⎬ 24 GA. Sheet
　 Full Palatal Castings ⎭
4. Guiding Plane Minor Connector – 22 GA. Sheet
5. Indirect Retainer – 10 GA. ½ RD. Strip

6. Wrought Wire Components – 18 GA. RD. Type II Wire
7. Finishing Lines – 12 GA. ½ RD. Strip Inverted
8. Direct Retainers – Molars, Large Plastic Patterns; Premolars and Canines, Medium Plastic Patterns
9. Master Cast Relief for Retention Mesh – One 20 GA. Sheet
10. Base Retention Mesh – 12 GA. ½ RD. Strip
11. Borders for Cast Base – 14 GA. RD. Strip

Student Dentist's Sig. _____ Instr. Sig. & No. _____

Fig. 18-1. Work authorization form used in undergraduate clinic designed specifically for removable partial dentures to furnish detailed information to laboratory technician. It is available in tablet form so that a carbon copy of work authorization can be conveniently made. Original copy is white and goes to laboratory technician. Carbon copy is yellow and is retained in files of dentist.

DENTISTRY 16

WORK AUTHORIZATION – REMOVABLE PARTIAL DENTURES
University of Florida College of Dentistry

To: *Central Laboratory UFCD*   Date: *6-11-76*

From: *John Resin Stn. # 92*

Patient Identification: *# 406*

General Request: *Please fabricate a maxillary removable partial denture framework*

Date and Time Required: *6-18-76 10 a.m.*

Alloy for Framework: (specific by trade name) *Jelenko # 7 gold*

Denture Base: ( ) Acrylic Resin   ( ) Metal   ( ) Combination

   Specific by Trade Name: _____

Tooth Selection:

   Anterior: Make _____ Mold _____ Shade _____

   Posterior: Make _____ Mold _____ Shade _____

Specific Instructions: *Orient master cast to surveyor by tripod marks. Block out all undercuts parallel to path of placement (except retentive terminals). Provide indices to transfer design to refractory cast. Wax pattern to below specs. Cast and finish. ANATOMIC REPLICA PATTERN. Please return finished framework and blocked out master cast. Thank you.*

COLOR CODE ON CAST: Design – Green; Survey Lines – Black; Finishing Lines – Red
PLEASE WAX TO FOLLOWING SPECIFICATIONS – TYPE "D" GOLD: COBALT-CHROME IN PARENTHESIS

1. Lingual Bar – 6 GA. ½ Pear i 24 GA. Sheet
2. Anterior, Posterior, and Single Palatal Bars – Two 26(28) GA. Sheet
3. Linguoplate Aprons
   Cast Bases   } 24 GA. Sheet
   Full Palatal Castings }
4. Guiding Plane Minor Connector – 22 GA. Sheet
5. Indirect Retainer – 10 GA. ½ RD. Strip

6. Wrought Wire Components – 18 GA. RD. Type II Wire
7. Finishing Lines – 12 GA. ½ RD. Strip Inverted
8. Direct Retainers – Molars, Large Plastic Patterns; Premolars and Canines, Medium Plastic Patterns
9. Master Cast Relief for Retention Mesh – One 20 GA. Sheet
10. Base Retention Mesh – 12 GA. ½ RD. Strip
11. Borders for Cast Base – 14 GA. RD. Strip

Student Dentist's Sig. *John Resin #92*   Instr. Sig. & No *A.E. Maser 116*

Fig. 18-2. This work authorization accompanies master cast upon which *dentist* has designed and drawn outline for removable partial denture framework. It is simple and non-time-consuming to execute, yet furnishes detailed information so that request can be properly fulfilled.

DEFINITIVE INSTRUCTIONS BY WORK AUTHORIZATIONS

Work authorization forms may be designed so that only a minimum of writing is necessary to relay thorough instructions (Fig. 18-2). The form can contain printed listings of materials and specifications that require either a *check mark* or a *fill-in* for authorizing their use.

A reminder space to designate the choice of metal for the framework is included. Frameworks for removable partial dentures are usually cast in either a type "D" gold or a chrome-cobalt alloy. The nature of the material of the denture base may be indicated by check mark. It is difficult to elicit this information from the markings on master casts.

Space is reserved on the work authorization form to furnish the technician with information on the dentist's selection of teeth. The responsibility for tooth selection must remain with the dentist. Success of the removable partial denture partly depends on the consideration given to the size, number, and placement of the artificial teeth as well as the material from which they are made.

A display of courtesy deserved by, and a demonstration of respect for, the laboratory technician are indicated. The general request is prefaced by *please* and the specific instructions are ended with *thank you*. Do any other three words promote better relations?

A good work authorization form not only assures clarity, but it also simplifies correct execution. Figures can be provided on which diagrams may be drawn to enhance written descriptions when necessary. These diagrams may show the occlusal and lingual surfaces of the posterior teeth and the lingual surfaces of the anterior teeth. The palatal region of the upper dental arch and the lingual slopes of the mandibular alveolar ridge also can be included. These features allow a clear, diagrammatic representation of the location of major connectors, which will complement the outline of the framework on the master cast.

A color code index can be used to explain the markings on the master cast when it is submitted to the laboratory for the fabrication of a framework. A green pencil is used to outline the framework; red designates the desired location of finishing lines on the framework; and black lines denote the height of contour on teeth and soft tissues created during the survey of the cast. The color code eliminates confusion in interpreting the markings on the master cast.

Specifications for waxing the framework components for gold or chrome-cobalt alloy castings must be furnished the technician and are an integral part of the work authorization form. Specifications that are adequate for most removable partial denture frameworks may be listed. This feature alone saves time and effort in preparing the work authorization and *is also a handy reference for the laboratory technician*. The listing of average specifications does not preclude altering a specification when the situation requires other characteristics in a given component.

The specific instructions in a work authorization must be so constructed that they will be a constant source of direction and supervision for the laboratory phases of a removable partial denture service. Instructions should leave no doubt of the dentist's requirements in a request for laboratory services. It is foolish to use undercut dimensions of 0.25 to 0.50 mm (0.01 to 0.02 in) when surveying a master cast unless directions for incorporating these dimensions in the finished framework are included.

Work authorization blanks should be available in tablet form so that a carbon duplicate can be conveniently made, supplying a copy for both the dentist and the dental laboratory technician. The original may be of a different color than is the carbon copy for ready identification.

LEGAL ASPECTS OF WORK AUTHORIZATIONS

No national statutory restrictions exist on dental laboratory operations. Regulation of dental laboratories and dental laboratory technicians is invested in the states. Fortunately all states exercise this control.

Interpretations of acts constituting the practice of dentistry are moderately uniform. However, statutory restrictions on dental laboratory operations vary widely from state to state in stringency and requirements for legal operations.

Prosecution and conviction of persons engaged in the illegal practice of dentistry is a time-consuming and difficult proceeding. This situation could be alleviated if duly executed work authorizations were required to be presented by all dental laboratories or dental technicians on demand of a duly authorized agency.

Many states require that work authorizations be made in duplicate and that both the dentist and dental laboratory technician retain a copy for a period of two years or more from the date of the work authorization. Thus documents are available to substantiate or refute claims and counterclaims concerning the illegal practice of dentistry or to aid in the settlement of misunderstandings between a dentist and a dental laboratory technician.

DELINEATION OF RESPONSIBILITIES BY WORK AUTHORIZATIONS

The dentist is responsible for all phases of a removable partial denture service in the strict sense of the word. He may request the dental laboratory technician to perform certain mechanical phases of the service; *however, the laboratory technician is responsible to the dentist and never to the patient.* A dentist who relegates the design of a removable partial denture to a less qualified individual immediately eliminates the opportunity for a preventive removable partial denture service.

A dentist who imposes on auxiliary personnel responsibilities that are legally and morally his own does a great injustice to his patients, his technicians, and the dental profession. There is little doubt that the illegal practice of dentistry and the presently existing impasse between dentist and some dental laboratory technicians are due, in part, to many individual dentists' imposing unrealistic responsibility on their laboratory technicians. Furthermore, this unwelcome relationship is partly due to the submission of poor impressions, casts, records, and instructions to the laboratory technician with the demand of impossible quality in the returned restoration under threat of economic boycott.

Most dental laboratory technicians are ethical and earnestly desire to contribute their talents to the dental profession. The dental profession is vitally interested in increasing the numbers of serious-minded dental auxiliary personnel to share in providing oral health. However, until such time as the dental profession elevates itself in the eyes of

laboratory technicians and also elevates the stature of dental laboratory technology, greater availability of responsible auxiliary personnel is more fancied than real.

The dental laboratory technician is a member of a team whose objectives are the prevention of oral disease and the maintenance of oral health as adjuncts to the physical and mental well-being of the public. A good dental laboratory technician is a valuable asset to the dentist and contributes much to the team effort in providing oral health for patients. To paraphrase statements by Dr. G. P. Smith, the degree and quality of the team effort is the responsibility of the dentist and depends on his knowledge, experience, technical skill, administrative ability, integrity, and ability to communicate effectively.

Much of the laboratory phase of a removable partial denture service may be delegated by a dentist. Work authorizations help to fulfill the moral obligation to supervise and direct those technical phases that can be accomplished by dental laboratory technicians.

There are substantial indications that many members of the dental profession either are not cognizant of the rewards of writing good work authorizations or are not proficient in their execution. It is not a secret that some dentists submit no instructions when availing themselves of commercial dental laboratory services.

If the practice of prosthodontics is to remain in the control of dentists, each member of the dental profession must avoid delegating responsibility to those who are less qualified to accept the responsibility.

Movements to legalize illegal dentistry (denturism) are seemingly becoming more prevalent and are being instituted by ill-advised and uninformed persons. Perhaps this current trend could have been avoided had dentists expended as much effort to communicate with technicians in the past as they are now to prevent illegal dentistry.

SELF-ASSESSMENT AIDS

1. What is a work authorization?
2. What are the national (U.S.) statutory regulations regarding work authorizations?
3. Work authorizations go by different names in various parts of the country, such as work order or work order form. What is it called in your state?
4. Do you know of any state dental practice acts that do not include a requirement for

work authorizations from dentists to dental laboratory technicians?

5. Are work authorizations legal documents?

6. Properly executed work authorizations are effective channels of communication between a dentist and a dental laboratory technician. What accrues to a dentist who always furnishes his dental laboratory or dental laboratory technician a clear work authorization?

7. The contents of a properly executed work authorization will include eight categories of transmitted data. Do you know what information these eight areas include?

8. A dental work authorization performs four distinct functions. What are they?

9. If you were a dental laboratory technician, what characteristics would you like to see in a work authorization from a dentist?

10. A dentist has a responsibility to his patient and to the dental laboratory technician. A dental laboratory technician has a responsibility to the dentist, never to a patient. True or false?

11. If you, the dentist, present clear instructions and other information to a good dental laboratory technician, should you not expect to receive quality performed laboratory services? What would you expect if your instructions were vague?

12. Whose responsibility is it to select artificial teeth, denture base materials, and metal alloys for frameworks—The dentist or the technician?

13. Would you believe that the definitive instructions contained on a work authorization form have been reduced to "make partial" by some dentists? Believe it!

14. Do you feel that a dentist must be responsible for the physical characteristics of framework components? If so, how do you relate your requirements or specifications to the dental laboratory technician?

15. A work authorization, properly executed, will delineate responsibilities. Can you expand this statement in your own words?

16. Do you consider a dental laboratory technician a dental health team member?

17. Should you and your dental laboratory technician have some differences over work returned from the laboratory, would you "second thought" your work authorization for the returned work?

18. Why do states require that a copy of the work authorization be retained by the dentist and dental laboratory technician for certain lengths of time?

19. Do you feel that the words "please" and "thank you" have a place in writing authorizations?

20. Take a good look at the work authorization forms illustrated in this chapter. Do you have suggestions for their improvement?

19 INITIAL PLACEMENT, ADJUSTMENT, AND SERVICING OF THE REMOVABLE PARTIAL DENTURE

Initial placement of the completed partial denture, the fifth phase of service, should never be sandwiched in between other scheduled appointments. Too often this is done in the appointment for initial placement of both complete and removable partial denture restorations. Both, being removable restorations not requiring the elaborate preparations common to the cementation of fixed restorations, can be quickly placed and the patient dismissed with instructions to return when soreness or discomfort develops. Perhaps this is where the word *patient* originated, because of the patience required in accommodating to a new denture.

Although it is true that this is a necessary part of adjusting to new dentures, many other factors are also pertinent. Among these are how well the patient has been informed as to the mechanical and biologic problems involved in the fabrication and wearing of a removable prosthetic restoration and how much confidence he has acquired in the excellence of the finished product through his own observation of the various steps in its construction. Knowing in advance that every step has been carefully planned and executed with skill and having acquired confidence both in the dentist and in the excellence of the restoration, the patient is better able to accept the adjustment period as a necessary, but transient, step in learning to wear the prosthesis. Much of this confidence can be dissipated when the dentist places the prosthesis with an air of finality as though to imply that "my part in the fabrication of this restoration is now completed. The rest is up to you, including payment of the fee on your way out of the office."

The term *adjustment* has two connotations, each of which must be considered separately. First are the adjustments to the bearing surfaces of the denture and the occlusion made by the dentist at the time of initial placement and thereafter. Second is the adjustment or accommodation by the patient, psychologically and biologically, to the presence of a foreign body, which is to serve as a prosthetic restoration of some missing part or parts of the body, in this particular instance, an oral prosthesis.

It must be presumed that the partial denture has been fabricated with care and that the prosthesis is representative of the best that the dentist is capable of producing. Certainly it is not within the scope of this book to suggest ways and means of adjusting a faulty designed or poorly fabricated prosthesis to fit the patient's mouth. But, as in industry, a casting is rarely, if ever, considered a precision product. Certain machining operations are necessary before the casting is considered finished and acceptable. So it is with a partial denture restoration. First the rough metal alloy casting must be finished and polished to fit an accurate stone cast of the patient's mouth. After the processing of resin bases the occluding teeth must be altered to perfect the occlusal relationship between opposing artificial dentition or between artificial dentition and an opposing cast or template. Denture bases then must be finished to eliminate excess and to perfect the contours of polished surfaces for the best functional and esthetic result. All these are machining operations made necessary by the inadequacies of casting procedures, for actually both the metal and resin parts of a prosthetic restoration are produced by casting methods. Unfortunately such machining operations in the laboratory rarely eliminate the need for final adjustment in the mouth, which is also, in effect, a machining process to perfect the fit of the restoration to the oral tissues.

Included in this final step in a long sequence of machining procedures necessary to produce a biologically acceptable prosthetic restoration are the adjustment of the occlusion to accommodate the occlusal rests and other metal parts of the denture, the adjustment of the bearing surfaces of the denture bases in harmony with the supporting soft tissues, and the final adjustment of occlusion on the artificial dentition to harmonize with natural occlusion in all mandibular positions.

Occlusal interference from denture framework. Any occlusal interference from occlusal rests and other parts of the denture framework should have been eliminated prior to or during the establishment of occlusal relations. Assuming that the denture framework will have been tried in the mouth before a final jaw relation is established, any such interference should have been detected and eliminated. *Much of this need not exist at all if mouth preparations and the design of the denture framework are carried out with a specific treatment plan in mind.* In any event, occlusal interference from the framework itself should not ordinarily require further adjustment at the time the finished denture is initially placed. *For the dentist to have sent an impression or casts of the patient's mouth to the laboratory and to receive a finished partial denture prosthesis without having once tried the cast framework in the mouth is not only a dereliction of his responsibility to the patient but is also, in effect, handing the practice of prosthetic dentistry over to the dental laboratory technician.* However, when such is done, it is obvious that occlusal interference from the casting itself must be detected and eliminated before proceeding with other adjustments to the denture.

Adjustments to bearing surfaces of denture bases. The machining of bearing surfaces to perfect the fit of the denture to the supporting tissues should be accomplished by the use of some indicator paste. The paste must be one that will be readily displaced by positive tissue contact and will not adhere to the tissues of the mouth. An area of the denture base showing through the film of indicator paste may be erroneously interpreted as a pressure spot, when actually the paste had adhered to the tissues in that area. Therefore only those areas showing through an intact film of indicator paste should be interpreted as pressure areas and be relieved accordingly.

Rather than dismiss the patient with instructions to return when soreness develops and then overrelieve the denture over a traumatized area to restore patient comfort, the use of pressure indicator paste should be routine with any tissue-bearing prosthetic restoration. The paste should be applied in a thin layer over the bearing surfaces and then both occlusal and digital pressure applied to the denture. The patient cannot be expected to apply a heavy enough force to the new denture to register all of the pressure areas present. Therefore the dentist should apply both vertical and horizontal forces with his fingers in excess of that which might be expected of the patient. The denture is then removed and inspected. Any areas heavy enough to displace a thin film of indicator paste should be relieved and the procedure repeated with a new film of indicator until excessive pressure areas have been eliminated.

Pressure areas most frequently encountered are as follows: in the mandibular arch—the lingual slope of the mandibular ridge in the premolar area, the mylohyoid ridge, the border extension into the retromylohyoid space, and the distobuccal border in the vicinity of the ascending ramus and the external oblique ridge; and in the maxillary arch—the inside of the buccal flange of the denture over the tuberosities, the border of the denture lying at the molar prominence, and at the pterygomaxillary notch where the denture may impinge on the pterygomandibular raphe or the pterygoid hamulus itself. In addition, in either arch there may be bony spicules or spicules of the denture base itself that will require specific relief.

The amount of relief by machining that will be necessary will depend on the accuracy of the impression registration, the master cast, and the denture base. Despite the accuracy of modern impression and cast materials, many denture base materials leave much to be desired in this regard, and the element of technical errors is also always present. It is therefore essential that discrepancies in the denture base be detected and corrected before the tissues of the mouth are subjected to the stress of supporting a prosthetic restoration. This is one of our major responsibilities to the patient, that trauma be always held to a minimum. *Therefore the appointment time for the initial placement of the denture must be adequate to permit such adjustment.*

Adjustment of occlusion in harmony with natural and artificial dentition. The final step in the adjustment of the partial denture at the time of initial placement is the adjustment of the occlusion to harmonize with the natural occlusion in all mandibular excursions. When opposing partial dentures are placed concurrently, the adjustment of the occlusion will parallel, to some extent, the adjustment of occlusion on complete dentures. This is particularly true when the few remaining natural teeth are out of occlusion. But where *one or more* natural teeth may occlude in any mandibular position, those teeth will influence mandibular movement to some extent. It is necessary, therefore, that the artificial dentition on the partial denture be made to harmonize with whatever natural occlusion remains.

Occlusal adjustment of tooth-borne removable partial dentures may be performed accurately by any of several intraoral methods. *It has been our experience, however, that occlusal adjustment of distal extension removable partial dentures is accomplished more conveniently and accurately by using an articulator than by any intraoral method.* Since distal extension denture bases will exhibit some movement under a closing force, intraoral indications of occlusal discrepancies, whether by inked ribbon or disclosing waxes, are difficult to interpret. Distal extension dentures, positioned on remounting casts, can conveniently be related to the articulator with new, nonpressure interocclusal records, and the occlusion can be adjusted accurately at the appointment for initial placement of the dentures (Fig. 19-1).

The methods by which occlusal relations may be established and recorded have been discussed in Chapter 16. In this chapter the advantages of establishing a functional occlusal relationship with an intact opposing arch have been discussed and also the limitations

that exist to the perfecting of harmonious occlusion on the finished prosthesis by intraoral adjustment alone. Even when the occlusion on two opposing partial dentures is being adjusted entirely in the mouth, it is best that one arch be considered an intact arch and the other one adjusted to it. This is accomplished by first eliminating any occlusal interference to mandibular movement imposed by one denture and adjusting any opposing natural dentition to accommodate to the prosthetically supplied teeth. Then the opposing partial denture is placed, and occlusal adjustments are made to harmonize with both the natural dentition and the opposing denture, which is now considered part of an intact dental arch. Which denture is adjusted first and which one is made to occlude with it is somewhat arbitrary, with the following exceptions: If one partial denture is entirely tooth supported and the other has a tissue-supported base, the tooth-supported denture is adjusted to final occlusion with any opposing natural teeth and then that arch is treated as an intact arch and the opposing denture adjusted to occlude with it. If both partial dentures are entirely tooth borne, the one occluding with the most natural teeth is adjusted first and the second denture then adjusted to occlude with an intact arch. Tooth-borne segments of a composite (tooth- and tissue-supported) partial denture are likewise adjusted first to harmonize with any opposing natural dentition. The final adjustment of occlusion on opposing tissue-supported bases is usually done on the mandibular denture, since this is the moving member, and the occlusion is made to harmonize with the maxillary denture, which is treated as part of an intact arch.

Intraoral occlusal adjustment is accomplished by using some kind of indicator and suitable mounted points and burs. Diamond or other abrasive points must be used to reduce enamel and metal contacts. These also may be used to reduce plastic tooth surfaces, but burs may be used for plastic with greater effectiveness. Articulation paper may be used as an indicator if one recognizes that heavy interocclusal contacts may become perforated, leaving only a light mark, while secondary contacts, being lighter and frequently sliding, may make a heavier mark. Although articulation ribbon does not become perforated, it is not easy to use in the

Fig. 19-1. A sequence of laboratory and clinical procedures for correction of occlusal discrepancies as a result of processing restorations. **A,** Maxillary master cast has been removed from indexed mounting on articulator, and base of cast has been covered with tinfoil prior to investing procedure. **B,** Processed maxillary restoration and master cast is recovered intact from investing medium. **C,** Restoration and indexed cast is attached to original mounting with sticky wax. Remounting jig is attached to lower member of articulator. **D,** Patty of quick-setting stone is placed on remount jig just thick enough so that occlusal and incisal surfaces will be recorded when articulator is closed. Original face-bow record is thus preserved. **E,** Face-bow record is trimmed and identified with patient's name, articulator number, horizontal and lateral condylar adjustments, and the date. **F** and **G,** Maxillary and mandibular restorations are recovered, finished, and polished.

Fig. 19-1, cont'd. H and **I,** After restorations are tried in and adjusted to basal seats, an impression is made of placed restorations using a perforated stock tray and irreversible hydrocolloid. **J** and **K,** Casts are poured in impressions after undercuts in denture bases are blocked out with wet facial tissue. Dentures are readily removed and replaced on mounting casts. **L,** Maxillary denture and remounting cast is placed in face-bow record on mounting jig, and maxillary cast is attached to upper arm of articulator with stone. **M,** Centric relation is recorded as near the vertical dimension of occlusion as possible, avoiding contact of opposing teeth. Recording medium is a fast-setting impression plaster. **N,** Mandibular restoration and remounting cast is attached to lower member of articulator with stone using just made centric relation record. **O,** Another intraoral recording of centric relation is made. *Continued.*

Fig. 19-1, cont'd. P, Restorations and attached record are returned to articulator. If condylar elements are snug against condylar housings, it can be safely assumed that centric relation has been recorded and that casts have been accurately mounted to this maxillomandibular relationship. **Q,** Occlusion may now be harmonized as a laboratory procedure on articulator. Original condylar settings may be used since original face-bow transfer record was duplicated. **R,** Patient is not given possession of restorations until occlusion has been refined and occlusal harmony is obtained.

mouth, and the differentiation between primary and secondary contacts is difficult to ascertain.

In general, occlusal adjustment of multiple contacts between natural and artificial dentition when tooth-borne partial dentures are involved follows the same principles as those for natural dentition alone. This is because the partial dentures are retained by devices attached to the abutment teeth, whereas with complete dentures no mechanical retainers are present. The use of more than one color of articulation paper or ribbon to record and differentiate between centric and eccentric contacts is just as helpful in adjusting partial denture occlusion as natural occlusion, and for the initial adjustment this method may be used.

For final adjustment, however, since one denture will be adjusted to occlude with an intact arch, the use of an occlusal wax may be necessary to establish points of excessive contact and interference. This cannot be done by articulation paper alone. An occlusal wax, such as Kerr occlusal indicator, which is adhesive on one side, or strips of 28-gauge

Kerr green casting wax or other similar soft wax, may be used. It should always be used bilaterally, with two strips folded together at the midline. Thus the patient is not as likely to deviate to one side as he is when wax is introduced unilaterally. (See Fig. 19-2).

For centric contacts the patient is guided to tap into the wax and then the wax is removed and inspected under transillumination for perforations. All perforated areas are either premature contacts or excessive contacts and must be adjusted. One of two methods may be used to locate specific areas to be relieved. Articulation ribbon may be used to mark the occlusion, and then those marks representing areas of excessive contact are identified by referring to the wax record and are relieved accordingly. A second method is to introduce the wax strips a second time, this time adapting them to the buccal and lingual surfaces for retention. After having the patient tap into the wax, perforated areas are marked with waterproof pencil. The wax is then stripped off and the penciled areas are relieved. This procedure has been outlined in some detail by Jankelson.

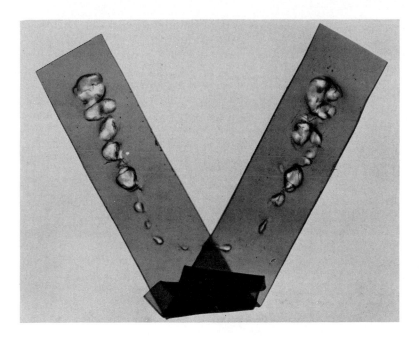

Fig. 19-2. Two strips of 28-gauge soft green (casting) wax are placed in mouth between opposing dentition. These are first folded over anteriorly to unite two halves, and then patient is guided to tap in centric occlusion two or three times. Viewed out of the mouth, against a source of light, uniform contacts free of perforations may be considered to be simultaneous contacts. Perforations in wax represent occlusal prematurities that should be relieved. Accuracy of this method or any other intraoral method is dependent not only on dentist's interpretation of marks (perforations) but also on stability of denture bases.

Whichever method is used, it must be repeated until occlusal balance in centric occlusion has been established and more uniform contacts without perforations are evident from a final interocclusal wax record. After adjustment in centric occlusion has been completed, Jankelson suggests that the patient should be asked to "open and eat the wax lightly" several times. Any remaining areas of interference are then reduced, thus assuring that there is no interference during the chewing stroke. Adjustments to relieve interference during the chewing stroke should be confined to buccal surfaces of mandibular teeth and lingual surfaces of maxillary teeth. This serves to narrow the cusps so that they will go all the way into the opposing sulci without wedging as they travel into centric contact. Skinner proposed that the patient be given a small bite of soft banana to chew rather than to expect him to chew without food actually being present. The small bolus of banana promotes normal functional activity of the chewing mech-

anism, yet by its soft consistency does not itself cause indentations in the soft wax. Any interfering contacts encountered during the chewing stroke are thus detected as perforations in the wax, which are marked with pencil and relieved accordingly.

Adjustments to occlusion should be repeated at a reasonable interval after the dentures have reached a point of equilibrium and the musculature has become adjusted to the changes brought about by restoration of occlusal contacts. This second occlusal adjustment usually may be considered sufficient until such time as tissue-supported denture bases no longer support the occlusion and corrective measures, either by reoccluding the teeth or relining the denture, must be employed. *However, a periodic recheck of occlusion at intervals of six months is advisable to avoid traumatic interference resulting from changes in denture support or tooth migration.*

After the adjustment of occlusion the anatomy of the artificial teeth should be restored to maximum efficiency by restoring grooves and spillways (food escapeways) and by narrowing the teeth buccolingually to increase the sharpness of the cusps and reduce the width of the food table. Mandibular buccal and maxillary lingual surfaces in particular should be narrowed to assure that these areas will not interfere with closure into the opposing sulci. Since artificial teeth used on partial dentures opposing natural or restored dentition should always be considered *material* out of which a harmonious occlusal surface is created, final adjustment of the occlusion always should be followed by the meticulous restoration of the most functional occlusal anatomy possible. Although this may be done after a subsequent occlusal adjustment at a later date, the possibility that the patient may fail to return on schedule is always present, and in the meantime, broad and inefficient occlusal surfaces may cause an overloading of the supporting structures, which would be traumatogenic. Therefore the restoration of an efficient occlusal anatomy is an essential part of the denture adjustment at the time of placement. Again, this requires that sufficient time be allotted for the initial placement of the partial denture to permit all necessary occlusal corrections to be accomplished.

Instructions to the patient. Finally, before you dismiss the patient the difficulties that may be encountered and the care that must be given the prosthesis and the abutment teeth must be reviewed with the patient.

The patient should be advised that he will probably experience some discomfort or minor annoyance initially. Whereas this is to some extent due to the presence of bulk, which the tongue in particular must become accustomed to, any foreign object, however comfortable, must be accepted biologically and psychologically before it can become an integral part of the oral mechanism.

The patient must be advised also of the possibility of soreness's developing despite every attempt on the part of the dentist to prevent its occurrence. Since patients vary widely in their ability to tolerate discomfort, it is perhaps best to advise every patient as though soreness is inevitable, with every assurance that any needed adjustments will be made. On the other hand, the dentist himself should be aware of the fact that some patients are unable to accommodate ever to the pres-

ence of a removable prosthesis. Fortunately these are few in any practice. However, the dentist must avoid any positive statements that might be interpreted or construed by the patient to be positive assurance tantamount to a guarantee that he will be able to use the prosthesis with comfort and acceptance. Too much depends on the patient's ability to accept a foreign object and to tolerate reasonable pressures to make such assurance possible.

Discussing phonetics with the patient in regard to his new dentures may indicate that this is a unique problem to be overcome because of the influence of the prosthesis on speech. With few exceptions, which are usually due to excessive and avoidable bulk in the denture design or to improper placement of teeth and the contour of denture bases, the average patient will experience little difficulty in wearing the partial denture. Most of the hindrances to normal speech will disappear in a few days.

Similarly, perhaps little or nothing should be said to the patient about the possibility of his gagging or the tongue's reaction to a foreign object. Most patients will experience little or no difficulty in this regard, and the tongue will normally accept smooth, nonbulky contours without objection. Contours that are too thick, too bulky, or improperly placed should be avoided in the construction of the denture, but if present, these should be detected and eliminated at the time of placement of the denture. The dentist should palpate the prosthesis in the mouth and reduce excessive bulk accordingly before the patient has an opportunity to object to it. The area most frequently needing thinning is the distolingual flange of the mandibular denture. Here the denture flange should almost always be thinned during the finishing and polishing of the denture base. Sublingually the denture flange should be reproduced as recorded in the impression, but distal to the second molar the flange should be trimmed somewhat thinner. Then, on placing the denture, the dentist should palpate this area to ascertain that a minimum of bulk exists that might be encountered by the side and base of the tongue. If this needs further reduction, it should be done and the denture repolished before dismissing the patient.

The patient should be advised of the need for keeping the dentures and the abutment teeth meticulously clean. If cariogenic processes are to be prevented, the accumulation of debris should be avoided as much as possible, particularly around abutment teeth and beneath minor connectors. Furthermore, inflammation of gingival tissues is prevented by removing accumulated debris and by substituting toothbrush massage for the normal stimulation of tongue and food contact with areas that will be covered by the denture framework.

The mouth and partial denture should be cleaned after eating and before retiring. Brushing before breakfast also may be effective in reducing the bacterial count, which may help to lessen acid formation in the caries-susceptible individual after eating. A partial denture may be effectively cleaned by the use of a small, stiff-bristle brush. Debris may be effectively removed through the use of dentifrices, since they contain the essential elements for cleaning. Household cleaners should not be used because they are too abrasive for use on resin surfaces. The patient, and the elderly or handicapped patient in particular, should be advised to clean the denture over a basin partially filled with water so that the fall will be broken if the denture is dropped accidentally during cleaning.

In addition to brushing with a dentifrice, additional cleaning may be accomplished by the use of a proprietary denture cleaning solution. The patient should be advised to soak the dentures in the solution for fifteen minutes once daily, followed by a thorough brushing with a dentifrice. Although hypochlorite solutions are effective denture cleansers, they have a tendency to tarnish chrome-cobalt frameworks and should be avoided.

In some mouths the precipitation of salivary calculus on the partial denture necessitates the taking of extra measures for its removal. Thorough daily brushing of the denture will avoid deposits of calculus for many patients. However, any build-up of calculus noted by the patient between scheduled recall appointments should be removed in the dental office. This can be quickly and readily accomplished by using an ultrasonic cleaner.

Since many patients will dine away from home, the informed patient should provide some means of carrying out midday oral hygiene. Simply rinsing the partial denture and the mouth with water after eating is beneficial if brushing is not possible.

Opinion is divided on the question of whether or not a partial denture should be worn during sleep. Conditions should determine the advice given the patient, *although generally the tissues should be allowed to rest by removing the denture at night.* In such a case the denture should be placed in a container and covered with water to prevent its dehydration, with subsequent dimensional change. About the only situation that possibly justifies the wearing of partial dentures at night is when stresses generated by bruxism would be more destructive since they then would be concentrated on fewer teeth. Broader distribution of the stress load, plus the splinting effect of the partial denture, may make the wearing of the denture at night advisable. However, an individual, latex rubber mouth protector should be worn at night until the cause of the bruxism is eliminated.

Frequently the question arises of whether an opposing complete denture should be worn when a partial denture in the other arch is out of the mouth. The answer is that if the partial denture is to be removed at night, the opposing complete denture should not be left in the mouth. There is no more certain way of destroying the alveolar ridge, which supports a maxillary complete denture, than to have it occlude with a few remaining anterior mandibular teeth.

The partial denture patient should not be dismissed as completed without at least one subsequent appointment for evaluation of the response of oral structures to the restorations and minor adjustment if needed. This should be made at an interval of twenty-four hours after initial placement of the denture. It need not be a lengthy appointment but should be made as a definite rather than a drop-in appointment. Not only does this give the patient assurance that any necessary adjustments will be made and provide the dentist with an opportunity to check on the patient's acceptance of the prosthesis, but it also avoids giving the patient any idea that he may break into the dentist's schedule at will and serves to give notice that an appointment is necessary for future adjustments.

Follow-up services. The sixth phase of removable partial denture service (periodic recall) and its rationale must be understood by the patient. Patients will probably experience only limited success with the treatment and restorations so meticulously accomplished by the dentist unless they return for periodic oral evaluations.

After all necessary adjustments to the partial denture have been made and the patient has been advised as to the proper care of the denture, he must also be advised as to the future care of the mouth to ensure health and longevity of the remaining structures. How often the mouth and denture should be examined by the dentist depends on the oral and physical condition of the patient. If the patient is caries-susceptible or has tendencies toward periodontal disease or alveolar atrophy, his mouth should be examined more frequently. Every six months should be the rule if conditions are normal. At least once a year a roentgenographic examination should supplement clinical examination and oral prophylaxis.

The need for increasing retention on clasp arms to make the denture more secure will depend on the type of clasp that has been used. Increasing retention should be accomplished by adjusting the clasp arm to engage a deeper part of the retention undercut rather than by bending the clasp in toward the tooth. The latter creates only frictional retention, which violates the principle of clasp retention. Being an active force, such retention contributes to tooth or restoration movement or both in a horizontal direction, disappearing only when either the tooth has been moved or the clasp arm returns to a *passive* relationship with the abutment tooth. Unfortunately this is almost the only adjustment that can be made to a half-round cast clasp arm. On the other hand, the round wrought-wire clasp arm may be adjusted cervically and brought into a deeper part of the retentive undercut. Thus the passivity of the clasp arm in its terminal position is maintained, but retention is increased by its being forced to flex more to withdraw from the deeper undercut. The patient should be advised that the abutment tooth and the clasp will serve longer if the retention is held to a minimum, which is only that amount necessary to resist reasonable dislodging forces.

Development of denture rocking or looseness in the future may be due to a change in the form of the supporting ridges rather than to a lack of retention. This should be detected as early as possible after it occurs and corrected by relining or rebasing. The loss of tissue support is usually so gradual that the patient may be unable to detect the need for relining. This usually must be determined by the dentist at subsequent examinations as evidenced by rotation of the distal extension denture about the fulcrum line. If the partial denture is opposed by natural dentition, the loss of base support causes a loss of occlusal contact, which may be detected by having the patient close on wax strips placed bilaterally. If, however, a complete denture or distal extension partial denture opposes the partial denture, the interocclusal wax test is not dependable, since occlusal contact may have been maintained by posterior closure, changes in the temporomandibular joint, or migration of the opposing denture. In such case, evidence of loss of ridge support is determined solely by the indirect retainer leaving its seat as the distal extension denture rotates about the fulcrum line.

No assurance can be given to the patient that uncrowned abutment teeth will not decay at some future time. Even with full cast crowns there can be no positive assurance that the tooth will not ever decay gingival to the crown, as a result of gingival recession and caries attack of exposed cementum. The patient can be assured, however, that prophylactic measures in the form of meticulous oral hygiene, coupled with routine care by the dentist, will be rewarded by greater health and longevity of the remaining teeth.

The patient should be advised that maximum service may be expected from the partial denture if he observes the following rules:

1. Avoid careless handling of the denture, which may lead to distortion or breakage. Damage to the partial denture occurs while it is out of the mouth, as a result of dropping it during cleaning or an accident's occurring when the denture is not being worn. Fractured teeth and denture bases can be repaired, as can broken clasp arms, but a distorted framework can rarely, if ever, be satisfactorily readapted or repaired.

2. Teeth should be protected from caries by proper oral hygiene, proper diet, and frequent dental care. The teeth will be no less susceptible to caries when a partial denture

is being worn but may be more so because of the retention of debris. At the same time, the remaining teeth have become all the more important as a result of oral rehabilitation, and abutment teeth have become even more valuable because of their importance to the success of the partial denture. Therefore the need for a rigid regimen of *oral hygiene, diet control*, and *periodic clinical observation and treatment* is essential to the future health of the entire mouth. *Also the patient must be more conscientious about responding to being recalled at stated intervals by the dentist for examination and necessary treatment.*

3. Periodontal damage to the abutment teeth can be avoided by maintaining tissue support of any distal extension bases. As a result of periodic examination this can be detected and corrected by relining or whatever procedure is indicated.

4. Partial denture treatment must be accepted as something that cannot be considered permanent but must receive regular and continuous care by both the patient and the dentist. The obligations for maintaining caries control and for returning at stated intervals for treatment must be clearly understood, as well as the fact that regular charges will be made by the dentist for whatever treatment is rendered.

SELF-ASSESSMENT AIDS

1. The term *adjustment* has two connotations in relation to removable partial dentures. Do you know these two connotations?
2. At what stage of treatment should any occlusal interference by a framework have been corrected?
3. What is meant by adjustments to the bearing surfaces of denture bases?
4. How do you detect areas of the denture base that may contribute to soreness if not relieved?
5. What is a pressure indicator paste? Can you give a detailed procedure for using a pressure indicator paste? How do you interpret prospective pressure spots when using a pressure indicator paste?
6. A silicone spray should be sprayed on the surface of the denture brushed with pressure indicator paste before placing it in the patients mouth to ascertain pressure spots. What purpose does the silicone spray serve?
7. Can you interpret overextension or underextension of borders of the denture base with the use of a pressure indicator paste?
8. Can the pterygomandibular raphe be impinged by the borders of either maxillary or madibular distal extension bases?
9. Some occlusal discrepancies are bound to occur in dentures as a result of the processing of acrylic resin. True or false?
10. The dentist must correct any and all occlusal discrepancies to the best of his ability before the patient is given possession of the restorations. True or false?
11. You are initially placing a tooth-borne removable partial denture. How do you correct occlusal discrepancies and assure yourself that occlusal harmony exists?
12. What is the danger in trying to correct occlusal discrepancies of distal extension dentures by an intraoral technique?
13. What is a remount cast? How is it made?
14. Can you give a detailed procedure for correction of occlusal discrepancies by remounting distal extension removable partial dentures on an articulator?
15. What are the several advantages in using an articulator to correct occlusal discrepancies?
16. After correction of occlusal discrepancies, should the occlusal anatomy of prosthetically supplied teeth be restored by ensuring that adequate grooves and spillways are present? How do you determine where and where not to recontour?
17. By what procedures do you restore the "glaze" on occlusal surfaces of vacuum-fired porcelain artificial teeth attached to an acrylic resin denture base?
18. An informed patient will adjust to new restorations better than an uninformed patient. At what phase of treatment should "patient education" begin?
19. What instructions do you review with the patient prior to ending the initial placement appointment?
20. Why should appointments be made for twenty-four and forty-eight hours after the initial placement of restorations?
21. Does your responsibility in the treatment of a patient end after the forty-eight hour evaluation appointment?
22. How do you feel about providing the patient with printed suggestions relative to the care and use of restorations before the initial placement appointment?
23. What length of time should you schedule for the initial placement of distal extension removable partial dentures?

20 RELINING AND REBASING THE REMOVABLE PARTIAL DENTURE

Differentiation between relining and rebasing has been discussed previously in Chapter 1. Briefly, *relining* is the resurfacing of a denture base with new material to make it fit the underlying tissues more accurately, whereas *rebasing* is the replacement of a denture base with new material without changing the occlusal relations of the teeth. Relining removable restorations is a frequent occurrence in many dental practices; however, rebasing is seldom performed, comparatively speaking.

In either case a new impression registration is necessary, using the existing denture base as an impression tray for either a closed-mouth or an open-mouth impression procedure. One of several types of impression materials may be used. The impression may be made with a metallic oxide impression paste, with one of the rubber-base or silicone impression materials, with an activated resin used as an impression material, or with a mouth-temperature wax.

In making the decision between a closed-mouth and an open-mouth impression method for relining, one must first consider the reasons for doing so and the objectives to be obtained. Again, it is necessary to differentiate between the two basic types of partial dentures, one being the all–tooth-borne restoration and the other being the tooth- and tissue-supported restoration.

RELINING TOOTH-BORNE DENTURE BASES

When total abutment support is available, but for one reason or another a removable partial denture has been the restoration of choice, support for that restoration is derived entirely from the abutment teeth at each end of each edentulous span. This support may be effective through the use of occlusal rests, boxlike internal rests, internal attachments, or supporting ledges on abutment restorations. Except for intrusion of abutment teeth under functional stress, settling of the restoration toward the tissues of the residual ridge is prevented by the supporting abutments. Tissue changes occurring beneath tooth-borne denture bases do not affect the support of the denture, and therefore relining or rebasing is usually done for other reasons: (1) unhygienic conditions and the trapping of debris between the denture and the residual ridge, (2) an unsightly condition due to the space that has developed, or (3) patient discomfort associated with lack of tissue contact arising from open spaces between the denture base and the tissues. Anteriorly, some loss of support beneath a denture base may lead to some denture movement, despite occlusal support and direct retainers located posteriorly. Rebasing might be the treatment of choice if the artificial teeth are to be replaced or rearranged, or if the denture base needs to be replaced for esthetic reasons or because it has become defective.

For either relining or rebasing to be accomplished, the original denture base must have been made of a resin material that can be relined or replaced. Frequently tooth-borne partial denture bases are made of metal as part of the cast framework. These cannot be satisfactorily relined, although they may sometimes be altered by drastic grinding to provide mechanical retention for the attachment of an entirely new resin base. Ordinarily a metal base, with its several advantages, is not used in a tooth-borne area in which early tissue changes are anticipated. A metal base should not be used after recent extractions or other surgery, nor for a long span when relining to provide secondary tissue support may become necessary. (A distal extension metal base is ordinarily used only when a partial denture is being made over tissues that have become conditioned to supporting a previous denture base.)

Since the tooth-borne denture base cannot be depressed beyond its terminal position with the occlusal rests seated and the teeth in occlusion and since it cannot rotate about a fulcrum, a closed-mouth impression method is used. Virtually any impression material may be used, provided sufficient space is allowed beneath the denture base to permit the excess material to flow to the borders, at which it is either turned by the bordering tissues or, as in the palate, is allowed to escape through holes without unduly displacing the underlying tissues. The qualities of each type of impression material must be kept in mind when one is selecting the material to be used for this purpose. Ordinarily an impression material is used that will record the anatomic form of the oral tissues.

A word should be said in favor of relining a tooth-borne resin base with autopolymerizing acrylic resin as an intraoral procedure. When one or more relatively short spans are to be relined, the making of an impression for that purpose requires that the denture be flasked and processed. The possibility that the vertical dimension of occlusion may be increased and that the denture may be distorted during laboratory procedures must be weighed against the disadvantages of using a direct reline material. Fortunately these materials are constantly being improved with greater predictability and color stability. The possibility that the original denture base will become crazed or distorted by the action of the activated monomer is minimal when the base is made of modern cross-linked resin. However, for this reason, earlier resin bases should not be subjected to relining with direct reline resins.

When relining in the mouth with a resin reline material is done with a definite technique, the results can be quite satisfactory, with complete bonding to the existing denture base, with good color stability, and with permanence and accuracy. The procedure for applying a direct reline of an existing resin base is as follows:

1. Relieve generously the tissue side of the denture base and just over the borders. This not only provides space for an adequate thickness of new material but also eliminates the possibility of tissue impingement because of confinement of the material.

2. Apply masking or adhesive tape over the polished surfaces from the relieved border to the occlusal surfaces of the teeth.

3. Mix the powder and liquid in a glass jar according to the proportions recommended by the manufacturer.

4. While the material is reaching the desired consistency, have the patient rinse the mouth with cold water. At the same time, wipe the fresh surfaces of the dried denture base with a cotton pellet saturated with some of the monomer. This facilitates bonding and makes sure that the surface is free of any contamination.

5. When the material has first begun to take on some body, but while it is still quite fluid, apply it to the tissue side of the denture base and over the borders. Immediately place the denture in the mouth in its terminal position and have the patient close into occlusion. Then, with the patient's mouth open, manipulate the cheeks to turn the excess at the border and establish harmony with bordering attachments. If a mandibular denture is being relined, have the patient move the tongue into each cheek and then against the anterior teeth to establish a functional lingual border. It is necessary that the direct retainers be effective to prevent displacement of the denture while molding of the borders is accomplished. Otherwise the denture must be held in its terminal position with finger pressure on the occlusal surfaces.

6. Immediately remove the denture from the mouth and with fine curved iris scissors trim away gross excess material and any material that has flowed onto proximal tooth surfaces and other components of the denture framework. While this is being done, have the patient again rinse the mouth with cold water. Then replace the denture in its terminal position, bringing the teeth into occlusion. Then repeat the border movements with the patient's mouth open. By this time or soon thereafter the material will have become firm enough to maintain its form out of the mouth.

7. Remove the denture, rinse it quickly in water, and dry the relined surface with com-

pressed air. Apply a generous coating of glycerine or Tect-ol with a brush or cotton pellet to prevent frosting of the surface because of evaporation of monomer. The material is then allowed to bench cure, thus eliminating patient discomfort and tissue damage from exothermic heat or prolonged contact with raw monomer. Although it is preferable that twenty to thirty minutes elapse before trimming and polishing, it may be done as soon as the material hardens. The masking tape must be removed before trimming is done but should be replaced over the teeth and polished surfaces below the junction of the new and old materials to protect those surfaces during final polishing.

Properly done, a direct reline is entirely acceptable for most tooth-borne partial denture bases made of a resin material, except when some tissue support is desired for long spans between abutment teeth. In the latter case a reline impression in wax may be accomplished, the denture may then be flasked, and a processed reline may be added for optimal tissue contact and support.

RELINING DISTAL EXTENSION PARTIAL DENTURE BASES

A distal extension partial denture, deriving its major support from the tissues of the residual ridge, requires relining much more frequently than does a tooth-supported denture. Because of this, distal extension bases are usually made of a resin material that can be relined to compensate for loss of support because of tissue changes. Whereas tooth-supported areas are relined for other reasons, the sole reason for relining a distal extension base is to reestablish tissue support for that base.

The need for relining a distal extension base is determined by evaluating the stability and occlusion at reasonable intervals after initial placement of the denture. Prior to the time of initial placement the patient must be advised (1) that periodic examination and also relining, when it becomes necessary, are imperative, (2) that the success of the partial denture and the health of the remaining tissues and abutment teeth depend on periodic examination and servicing of both the denture and the abutment teeth, and (3) that a charge will be made for these visits in proportion to the treatment required.

There are two indications of the need for relining a distal extension partial denture base. First a loss of occlusal contact between opposing dentures or between the denture and opposing natural dentition may be evident. This is determined by having the patient close on two strips of 28-gauge soft green or blue (casting) wax. If occlusal contact between artificial dentition is weak or lacking while the remaining natural teeth in opposition are making firm contact, the distal extension denture needs to have occlusion reestablished on the present base either by altering the occlusion, or by reestablishing the original position of the denture framework and base, or sometimes both. In most instances, reestablishing the original relationship of the denture is necessary, and the occlusion will automatically be reestablished.

Second a loss of tissue support causing rotation and settling of the distal extension base or bases is obvious when alternate finger pressure is applied on either side of the fulcrum line. Although checking for occlusal contact alone may be misleading, such rotation is positive proof that relining is necessary. If occlusal inadequacy is detected without any evidence of denture rotation toward the residual ridge, all that needs be done is to reestablish occlusal contact by rearranging the teeth or by adding to the occlusal surfaces with resin or cast gold onlays. On the other hand, if occlusal contact is adequate but denture rotation can be demonstrated, it is usually due to migration or extrusion of opposing teeth or to a shift in position of an opposing maxillary denture, thus maintaining occlusal contact at the expense of the stability and tissue support of that denture. This is frequently the situation when a partial denture is opposed by a maxillary complete denture. It is not unusual for a patient to complain of looseness of the maxillary complete denture and request relining of that denture when actually it is the partial denture that needs relining. Relining and thus repositioning the partial denture results in repositioning of the maxillary complete denture with a return of stability and retention in that denture. Therefore evidence of rotation of a distal extension partial denture about the fulcrum line must be the deciding factor as to whether relining needs to be done.

Rotation tissueward about the fulcrum line always results in a lifting of the indirect retainer(s). The framework of any distal extension partial denture must be in its original terminal position with indirect retainers fully seated during and at the end of any relining procedure. Any possibility of rotation about the fulcrum line because of occlusal influence must be prevented, and therefore the framework must be held in its original terminal position during the time the impression is being made. This all but eliminates the practicability of using a closed-mouth impression procedure effectively when relining unilateral or bilateral distal extension bases. Steffel has outlined in detail one procedure for making a functional reline impression (see Chapter 15). The use of posterior stops of modeling plastic does not entirely eliminate the possibility that tissue displacement and denture rotation will occur when the mouth is closed and the teeth are in occlusion. Although adjusting the occlusion helps to prevent such rotation when the final impression is being made, one cannot always be sure that some rotation and lifting of the indirect retainers does not occur.

The only sure method, therefore, of making a reline impression for a distal extension partial denture is with an open-mouth procedure done in exactly the same manner as the original secondary impression. The denture to be relined is first relieved generously on the tissue side and then is treated the same as the original impression base for a functional impression. The step-by-step procedure is the same, with the dentist's three fingers placed on the two principal occlusal rests and at a third point between, preferably at an indirect retainer farthest from the axis of rotation. The framework is thus returned to its original terminal position, with all tooth-supported components fully seated. The tissues beneath the distal extension base are then registered in a relationship to the original position of the denture that will assure (1) the denture framework's being returned to its intended relationship with the supporting teeth, (2) the reestablishment of optimal tissue support for the distal extension base, and (3) the restoration of the original occlusal relationship with the opposing teeth.

Although it is true that the teeth are not allowed to come into occlusion during an open-mouth impression procedure, the original position of the denture is positively determined by its relationship with the supporting abutment teeth. Since this is the relationship on which the original occlusion was established, returning the denture to that position should bring about a return to the original occlusal relationship if two conditions are satisfied. First of these is that the laboratory procedures during relining must be done accurately without any increase in vertical dimension. This is essential with any reline procedure, but particularly with a partial denture because any change in vertical dimension will prevent occlusal rests from seating and will result in overloading and trauma to the underlying tissues. The second condition is that the opposing teeth have not extruded or migrated or that the position of an opposing denture has not become irreversibly altered. In the latter situation some adjustment of the occlusion will be necessary, but this should be deferred until the opposing teeth or denture and the structures associated with the temporomandibular joint have had a chance to return to their original position before denture settling occurred. One of the greatest satisfactions of a job well done is to be found in the execution of an open-mouth reline procedure as described above, which results in the restoration not only of the original denture relationship and tissue support but the original occlusal relationship as well.

In rare instances, after the relining of a distal extension partial denture by this method, the occlusion is found to be negative rather than positive or the same as it was before relining. This may be due to wear of occlusal surfaces over a period of time, to the original occlusion's being high with resulting depression of opposing teeth, or to other reasons. In such case, occlusion on the denture must be restored to reestablish an even distribution of occlusal loading over both natural and artificial dentition. Otherwise the natural dentition must carry the burden of mastication unaided, and the denture becomes only a space-filling or cosmetic device.

METHODS OF REESTABLISHING OCCLUSION ON A RELINED PARTIAL DENTURE

Occlusion on a relined partial denture may be reestablished by one of several methods.

One method involves making a remounting cast, as previously described, and correctly relating the opposing casts to an articulator. The articulator then may be adjusted by interocclusal records. If the artificial teeth to be corrected are acrylic resin, the occlusion can be reestablished either by adding autopolymerizing acrylic resin to occlusal surfaces or by fabricating gold occlusal surfaces, which can be attached to the original replaced teeth. The original teeth also may be removed from the denture base and replaced by new teeth arranged to harmonize with the opposing occlusal surfaces. Baseplate wax may be used to support the teeth as they are being arranged. The wax should be carved to restore the lingual anatomy of the teeth and the portion of the denture base that was eliminated when the original teeth were removed. A stone matrix is made covering the occlusal and lingual surfaces of the teeth and denture flange. Then wax may be removed from the denture base and teeth. Those areas on the stone matrix, intimate to the new acrylic resin to be added, should be painted with a tinfoil substitute. The new teeth are placed in the stone matrix, and the matrix is accurately attached to the denture base with sticky wax. Autopolymerizing acrylic resin is then used to attach the teeth and is conveniently sprinkled on by a buccal approach. The buccal surface of the denture base adjacent to the teeth should be overfilled slightly so that the correct shape may be restored to this portion of the base during finishing and polishing procedures. Occlusal discrepancies as a result of this procedure should be corrected on the articulator by new jaw relation records if the denture involved has a distal extension base.

A second method is to remove the original teeth and replace them with a hard inlay wax occlusion rim on which a functional registration of occlusal pathways is then established (Chapter 16). Either the original teeth or new teeth may then be arranged to occlude with the template thus obtained and subsequently attached to the denture base with processed or self-curing resin. If the latter is used, the need for flasking may be eliminated by securing the teeth to a stone matrix while the resin attachment is applied with a brush technique. Regardless of the method used for reattaching the teeth, the occlusion thus established should require little adjustment in the mouth and should be typical of the occlusal harmony that is possible by this method.

The third method is a functional method obtained by establishing occlusal pathways in wax, but it results in cast gold onlays being cemented to the original replacement teeth.

Recesses must be ground into the occlusal surfaces that are to be restored, and some lubricant must be used to ensure removal of the wax patterns. A hard inlay wax is used to record functional occlusion in all excursions, preferably over a period of twenty-four hours or more. The wax record is then carved as for full coverage inlay patterns, except that they are left in one piece for all adjacent teeth. Some occlusal anatomy should be carved into the patterns to provide escapeways and promote greater efficiency and less occlusal loading than do the broad occlusal contacts registered in wax. The inlays are then cast in a C-type gold and cemented to the artificial teeth.

Tissue conditioning prior to relining a partial denture base. Distal extension partial denture bases frequently need relining within a few months because of initial tissue changes after the placement of a first partial denture. This is not usually observed when the patient has previously worn a partial denture. Applegate has shown the beneficial effects of a treatment base prior to completion of the final base. Whether as a result of wearing a treatment base or of having worn a partial denture, gross tissue changes are not as likely to occur once the tissues have become conditioned to supporting a denture base.

There is much interest in the use of fluid resins for tissue-conditioning purposes prior to relining of a removable denture. This is due to the stabilizing effect of a soft resin reline rather than to any medicinal action of the treatment material. It has been clearly shown that tissues that are unhealthy and edematous because of an ill-fitting denture base may be returned to a normal, healthy state by repeated applications of a soft relining material in conjunction with sound prosthodontic principles.

Tissues under a partial denture base generally remain healthy because of the supporting and stabilizing effect of the denture framework. Therefore treatment with tissue-conditioning material is not usually indicated if the denture can be conveniently removed from the mouth for varying periods prior to relining. On the other hand, utilizing one of the tissue treatment materials for stabilizing the denture is indicated—but only for treatment purposes. These are not meant to be impression materials, nor can they provide the support necessary to restore the proper relationship of the denture framework to the supporting teeth. An open-mouth relining procedure as outlined previously in the chapter should follow any tissue treatment procedures. However, all restorations to be relined should remain out of the mouth twenty-four hours prior to the relining procedures to permit the tissues to return to as near a normal state as possible.

SELF-ASSESSMENT AIDS

1. What is the difference between relining and rebasing an acrylic resin denture base?
2. On occasion, tissue changes beneath tooth-borne denture bases require correction of the bases to reestablish intimate contact of the base and residual ridge. Can you think of three indications which would lead you to believe that intimate contact must be restored?
3. In any relining procedure, sufficient space between the denture base and residual ridge must be provided to accommodate new material. True or false?
4. Tooth-borne removable partial denture bases may often be relined with a color-matching, autopolymerizing acrylic resin as a chairside procedure. Can you give such a procedure, including preparation of the bases as well as the precautions that must be observed for patient comfort?
5. When relining a tooth-borne base, should the anatomic or functional form of the ridge be utilized?
6. Suppose you discover that rests are not correctly seated in their prepared seats when you are accomplishing a chairside reline procedure. What must you do?
7. Suppose you must reline a Class III, modification 1, type of removable restoration and the edentulous areas of the residual ridge are from canine to third molar on each side and you desire some support of the bases by the residual ridges. What procedure should you then undertake to acceptably reline the restoration? Include your impression procedure, impression material, processing, and correction of any occlusal discrepancies encountered.
8. There are two indications of the need for relining a distal extension removable partial denture. Can you state these two indications?
9. There is little difference in relining a distal extension denture base and making a secondary impression with a tray attached to the framework. Can you describe the procedures, both clinical and laboratory, that must be performed in relining a distal extension base?
10. After completion of the reline procedure and finishing of the restoration, occlusal discrepancies invariably occur. They, of course, must be corrected before the patient is given possession of the restoration. How do you go about correcting occlusal discrepancies for a relined distal extension denture?
11. Should the same adjustment procedures of the denture base to residual ridge be undertaken for a relined base as was performed for initial placement of a new denture?
12. Does adjustment of the denture base to the basal seat precede or come after correction of occlusal discrepancies?
13. Suppose that after relining a distal extension denture base you find that occlusal contacts of opposing posterior artificial teeth are minimal or nonexistent. What then?
14. Tissue conditioning of basal seats, especially in maxillary arches, to eliminate inflammatory responses of the tissues prior to relining the base is sometimes required. How do you handle the fluid resins when such a procedure is required?
15. What is the quickest way to resolve inflammatory responses of oral tissues to a removable restoration?

21 REPAIRS AND ADDITIONS TO REMOVABLE PARTIAL DENTURES

The need for repairing or adding to a partial denture will occasionally arise. However, the frequency of this occurring should be held to a minimum by careful diagnosis, intelligent treatment planning, adequate mouth preparations, and by carrying out an effective partial denture design with all component parts properly constructed. Any need for repairs or additions will then be due to unforeseen complications arising in abutment or other teeth in the arch or to breakage or distortion of the denture through accident or careless handling by the patient rather than to faulty design or construction.

It is important that the patient be instructed in the proper placement and removal of the restoration so that undue strain is not placed on clasp arms or other parts of the denture nor on the abutment teeth contacted. The patient also should be advised that care must be given the restoration when it is out of the mouth and that any distortion may be irreparable. It should be made clear that there can be no guarantee against breakage or distortion from causes other than obvious structural defects.

CLASSIFICATION OF REPAIRS AND ADDITIONS

Repairs and additions to partial dentures may be classified according to what occasioned their necessity: broken clasp arms, fractured rests, distortion or breakage of other components, loss of an additional tooth, and miscellaneous causes.

Broken clasp arms. There are several reasons for breakage of clasp arms:

1. Breakage may result from repeated flexure into and out of too severe an undercut. If the periodontal support is greater than

the fatigue limit of the clasp arm, failure of the metal occurs first; otherwise the abutment tooth is loosened and eventually lost because of the persistent strain placed on it. This type of breakage can be avoided by locating clasp arms only where an acceptable minimum of retention exists, as determined by an accurate survey of the master cast. The amount of retention is predictable only by the proper utilization of guiding planes during placement and removal.

2. Breakage may occur because of structural failure of the clasp arm itself. A cast clasp arm that is not uniformly tapered because the pattern was not properly formed or because of careless finishing and polishing will eventually break at its weakest point because of repeated flexure at that point. This can be avoided by providing a uniform taper to flexible retentive clasp arms and uniform bulk to all rigid nonretentive clasp arms.

Wrought-wire clasp arms may eventually fail because of repeated flexure at the point at which a nick or constriction occurred because of careless use of the contouring pliers. They also may break at the point of origin from the casting because of excessive manipulation during initial adaptation to the tooth or subsequent readaptation. The latter can best be avoided by cautioning the patient against repeatedly lifting the clasp arm away from the tooth by application of the fingernail during removal of the denture. A wrought-wire clasp arm can normally be adjusted several times over a period of years without failure. It is only when the number of adjustments are excessive that breakage is likely to occur.

Wrought-wire clasp arms also may break

at the point of origin because of recrystallization of the metal. It can be prevented by proper selection of the wrought wire used and by avoiding burnout temperatures exceeding 1300° F and excessive casting temperatures when a cast-to method is used. When the wrought wire is attached to the framework by soldering, as must be done with all but one of the chromium-cobalt alloys, the soldering technique must avoid recrystallization of the wire. For this reason, it is best that soldering be done electrically to prevent overheating the wrought wire. A low-fusing (1420° to 1500° F) triple thick, color-matching gold solder should be used rather than a solder possessing a higher fusing temperature.

3. Breakage may occur because of careless handling by the patient. Any clasp arm will become distorted or will break if subjected to excessive abuse by the patient. The most common cause of failure of a cast clasp arm is distortion caused by accidentally dropping the denture into the lavatory basin or onto other hard surfaces. The most common cause of failure of a wrought-wire clasp is repeated readjustments made necessary by the patient's lifting improperly against the wrought wire during removal of the denture. This is avoided by instructing the patient before a mirror in how to remove the denture without distorting the wrought-wire clasp arms. Removal should be accomplished by lifting against some other part of the framework or at the point of origin of the wrought-wire clasp arm rather than along its course. Breakage is also avoided by placing wrought-wire clasp arms on the lingual surface of abutment teeth whenever possible, where they are inaccessible to the fingernail during removal.

Fractured occlusal rests. Breakage of an occlusal rest almost always occurs at the point at which it crosses the marginal ridge because of weakness at this point. Improperly prepared occlusal rest seats are usually the cause of such weakness: an occlusal rest crossing a marginal ridge that was not lowered sufficiently during mouth preparations is either made too thin or is thinned by adjustment in the mouth to avoid occlusal interference. Failure of an occlusal rest is rarely due to a structural defect in the metal and rarely if ever due to accidental distortion. Therefore the blame for such failure

must frequently be assumed by the dentist for not having provided sufficient space during mouth preparations for the placement of an occlusal rest of adequate bulk.

Distortion or breakage of other components, such as major and minor connectors. Assuming that these components were made with adequate bulk originally, distortion can occur only from abuse by the patient. All such components should be designed and fabricated with sufficient bulk to assure their rigidity and permanence of form under normal circumstances. In such cases any distortion or breakage occurring when the restoration is out of the mouth is then the fault and obligation of the patient, the dentist's responsibility being limited to its repair or replacement at a reasonable fee.

Major and minor connectors occasionally become weakened by adjustment to avoid or eliminate tissue impingement. Such adjustment at the time of initial placement is due to inadequate survey of the master cast or to faulty design or fabrication of the casting. This is inexcusable and reflects on the dentist; such a restoration should be remade rather than further weakening the restoration by attempting to compensate for its inadequacies by relieving the metal. Similarly, tissue impingement arising from inadequately relieved components is due to faulty construction, and the casting should be remade with enough relief to avoid impingement. Failure of any component that was weakened by adjustment at the time of initial placement is the responsibility of the dentist. However, adjustment made necessary by settling of the restoration because abutment teeth have become intruded under functional loading may be unavoidable, and subsequent failure due to the weakening effect of such adjustment may necessitate the making of a new restoration as a consequence of tissue changes. Frequently, repeated adjustment to a major or minor connector to relieve tissue impingement may not result in actual breakage but results in a loss of rigidity to the point that the connector can no longer function effectively. In such cases either a new restoration must be made or that part replaced by casting a new section and then reassembling the denture by soldering. This occasionally requires disassembly of denture base areas and replaced teeth, and the cost and probable success must then be weighed against the cost of an entirely new restoration. Frequently the latter course is advisable.

Loss of an additional tooth or teeth not involved in the support or retention of the restoration. Such additions to a partial denture are usually simply made when the bases are made of resin. The addition of teeth to metal bases is more complex and necessitates either casting a new component, and attaching it by soldering, or creating retentive elements for the attachment of a resin extension. In most instances, when a distal extension denture base is extended, the need for subsequent relining of the entire base should be considered. After the extension of the denture base, a relining procedure of both the new and old base then should be carried out to provide optimal tissue support for the restoration.

Loss of an abutment tooth necessitating not only its replacement but also the substitution of a new clasp assembly on another abutment. This is usually the next adjacent tooth, which may or may not have to undergo restorative treatment. In the latter case, any new restoration should be done to conform to the original path of placement, with proximal guiding plane, occlusal rest seat, and suitable retentive areas. Otherwise, modifications to the existing tooth should be done the same as would be done during any other mouth preparations, with proximal disking, preparation of an adequate occlusal rest seat, and any reduction in tooth contours necessary to accommodate retentive and stabilizing components. A new clasp assembly then may be cast for this tooth and the denture reassembled with the new replacement tooth added.

The most frequent cause of the loss of an abutment tooth is periodontal involvement. If an abutment tooth becomes carious or fractures, it can frequently be restored with a crown made to fit the existing denture clasp. Early pulpal involvement is usually amenable to endodontic treatment, gained by access through the existing restoration. However, an abutment tooth that becomes periodontally involved is too often lost. In many instances this could have been avoided initially by more careful evaluation of the periodontal support of a tooth that is to serve as an abutment and by the use of multiple abutments by splinting whenever advisable. When an adjacent tooth must be substituted as the new abutment, it must be considered

as potentially a periodontally weakened tooth and treated accordingly. Occasionally, splinting of two teeth with double restorations is necessary before the denture is extended to include the new abutment. This is often made more necessary by the fact that the edentulous area is increased by one tooth, and in a distal extension situation the leverage on the abutment is increased correspondingly.

Other types of repairs. Included in this category is the replacement of a broken or lost prosthetically supplied tooth, the repair of a broken resin base, or the reattachment of a loosened resin base to the metal framework. Breakage is sometimes due to poor design, faulty construction, or the use of the wrong material for a given situation. Other times it is due to an accident that will not necessarily repeat itself. If the latter occurs, repair or replacement usually suffices. On the other hand, if fracture has occurred because of structural defects or if it occurs a second time after the denture's having been repaired once before, then some change in the design, either by modification of the original denture or with a new denture, may be necessary. Usually the share of responsibility by dentist and patient will depend on the length of service given by the denture before breakage occurred and on other contributing factors, such as the existence of an abnormal occlusion. Such matters are best approached by a frank and honest appraisal of all the factors involved, based on the patient's understanding that the permanence or longevity of any prosthetic restoration, since it is dependent on the changing characteristics of living tissues, can never be assured.

PROCEDURES FOR MAKING REPAIRS AND ADDITIONS

Although some repairs or additions to partial dentures may be done by the laboratory technician through properly executed work authorizations, impressions and other chairside procedures must be done in accordance with the laboratory procedures to follow.

If a new clasp assembly is to be made, an impression is made for a new master cast. This is poured and surveyed, and the design of the new clasp outlined. The same applies to the making of any new component part to be cast and subsequently attached to the original framework. Frequently the patient can continue to wear the denture while the new part is being made and must be without it only for the brief period of time it takes to reassemble the parts. Jaw relations are usually made with the original denture in the mouth, and at the same time an impression is made for an occluding cast.

For more simple repairs and additions, it is usually preferable that the impression be made with the denture in place, the denture being removed in the impression. An alginate hydrocolloid impression material should be used that has sufficient toughness on setting to permit withdrawal of the denture in the impression.

The cast should be poured immediately in stone. If an occlusal rest or some soldered clasp assembly is to be made, the soldering will be done on a refractory duplicate of the stone cast, and the original stone cast will be used for the final fitting and finishing.

REPLACING A BROKEN CLASP ARM WITH A WROUGHT-WIRE RETENTIVE ARM

A broken retentive clasp arm, regardless of its type, may be replaced with a wrought-wire retentive arm embedded in a resin base or attached to a metal base by electric soldering. Frequently this avoids the necessity of constructing an entirely new clasp assembly. Eighteen-gauge wrought wire is used to replace the original clasp arm.

When a resin base is present, the wire may be embedded into it with repair resin, thus eliminating the need for soldering (Fig. 21-1). The method for replacing a clasp in this manner is as follows:

The remainder of the original clasp arm is cut off flush with its point of origin. A hole is then drilled just below the adjacent artificial tooth as close as possible to the minor connector from which the clasp arm originated. This hole must be angled downward toward the opposite side, emerging approximately midway on the opposite side of the resin base. From this hole a groove is cut in the resin base long enough to accommodate a sufficient length of the wrought wire for adequate retention. At the opposite end of this groove a hole is made that will accommodate a right-angle turn in the wire. A piece of 18-gauge wrought wire to be used as a clasp arm is shaped with a right-angle bend at one end, adapted to fit the lingual groove, and then

Fig. 21-1. Lingual view of technique for replacing a broken retentive clasp arm with an 18-gauge wrought wire. Wrought wire is embedded securely with self-curing repair resin in a groove cut in resin base.

bent to fit the hole passing through to the opposite side. A straight portion sufficient to be adapted later as a clasp arm is left emerging from the resin base at the point of origin of the new clasp arm.

After the projecting wrought wire is secured with sticky wax, self-curing repair resin is painted into the resin base until the defect is overfilled. After polymerizing is done, this is trimmed and polished. The projecting wrought wire is then cut off to the required length, tapered as discussed earlier, and adapted to serve as a new retentive clasp arm. The abutment tooth must be surveyed to determine the location of the desired undercut. The terminal portion of the adapted clasp arm is then rounded and tapered slightly.

This method is suitable any time a retentive clasp arm must be replaced and avoids any disassembly of the original denture. Because of the flexibility of wrought wire, it cannot be used to replace a stabilizing arm when rigidity is needed. In such cases, when a rigid clasp arm has been lost, it is best that an entirely new clasp assembly be cast and attached to the framework by soldering.

REPAIRING BY SOLDERING

It has been said that 80% of all soldering in dentistry can be done electrically. Electric soldering units are available for this purpose, and most dental laboratories are so equipped (Fig. 21-2). Electric soldering permits soldering close to a resin base without removing that base, because of the rapid localization of heat at the electrode. The resin

Fig. 21-2. Electric soldering machine with capability of heat adjustment of low, medium, medium high, and high. Carbon electrode that furnishes heat for soldering is on right. Electrode on left completes electric circuit when touched to framework being soldered. Carbon electrode should be placed first on framework and removed last when soldering.

base needs only to be protected with wet asbestos during soldering.

Color-matching gold solder may be used for soldering both gold and chromium-cobalt alloys. A solder for gold alloys that melts between 1420° and 1500° F is entirely adequate to solder gold alloys to chrome-cobalt alloys, thereby lessening the chance of recrystallizing gold wrought wire by excessive and prolonged heat. For electric soldering, triple-thick solder should be used so that the additional bulk of the solder will retard melting momentarily while the carbon electrode conducts heat to the area being soldered. For soldering chromium-cobalt alloys a color-matching white 19K gold solder, which melts at about 1676° F, is used. An application of flux is essential to the success of any soldering operation to prevent oxidation of the parts being joined as well as the solder itself. A borax-type flux is used when soldering gold alloys. Fluoride type flux must be used when soldering chrome-cobalt alloys. When a gold alloy is to be soldered to a chrome-cobalt alloy, a fluoride-type flux should be chosen.

Following is a procedure for electric soldering:

1. Roughen both sections to be joined.

2. Adapt platinum foil to the master cast to serve as a backing upon which the solder will flow. Lift the edges of the foil to form a trough to confine the flow of the solder.

3. Seat the pieces to be soldered onto the master cast and secure them temporarily with sticky wax. Over each piece add enough soldering investment to secure them after the sticky wax is eliminated, but leave as much metal exposed as possible.

4. After flushing off the sticky wax with hot water, secure the cast to the soldering stand. Cut sufficient solder and place conveniently nearby.

5. Flux both sections. Put sufficient triple-thick solder on or in the joint to complete the soldering in one operation, always starting with enough solder to complete the job.

6. Wet the carbon tip with water to aid conduction of the current and then touch the carbon tip to the solder. Place the other electrode on any portion of the framework to complete the electric circuit and heat the carbon electrode. Do not push the solder with the carbon tip, but let the heat alone make the solder flow. Do not remove the carbon from the solder while the soldering operation is in progress, as this will cause surface pitting because of arcing as the carbon is removed. After the solder has flowed, remove the electrodes, *removing the carbon tip electrode last*, and proceed to remove the work from the cast for finishing.

Torch soldering requires an entirely different approach. It is used when the solder joint is long or unusually bulky and when a larger quantity of solder has to be used. Torch soldering cannot be undertaken to repair a removable restoration having acrylic resin denture bases or artificial teeth supported by acrylic resin. The procedure for torch soldering is as follows:

1. Roughen both sections to be joined.

2. Adapt platinum foil to the master cast so that it extends under both sections.

3. Seat the sections on the master cast in the correct relationship and secure them temporarily with sticky wax. Flow sticky wax also into the joint to be soldered.

4. Attach a dental bur or nail over the two sections with a liberal amount of sticky wax. Attach a second and even a third nail or bur across other areas to lend additional support. Never use pieces of wood for this purpose because the wood will swell if it gets wet, thus distorting the relationship of the two sections.

5. Remove the assembled casting from the master cast carefully. Adapt a stock of utility wax directly under each section, on either

side of the platinum foil. After boilout is done, investment will remain in the center to support the platinum foil.

6. Invest the casting in sufficient soldering investment to secure it, leaving as much of the area to be soldered exposed as possible. When the investment has set, boil out the sticky and utility waxes. Then place the investment in a drying oven at a temperature not exceeding 200° F until the contained moisture has been eliminated. Do not preheat the investment with a torch, or oxides will be formed that will interfere with the flow of the solder.

7. Use the reducing part of the flame, which is that feathery part just outside the blue inner cone. Flux the joint thoroughly and dry out the flux with the outer part of the flame until it has a powdery appearance. Heat the casting until it is dull red and then, holding a strip of solder in the soldering tweezers, dip it into the flux and feed it into the joint while the casting is being held at a dull red heat with the torch. Once the soldering operation has begun, do not remove the flame, as any cooling will cause oxides to be formed. The heat from the casting should be sufficient to melt the solder; therefore do not put the flame directly on the solder or it will become overheated, resulting in pitting.

8. After the soldering has been completed, allow the investment to cool slowly before quenching and proceeding with finishing. Remember that any soldering operation that heats the entire casting is in effect a heat-treating operation, and heat-hardening of a repaired gold alloy casting is desirable to restore its optimal physical properties.

SELF-ASSESSMENT AIDS

1. The need for repairing a component of a removable partial denture may arise occasionally. How may the frequency of breakage of a component be minimized?
2. For what three reasons may breakage of a direct retainer arm occur?
3. An occlusal or incisal rest may fracture in use and invariably occurs at marginal ridge or incisal areas. What is the predominant reason for lack of strength at the junction of the rest and minor connector?
4. Have you ever tried to adjust a distorted major connector? If yes, how did it work out?
5. Other than by accident, for what reasons could a major connector become distorted?
6. An abutment with a guarded prognosis is sometimes utilized to avoid an extension-type denture. Loss of such abutments requires extension of denture bases and inclusion of an artificial tooth replacing the abutment. Suppose the denture was not designed anticipating eventual loss of the posterior abutment. Would this influence your decision to repair or remake the denture?
7. What is the most frequent cause for the loss of an abutment tooth?
8. When a terminal abutment for a distal extension removable partial denture is lost, can the existing denture be modified with a new clasp assembly on another abutment?
9. Porcelain artificial teeth that have been excessively ground or that were not arranged in occlusal harmony sometimes fracture in use and have to be replaced. Can you perform this procedure? Is an impression necessary? If the replaced tooth is on an extension base, how do you adjust the occlusion?
10. Most repairs to removable partial dentures require than an impression of the arch be made with the restoration in place to recover a working cast. True or false?
11. What procedures are necessary to replace a broken retentive arm of a direct retainer with a wrought-wire arm?
12. What is a distinct advantage of electric soldering over torch soldering for the repair of a metallic element of a removable partial denture?
13. Suppose a rest broke at its junction with the minor connector. How could you create a new rest by soldering? Would you perform a clinical procedure on the old rest seat preparation first?
14. You are soldering chromium-cobalt alloy. What solder should you use? Any special type of flux required?
15. What solder and flux would you use to repair a Type IV gold alloy framework by soldering?
16. When using an electric soldering unit, why must the carbon electrode be removed from the work last?
17. What is the purpose of using a flux when performing soldering operations?
18. Should torch soldering be attempted on a restoration with acrylic resin bases?
19. After you have repaired a framework by either electric or torch soldering, should a heat-hardening treatment be performed? Why or why not?

22 INTERIM, TRANSITIONAL, AND TREATMENT REMOVABLE PARTIAL DENTURES

Removable partial dentures designed to be used for short intervals often must be fabricated as a part of a total prosthodontic treatment. Such restorations serve many useful purposes and may be classified according to the purpose for which they are used. It is not our intent to introduce new terminology; however, for the sake of clarity it seems justifiable to discuss these restorations under three headings.

Interim partial dentures. Interim partial dentures are made for economic or other reasons when the use of such a restoration is justified. For example, a patient may be preparing to take a trip and time does not permit the making of adequate mouth preparations and the rendering of a more complete partial denture service. Another example is that the patient may be in poor health or may be facing some medical or surgical emergency. Also, a young person may have lost teeth prematurely through an accident or for other reasons. Either for the sake of appearance, or for the purpose of maintaining a space, or both, an interim partial denture must be made until such time as fixed restorations can be fabricated or more definitive partial denture service is possible.

When recent extractions must be replaced temporarily while tissues heal or, in younger patients, until the adjacent teeth have reached sufficient maturity to be used as abutments for fixed restorations, the use of an interim partial denture maintains mesiodistal and occlusal relations until other restorative treatment can be done. An acceptable esthetic result usually can be obtained. It is important, however, that the patient or the parents of the younger patient be made aware that any such removable restoration is *temporary*

and may jeopardize the integrity of the adjacent teeth and the health of the supporting soft tissues if worn for extended periods without supportive care. The need for strict oral hygiene and diet control also must be clearly understood and such provisions made while an interim partial denture is being worn. Generally the younger patient is even more susceptible to caries when wearing a removable restoration, and adequate prophylactic measures must be taken to prevent decalcification and caries in the teeth contacted.

An interim partial denture may replace only one or more missing anterior teeth, or it may replace several teeth, both anterior and posterior, in a partially edentulous dental arch. Such a restoration is usually made of acrylic resin, either by a sprinkling method or by waxing, flasking, and processing with either self-curing or thermal-curing resin. It may be retained by wrap-around wrought-wire clasps, Crozat-type clasps, interproximal spurs, or wire loops. In rare instances, separate cast circumferential type clasps may be used, attached to the resin base by a retaining lug.

Whatever the materials and methods of retention used, such partial dentures are *temporary*, and a distinction must be made between this type of restoration and a partial denture prosthesis with prepared abutments and rigid all-cast framework construction. *Too frequently a partial denture is constructed by dental laboratories on order from the dentist, who then represents it to the patient as a "partial denture," with a fee that is a multiple of the laboratory cost. However, it should be considered nothing more than a temporary restoration. The patient is being* misled (perhaps the word "fleeced" is more appropriate) when such a temporary restoration is purported to be representative of modern restorative dentistry.

Interim partial dentures are made for one or more of the following reasons: (1) to maintain a space, (2) to reestablish occlusion, (3) to replace visible missing teeth while definitive restorative procedures are being accomplished, (4) to serve while the patient is undergoing periodontal or other treatment, and (5) to condition the patient to wearing a removable prosthesis. In the latter instance the patient's response to wearing a more costly restoration may be evaluated, and on some rare occasions, further treatment may be interrupted while the patient becomes conditioned to the wearing of a removable restoration.

In some instances an existing partial denture can be used with modifications as an interim partial denture. Such modifications may include relining and the adding of teeth and clasps to an existing denture. In other instances an existing partial denture may be converted to a transitional complete denture for immediate placement while tissues heal and an opposing arch is prepared to receive a partial denture. Sometimes an interim partial denture must be made to replace missing anterior teeth in a partially edentulous arch, which are ultimately to be replaced with fixed restorations. On occasion the anterior portion of the restoration is cut away when the fixed restorations are placed, leaving the remainder of the denture to be worn while posterior abutment teeth are being prepared.

Still another type of interim denture is one on which missing posterior teeth are replaced temporarily with a resin occlusion rim rather than with occluding teeth. In dental school clinics it is sometimes impossible to complete treatment in a school year, and the continuing student may desire to resume treatment after the summer recess. In such instances, occlusion may be maintained, and, as in the case of treatment dentures, the tissues may be conditioned by having the patient wear a temporary restoration with posterior occlusion rims that have been adjusted to occlusal harmony.

Transitional partial dentures. A transitional partial denture is made to aid the patient in making the transition to complete dentures when total loss of teeth is inevit-able. Such a partial denture also may be considered a treatment restoration, since the patient is at the same time being conditioned to the wearing of a removable prosthesis. It should be considered strictly a temporary measure that provides the patient with a restoration for the remaining life of the natural teeth when further restorative treatment of those teeth is impractical or economically or technically impossible.

Such a partial denture may be worn for prolonged periods, in the meantime undergoing revision, modification to include additional teeth lost, or relining when such becomes necessary or advisable. The dentist should agree to provide such a partial denture only under the following conditions: (1) that a definite fee for the treatment is impossible to predict and that the cost will depend on the servicing necessary and (2) that when, in his opinion, further wearing of the transitional denture is unwise and jeopardizes the health of the remaining tissues, the transition to complete dentures will proceed.

Treatment partial dentures. Treatment partial dentures are used for the following reasons: (1) to establish a new occlusal relationship or vertical dimension and (2) to condition teeth and ridge tissues to support better the partial denture to follow.

Treatment partial dentures may be used as occlusal splints in much the same manner as cast or resin occlusal splints are used on natural teeth (Figs. 22-1 and 22-2). When total tooth support is available, there is little difference between a fixed and a removable occlusal splint, except that a removable splint is too likely to be left out of the mouth unless the patient is actually made more comfortable by its presence. This is usually true when temporomandibular joint pathology is alleviated by the wearing of an occlusal splint. In other situations it may be advisable to cement the removable restoration to the teeth until such time as the patient has become accustomed to, and dependent on, the jaw relationship provided by the splint.

Both fixed and removable tooth-supported occlusal splints have much in common. Either of them may be eliminated sectionally as restorative treatment is being done, thus maintaining the established jaw relation until all restorative treatment has been completed. The dentist usually decides whether these

Fig. 22-1. Four views showing use of a removable occlusal splint. **A,** Evidence of overclosure to be corrected by occlusal reconstruction. **B,** Removable occlusal splint for lower arch, using tooth-colored acrylic resin for occlusal surfaces. **C,** Removable splint in mouth. Occlusal anatomy is result of an occlusal registration done in wax on resin base, which is then invested, and to which tooth-colored resin is added to reproduce functional occlusal surfaces that were recorded in wax. **D,** Resulting occlusion with removable splint. This may be adjusted until satisfactory, and then it signifies the vertical dimension, to be maintained by oral rehabilitation.

Fig. 22-2. Cast gold occlusal splints. Following occlusal adjustment, splints are cemented to teeth. Since these are made to fit unprepared natural teeth, they cannot extend beyond height of contour of each tooth. Surveying is therefore necessary prior to their construction. Splints may be eliminated tooth by tooth as subsequent restorations are being done, thus maintaining established vertical relationship.

are to be fixed or removable and whether they are made of a cast (silver or gold) alloy or of a resin material.

When one or more distal extension bases exist on an occlusal splint, a different situation exists. The establishment of a new occlusal or vertical relation depends too much on the quality of support the splint receives to ignore the need for the best possible support for any existing distal extension base. Both broad coverage and functional basing of tissue-supported bases are desirable, as well as some type of occlusal rest on the nearest abutments. Any tissue-supported occlusal splint should at least be relined in the mouth with a self-curing reline resin to afford optimal coverage and support for the distal extension base.

O. C. Applegate, in an article on the choice of partial or complete denture treatment, has emphasized the advantages of conditioning edentulous areas to provide stable support for distal extension partial dentures. This is accomplished by having the patient wear a treatment partial denture for a period of time prior to construction of the final base. In the absence of opposing occlusion, stimulation of the underlying tissues by applying intermittent finger pressure to the denture base is advised. Whether the stimulation is from occlusal or finger pressure, there seems to be little doubt that the tissues of the residual ridge become more capable of supporting a distal extension partial denture when they have been conditioned by the wearing of a previous restoration.

Abutment teeth also benefit from the wearing of a treatment restoration when such a restoration applies an occlusal load to those teeth, either through occlusal coverage or through occlusal rests. Frequently a tooth that is to be used as an abutment for a partial denture has been out of occlusion for some time. Immediately on applying an occlusal load to that tooth sufficient to support any type of removable prosthesis, some intrusion of the tooth will occur. If such intrusion is allowed to occur after initial placement of the final prosthesis, the occlusal relationship of the prosthesis and its relation to the adjacent gingival tissues will be altered. Perhaps this is one reason for gingival impingement, which occurs after the denture has been worn for some time, even though seemingly adequate relief had been provided

initially. When a treatment partial denture is worn, such abutment teeth have an opportunity to become stabilized under the loading of the treatment restoration, and intrusion will have occurred prior to the making of the impression for the master cast. There is sufficient reason to believe that both abutment teeth and supporting ridge tissues are better capable of providing continuing support for the partial denture when they have been previously conditioned by the wearing of a treatment restoration.

Another example of the use of a treatment partial denture is to facilitate the eruption of posterior teeth through the use of an acrylic resin bite plane. Particularly in the younger patient, early loss of some posterior teeth results in either depression or incomplete eruption of the remaining teeth. The most frequently seen example of this is when the molar teeth in one arch are missing and the premolar teeth remain in occlusion. These are then either depressed or were never able to erupt fully because of excessive occlusal loading. Overclosure results, with anterior teeth likewise in excessive contact, leading to orthodontic movement of these teeth or excessive vertical overlap or both. Prosthetic replacement of missing teeth with a partial denture can thus only perpetuate an overclosed relationship unless one of two objectives is accomplished first: (1) to increase the occlusal height of the remaining teeth arbitrarily with restorations or (2) to permit the remaining posterior teeth to attain full eruption by increasing the vertical dimension of occlusion. Usually the latter method is preferable.

For such treatment an acrylic resin restoration is made that causes the lower anterior teeth to close against an acrylic resin plane while the posterior teeth remain out of occlusion. Some depression of the lower anterior teeth may occur, but without ill effect. More important, posterior teeth that have become depressed or were not fully erupted may migrate into a new vertical occlusion as dictated by the amount of opening anteriorly. Once this has occurred, prosthetic replacement of the missing teeth may proceed and the established vertical dimension be maintained with fixed or removable restorations or a combination of both.

• • •

These are the various types of prosthetic restorations for the partially edentulous mouth that are, and must be, considered temporary restorations. It is imperative that a distinction be made between these and a true partial denture service and that the patient be advised of the purposes and limitations of such restorations. In no instance should the patient be misled into believing that an inadequate, interim partial denture is representative of modern prosthetic dentistry.

SELF-ASSESSMENT AIDS

1. Removable partial dentures designed to be used for short intervals are temporary restorations and serve definite purposes. They must not be represented to the patient as other than temporary. True or false?
2. There are three basic types of removable partial dentures of a temporary nature: *interim*, *transitional*, and *treatment*. In each of the following uses, please categorize the type of temporary restoration.
   a. A young adult lost a maxillary central incisor by accident and was getting married in three days. The incisor was replaced with a temporary removable restoration to restore appearance.
   b. A patient had a few remaining teeth that could not even be retained for overdentures. The patient had never worn a removable restoration and was very apprehensive about the ability to do so. Temporary removable partial dentures were placed to allay the patient's apprehension.
   c. A 12-year-old child lost a maxillary right central and lateral incisor. The dentist maintained the space with a temporary restoration replacing the missing teeth until fixed restorations could be used on matured teeth.
   d. An adult patient having badly abraded anterior and posterior opposing teeth was treated with a removable silver splint on the mandibular posterior teeth to increase the vertical dimension of occlusion prior to his being treated with fixed restorations.
   e. An adult patient's mandibular molars and second premolars had been missing for two years without any restoration replacing the mandibular teeth. The patient's maxillary premolars were missing and without replacement. An exercise prosthesis was placed on the lower arch and used for two months to condition the residual ridges and first premolars.
3. Interim removable partial dentures are made for several reasons. Can you give four reasons?
4. Under what circumstances would you treat a patient with a transitional partial denture?
5. There are two indications for the use of a treatment prosthesis. What are they?
6. The construction of temporary removable partial dentures needs only that prosthodontic principles not be violated and that procedures are meticulously executed. True or false?

23 MISCELLANEOUS PARTIAL PROSTHODONTICS

JOHN J. SHARRY, B.S., D.M.D.*

The prosthetic replacement of tissue defects, which were either traumatically or developmentally acquired, often depends on removable prostheses that are retained by clasps on the teeth.

Certain considerations will be discussed that do not supplant but rather supplement those general principles of design that apply to the usual removable partial denture. Such components as the pharyngeal portion of a cleft palate prosthesis and the obturator that closes the defect resulting from a hemisection of the maxilla impose further burdens on the usual designs. Resultant dislodging forces must be considered and included in the design that will be used for any particular patient.

Several types of prostheses depend on a partial denture framework for their retention. An attempt to describe only a representative few is made, since the variations are myriad and do not lend themselves to easy classification.

CLEFT PALATE PROSTHESES

The cleft palate obturator is one of the most common obturators and is the one about which most has been written. (Various other restorations, often referred to as maxillofacial prostheses, will be discussed later in general rather than specific terms.)

Classification. Cleft palates lend themselves to morphologic classifications. The simplest and perhaps the most easily remembered is that of Veau. He proposed four classes: Class I, in which the cleft involves only the soft palate; Class II, which involves

the soft and hard palates but not the alveolus; Class III, which involves the soft and hard palates, continuing through the alveolus on one side of the premaxillary area; and Class IV, which involves the soft and hard palates, the cleft continuing through the alveolus on both sides, leaving a free premaxilla (Fig. 23-1). The latter two classes are usually, though not always, associated with a cleft lip. The cleft lip is usually closed within a matter of weeks or months. The prosthodontist can make impressions of the newborn's lip and palate in order to construct a feeding aid of soft plastic.

Etiology. The etiology of cleft palate is not clear but seems at the present time to have some basis in heredity, although many other factors have been mentioned, such as infectious diseases of the mother, nutritional inadequacies, and various other changes in the intrauterine environment.

Personality evaluation. The personality range of individuals with a cleft palate is not much different from that of the general population. Perhaps more of them fall into the quiet, unresponsive, withdrawn category and a few exhibit a brashness or bravado (which generally disappears on continued association with them). However, a large share are well-adjusted, pleasant people. Sometimes one wonders how so many can be happy when the attitude of the parents and the public is often such that a considerable degree of overprotection or rejection is the fate of these individuals when they are children.

It should be noted here that so many factors influence diagnosis and treatment of these patients that a "team approach" (dentist, surgeon, pediatrician, speech therapist,

*Dean, University of Texas Dental School at San Antonio.

Fig. 23-1. Veau's classification of cleft palates.

and so forth) to management of these patients is essential.

There are a few areas in which certain differences of approach are necessary in prosthetic treatment for such persons. For example, it is often found that their speaking habits are so poor that they cannot be understood. This difficulty will usually disappear with continued association, but initially a relative can interpret for them. If they are alone, then a paper and pencil will solve the problem. But speech therapy should begin at once and proceed parallel with prosthetic treatment.

Anatomy. During the examination of clefts that have not been treated surgically, the dentist should examine the nasal and pharyngeal cavities and their component structures and, using a blunt instrument or finger, ascertain the tissue consistency of various areas. It should be noted here that the gag reflex of the person with a cleft palate is markedly diminished and does not usually hinder palpatory examination.

Knowledge of the anatomic structure of these cavities serves not merely to satisfy intellectual curiosity but, more important, to place the dentist on familiar ground when and if it becomes necessary to remove impression materials that may inadvertently be forced through the cleft or perforation while obtaining impressions of the dental arches.

The normal soft palate either closes the nasal cavity from the pharynx or the oral cavity from the pharynx, or it just relaxes as the occasion demands (Fig. 23-2). If this "valve" is not whole, then of course it cannot effectively perform these closing functions but rather allows food to enter the nasopharynx during deglutition and allows air to enter the nasal cavity during the production of those speech sounds wherein the air should be directed into the oral cavity. Further, it makes the production of such sounds as "puh" and "kuk" practically impossible.

A group of muscles is attached to the soft palate and is responsible for the closure of the nasal cavity. This total action (closing off the nasal cavity) is called the *velopharyngeal closure*. To accomplish this the following, more or less simultaneous, muscular contractions take place.

The levator veli palatini (levator palatini) muscle, which originates on the petrous portion of the temporal bone and the cartilage of the eustachian tube and runs downward and forward to insert into the palatine aponeurosis, contracts, pulling the soft palate upward and backward (Fig. 23-3). This is a paired muscle, and on entering the soft palate it merges with its fellow of the opposite side, forming a sling. At the same time, the tensor veli palatini (tensor palatini), which arises from the scaphoid fossa, the sphenoid

Fig. 23-2. Three positions of soft palate during normal activity.

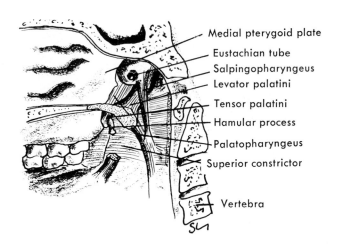

Medial pterygoid plate
Eustachian tube
Salpingopharyngeus
Levator palatini
Tensor palatini
Hamular process
Palatopharyngeus
Superior constrictor

Vertebra

Fig. 23-3. Dissection of velopharyngeal area as seen from side.

spine, and eustachian cartilage, travels downward and forward to the lateral aspect of the hamulus (which is used as a pulley), swings medially to enter the soft palate, contracts, and effects tension on the soft palate. Now the soft palate has been pulled backward and upward.

However, the pull is not sufficient to close the gap between the distal limits of the soft palate and the pharynx, and so the pharynx accommodates by moving forward and medially. This is accomplished by the joint action of three muscles. The pterygopharyngeal portion of the superior constrictor, which

originates usually on the medial pterygoid plate, travels backward fanwise to terminate in a median raphe in the posterior pharynx. It contracts and pulls the posterior pharyngeal wall forward to meet the soft palate. (See Fig. 23-4.) Meanwhile, since this action may not be quite enough in certain instances, the palatopharyngeus muscle, which can be seen in the throat as the posterior pillars of the tonsils and which has two parts, the thyropalatal and pharyngopalatal portions, comes into play. This latter part, which arises in the palatal aponeurosis and travels backward and downward to insert in a fanwise

Fig. 23-4. Musculature of soft palate as seen from above. **A,** Area of section. **B,** Portion of section used. **C,** Detail of section.

Tenso veli palatini

Levator veli palatini

Salpingopharyngeus

Azygos uvulae

Superior constrictor

Fig. 23-5. Passavant's cushion in posterior pharyngeal wall.

fashion in the posterior pharynx anterior to, but interlaced with, the superior constrictor fibers, contracts strongly. It is more or less circular, and it further attempts to approximate the soft palate and pharynx and, in doing so, produces a ridge or "bunching up" of the posterior pharyngeal musculature, called Passavant's cushion (Fig. 23-5). This is usually, though not always, visible in the patient with a cleft palate. It is located at levels varying from as high as the region of the atlas to as low as the level of the distally projected mandibular occlusal plane. Now the soft palate is touching the posterior pharyngeal wall, but there is a leak when the lateral aspect of the soft palate does not meet the lateral aspect of the pharynx. This will be closed by the salpingopharyngeus muscle. This muscle rises from the cartilage of the eustachian tube and travels downward and laterally to fan out and insert in the lateral pharyngeal wall. When it contracts it pulls the lateral wall medially, thus closing the last gap in velopharyngeal closure. All these muscle contractions take place almost simultaneously. The velopharyngeal mechanism has now closed the nasal cavity from the oral cavity and pharynx. This movement is used in deglutition to prevent food from entering the nose and in speech when pronouncing the so-called plosive sounds—puh, buh, tuh, duh, kuh, guh. These sounds are produced by closing off the nose and building up pressure in the mouth and suddenly releasing it. Thus the name "plosive."

The second position, the closure of the oral cavity, is a result of the contraction of the following. The thyropalatal portion of the palatopharyngeus muscle arises from the posterolateral rim of the thyroid cartilage and courses upward through the posterior pillar to insert into the palatine aponeurosis, where it merges with its fellow of the opposite side, forming an inverted U. When it contracts it pulls the soft palate down toward the tongue. Meanwhile the tensor is flattening the dome of the soft palate to bring down the portion of the structure that may not come down with the action of the thyropalatal muscle. Concurrently the tongue is forced upward and backward. To finally eliminate the possibility of a leak, the palatoglossus muscle, which is attached superiorly to the palate and inferiorly to the tongue, forming more or less a sphincteric structure in this motion, contracts and completes the approximation. Therefore it can now be seen that velopharyngeal closure *is not* a simple sphincteric action of the superior constrictor and palatopharyngeus muscles (which run in a nearly horizontal direction) but is instead the resultant contraction of these and others running in a vertical direction, such as the levator, the tensor, and the salpingopharyngeus muscles. This second position is used in sucking and in the pronunciation of sounds such as "ng" in the word sing. The third position finds the palate relaxed as in normal breathing.

Pathology. The patient with a cleft palate, because of his inability to close off the nose, is constantly the victim of nasal infections and middle ear infections sometimes resulting in deafness. He cannot pronounce correctly the plosive sounds and tries to overcompensate with his tongue. He tries to

make the latter obturate the cleft and articulate at the same time. These habits are an obstacle to the speech therapist who must attempt to train the patient to forget these habits and learn a new set of movements.

Despite some of these difficulties, the patient can be nourished adequately, and aside from the possibility of constant nasal and pharyngeal infections, he may be generally quite healthy, although many cleft palate patients have other defects also, such as heart and skeletal congenital abnormalities. The inability to speak properly constitutes his greatest problem. The prosthesis itself, while aiding in velopharyngeal closure, has, for a short while, a harmful effect on articulation by virtue of its impairment of oral sensory stimuli.

Physiology of speech. Speech is a function of respiration, phonation, resonation, articulation, and integration. Respiration is, of course, concerned with the exchange of air by the lungs; phonation is accomplished by the abduction and adduction of the vocal cords, which change the pitch of the voice; resonation is realized in the nasal, oral, and pharyngeal cavities, which are the prime resonation chambers. The teeth, tongue, lips, and palate serve as articulatory mechanisms, and all, of course, would be nothing without the integrating facilities of the human brain. (See Fig. 23-6).

The soft palate performs any one of the following basic functions in speech. It closes off the nasal cavity, as in producing "k" and hard "g"; it closes off the oral cavity for production of the sounds "m," "n," and "ng" (as in "ring"), or it may close neither cavity completely but allow varying portions of the airstream to enter the appropriate resonating chambers.

Although the soft palate is but one part of the velopharyngeal mechanism (the other part being the pharyngeal muscles), it is of such importance that when cleft, the individual cannot effect velopharyngeal closure.

Surgical treatment. Two general types of physical treatment can restore partially or completely the function of the soft palate. The first concerns surgical procedures to close the soft palate (and the hard palate when involved). The other utilizes an artificial restoration, called an *obturator*, which serves not to close the soft palate but rather to fill the space between the two halves of the palate. (Both the surgical and prosthetic ap-

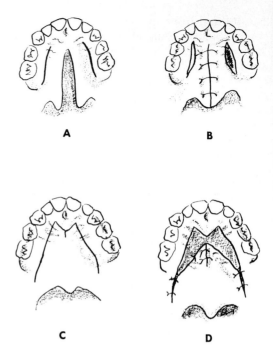

Fig. 23-6. Mechanisms of speech. **A,** Respiratory organ (lungs). **B,** Phonating organ (vocal cords). **C,** Resonating chambers (oral and nasal cavities). **D,** Articulating organs (lips, tongue, and teeth). **E,** Integrating center (brain).

Fig. 23-7. Surgical procedures in cleft palate therapy. **A,** Relaxing incisions in palatal mucosa. **B,** Mucosa elevated and displaced medially where freshened edges of cleft are sutured together. **C,** Incision for push-back operation. **D,** Push-back completed and sutured.

proaches are usually of little avail without speech therapy, given previously, conjointly, or subsequently. It must be noted here that given the choice of a highly skilled surgeon's efforts or those of an equally skilled prosthodontist, the surgeon is to be preferred, for if he is highly skilled, he will know whether he can or cannot succeed and will recommend his prosthodontist counterpart if it is in the best interest of the patient. The surgical approach is generally concerned with the closure and, in many instances, the lengthening of the palate. Closure is achieved by denuding the opposing edges of the two halves of the cleft palate and suturing them together. This may necessitate lateral relaxing incisions parallel to the long axis of the cleft, which will allow it to be apposed and sutured together (Fig. 23-7, *A* and *B*). Lengthening of the palate may be accomplished by an anterior incision of the palatine mucosa, which may run from the area of the molars on one side around back of the anterior teeth (avoiding the anterior palatine foramen) to the molars on the opposite side

(Fig. 23-7, *C* and *D*). The palatine mucosa posteriorly and medially to this incision is dissected from the palatine bone and displaced backward, thus lengthening the soft palate. The denuded palatine bone anteriorly becomes epithelized via granulation tissue.

When the palatal types of operation are not feasible, the surgeon may perform a pharyngeal flap operation, wherein a longitudinal flap is dissected from the posterior pharyngeal wall (its attachment being located either below or above) and is brought forward and sutured to the denuded posterior edge of the soft palate (Fig. 23-8). This then forms a continuous tissue bridge between the soft palate and the pharynx, which functions well as part of the velopharyngeal mechanism. The flap, as dissected, tends to curl medially, leaving lateral space for air transmission through the nasal cavity. Since much of the pharyngeal closing movement is in a medial direction, one can see that this action can aid in velopharyngeal closure because the lateral walls converge medially toward the flap.

Fig. 23-8. Pharyngeal flap operation viewed from side. Flap is based below.

Fig. 23-9. Ladderlike extension of framework into area of cleft (arrow).

There are more definitive surgical approaches to the cleft palate, but they are generally concerned with either of these two aims.

Prosthetic treatment. The prosthetic approach utilizes a metal framework that is similar to a partial denture framework in which is included a posterior latticework extension into the area of the cleft (Fig. 23-9). This extension supports an acrylic resin bulb, which is the obturator.

The *preservation* of the patient's teeth is of *prime importance*, because although obturators have been made for edentulous patients, they can never be as efficient as those that utilize the teeth for stabilization. Therefore all necessary restorative dentistry must be accomplished immediately. In a large percentage of patients the dentist is faced with the problem of restoring occlusal harmony, and therefore the patient may first require orthodontic treatment. However, an obturator often can be combined with the orthodontic appliance. When a patient has good occlusion, no active caries, and no periodontal disease or other oral lesions, construction of the permanent prosthetic restoration may be undertaken. It is imperative that these patients be recalled for examination every four or five months and signs of disease be treated

immediately. Obturators suspected of contributing to disease must be redesigned.

Impressions with alginate hydrocolloid impression materials. The examination will reveal the nature of the unrepaired cleft or, if repaired, those perforations that sometimes result from tissue breakdown. One should look particularly in the anterior mucobuccal fold for minute oronasal perforations after the repair of Classes III and IV clefts.

A resilient impression material must be used because of the many tissue undercuts. The alginate hydrocolloid impression materials serve this purpose adequately.

The problems incident to impressions are divided into two groups, the unrepaired cleft presenting one situation and the repaired cleft another. The unrepaired cleft palate, Classes II, III, and IV, will be considered first. (The method of obtaining impressions of the teeth are not modified by Class I clefts.) When one is using a hydrocolloid impression material, the posterior portion of the tray should be modified with boxing or utility wax to prevent material from flowing down the patient's throat. In addition the use of this wax adjacent to the cleft or perforation will record more accurately the mucosal detail by confining the impression material to those areas. (See Fig. 23-10.)

Fig. 23-10. Use of utility wax to confine impression material to tissues.

The material should be prevented from entering the nasal cavity in such a large quantity that it may fracture from the main body of material. Such an accident requires a tedious process of fragmentation and removal. To prevent this, simply underload the tray in the area of the cleft. The tooth-bearing section of the tray is completely filled with the alginate, but the area corresponding to the cleft is loaded to a height of only 2 to 3 mm. Thus, when the tray is seated, the material is not likely to be forced upward into the cleft in sufficient quantity to "lock."

Cleft palates previously repaired present slightly different problems. The palatal repair itself may look adequate, and yet an oronasal perforation may exist in the labial mucobuccal fold, as previously mentioned. If it is present, either pack this perforation with wet gauze (in many instances the perforations are too small for this approach) or else the tray must be "underloaded" in this area so that a large amount of the impression material will not be forced into the nasal cavity.

Amounts small enough to be dislodged by blowing the nose should not be of concern. Larger amounts, however, require a considerable degree of skill in their fragmentation and removal: *they cannot be pushed into the mouth as in unrepaired defects and must be manipulated within the nasal cavity.*

Those perforations that may exist on the palate itself should be approached in a similar manner. If the area is large enough to pack off with wet gauze, then this is the method of choice. If the diameter is 12 mm or more, then perhaps it is better to handle it like an open cleft, using utility wax damming and underloading the tray in that area.

Framework. The design of the framework is of primary importance, as it must be balanced to eliminate, as much as possible, harmful torque effects on the teeth. The essential requirements for the casting consist of the following: (1) The metal to be used should be as thin as possible commensurate with strength so that metal bulk does not present an added obstacle to speech. (2) The tip of the clasp should engage a distal undercut on the posterior abutments to support the obturator. On abutments further anterior the clasp should engage mesial undercuts when anterior replacements are necessary (Fig. 23-11). If proper undercuts are not present or if the teeth must be restored with full crowns because of caries or for other reasons such as fixed splinting, adequate embrasure crossing space must be planned in the restorations. It is wise to utilize continuous lingual stabilization, even on teeth not used for retentive clasps, in order to distribute widely the torquing forces often developed by these restorations.

The pharyngeal portion is usually attached to the framework by a distal loop or "ladder" from the casting. The superoinferior position of the loop will vary according to the type of prosthesis.

Obturator design. Following are the three main types of obturators: the so-called hinge or movable type, the fixed type, and the meatus type (Fig. 23-12). The hinged type is connected to the main framework by means of a hinge. Its bulk is located above the cleft edges and supposedly serves an anatomic purpose in that it moves up and back, supported by the soft palate edges, as does the normal soft palate to effect velopharyngeal closure. Theoretically this is workable, but in practice it is not quite true because many cleft palates have limited motion, and many authors believe that this type of obturator is limited in use except for a few patients. The fixed type is stationary and is directed toward Passavant's pad. It depends on the forward movement of the pad and lateral movement of the pharynx to effect closure. This is the

Fig. 23-11. When anterior replacements are necessary (shaded teeth), clasp on anterior abutments should engage a mesial undercut. Clasp on distal abutments should engage a distal undercut.

Fig. 23-12. Location of pharyngeal portion of several obturators. **A,** Hinge type. **B,** Fixed type. **C,** Meatus type.

obturator in most general use today and, if made well, is relatively efficient. The meatus obturator will be discussed later because of the difference in construction.

Pharyngeal impressions. The method of obtaining impressions for the hinge type or the fixed type is essentially the same. It involves the following steps: A mound of modeling plastic approximating the pharyngeal defect in shape and size is placed on the distal extension and warmed. This bulk is directed as high above the area of Passavant's pad as feasible and is placed into the patient's mouth while still warm. When the framework is seated properly on the teeth, the patient is instructed to swallow, tilt the head back, and then place the chin on the chest. Keeping it there, he should turn the head from left shoulder to right shoulder. (See Fig. 23-13.) This total routine should be accomplished quickly to mold the modeling

plastic while it is still warm. The resultant impression is then removed from the mouth and compared with the defect. Gross inadequacies are noted, and if necessary, more material is added. The modeling plastic impression is then removed and all excess trimmed. It should have a superoinferior thickness of not more than 5 to 6 mm to keep it as lightweight as possible.

Experience in making impressions for a fixed type of restoration (and occasionally the hinge type) has demonstrated that attempts to obtain accurate detail in impressions by means of the "wash" materials may be abandoned. There is a certain amount of leakage that will occur around any obturator, and this leakage does not materially affect the efficiency of the restoration. When the patient swallows, there is a vigorous excursion of the pharyngeal musculature; when he talks, there is less movement. Because the

Fig. 23-13. Positions of head for border-molding pharyngeal impressions.

restoration must be made comfortable enough to enable the patient to swallow, an air leak will occur during ordinary speech. Furthermore the musculature changes its shape, and the detail obtained from a wash impression will not be maintained on tissue topography for any length of time.

The procedures used for making impressions for cleft palate prostheses may well be due for reevaluation. Recently, several children for whom orthodontic appliances were to be constructed were examined jointly by an orthodontist and a prosthodontist. It was decided that removable appliances which combined orthodontic and prosthodontic treatment should be constructed. However, it was believed that it would be wise to provide the prosthodontic treatment in several progressing steps to avoid any antagonism on the part of the child toward the obturating section.

Accordingly, impressions of the pharyngeal area were avoided, and some firm wax was attached to the palatal portion of the arcylic resin appliance, which had been finished. The wax extension was constructed initially to such a dimension that it would not contact the pharyngeal tissues at any time. Acrylic resin was then substituted for the wax, and the patient wore this "bulb" for one week. The next week the bulb was enlarged to contact one or two small areas during swallowing. It was planned to accustom the child gradually to a mass of material in the nasopharynx and then to obtain an impression of the tissues in that region. However, it was noted that when the bulb was enlarged (by means of hand molding), there was a marked improvement in the nasal quality of the voice.

Further empirical enlargement of the bulb was made at the next appointment. There was some further improvement of the voice, but it was not as dramatic as that of the second appointment. Finally the pharyngeal impression was made, and the finished restoration was placed. The voice quality was not improved over that of the previous week. The results in several succeeding patients treated in this same manner suggested that it may not be necessary to obtain detailed impressions for pharyngeal obturators.

It has been interesting to note again and again the secondary role that surgical and prosthetic procedures play in the correction of cleft palate speech. We may work hard and provide our patients with an excellent technical result, but even with our understandable enthusiasm, we are not entirely satisfied with the vocal results. Conversely, we often see patients for whom relatively little has been done, and yet with all their lack of physical equipment, they speak reasonably well. We are convinced that the procedures per se do not always make the correction. They merely provide the equipment: personality—either the patient's, the therapist's, or both—heals. Nevertheless we need to provide the best equipment possible.

Meatus obturator. The pharyngeal impression for a meatus obturator is considered as a separate section here. It is rarely used; the classic design is difficult to achieve in most patients but, when achieved, has dramatic results. As will be discussed later, a compromise form is quite effective. The meatus obturator is formulated on the presumption that complete occlusion of the oropharynx from the nasopharynx is not necessary for good cleft palate speech. It is believed, rather, that the partial occlusion of the nasal cavity will result in a marked diminution and, in many instances, complete elimination of the nasal sound that is so apparent and so objectionable in the patient with a cleft palate. If the restoration fulfills this objective, the logopedist, who when using other appliances has to train certain muscles to reduce the hypernasality and others to conquer the articulative defects, need direct his efforts only toward correcting the latter. He need not concern himself with the muscle-training incident to reducing nasality. This in turn should reduce the number of training sessions necessary to improve speech for any particular patient.

This type of obturator ignores Passavant's pad and the posterior pharyngeal wall. Instead it makes contact with the superior aspect of the nasal cavity at the junction of nasal and pharyngeal cavities.

In other words, whereas the usual fixed type of obturator is directed in a line more or less parallel to, and continuous with, the palate, this type is inclined perpendicularly to the palate (Fig. 23-14).

The construction is not complicated. The upper casting is finished with the usual loop projecting into the cleft and is checked in the mouth for accuracy. With this framework as a vehicle, softened modeling plastic is molded around the distal loop with its greatest bulk directly above the loop. When the modeling plastic is hard, it is removed. More softened material is added, and the denture framework is repositioned in the mouth. Then an attempt by the patient is made to blow air through the nose. If air escapes, then small amounts of modeling plastic are added in likely areas until no air escapes through the nose and the patient talks as though he had a bad cold (the so-called rhinolalia clausa). The impression is removed from the mouth, and at this time any projection of material into the eustachian tubes should be cut from the impression to allow free interchange of air.

The completed impression is invested, boiled out, and processed in acrylic resin. After being polished, it is placed in the patient's mouth to check for gross errors in processing. When it is satisfactory, a vent about 3 mm in diameter is cut in an anteroposterior direction, approximately in the center and free of turbinates and vomer. If the latter is very large, it may be necessary to make two smaller holes on either side. (See Fig. 23-15.)

This opening serves as a means of breathing through the nose. The restoration is put back into the mouth, and the patient is instructed to speak. If the voice sounds "closed," the aperture is enlarged until a balance between the closed and open "nose" is reached. Immediately on placing the prosthesis and balancing the size of the hole, the resultant nasality should improve. Only the articulative defects remain, and these are not as unpleasant because of the normal nasal quality. There is usually no gagging tendency and no irritation of the mucous membrane. When the physical situation permits the use of any type of obturator, the decision as to which should be used must be determined by individual preference rather than by intrinsic value.

It was apparent early that a classic meatus type could be constructed in too few instances. Therefore a compromise between the fixed type and the meatus type is now attempted, rarely getting the impression as high as the latter and never as low as the former. It is my opinion that the obturator should be as high in the pharynx as is feasible. This compromise obturator does not usually require vents.

Fig. 23-14. Side view of a meatus obturator showing its relation to framework.

Fig. 23-15. Frontal view of meatus obturator showing vents.

Fig. 23-16. Model of repaired cleft palate with its restoration. Four remaining maxillary teeth, which do not occlude with manidublar teeth, are crowned and act as a retentive mechanism for an overdenture. Occlusion is established entirely on denture.

Psychologic aspects. The psychologic aspects of cleft palate prostheses cannot be overemphasized. Underdeveloped maxillary dental arches are often see in those patients who have had early surgical closure. If the orthodontist is unable for any reason to correct these malocclusions, the patient is left with an underdeveloped middle third of the face. This pseudo–Class III appearance can be somewhat diminished by a facade prosthesis. In these instances all teeth have to be crowned, and the prosthesis is fashioned anterior to these teeth for proper appearance. Fig. 23-16 shows an extreme situation in which only four teeth remained, and these were not occluding with any of the mandibular teeth. The overdenture was fashioned to improve the appearance and also to provide a masticating unit.

MAXILLOFACIAL PROSTHESIS

Many oral defects are the result of neoplasms or of accidental trauma. The prosthetic replacement of lost oral structure has to be approached with some caution, since the remaining tissues are often scarred and more reactive to pressures. The presence of teeth is a great boon to the prosthodontist who may treat such persons. It is well known that attempts to replace the tissue lost in a hemisection of the palate is extremely difficult *in the edentulous patient.* If worn at all, such prostheses are maintained largely by the active will of the patient and to a lesser degree by the usual biophysical factors.

When teeth are present in the mouth, the construction of the prosthesis is divided into three phases: (1) the complete and perfect restoration of all the remaining teeth and periodontal tissues, (2) the design and construction of the metal framework, and (3) the construction of the tissue replacement section. The first phase should include full crown coverage if necessary for restoration of carious areas, for protection from carious processes, and to provide optimal location of retentive components.

As in cleft palate therapy, the loss of any of the teeth places a burden on remaining teeth, and the loss of all teeth is catastrophic. The dentist should resort to any measures that will preserve the integrity of the remaining teeth, including the splinting together of several teeth.

Although the detailed design of the metal framework will vary for each patient, two general principles must be considered. First, the stabilizing aspects of the design must be emphasized. For example, every molar and premolar tooth remaining after a hemisection of the maxilla should have a stabilizing arm, to distribute torque forces adequately (Fig. 23-17). Second, retentive clasp arms should be designed so that they resist the displace-

Fig. 23-17. Prosthetic treatment of maxillary hemisection. **A,** All posterior teeth remaining after a hemisection of maxilla should have reciprocal arms to distribute widely the downward dislodging force of unsupported side. **B,** When corrected impression is obtained, all original cast except teeth and adjacent gingival tissues is cut away, and a new cast is poured into corrected impression. Dotted line separates new section from original section of cast.

ment forces of the finished restoration. It must be remembered that weight alone is often an important displacing force for these restorations.

The tissue replacement section of the prosthesis is important because, of course, it serves the primary function of this type of restoration. When the framework has been checked in the mouth for accurate fit, an acrylic resin impression tray is fashioned as part of the framework. This impression tray is underextended at least 1 mm in all directions. The border is now accurately recorded in a low-fusing stick modeling plastic. When this is done, all modeling plastic areas that contact tissue are scraped 0.5 mm, and the final impression is obtained in a rubber-base impression material.

The original cast is now altered by removing all the tissue-borne section, retaining only the teeth and the adjacent gingival portion. The impression and framework are replaced accurately on the remainder of the cast, and a new tissue section is poured into the final impression. Thus a corrected cast is available for processing.

The utmost care must be exercised to avoid even the slightest displacement of remaining soft tissue. This is extremely important in patients whose defects are due to cancer surgery because any tissue irritation in these areas is potentially dangerous. This is especially true if irradiation therapy followed surgery. Mechanical attempts to lock restorations into tissue undercuts by ingenious sectional devices are hazardous.

Many of the patients who have a defect that is the result of cancer therapy have received radiation therapy in combination with the surgical procedures. This therapy greatly diminishes the normal blood supply and makes the tissues particularly susceptible to infections and traumatic injury. Because the original blood supply to the maxilla is greater than that to the mandible, the effects of radiation are more common on the mandible. Patient responses to a therapeutic dose of 5,000 roentgens vary considerably so that an individual assessment of the patient should guide the placement of a prosthesis. The degree and duration of the acute reaction to the therapy along with the appearance of the tissues (particularly color) as it relates to blood supply dictate the prosthetic treatment. The surgery usually diminishes the sensory nerve supply to the area so that these patients may

develop a mucosal ulcer without the usual symptom of pain. Therefore all patients who have been irradiated should be closely followed for possible trauma caused by the prosthesis.

It follows naturally that there is a correlation between the tissue resistance and the amount of trauma required to produce a breakdown in the tissues. The amount of time the denture is worn and the way it is used (speech, deglutition, mastication) will influence the total amount of trauma produced. Each patient should therefore gradually increase the time and activities performed with the prosthesis until it is determined how much trauma he can safely tolerate.

As was mentioned previously, weight is a considerable displacing factor, and when prostheses demand thickness and bulk, they should be constructed in such a way that they are hollow. This is an easy process today with the autopolymerizing resins. These resins enable us to process hollow restorations, which may be capped and sealed with additional autopolymerizing resin.

When constructing prostheses after radical surgery of the face and neck, one must be prepared to alter them to accommodate for changes in tissue topography. The latter result from altered physiology in connection with lymph drainage in general. Sometimes these patients will have a marked difference in the tissue-fluid content of their facial tissues from morning to night. This may prove difficult for the prosthodontist because if the prosthesis fits in the morning, it will be loose in the afternoon, and if it fits in the afternoon, it may cause sore spots in the morning. In general the former situation is to be preferred. Accordingly it may be better to make all impressions in the morning.

Furthermore the process of scar contraction may continue for several weeks or months, which will demand continual revision of the prosthesis.

One final word should be added about scarring. Restoration of facial contour should never be attempted when considerable pressure against scar tissue is required to do so. This again may cause ulceration, displacement of the restoration, movement of the teeth, or all three.

When arranging teeth for a restoration, replacing a hemisection of the maxilla, it should be remembered that the remaining tissue bearing the force of occlusion is of poor quality. Therefore the occlusion should be arranged to contact just lightly on the affected side. In some instances it may be preferable to eliminate occlusal contact entirely, to avoid any pressure. The patient should be instructed to avoid chewing on the affected side. He now has a difficult situation, but it is better for him to eat only on one side without soreness than to eat on both and develop constantly irritated tissue areas.

It must be realized that these particular patients have been through a difficult period. The thoughts of losing large parts of the face are matters of concern to even the most callous. The realization that the resultant defects in speech or appearance may be permanent does not encourage the patient. Therefore he should be informed that the prostheses are available, and a clear assessment of their role should be offered to him.

The dentist should neither dispel hope with talk of failure nor build false hope with talk of great success. Rather he should consider his own chances of creating a successful prosthesis. Then the patient should be encouraged to cooperate in the construction of the restoration and be encouraged to wear it. Negative approaches are poor. If one dwells unduly on the chance of failure, he is making a bad mistake. Instead, tell the truthful story of the many people who wear these restorations successfully.

It occurs to me that there is a great deal of difference between the following statements:

1. There are many people who wear these restorations happily and successfully.

2. There are many people who cannot wear these restorations.

The former is encouraging, the latter deadening. Use a positive bright approach, being careful not to build up false hopes. Building a bleak picture can seriously affect the patient's attitude toward the prosthesis.

Years of constructing these cleft palate and surgical prostheses have convinced me that it is perhaps the most rewarding branch of prosthetic dentistry. These patients are not petty, arrogant people; they are appreciative, cooperative, and a pleasure to know.

The patient can often tell the dentist much about how the restoration should serve and can offer constructive suggestions concerning its design. Always listen to, and weigh carefully, these suggestions. It has been my experience that near failures have been converted to successful restorations by following the patient's directions in certain aspects of construction.

In addition, denture adhesives have improved a great deal in the last several years. They can be healthy aids to retention, partially relieving the teeth of burden, thus extending tooth longevity. Of course, scrupulous cleansing of oral tissues and restorations must be maintained.

SELECTED REFERENCES

TEXTBOOKS

Applegate, O. C.: Essentials of removable partial denture prosthesis, Philadelphia, 1965, W. B. Saunders Co.

Beumer, J., Curtis, T. A., and Firtell, D. N.: Maxillofacial prosthetics, St. Louis, 1979, The C. V. Mosby Co.

Brewer, A. A., and Morrow, R. M.: Overdentures, ed. 2, St. Louis, 1980, The C. V. Mosby Co.

Craig, R. G.: Restorative dental materials, ed. 6, St. Louis, 1980, The C. V. Mosby Co.

Dolder, E. J., and Durrer, G. T.: The bar-joint denture, Chicago, 1978, Quintessence Publishing Company, Inc.

Dubrul, E. L.: Sicher's oral anatomy, ed. 7, St. Louis, 1980, The C. V. Mosby Co.

Dykema, R. W., Cunningham, D. M., and Johnston, J. F.: Modern practice in removable partial prosthodontics, Philadelphia, 1969, W. B. Saunders Co.

Ellinger, C. W., Rayson, J. H., Terry, J. M., and Rahn, A. O.: Synopsis of complete dentures, Philadelphia, 1975, Lea & Febiger.

Farrell, J.: Partial denture designing, London, 1970, Henry Kimpton Medical Publisher and Bookseller.

Gaerny A.: Removable closure of the interdental space (C.I.S.), Berlin and Chicago, 1972, Quintessence Publishing Company, Inc.

Goldman, H. M., and Cohen, D. W.: Periodontal therapy, ed. 6, St. Louis, 1979, The C. V. Mosby Co.

Heartwell, C. M., Jr., and Rahn, A. O.: Syllabus of complete dentures, ed. 3, Philadelphia, 1980, Lea & Febiger.

Hickey, J. C., and Zarb, G. A.: Boucher's prosthodontic treatment for edentulous patients, ed. 8, St. Louis, 1980, The C. V. Mosby Co.

Johnson, D. L., and Stratton, R. J.: Fundamentals of removable prosthodontics, Chicago, 1980, Quintessence Publishing Company, Inc.

Johnston, J. F., Phillips, R. W., and Dykema, R. W.: Modern practice in crown and bridge prosthodontics, Philadelphia, 1971, W. B. Saunders Co.

Laney, W. R., Desjardins, R. P., Chalian, V. A., and Gillis, R. E., Jr.: Maxillofacial prosthetics, Littleton, Mass., 1979, PSG Publishing Co.

Miller, E. L.: Removable partial prosthodontics, Baltimore, 1972, The Williams and Wilkins Co.

Osborne, J., and Lammie, G. A.: Partial dentures, ed. 4, Oxford, 1974, Blackwell Scientific Publications.

Phillips, R. W.: Skinner's science of dental materials, ed. 7, Philadelphia, 1973, W. B. Saunders Co.

Preiskel, H. W.: Precision attachments in dentistry, ed. 3, St. Louis, 1980, The C. V. Mosby Co.

Ramfjord, S. P., and Ash, M. M., Jr.: Occlusion, ed. 2, Philadelphia, 1971, W. B. Saunders Co.

Sharry, J. J., editor: Complete denture prosthodontics, ed. 3, New York, 1974, McGraw-Hill Book Co.

Singer, F., and Schön, F.: Partial dentures, Chicago, 1973, Quintessence Publishing Company, Inc.

Tylman, S. D., and Malone, W. P. F.: Tylman's theory and practice of fixed prosthodontics, ed. 7, St. Louis, 1978, The C. V. Mosby Co.

Yalisove, I. L., and Dietz, J. B., Jr.: Telescopic prosthetic therapy, Philadelphia, 1979, George F. Stickley Co.

Zarb, G. A., Bergman, B., Clayton, J. A., and MacKay, H. F.: Prosthodontic treatment for partially edentulous patients, St. Louis, 1978, The C. V. Mosby Co.

ABUTMENT RETAINERS: EXTERNAL AND INTERNAL ATTACHMENTS

Adisman, I. K.: The internal clip attachment in fixed-removable partial denture prosthesis, N.Y. J. Dent. 32:125-129, 1962.

Ainamo, J.: Precision removable partial dentures with pontic abutments, J. Prosthet. Dent. 23:289-295, 1970.

Augsburger, R. H.: The Gilmore attachment, J. Prosthet. Dent. 16:1090-1102, 1966.

Becker, C. M., Campbell, M. C., and Williams, D. L.: The Thompson dowel-rest system modified for chrome-cobalt removable partial denture frameworks, J. Prosthet. Dent. 39:384-391, 1978.

Blatterfein, L.: Study of partial denture clasping, J. Am. Dent. Assoc. 43:169-185, 1951.

Blatterfein, L.: Design and positional arrangement of clasps for partial dentures, N.Y. J. Dent. 22:305-306, 1952.

Breisach, L.: Esthetic attachments for removable partial dentures, J. Prosthet. Dent. 17:261-265, 1967.

Brodbelt, R. H. W.: A simple paralleling template for precision attachments, J. Prosthet. Dent. 27:285-288, 1972.

Brudvik, J. S., and Wormley, J. H.: Construction techniques for wrought wire retentive clasp arms are related to clasp flexibility, J. Prosthet. Dent. 30:769-774, 1973.

Caldarone, C. V.: Attachments for partial dentures without clasps, J. Prosthet. Dent. 7:206-208, 1957.

Clayton, J. A.: A stable base precision attachment removable partial denture (PARPD): theories and principles, Dent. Clin. North Am. 24:3-29, 1980.

Cooper, H.: Practice management related to precision attachment prostheses, Dent. Clin. North Am. 24:45-61, 1980.

DeVan, M. M.: Fortn. Rev. Chic. Dent. Soc. 27:7-12 (portrait), 1954.

DeVan, M. M.: Preserving natural teeth through the use of clasps, J. Prosthet. Dent. 5:208-214, 1955.

Dietz, W. H.: Modified abutments for removable and fixed prosthodontics, J. Prosthet. Dent. **11**:1112-1116, 1961.

Dolder, E. J.: The bar joint mandibular denture, J. Prosthet. Dent. **11**:689-707, 1961.

Farrell, J.: Wrought wire retainers—a method of increasing their flexibility, Br. Dent. J. **131**:327, 1971.

Garver, D. G.: A new clasping system for unilateral distal-extension removable partial dentures, J. Prosthet. Dent. **39**:268-273, 1978.

Gilson, T. D.: A fixable-removable prosthetic attachment, J. Prosthet. Dent. **9**:247-255, 1959.

Gindea, A. E.: A retentive device for removable dentures, J. Prosthet. Dent. **27**:501-508, 1972.

Green, J. H.: The hinge-lock abutment attachment, J. Am. Dent. Assoc. **47**:175-180, 1953.

Handlers, M., Lenchner, N. H., and Weissman, B.: A retaining device for partial dentures, J. Prosthet. Dent. **7**:483-488, 1957.

Hekneby, M.: The spring-slide joint for lower free end removable partial dentures, J. Prosthet. Dent. **11**:256-263, 1961.

Isaacson, G. O.: Telescope crown retainers for removable partial dentures, J. Prosthet. Dent. **22**:436-448, 1969.

James, A. G.: Self-locking posterior attachment for removable tooth-supported partial dentures, J. Prosthet. Dent. **5**:200-205, 1955.

Johnson, J. F.: The application and construction of the pinledge retainer, J. Prosthet. Dent. **3**:559-567, 1953.

Knodle, J. M.: Experimental overlay and pin partial denture, J. Prosthet. Dent. **17**:472-478, 1967.

Knowles, L. E.: A dowel attachment removable partial denture, J. Prosthet. Dent. **13**:679-687, 1963.

Koper, A.: Retainer for removable partial dentures—the Thompson dowel, J. Prosthet. Dent. **30**:759-768, 1973.

Kotowicz, W. E.: Clinical procedures in precision attachment removable partial denture construction, Dent. Clin. North Am. **24**:143-164, 1980.

Kotowicz, W. E., Fisher, R. L., Reed, R. A., and Jaslow, C.: The combination clasp and the distal extension removable partial denture, Dent. Clin. North Am. **17**:651-660, Oct., 1973.

Krol, A. J.: Clasp design for extension base removable partial dentures, J. Prosthet. Dent. **29**:408-415, 1973.

Krol, A. J.: RPI clasp retainer and its modifications, Dent. Clin. North Am. **17**:631-649, 1973.

Langer, A.: Combinations of diverse retainers in removable partial dentures, J. Prosthet. Dent. **40**:378-384, 1978.

Lubovich, R. P., and Peterson, T.: The fabrication of a ceramic-metal crown to fit an existing removable partial denture their clasp, J. Prosthet. Dent. **37**:610-614, 1977.

Mann, A. W.: The lower distal extension partial denture using the Hart-Dunn attachment, J. Prosthet. Dent. **8**:282-288, 1958.

McLeod, N. S.: A theoretical analysis of the mechanics of the Thompson dowel semiprecision intracoronal retainer, J. Prosthet. Dent. **37**:19-27, 1977.

McLeod, N. S.: Improved design for the Thompson dowel rest semiprecision intracoronal retainer, J. Prosthet. Dent. **40**:513-516, 1978.

Mensor, M. C., Jr.: Attachment fixation for overdentures. I. J. Prosthet. Dent. **37**:366-373, 1977.

Mensor, M. C., Jr.: Attachment fixation of the overdenture. II. J. Prosthet. Dent. **39**:16-20, 1978.

Morrison, M. L.: Internal precision attachment retainers for partial dentures, J. Am. Dent. Assoc. **64**:209-215, 1962.

Morrow, R. M.: Tooth-supported complete dentures: an approach to preventive prosthodontics, J. Prosthet. Dent. **21**:513-522, 1969.

Myers, G. E., Wepfer, G. G., and Peyton, F. A.: The thiokol rubber base impression materials, J. Prosthet. Dent. **8**:330-339, 1958.

Oddo, V. J., Jr.: The movable-arm clasp for complete passivity in partial denture construction, J. Am. Dent. Assoc. **74**:1009-1015, 1967.

Plotnick, I. J.: Internal attachment for fixed removable partial dentures, J. Prosthet. Dent. **8**:85-93, 1958.

Pound, E.: Cross-arch splinting vs. premature extractions, J. Prosthet. Dent. **16**:1058-1068, 1966.

Preiskel, H.: Precision attachments for free-end saddle prostheses, Br. Dent. J. **127**:462-468, 1969.

Preiskel, H.: Screw retained telescopic prosthesis, Br. Dent. J. **130**:107-112, 1971.

Prince, I. B.: Conservation of the supportive mechanism, J. Prosthet. Dent. **15**:327-338, 1965.

Singer, F.: Improvements in precision—attached removable partial dentures, J. Prosthet. Dent. **17**:69-72, 1967.

Smith, R. A., and Rymarz, F. P.: Cast clasp transitional removable partial dentures, J. Prosthet. Dent. **22**:381-385, 1969.

Stansbury, B. E.: A retentive attachment for overdentures, J. Prosthet. Dent. **35**:228-230, 1976.

Strohaver, R. A., and Trovillion, H. M.: Removable partial overdentures, J. Prosthet. Dent. **35**:624-629, 1976.

Tautin, F. S.: Abutment stabilization using a nonresilient gingival bar connector, J. Am. Dent. Assoc. **99**:988-989, 1979.

Vasic, S., et al.: An aesthetic clasp for acrylic partial dentures, J. Can. Dent. Assoc. **37**:38-39, 1971.

Vig, R. G.: Splinting bars and maxillary indirect retainers for removable partial dentures, J. Prosthet. Dent. **13**:125-129, 1963.

Walter, J. D.: Anchor attachments used as locking devices in two-part removable prostheses, J. Prosthet. Dent. **33**:628-632, 1975.

Waltz, M. E.: Ceka extracoronal attachments, J. Prosthet. Dent. **29**:167-171, 1973.

White, J. T.: Visualization of stress and strain related to removable partial denture abutments, J. Prosthet. Dent. **40**:143-151, 1978.

Williams, A. G.: Technique for provisional splint with attachment, J. Prosthet. Dent. **21**:555-559, 1969.

Zakler, J. M.: Intracoronal precision attachments, Dent. Clin. North Am. **24**:131-141, 1980.

Zinner, I. D.: Semiprecision rest system for distal-extension removable partial denture design, J. Prosthet. Dent. **42**:131-134, 1979.

ANATOMY

Barker, B. C. W.: Dissection of regions of interest to the dentist from a medical approach, Aust. Dent. J. **16**:163-171, 1971.

Bennett, N. G.: A contribution to the study of the movements of the mandible, J. Prosthet. Dent. **8**:41-54, 1958.

Boucher, C. O.: Anatomy of the mouth in relation to complete dentures, J. Wis. State Dent. Soc. **19:**161-166, 1943.

Boucher, C. O.: Complete denture impressions based upon the anatomy of the mouth, J. Am. Dent. Assoc. **31:**1174-1181, 1944.

Brodie, A. G.: Anatomy and physiology of head and neck musculature, Am. J. Orthod. **36:**831-844, 1950.

Craddock, F. W.: Retromolar region of the mandible, J. Am. Dent. Assoc. **47:**453-455, 1953.

Haines, R. W., and Barnett, S. G.: The structure of the mouth in the mandibular molar region, J. Prosthet. Dent. **9:**962-974, 1959.

Last, R. J.: The muscles of the mandible, Dent. Dig. **61:**165-169, 1955.

Martone, A. L., et al.: Anatomy of the mouth and related structures. I. J. Prosthet. Dent. **11:** 1009-1018, 1961; II. **12:**4-27, 1962; III. **12:**206-219, 1962; IV. **12:**409-419, 1962; V. **12:**629-636, 1962; VI. **12:**817-834, 1962; VII. **13:**4-33, 1963; VIII. **13:**204-228, 1963.

Merkeley, H. J.: The labial and buccal accessory muscles of mastication, J. Prosthet. Dent. **4:**327-334, 1954.

Merkeley, H. J.: Mandibular rearmament. I. Anatomic considerations, J. Prosthet. Dent. **9:**559-566, 1959.

Pendleton, E. C.: Anatomy of the face and mouth from the standpoint of the denture prosthetist, J. Am. Dent. Assoc. **33:**219-234, 1946.

Pendleton, E. C.: Changes in the denture supporting tissues, J. Am. Dent. Assoc. **42:**1-15, 1951.

Pietrokovski, J.: The bony residual ridge in man, J. Prosthet. Dent. **34:**456-462, 1975.

Pietrokovski, J., Sorin, S., and Zvia, H.: The residual ridge in partially edentulous patients, J. Prosthet. Dent. **36:**150-158, 1976.

Roche, A. F.: Functional anatomy of the muscles of mastication, J. Prosthet. Dent. **13:**548-570, 1963.

Silverman, S. I.: Denture prosthesis and the functional anatomy of the maxillofacial structures, J. Prosthet. Dent. **6:**305-331, 1956.

BIOMECHANICS

Applegate, O. C.: Use of the paralleling surveyor in modern partial denture construction, J. Am. Dent. Assoc. **27:**1397-1407, 1940.

Avant, W. E.: Factors that influence retention of removable partial dentures, J. Prosthet. Dent. **25:**265-270, 1971.

Avant, W. E.: Fulcrum and retention lines in planning removable partial dentures, J. Prosthet. Dent. **25:** 162-166, 1971.

Brudevold, F.: Basic study of the chewing forces of a denture wearer, J. Am. Dent. Assoc. **43:**45-51, 1951.

Cecconi, B. T.: Effect of rest design on transmission of forces to abutment teeth, J. Prosthet. Dent. **32:**141-151, 1974.

Cecconi, B. T., Asgar, K., and Dootz, E.: The effect of partial denture clasp design on abutment tooth movement, J. Prosthet. Dent. **25:**44-56, 1971.

Cecconi, B. T., Asgar, K., and Dootz, E.: Removable partial denture abutment tooth movement as affected by inclination of residual ridges and types of loading, J. Prosthet. Dent. **25:**375-381, 1971.

Cecconi, B. T., Asgar, K., and Dootz, E.: Clasp assembly modifications and their effect on abutment tooth movement, J. Prosthet. Dent. **27:**160-167, 1972.

Clayton, J. A., and Jaslow, C.: A measurement of clasp forces on teeth, J. Prosthet. Dent. **25:**21-43, 1971.

Craig, R. G., and Farah, J. W.: Stresses from loading distal extension removable partial dentures, J. Prosthet. Dent. **39:**274-277, 1978.

DeVan, M. M.: The nature of the partial denture foundation: suggestions for its preservation, J. Prosthet. Dent. **2:**210-218, 1952.

Frechette, A. R.: The influence of partial denture design on distribution of force to abutment teeth, J. Prosthet. Dent. **6:**195-212, 1956.

Goodkind, R. J.: The effects of removable partial dentures on abutment tooth mobility, J. Prosthet. Dent. **30:**139-146, 1973.

Goodman, J. J., and Goodman, H. W.: Balance of force in precision free-end restorations, J. Prosthet. Dent. **13:**302-308, 1963.

Hall, W. A.: Variations in registering interarch transfers in removable partial denture construction, J. Prosthet. Dent. **30:**548-553, 1973.

Harrop, J., and Javid, N.: Reciprocal arms of direct retainers in removable partial dentures, J. Canad. Dent. Assoc. **4:**208-211, 1976.

Henderson, D., and Seward, T. E.: Design and force distribution with removable partial dentures; a progress report, J. Prosthet. Dent. **17:**350-364, 1967.

Hindels, G. W.: Stress analysis in distal extension partial dentures, J. Prosthet. Dent. **7:**197-205, 1957.

Kaires, A. K.: Partial denture design and its relation to force distribution and masticatory performance, J. Prosthet. Dent. **6:**672-683, 1956.

Knowles, L. E.: The biomechanics of removable partial dentures and its relationship to fixed prosthesis, J. Prosthet. Dent. **8:**426-430, 1958.

Kratochvil, F. J.: Influence of occlusal rest position and clasp design on movement of abutment teeth, J. Prosthet. Dent. **13:**114-124, 1963.

Lowe, R. O., et al.: Swallowing and resting forces related to lingual flange thickness in removable partial dentures, J. Prosthet. Dent. **23:**279-288, 1970.

MacGregor, A. R., Miller, T. P. G., and Farah, J. W.: Stress analysis of partial dentures, J. Dent. **6:**125-132, 1978.

McCartney, J. W.: Motion vector analysis of an abutment for a distal-extension removable partial denture, J. Prosthet. Dent. **43:**15-21, 1980.

McDowell, G. C.: Force transmission by indirect retainers during unilateral loading, J. Prosthet. Dent. **39:** 616-621, 1978.

Plotnick, I. J., Beresin, V. E., and Simkins, A. B.: The effect of variations in the opposing dentition on changes in the partially edentulous mandible. I. J. Prosthet. Dent. **33:**278-286, 1975; II. **33:**403-406; III. **33:**529-534.

Shohet, H.: Relative magnitudes of stress on abutment teeth with different retainers, J. Prosthet. Dent. **21:** 267-282, 1969.

Smith, B. H.: Changes in occlusal face height with removable partial dentures, J. Prosthet. Dent. **34:**278-285, 1975.

Smith, B. J., and Turner, C. H.: The use of crowns to modify abutment teeth of removable partial dentures, J. Dent. **7:**52-56, 1979.

Smyd, E. S.: Bio-mechanics of prosthetic dentistry, J. Prosthet. Dent. **4:**368-383, 1954.

Smyd, E. S.: The role of tongue, torsion, and bending in prosthodontic failures, J. Prosthet. Dent. **11:**95-111, 1961.

Stern, W. J.: Guiding planes in clasp reciprocation and retention, J. Prosthet. Dent. **34:**408-414, 1975.

Wills, D. J., and Manderson, R. D.: Biomechanical aspects of the support of partial dentures, J. Dent. **5**:310-318, 1977.

Yurkstas, A., Fridley, H. H., and Manly, R. S.: A functional evaluation of fixed and removable bridgework, J. Prosthet. Dent. **1**:570-577, 1951.

Zoeller, G. N.: Block form stability in removable partial dentures, J. Prosthet. Dent. **22**:633-637, 1969.

Zoeller, G. N., and Kelly, W. J., Jr.: Block form stability in removable partial prosthodontics, J. Prosthet. Dent. **25**:515-519, 1971.

CLASSIFICATION

Applegate, O. C.: The rationale of partial denture choice, J. Prosthet. Dent. **10**:891-907, 1960.

Avant, W. E.: A universal classification for removable partial denture situations, J. Prosthet. Dent. **16**:533-539, 1966.

Bailyn, M.: Tissue support in partial denture construction, Dent. Cosmos **70**:988-997, 1928.

Beckett, L. S.: The influence of saddle classification on the design of partial removable restoration, J. Prosthet. Dent. **3**:506-516, 1953.

Costa, E.: A simplified system for identifying partially edentulous arches, J. Prosthet. Dent. **32**:639-645, 1974.

Cummer, W. E.: Partial denture service. In Anthony, L. P., editor: American textbook of prosthetic dentistry, Philadelphia, 1942, Lea & Febiger.

Friedman, J.: The ABC classification of partial denture segments, J. Prosthet. Dent. **3**:517-524, 1953.

Godfrey, R. J.: Classification of removable partial dentures, J. Am. Coll. Dent. **18**:5-13, 1951.

Mensor, M. C.: Classification and selection of attachments, J. Prosthet. Dent. **29**:494-497, 1973.

Miller, E. L.: Systems for classifying partially dentulous arches, J. Prosthet. Dent. **24**:25-40, 1970.

Skinner, C. N.: A classification of removable partial dentures based upon the principles of anatomy and physiology, J. Prosthet. Dent. **9**:240-246, 1959.

CLEFT PALATE

Aram, A., and Subtelny, J. D.: Velopharyngeal function and cleft palate prostheses, J. Prosthet. Dent. **9**:149-158, 1959.

Baden, E.: Fundamental principles of orofacial prosthetic therapy in congenital cleft palate, J. Prosthet. Dent. **4**:420-433, 1954.

Bixler, D.: Heritability of clefts of the lips and palate, J. Prosthet. Dent. **33**:100-108, 1975.

Buckner, H.: Construction of a denture with hollow obturator, lid and soft acrylic lining, J. Prosthet. Dent. **31**:95-99, 1974.

Calvan, J.: The error of Gustan Passavant, Plast. Reconstr. Surg. **13**:275-289, 1954.

Cooper, H. K.: Integration of service in the treatment of cleft lip and cleft palate, J. Am. Dent. Assoc. **47**:27-32, 1953.

Dalston, R. M.: Prosthodontic management of the cleft-palate patient: a speech pathologist's view, J. Prosthet. Dent. **37**:327-329, 1978.

Ettinger, R. L.: Use of teeth with a poor prognosis in cleft palate prosthodontics, J. Am. Dent. Assoc. **94**:910-914, 1977.

Fox, A.: Prosthetic correction of a severe acquired cleft palate, J. Prosthet. Dent. **8**:542-546, 1958.

Gibbons, P., and Bloomer, H.: A supportive-type prosthetic speech aid, J. Prosthet. Dent. **8**:362-369, 1958.

Graber, T. M.: Oral and nasal structures in cleft palate speech, J. Am. Dent. Assoc. **53**:693-706, 1956.

Harkins, C. S.: Modern concepts in the prosthetic rehabilitation of cleft palate patients, J. Oral Surg. **10**:298-312, 1952.

Harkins, C. S., and Ivy, R. H.: Surgery and prosthesis in the rehabilitation of cleft palate patients, J. South. Calif. Dent. Assoc. **19**:16-24, 1951.

Immekus, J. E., and Aramy, M. A.: A fixed-removable partial denture for cleft palate patients, J. Prosthet. Dent. **34**:286-291, 1975.

Landa, J. S.: The prosthodontist views the rehabilitation of the cleft palate patient, J. Prosthet. Dent. **6**:421-427, 1956.

Lavelle, W. E., and Zach, G. E.: The tissue bar and Ceka anchor as aids in cleft palate rehabilitation, J. Prosthet. Dent. **30**:321-325, 1973.

Lloyd, R. S., Pruzansky, S., and Subtelny, J. D.: Prosthetic rehabilitation of a cleft palate patient subsequent to multiple surgical and prosthetic failures, J. Prosthet. Dent. **7**:216-230, 1957.

Merkeley, H. J.: Cleft palate prosthesis, J. Prosthet. Dent. **9**:506-513, 1959.

Nidiffer, T. J., and Shipmon, T. H.: The hollow-bulb obturator for acquired palatal openings, J. Prosthet. Dent. **7**:126-134, 1957.

Olinger, N. A.: Cleft palate prosthesis rehabilitation, J. Prosthet. Dent. **2**:117-135, 1952.

Rosen, M. S.: Prosthetics for the cleft palate patient, J. Am. Dent. Assoc. **60**:715-721, 1960.

Rothenberg, L. I. A.: Overlay dentures for the cleft-palate patient, J. Prosthet. Dent. **37**:190-195, 1977.

Schneiderman, C. R., and Maun, M. B.: Air flow and intelligibility of speech of normal speakers and speakers with a prosthodontically repaired cleft palate, J. Prosthet. Dent. **39**:193-199, 1978.

Sharry, J. J.: The meatus obturator in cleft palate prosthesis, Oral Surg. **7**:852-855, 1954.

Sharry, J. J.: Meatus obturator in particular and pharyngeal impressions in general, J. Prosthet. Dent. **8**:893-896, 1958.

Tautin, F. S., and Schaaf, N. A.: Superiorly based obturator, J. Prosthet. Dent. **33**:96-99, 1975.

COMPLETE MOUTH AND OCCLUSAL REHABILITATION

Brewer, A. A., and Fenton, A. H.: The overdenture, Dent. Clin. North Am. **17**:723-746, 1973.

Bronstein, B. R.: Rationale and technique of biomechanical occlusal rehabilitation, J. Prosthet. Dent. **4**:352-367, 1954.

Cohn, L. A.: Occluso-rehabilitation. Principles of diagnosis and treatment planning, Dent. Clin. North Am., pp. 259-281, March, 1962.

Dubin, N. A.: Advances in functional occlusal rehabilitation, J. Prosthet. Dent. **6**:252-258, 1956.

Kazis, H.: Functional aspects of complete mouth rehabilitation, J. Prosthet. Dent. **4**:833-841, 1954.

Kornfeld, M.: The problem of function in restorative dentistry, J. Prosthet. Dent. **5**:670-676, 1955.

Landa, J. S.: An analysis of current practices in mouth rehabilitation, J. Prosthet. Dent. **5**:527-537, 1955.

Mann, A. W., and Pankey, L. D.: Oral rehabilitation utilizing the Pankey-Mann instrument and a functional bite technique, Dent. Clin. North Am., pp. 215-230, March, 1959.

Mann, A. W., and Pankey, L. D.: Oral rehabilitation. I. Use of the P-M instrument in treatment planning and restoring the lower posterior teeth, J. Prosthet. Dent. 10:135-150, 1960.

Mann, A. W., and Pankey, L. D.: Oral rehabilitation. II. Reconstruction of the upper teeth using a functionally generated path technique, J. Prosthet. Dent. 10: 151-162, 1960.

Rubinstein, M. N.: Approach to mouth reconstruction, Dent. Dig. 61:24-28, 1955.

Schuyler, C. H.: An evaluation of incisal guidance and its influence on restorative dentistry, J. Prosthet. Dent. 9:374-378, 1959.

Schweitzer, J. M.: Open bite from the prosthetic point of view, Dent. Clin. North Am., pp. 269-283, March, 1957.

CROWNS AND FIXED PARTIAL DENTURES

Alexander, P. C.: Analysis of the cuspid protective occlusion, J. Prosthet. Dent. 13:309-317, 1963.

Beeson, P. E.: The use of acrylic resins as an aid in the development of patterns for two types of crowns, J. Prosthet. Dent. 13:493-498, 1963.

Caplan, J.: Maintenance of full coverage fixed-abutment bridges, J. Prosthet. Dent. 5:852-854, 1955.

Coelho, D. H.: The ultimate goal in fixed bridge procedures, J. Prosthet. Dent. 4:667-672, 1954.

Coelho, D. H.: Criteria for the use of fixed prosthesis, Dent. Clin. North Am., pp. 299-311, March, 1957.

Collett, H. A.: Cast shell veneer crowns, J. Prosthet. Dent. 25:177-182, 1971.

Cooper, T. M., et al.: Effect of venting on cast gold full crowns, J. Prosthet. Dent. 26:621-626, 1971.

Cowgen, G. T.: Retention, resistance and esthetics of the anterior three-quarter crown, J. Am. Dent. Assoc. 62:167-171, 1961.

Culpepper, W. D., and Moulton, P. S.: Considerations in fixed prosthodontics, Dent. Clin. North Am. 23: 21-35, 1979.

Ewing, J. E.: Re-evaluation of the cantilever principle, J. Prosthet. Dent. 7:78-92, 1957.

Freese, A. S.: Impressions for temporary acrylic resin jacket crowns, J. Prosthet. Dent. 7:99-101, 1957.

Goldberg, A., and Jones, R. D.: Constructing cast crowns to fit existing removable partial denture clasps, J. Prosthet. Dent. 36:382-386, 1976.

Guyer, S. E.: Nonrigid subocclusal connector for fixed partial dentures, J. Prosthet. Dent. 26:433-436, 1971.

Hagerman, D. A., and Arnim, S. S.: The relation of new knowledge of the gingiva to crown and bridge procedures, J. Prosthet. Dent. 5:538-542, 1955; Dent. Abstr. 1:44, 1956.

Henderson, D., et al.: The cantilever type of posterior fixed partial dentures: a laboratory study, J. Prosthet. Dent. 24:47-67, 1970.

Hill, G. M.: Construction of a crown to fit a removable partial denture clasp, J. Prosthet. Dent. 38:226-228, 1977.

Johnson, E. A., Jr.: Combination of fixed and removable partial dentures, J. Prosthet. Dent. 14:1099-1106, 1964.

Johnston, J. F., Dykeman, R. W., Mumford, G., and Phillips, R. W.: Construction and assembly of porcelain veneer gold crowns and pontics, J. Prosthet. Dent. 12:1125-1137, 1962.

Kahn, A. E.: Reversible hydrocolloids in the construction of the unit-built porcelain bridge, J. Prosthet. Dent. 6:72-79, 1956.

Leff, A.: New concepts in the preparation of teeth for full coverage, J. Prosthet. Dent. 5:392-400, 1955.

Leff, A.: Reproduction of tooth anatomy and positional relationship in full cast or veneer crowns, J. Prosthet. Dent. 6:550-557, 1956.

Malson, T. S.: Anatomic cast crown reproduction, J. Prosthet. Dent. 9:106-112, 1959.

Nuttal, E. B.: Clinical and technical aspects of crown and bridge prosthesis, Bull. Phila. Cty. Dent. Soc. 14:128-133, 1950.

Patur, B.: The role of occlusion and the periodontium in rsetorative procedures, J. Prosthet. Dent. 21:371-379, 1969.

Phillips, R. W., and Biggs, D. H.: Distortion of wax patterns as influenced by storage time, storage temperature, and temperature of wax manipulation, J. Am. Dent. Assoc. 41:28-37, 1950.

Phillips, R. W., and Price, R. R.: Some factors which influence the surface of stone dies poured in alginate impressions, J. Prosthet. Dent. 5:72-79, 1955.

Phillips, R. W., and Swartz, M. L.: A study of adaptation of veneers to cast gold crowns, J. Prosthet. Dent. 7:817-822, 1957.

Pound, E.: The problem of the lower anterior bridge, J. Prosthet. Dent. 5:543-545, 1955.

Preston, J. D.: Preventing ceramic failures when integrating fixed and removable prostheses, Dent. Clin. North Am. 23:37-52, 1979.

Pruden, K. C.: A hydrocolloid technique for pin-ledge bridge abutments, J. Prosthet. Dent. 6:65-71, 1956.

Pruden, W. H.: Full coverage, partial coverage, and the role of pins, J. Prosthet. Dent. 26:302-306, 1971.

Rubin, M. K.: Full coverage: the provisional and final restorations made easier, J. Prosthet. Dent. 8:664-672, 1958.

Sheets, C. E.: Dowel and core foundations, J. Prosthet. Dent. 23:58-65, 1970.

Shooshan, E. D.: The reverse pin-porcelain facing, J. Prosthet. Dent. 9:284-301, 1959.

Smith, G. P.: The marginal fit of the full cast shoulderless crown, J. Prosthet. Dent. 7:231-243, 1957.

Smith, G. P.: Objectives of a fixed partial denture, J. Prosthet. Dent. 11:463-473, 1961.

Staffanou, R. S., and Thayer, K. E.: Reverse pin-porcelain veneer and pontic technique, J. Prosthet. Dent. 12:1138-1145, 1962.

Talkov, L.: The copper band splint, J. Prosthet. Dent. 6: 245-251, 1956.

Thurgood, B. W., Thayer, K. E., and Lee, R. E.: Complete crowns constructed for an existing partial denture, J. Prosthet. Dent. 29:507-512, 1973.

Treppo, K. W., and Smith, F. W.: A technique for restoring abutments for removable partial dentures, J. Prosthet. Dent. 40:398-401, 1978.

Troxell, R. R.: The polishing of gold castings, J. Prosthet. Dent. 9:668-675, 1959.

Wagman, S. S.: Tissue management for full cast veneer crowns, J. Prosthet. Dent. 15:106-117, 1965.

Wagner, A. W., Burkhart, J. W., and Fayle, H. E., Jr.: Contouring abutment teeth with cast gold inlays for removable partial dentures, J. Prosthet. Dent. 201: 330-334, 1968.

Wallace, F. H.: Resin transfer copings, J. Prosthet. Dent. 8:289-292, 1958.

Welsh, S. L.: Complete crown construction for a clasp-bearing abutment, J. Prosthet. Dent. **34**:320-323, 1975.

Wheeler, R. C.: Complete crown form and the periodontium, J. Prosthet. Dent. **11**:722-734, 1961.

Yalisone, I. L.: Crown and sleeve-coping retainers for removable partial prostheses, J. Prosthet. Dent. **16**:1069-1085, 1966.

DENTAL LABORATORY PROCEDURES

Asgar, K., and Peyton, F. A.: Casting dental alloys to embedded wires, J. Prosthet. Dent. **15**:312-321, 1965.

Becker, C. M., Smith, E. E., and Nicholls, J. I.: The comparison of denture-base processing techniques. I. Material characteristics, J. Prosthet. Dent. **37**:330-338, 1977.

Benfield, J. W., and Lyons, G. V.: Precision dies from elastic impressions, J. Prosthet. Dent. **12**:737-752, 1962.

Blanchard, C. H.: Filling undercuts on refractory casts with investment, J. Prosthet. Dent. **3**:417-418, 1953.

Bolouri, A., Hilger, T. C., and Gowrylok, M. D.: Modified flasking technique for removable partial dentures, J. Prosthet. Dent. **34**:221-223, 1975.

Collett, H. A.: Casting chrome-cobalt alloys in small laboratories, J. Prosthet. Dent. **21**:216-266, 1969.

Dirksen, L. C., and Campagna, S. J.: Mat surface and rugae reproduction for upper partial denture castings, J. Prosthet. Dent. **4**:67-72, 1954.

Dootz, E. R., Craig, R. G., and Peyton, F. A.: Influence of investments and duplicating procedures on the accuracy of partial denture castings, J. Prosthet. Dent. **15**:679-690, 1965.

Dootz, E. R., Craig, R. G., and Peyton, F. A.: Aqueous acrylamide gel duplicating material, J. Prosthet. Dent. **17**:570-577, 1967.

Dootz, E. R., Craig, R. G., and Peyton, F. A.: Simplification of the chrome-cobalt partial denture casting procedure, J. Prosthet. Dent. **17**:464-471, 1967.

Elbert, C. A., and Ryge, G.: The effect of heat treatment on hardness of a chrome-cobalt alloy, J. Prosthet. Dent. **15**:873-879, 1965.

Elliott, R. W.: The effects of heat on gold partial denture castings, J. Prosthet. Dent. **13**:688-698, 1963.

Enright, C. M.: Dentist-dental laboratory harmony, J. Prosthet. Dent. **11**:393-394, 1961.

Gay, W. D.: Laboratory procedures for fitting removable partial denture frameworks, J. Prosthet. Dent. **40**:227-229, 1978.

Gilson, T. D., Asgar, K., and Peyton, F. A.: The quality of union formed in casting gold to embedded attachment metals, J. Prosthet. Dent. **15**:464-473, 1965.

Grunewald, A. H., Paffenbarger, G. C., and Dickson, G.: The effect of molding processes on some properties of denture resins, J. Am. Dent. Assoc. **44**:269-284, 1952.

Grunewald, A. H., Paffenbarger, G. C., and Dickson, G.: Dentist, dental laboratory, and the patient, J. Prosthet. Dent. **8**:55-60, 1958.

Grunewald, A. H., Paffenbarger, G. C., and Dickson, G.: The role of the dental technician in a prosthetic service, Dent. Clin. North Am., pp. 359-370, July, 1960.

Johnson, H. B.: Technique for packing and staining complete or partial denture bases, J. Prosthet. Dent. **6**:154-159, 1956.

Jones, D. W.: Thermal analysis and stability of refractory investments, J. Prosthet. Dent. **18**:234-241, 1967.

Lanier, B. R., et al.: Making chromium-cobalt removable partial dentures: a modified technique, J. Prosthet. Dent. **25**:197-205, 1971.

Mahler, D. B., and Ady, A. B.: The influence of various factors on the effective setting expansion of casting investments, J. Prosthet. Dent. **13**:365-373, 1963.

Morris, H. F., Asgar, K., Rowe, A. P., and Nasjleti, C. E.: The influence of heat treatments on several types of base-metal removable partial denture alloys, J. Prosthet. Dent. **41**:388-395, 1979.

Perry, C. K.: Transfer base for removable partial dentures, J. Prosthet. Dent. **31**:582-584, 1974.

Peyton, F. A., and Anthony, D. H.: Evaluation of dentures processed by different techniques, J. Prosthet. Dent. **13**:269-281, 1963.

Quinlivan, J. T.: Fabrication of a simple ball-socket attachment, J. Prosthet. Dent. **32**:222-225, 1974.

Reitz, P. V., and Weiner, M. G.: Fabrication of interim acrylic resin removable partial dentures with clasps, J. Prosthet. Dent. **40**:686-688, 1978.

Ryge, G., Kozak, S. F., and Fairhurst, C. W.: Porosities in dental gold castings, J. Am. Dent. Assoc. **54**:746-754, 1957.

Scandrett, F. R., Hanson, J. G., and Unsicker, R. L.: Layered silicone rubber technique for flasking removable partial dentures, J. Prosthet. Dent. **40**:349-350, 1978.

Schmidt, A. H.: Repairing chrome-cobalt castings, J. Prosthet. Dent. **5**:385-387, 1955.

Simmons, E. B., Wagner, A. G., and Traweek, F. C.: Processing acrylic resin bases for removable partial dentures on a hydrocolloid cast, J. Prosthet. Dent. **39**:692-696, 1978.

Smith, G. P.: The responsibility of the dentist toward laboratory procedures in fixed and removable partial denture prosthesis, J. Prosthet. Dent. **13**:295-301, 1963.

Smith, R. A.: Clasp repair for removable partial dentures, J. Prosthet. Dent. **29**:231-234, 1973.

Stankewitz, C. G.: Acrylic resin blockout for interim removable partial dentures, J. Prosthet. Dent. **40**:470-471, 1978.

Teppo, K. W., and Smith, F. W.: A method of immediate clasp repair, J. Prosthet. Dent. **30**:77-80, 1975.

Tuccillo, J. J., and Nielsen, J. P.: Compatibility of alginate impression materials and dental stones, J. Prosthet. Dent. **25**:556-566, 1971.

Ulmer, F. C., and Ward, J. E.: Simplified technique for production of a distal-extension removable partial denture remounting cast, J. Prosthet. Dent. **41**:473-474, 1979.

DENTURE ESTHETICS: TOOTH SELECTION AND ARRANGEMENT

Askinas, S. W.: Facings in removable partial dentures, J. Prosthet. Dent. **33**:633-636, 1975.

Culpepper, W. D.: A comparative study of shade-matching procedures, J. Prosthet. Dent. **24**:166-173, 1971.

DeVan, M. M.: The appearance phase of denture construction, Dent. Clin. North Am., pp. 255-268, March, 1957.

French, F. A.: The selection and arrangement of the anterior teeth in prosthetic dentures, J. Prosthet. Dent. **1**:587-593, 1951.

Frush, J. P., and Fisher, R. D.: Introduction to dentogenic restorations, J. Prosthet. Dent. **5:**586-595, 1955.

Frush, J. P., and Fisher, R. D.: How dentogenic restorations interpret the sex factor, J. Prosthet. Dent. **6:**160-172, 1956.

Frush, J. P., and Fisher, R. D.: How dentogenics interprets the personality factor, J. Prosthet. Dent. **6:**441-449, 1956.

Geiger, E. C. K.: Duplication of the esthetics of an existing immediate denture, J. Prosthet. Dent. **5:**179-185, 1955.

Hughes, G. A.: Facial types and tooth arrangement, J. Prosthet. Dent. **1:**82-95, 1951.

Krajicek, D. D.: Natural appearance for the individual denture patient, J. Prosthet. Dent. **10:**205-214, 1960.

Levin, E. I.: Dental esthetics and the golden proportion, J. Prosthet. Dent. **40:**244-252, 1978.

Lombardi, R. E.: Factors mediating against excellence in dental esthetics, J. Prosthet. Dent. **38:**243-248, 1977.

Myerson, R. L.: The use of porcelain and plastic teeth in opposing complete dentures, J. Prosthet. Dent. **7:**625-633, 1957.

Payne, A. G. L.: Factors influencing the position of artificial upper anterior teeth, J. Prosthet. Dent. **26:**26-32, 1971.

Pound, E.: Lost—fine arts in the fallacy of the ridges, J. Prosthet. Dent. **4:**6-16, 1954.

Pound, E.: Recapturing esthetic tooth position in the edentulous patient, J. Am. Dent. Assoc. **55:**181-191, 1957.

Pound, E.: Applying harmony in selecting and arranging teeth, Dent. Clin. North Am., pp. 241-258, March, 1962.

Roraff, A. R.: Instant photographs for developing esthetics, J. Prosthet. Dent. **26:**21-25, 1971.

Smith, B. J.: Esthetic factors in removable partial prosthodontics, Dent. Clin. North Am. **23:**53-63, 1979.

Tillman, E. J.: Molding and staining acrylic resin anterior teeth, J. Prosthet. Dent. **5:**497-507, 1955; Dent. Abstr. **1:**111, 1956.

Van Victor, A.: Positive duplication of anterior teeth for immediate dentures, J. Prosthet. Dent. **3:**165-177, 1953.

Van Victor, A.: The mold guide cast—its significance in denture esthetics, J. Prosthet. Dent. **13:**406-415, 1963.

Vig, R. G.: The denture look, J. Prosthet. Dent. **11:**9-15, 1961.

Wallace, D. H.: The use of gold occlusal surfaces in complete and partial dentures, J. Prosthet. Dent. **14:**326-333, 1964.

Wolfson, E.: Staining and characterization of acrylic teeth, Dent. Abstr. **1:**41, 1956.

Young, H. A.: Denture esthetics, J. Prosthet. Dent. **6:**748-755, 1956.

DIAGNOSIS AND TREATMENT PLANNING

Applegate, O. C.: Evaluating oral structures for removable partial dentures, J. Prosthet. Dent. **11:**882-885, 1961.

Bartels, J. C.: Diagnosis and treatment planning, J. Prosthet. Dent. **7:**657-662, 1957.

Bennett, C. G.: Transitional restorations for function and esthetics, J. Prosthet. Dent. **15:**867-872, 1965.

Blatterfein, L.: The planning and contouring of acrylic resin veneer crowns for partial denture clasping, J. Prosthet. Dent. **6:**386-404, 1956.

Bolender, C. L., Swenson, R. D., and Yamane, G.: Evaluation of treatment of inflammatory papillary hyperplasia of the palate, J. Prosthet. Dent. **15:**1013-1022, 1965.

Casey, D. M., and Lauciello, F. R.: A review of the submerged-root concept, J. Prosthet. Dent. **43:**128-132, 1980.

Contino, R. M., and Stallard, H.: Instruments essential for obtaining data needed in making a functional diagnosis of the human mouth, J. Prosthet. Dent. **7:**66-77, 1957.

Dreizen, S.: Nutritional changes in the oral cavity, J. Prosthet. Dent. **16:**1144-1150, 1966.

Dummer, P. M. H., and Gidden, J.: The upper anterior sectional denture, J. Prosthet. Dent. **41:**146-152, 1979.

Dunn, B. W.: Treatment planning for removable partial dentures, J. Prosthet. Dent. **11:**247-255, 1961.

Foster, T. D.: The use of the face-bow in making permanent study casts, J. Prosthet. Dent. **9:**717-721, 1959.

Frechette, A. R.: Partial denture planning with special reference to stress distribution, J. Prosthet. Dent. **1:**700-707 (disc., 208-209), 1951.

Friedman, S.: Effective use of diagnostic data, J. Prosthet. Dent. **9:**729-737, 1959.

Garver, D. G., et al.: Vital root retention in humans: a preliminary report, J. Prosthet. Dent. **40:**23-28, 1978.

Garver, D. G., and Fenster, R. K.: Vital root retention in humans: a final report, J. Prosthet. Dent. **43:**368-373, 1980.

Guyer, S. E.: Selectively retained vital roots for partial support of overdentures: a patient report, J. Prosthet. Dent. **33:**258-263, 1975.

Harvey, W. L.: A transitional prosthetic appliance, J. Prosthet. Dent. **14:**60-70, 1964.

Heintz, W. D.: Treatment planning and design: prevention of errors of omission and commission, Dent. Clin. North Am. **23:**3-12, 1979.

Henderson, D., Hickey, J. C., and Wehner, P. J.: Prevention and preservation—the challenge of removable partial denture service, Dent. Clin. North Am., pp. 459-473, July, 1965.

House, M. M.: The relationship of oral examination to dental diagnosis, J. Prosthet. Dent. **8:**208-219, 1958.

Kabcenell, J. L.: Planning for individualized prosthetic treatment, J. Prosthet. Dent. **34:**405-407, 1975.

Killebrew, R. F.: Crown construction and splinting of mobile partial denture abutments, J. Am. Dent. Assoc. **70:**334-338, 1965.

Krikos, A. A.: Preparing guide planes for removable partial dentures, J. Prosthet. Dent. **34:**152-155, 1975.

Lambson, G. O.: Papillary hyperplasia of the palate, J. Prosthet. Dent. **16:**636-645, 1966.

McCracken, W. L.: Differential diagnosis: fixed or removable partial dentures, J. Am. Dent. Assoc. **63:**767-775, 1961.

McGill, W. J.: Acquiring space for partial dentures, J. Prosthet. Dent. **17:**163-165, 1967.

Miller, E. L.: Planning partial denture construction, Dent. Clin. North Am. **17**:571-584, 1973.

Miller, E. L.: Critical factors in selecting removable prostheses, J. Prosthet. Dent. **34**:486-490, 1975.

Moulton, G. H.: The importance of centric occlusion in diagnosis and treatment planning, J. Prosthet. Dent. **10**:921-926, 1960.

Nassif, J., and Blumenfeld, W. L.: Joint consultation services by the periodontist and prosthodontist, J. Prosthet. Dent. **29**:55-60, 1973.

Nassif, J., Blumenfeld, W. L., and Tarsitano, J. T.: Dialogue—a treatment modality, J. Prosthet. Dent. **33**:696-700, 1975.

Payne, S. H.: Diagnostic factors which influence the choice of posterior occlusion, Dent. Clin. North Am., pp. 203-213, March, 1957.

Rudd, K. D., and Dunn, B. W.: Accurate removable partial dentures, J. Prosthet. Dent. **18**:559-570, 1967.

Saunders, T. R., Gillis, R. E., and Desjardins, R. P.: The maxillary complete denture opposing the mandibular bilateral distal-extension partial denture: treatment considerations, J. Prosthet. Dent. **41**:124-128, 1979.

Sauser, C. W.: Pretreatment evaluation of partially edentulous arches, J. Prosthet. Dent. **11**:886-893, 1961.

Seiden, A.: Occlusal rests and rest seats, J. Prosthet. Dent. **8**:431-440, 1958.

Turner, C. E., and Shaffer, F. W.: Planning the treatment of the complex prosthodontic case, J. Am. Dent. Assoc. **97**:992-993, 1978.

Uccellani, E. L.: Evaluating the mucous membranes of the edentulous mouth, J. Prosthet. Dent. **15**:295-303, 1965.

Wagner, A. G.: Instructions for the use and care of removable partial dentures, J. Prosthet. Dent. **26**:481-490, 1971.

Waldron, C. A.: Oral leukoplakia, carcinona, and the prosthodontist, J. Prosthet. Dent. **15**:367-376, 1965.

Walker, W. A., and Kramer, D. C.: Claspless chrome-cobalt transitional removable partial dentures, J. Am. Dent. Assoc. **96**:814-818, 1978.

Waller, M. I.: The root seat and the removable partial denture: a clinical investigation, J. Prosthet. Dent. **34**:1623, 1975.

Young, H. A.: Diagnostic survey of edentulous patients, J. Prosthet. Dent. **5**:5-14, 1955.

IMPRESSION MATERIALS AND METHODS; THE PARTIAL DENTURE BASE

Akerly, W. B.: A combination impression and occlusal registration technique for extension-base removable partial dentures, J. Prosthet. Dent. **39**:226-229, 1978.

Applegate, O. C.: The partial denture base, J. Prosthet. Dent. **5**:636-648, 1955.

Applegate, O. C.: An evaluation of the support for the removable partial denture, J. Prosthet. Dent. **10**:112-123, 1960.

Bailey, L. R.: Acrylic resin tray for rubber base impression materials, J. Prosthet. Dent. **5**:658-662, 1955.

Bailey, L. R.: Rubber base impression techniques, Dent. Clin. North Am., pp. 156-166, March, 1957.

Blatterfein, L., Klein, I. E., and Miglino, J. C.: A loading impression technique for semiprecision and precision removable partial dentures, J. Prosthet. Dent. **43**:9-14, 1980.

Chase, W. W.: Adaptation of rubber-base impression materials to removable denture prosthetics, J. Prosthet. Dent. **10**:1043-1050, 1960.

Chong, M. P., et al.: The tear test as a means of evaluating the resistance to rupture of alginate impression materials, Aust. Dent. J. **16**:145-151, 1971.

Clark, R. J., and Phillips, R. W.: Flow studies of certain dental impression materials, J. Prosthet. Dent. **7**:259-266, 1957.

Davis, M. C.: The use of rubber base impression materials in the construction of inlays, J. Prosthet. Dent. **8**:123-134, 1958.

Dootz, E. R.: Fabricating non-precious metal bases, Dent. Clin. North Am. **24**:113-122, 1980.

Frank, R. P.: Analysis of pressures produced during maxillary edentulous impression procedures, J. Prosthet. Dent. **22**:400-403, 1969.

Fusayama, T., and Nakazato, M.: The design of stock trays and the retention of irreversible hydrocolloid impressions, J. Prosthet. Dent. **21**:136-142, 1969.

Gilmore, W. H., Schnell, R. J., and Phillips, R. W.: Factors influencing the accuracy of silicone impression materials, J. Prosthet. Dent. **9**:304-314, 1959.

Harris, W. T., Jr.: Water temperature and accuracy of alginate impressions, J. Prosthet. Dent. **21**:613-617, 1969.

Harrison, J. D.: Prevention of failures in making impressions and dies, Dent. Clin. North Am. **23**:13-20, 1979.

Heartwell, C. M., et al.: Comparison of impressions made in perforated and nonperforated rimlocks trays, J. Prosthet. Dent. **27**:494-500, 1972.

Herfort, T. W., et al.: Viscosity of elastomeric impression materials, J. Prosthet. Dent. **38**:396-404, 1977.

Holmes, J. B.: Influence of impression procedures and occlusal loading on partial denture movement, J. Prosthet. Dent. **15**:474-481, 1965.

Hudson, W. C.: Clinical uses of rubber impression materials and electroforming of casts and dies in pure silver, J. Prosthet. Dent. **8**:107-114, 1958.

Johnston, J. F., Cunningham, D. M., and Bogan, R. G.: The dentist, the patient, and ridge preservation, J. Prosthet. Dent. **10**:288-295, 1960.

Koran, A., III: Impression materials for recording the denture bearing mucosa, Dent. Clin. North Am. **24**:97-111, 1980.

Kramer, H. M.: Impression technique for removable partial dentures, J. Prosthet. Dent. **11**:84-92, 1961.

Lee, R. E.: Mucostatics, Dent. Clin. North Am. **24**:81-96, 1980.

Leupold, R. J.: A comparative study of impression procedures for distal extension removable partial dentures, J. Prosthet. Dent. **16**:708-720, 1966.

Leupold, R. J., and Kratochvil, F. J.: An altered-cast procedure to improve support for removable partial dentures, J. Prosthet. Dent. **15**:672-678, 1965.

Mitchell, J. V., and Damele, J. J.: Influence of tray design upon elastic impression materials, J. Prosthet. Dent. **23**:51-57, 1970.

Morrow, R. M., et al.: Compatibility of alginate impression materials and dental stones, J. Prosthet. Dent. **25**:556-566, 1971.

Myers, G. E.: Electroformed die technique for rubber base impressions, J. Prosthet. Dent. **8**:531-535, 1958.

O'Brien, W. J.: Base retention, Dent. Clin. North Am. **24**:123-130, 1980.

Pfeiffer, K. A.: Clinical problems in the use of alginate hydrocolloid, Dent. Abstr. **2**:82, 1957.

Phillips, R. W.: Factors influencing the accuracy of reversible hydrocolloid impressions, J. Am. Dent. Assoc. **43**:1-17, 1951.

Phillips, R. W.: Factors affecting the surface of stone dies poured in hydrocolloid impressions, J. Prosthet. Dent. **2**:390-400, 1952.

Phillips, R. W.: Elastic impression materials—a second progress report of a recent conference, J. South. Calif. Dent. Assoc. **26**:150-153, 1958.

Phillips, R. W.: Physical properties and manipulation of rubber impression materials, J. Am. Dent. Assoc. **59**:454-458, 1959.

Prieskel, H. W.: Impression techniques for attachment-retained distal extension removable partial dentures, J. Prosthet. Dent. **25**:620-628, 1971.

Rapuano, J. A.: Single tray dual-impression technique for distal extension partial dentures, J. Prosthet. Dent. **24**:41-46, 1970.

Rehberg, H. J.: The impression tray—an important factor in impression precision, Int. Dent. J. **27**:146-153, 1977.

Rosenstiel, E.: Rubber base elastic impression materials, Dent. Abstr. **1**:55, 1956.

Rudd, K. D., et al.: Comparison of effects of tap water and slurry water on gypsum casts, J. Prosthet. Dent. **24**:563-570, 1970.

Rudd, K. D., Morrow, R. M., and Bange, A. A.: Accurate casts, J. Prosthet. Dent. **21**:545-554, 1969.

Rudd, K. D., Morrow, R. M., and Strunk, R. R.: Accurate alginate impressions, J. Prosthet. Dent. **22**:294-300, 1969.

Silver, M.: Impressions and silver-plated dies from a rubber impression material, J. Prosthet. Dent. **6**:543-549, 1956.

Smith, P. K.: The effect on the accuracy of polysulphide impression material after treating preparations with various agents, Aust. Dent. J. **16**:337-339, 1971.

Smith, R. A.: Secondary palatal impressions for major connector adaptation, J. Prosthet. Dent. **24**:108-110, 1970.

Stafford, G. D., and MacCulloch, W. T.: Radiopaque denture base materials, Br. Dent. J. **131**:22-24, 1971.

Steffel, V. L.: Relining removable partial dentures for fit and function, J. Prosthet. Dent. **4**:496-509, 1954; J. Tenn. Dent. Assoc. **36**:35-43, 1956.

Vahidi, F.: Vertical displacement of distal-extension ridges by different impression techniques, J. Prosthet. Dent. **40**:374-377, 1978.

Wilson, J. H.: Partial dentures—relining the saddle supported by the mucosa and alveolar bone, J. Prosthet. Dent. **3**:807-813, 1953.

Young, J. M.: Surface characteristics of dental stone: impression orientation, J. Prosthet. Dent. **33**:336-341, 1975.

MAXILLOFACIAL PROSTHESIS

Ackerman, A. J.: Maxillofacial prosthesis, Oral Surg. **6**:176-200, 1953.

Ackerman, A. J.: The prosthetic management of oral and facial defects following cancer surgery, J. Prosthet. Dent. **5**:413-432, 1955.

Brown, K. E.: Fabrication of a hollow-bulb obturator, J. Prosthet. Dent. **21**:97-103, 1969.

Cantor, R., et al.: Methods for evaluating prosthetic facial materials, J. Prosthet. Dent. **21**:324-332, 1969.

Curtis, T. A., and Cantor, R.: The forgotten patient in maxillofacial prosthesis, J. Prosthet. Dent. **31**:662-680, 1974.

Desjardins, R. P.: Prosthodontic management of the cleft palate patient, J. Prosthet. Dent. **33**:655-665, 1975.

Firtell, D. N., and Grisius, R. J.: Retention of obturator—removable partial dentures: a comparison of buccal and lingual retention, J. Prosthet. Dent. **43**:212-217, 1980.

Gay, W. D., and King, G. E.: Applying basic prosthodontic principles in the dentulous maxillectomy patient, J. Prosthet. Dent. **43**:433-435, 1980.

Immekus, J. E., and Aramy, M.: Adverse effects of resilient denture liners in overlay dentures, J. Prosthet. Dent. **32**:178-181, 1974.

Kelly, E. K.: Partial denture design applicable to the maxillofacial patient, J. Prosthet. Dent. **15**:168-173, 1965.

Metz, H. H.: Mandibular staple implant for an atrophic mandibular ridge: solving retention difficulties of a denture, J. Prosthet. Dent. **32**:572-578, 1974.

Monteith, G. G.: The partially edentulous patient with special problems, Dent. Clin. North Am. **23**:107-115, 1979.

Moore, D. J.: Cervical esophagus prosthesis, J. Prosthet. Dent. **30**:442-445, 1973.

Nethery, W. J., and Delclos, L.: Prosthetic stent for gold-grain implant to the floor of the mouth, J. Prosthet. Dent. **23**:81-87, 1970.

Smith, E. H., Jr.: Prosthetic treatment of maxillofacial injuries, J. Prosthet. Dent. **5**:112-128, 1955.

Strain, J. C.: A mechanical device for duplicating a mirror image of a cast or moulage in three dimensions, J. Prosthet. Dent. **5**:129-132, 1955.

Toremalm, N. G.: A disposable obturator for maxillary defects, J. Prosthet. Dent. **29**:94-96, 1973.

Young, J. M.: The prosthodontist's role in total treatment of patients, J. Prosthet. Dent. **27**:399-412, 1972.

MISCELLANEOUS

Abere, D. J.: Post-placement care of complete and removable partial dentures, Dent. Clin. North Am. **23**:143-151, 1979.

Academy of Denture Prosthetics: Principles, concepts and practices in prosthodontics, J. Prosthet. Dent. **37**:204-221, 1977.

Adisman, I. K.: What a prosthodontist should know, J. Prosthet. Dent. **21**:409-416, 1969.

Applegate, O. C.: Conditions which may influence the choice of partial or complete denture service, J. Prosthet. Dent. **7**:182-196, 1957.

Applegate, O. C.: The removable partial denture in the general practice of tomorrow, J. Prosthet. Dent. **8**:609-622, 1958.

Applegate, O. C.: Factors to be considered in choosing an alloy, Dent. Clin. North Am., pp. 583-590, Nov., 1960.

Asgar, K., et al.: A new alloy for partial dentures, J. Prosthet. Dent. **23**:36-43, 1970.

Atwood, D. A.: Practice of prosthodontics: past, present, and future, J. Prosthet. Dent. **21**:393-401, 1970.

Augsburger, R. H.: Evaluating removable partial dentures by mathematical equations, J. Prosthet. Dent. **22**:528-543, 1969.

Backenstose, W. M., and Wells, J. G.: Side effects of immersion-type cleansers on the metal components of dentures, J. Prosthet. Dent. **37**:615-621, 1977.

Baker, C. R.: Difficulties in evaluating removable partial dentures, J. Prosthet. Dent. **17**:60-62, 1967.

Baker, C. R.: Occlusal reactive prosthodontics, J. Prosthet. Dent. **17**:566-569, 1967.

Barrett, D. A., and Pilling, L. O.: The restoration of carious clasp-bearing teeth, J. Prosthet. Dent. **15**:309-311, 1965.

Barsby, M. J., and Schwarz, W. D.: A survey of the teaching of partial denture construction in dental schools in the United Kingdom, J. Dent. **7**:1-8, 1979.

Bates, J. F.: Studies related to fracture of partial dentures, Br. Dent. J. **120**:79-83, 1966.

Bauman, R.: Survey of dentists' attitudes regarding instructions for home care for patients who wear dentures, J. Am. Dent. Assoc. **100**:206-208, 1980.

Beck, H. O.: A clinical evaluation of the arcon concept of articulation, J. Prosthet. Dent. **9**:409-421, 1959.

Beck, H. O.: Alloys for removable partial dentures, Dent. Clin. North Am., pp. 591-596, Nov., 1960.

Beck, H. O., and Morrison, W. E.: Investigation of an arcon articulator, J. Prosthet. Dent. **6**:359-372, 1956.

Blatterfein, L.: Role of the removable partial denture in the restoration of lost vertical dimension, N.Y. Univ. J. Dent. **10**:274-276, 1952.

Blatterfein, L., et al.: Minimum acceptable procedures for satisfactory removable partial denture service, J. Prosthet. Dent. **27**:84-87, 1972.

Boucher, C. O., editor: Current clinical dental terminology, ed. 2, St. Louis, 1974, The C. V. Mosby Co.

Boucher, C. O.: Writing as a means for learning, J. Prosthet. Dent. **27**:229-234, 1972.

Boucher, L. J., et al.: Guidelines for advanced prosthodontic education, J. Prosthet. Dent. **23**:104-110, 1970.

Breitbart, A. R.: Converting a tooth-supported denture to a distal extension removable partial denture, J. Prosthet. Dent. **18**:233, 1967.

Brockhurst, P. J.: Comparison of the performance of materials for spring members in dental appliances, using the theory of simple bending, Aust. Dent. J. **15**:119-125, 1970.

Cavalaris, C. J.: Pathologic considerations associated with partial dentures, Dent. Clin. North Am. **17**:585-600, 1973.

Cecconi, B. C.: Removable partial denture research and its clinical significance, J. Prosthet. Dent. **39**:203-210, 1978.

Charbeneau, G. T., et al.: Report of the Committee on Scientific Investigation of the American Academy of Restorative Dentistry, J. Prosthet. Dent. **36**:441-467, 1976.

Cheraskin, E., and Ringsdorf, W. M., Jr.: The ecology of the prosthodontic problem, J. Am. Dent. Assoc. **92**:133-139, 1976.

Coy, R. E., and Arnold, P. D.: Survey and design of diagnostic casts for removable partial dentures, J. Prosthet. Dent. **32**:103-106, 1974.

Cunningham, D. M.: Comparison of base metal alloys and Type IV gold alloys for removable partial denture frameworks, Dent. Clin. North Am. **17**:719-722, 1973.

Cutright, D. E.: Morphogenesis of inflammatory papillary hyperplasia, J. Prosthet. Dent. **33**:380-385, 1975.

Dale, J. W.: A full and partial denture survey, Aust. Dent. J. **15**:225-227, 1970.

Derry, A., and Bertram, U.: A clinical survey of removable partial dentures after 2 years usage, Acta Odontol. Scand. **28**:581-598, 1970.

DeVan, M. M.: The additive partial denture: its principles and design (partial dentures), North West Dent. **35**:303-307, 312, 1956; Dent. Abstr. **2**:468, 1957.

Elliott, R. W.: The effects of heat on gold partial denture castings, J. Prosthet. Dent. **13**:688-698, 1963.

Ettinger, R. L.: The acrylic removable partial denture, J. Am. Dent. Assoc. **95**:945-949, 1977.

Ewing, J. E.: Temporary cementation in fixed partial prosthesis, J. Prosthet. Dent. **5**:388-391, 1955.

Ewing, J. E.: The construction of accurate full crown restorations for an existing clasp by using a direct metal pattern technique, J. Prosthet. Dent. **15**:889-899, 1965.

Farah, J. W., MacGregor, A. R., and Miller, T. P. G.: Stress analysis of disjunct removable partial dentures, J. Prosthet. Dent. **42**:271-275, 1979.

Federation of Prosthodontic Organizations: Guidelines for evaluation of completed prosthodontic treatment for removable partial dentures, J. Prosthet. Dent. **27**:326-328, 1972.

Fenton, A. H., and Jeffrey, J. D.: Allergy to a partial denture casting: case report, J. Canad. Dent. Assoc. **10**:446-468, 1978.

Fenton, A. H., Zarb, G. A., and MacKay, H. F.: Overdenture oversights, Dent. Clin. North Am. **23**:117-130, 1979.

Fields, H., and Campfield, R. W.: Removable partial prosthesis partially supported by an endosseous blade implant, J. Prosthet. Dent. **31**:273-278, 1974.

Fish, S. F.: Partial dentures, Br. Dent. J. **128**:243-246, 289-293, 339-344, 398-402, 446-453, 495-502, 547-551, 590-592, 1970.

Fish, S. F., et al.: A study of prosthetic dentistry, Br. Dent. J. **127**:59-70, 1969.

Frank, R. P.: Fabrication of temporary and treatment partial dentures, J. Prosthet. Dent. **30**:215-221, 1973.

Frank, R. P.: Evaluating refractory cast wax-ups for removable partial dentures, J. Prosthet. Dent. **35**: 388-392, 1976.

Gilmore, H. W., et al.: Report of the Committee on Scientific Investigation of the American Academy of Restorative Dentistry, J. Prosthet. Dent. **40**: 192-206, 1978.

Girardot, R. L.: The physiologic aspects of partial denture restorations, J. Prosthet. Dent. 3:689-698, 1953.

Glossary of prosthodontic terms, J. Prosthet. Dent. **38**:70-109, 1977.

Hamilton, A. I., et al.: Report of the Committee on Scientific Investigation of the American Academy of Restorative Dentistry, J. Prosthet. Dent. 34:86-110, 1975.

Hardcourt, H. J., et al.: The properties of nickel-chromium casting alloys containing boron and silicon, Br. Dent. J. **129**:419-423, 1970.

Harrison, W. M., and Stansbury, B. E.: The effect of joint surface contours on the transverse strength of repaired acrylic resin, J. Prosthet. Dent. **23**: 464-472, 1970.

Heintz, W. D.: Principles, planning, and practice for prevention, Dent. Clin. North Am. **17**:705-718, 1973.

Herlands, R. E.: Removable partial denture terminology, J. Prosthet. Dent. 8:964-972, 1958.

Hickey, J. C.: Responsibility of the dentist in removable partial dentures, J. Ky. Dent. Assoc. **17**: 70-87, 1965.

Hickey, J. C.: Charge to workshop on advanced prosthodontic training, J. Prosthet. Dent. **21**:388-392, 1969.

Hobdell, M. H., et al.: The prevalence of full and partial dentures in British populations, Br. Dent. J. **128**:437-442, 1970.

Jankelson, B. H.: Adjustment of dentures at time of insertion and alterations to compensate for tissue changes, J. Am. Dent. Assoc. 64:521-531, 1962.

Jones, R. R.: The lower partial denture, J. Prosthet. Dent. 2:219-229, 1952.

Kaires, A. K.: A study of partial denture design and masticatory pressures in a mandibular bilateral distal extension case, J. Prosthet. Dent. **8**: 340-350, 1958.

Kelly, E.: Fatigue failure in denture base polymers, J. Prosthet. Dent. 21:257-266, 1969.

Kelly, E.: Changes caused by a mandibular removable partial denture opposing a maxillary complete denture, J. Prosthet. Dent. 27:140-150, 1972.

Kelly, E. K.: The physiologic approach to partial denture design, J. Prosthet. Dent. 3:699-710, 1953.

Kessler, B.: An analysis of the tongue factor and its functioning areas in dental prosthesis, J. Prosthet. Dent. 5:629-635, 1955.

Klein, I. E., et al.: Minimum clinical procedures for satisfactory complete denture, removable partial denture, and fixed partial denture services, J. Prosthet. Dent. **22**:4-10, 1969.

Kratochvil, F. J.: Maintaining supporting structures with a removable partial prosthesis, J. Prosthet. Dent. 25:167-174, 1971.

Kratochvil, F. J., and Caputo, A. A.: Photoelastic analysis of pressure on teeth and bone supporting removable partial dentures, J. Prosthet. Dent. **32**: 52-61, 1974.

Landa, J. S.: The troublesome transition from a partial lower to a complete lower denture, J. Prosthet. Dent. 4:42-51, 1954.

Levin, B.: Removable prosthodontics in the United Kingdom and Scandinavia, J. Prosthet. Dent. **33**: 224-232, 1975.

Lewis, A. J.: Failure of removable partial denture castings during service, J. Prosthet. Dent. **39**:147-149, 1978.

Lewis, A. J.: Radiographic evaluation of porosities in removable partial denture castings, J. Prosthet. Dent. **39**:278-281, 1978.

Lorton, L.: A method of stabilizing removable partial denture castings during clinical and laboratory procedures, J. Prosthet. Dent. **39**:344-345, 1978.

Love, W. B.: Prosthodontics—past, present, and future, J. Prosthet. Dent. **36**:261-264, 1976.

Maison, W. G.: Instructions to denture patients, J. Prosthet. Dent. **9**:825-831, 1959.

Makrauer, F. L., and Davis, J. S.: Gastroscopic removal of a partial denture, J. Am. Dent. Assoc. **94**:904-906, 1977.

Margolese, S., Swoope, C. C., and Pettapiece, G.: Attitudes of dentists in British Columbia toward removable prosthodontics, J. Prosthet. Dent. **43**: 22-25, 1980.

Martone, A. L.: The fallacy of saving time at the chair, J. Prosthet. Dent. **7**:416-419, 1957.

Martone, A. L.: The effects of oral prostheses on the production of speech sounds, Ohio State Univ. Dent. Abstr. **2**:508, 1957.

Martone, A. L.: The challenge of the partially edentulous mouth, J. Prosthet. Dent. **8**:942-954, 1958.

Massler, M.: Geriatric nutrition: the role of taste and smell in appetite, J. Prosthet. Dent. **32**:247-250, 1980.

McCracken, W. L.: Auxiliary uses of cold-curing acrylic resins in prosthetic dentistry, J. Am. Dent. Assoc. **47**:298-304, 1953.

McCracken, W. L.: A comparison of tooth-borne and tooth-tissue–borne removable partial dentures, J. Prosthet. Dent. 3:375-381, 1953.

McCracken, W. L.: A philosophy of partial denture treatment, J. Prosthet. Dent. **13**:889-900, 1963.

Means, C. R., and Flenniken, I. E.: Gagging—a problem in prosthetic dentistry, J. Prosthet. Dent. 23:614-620, 1970.

Mehringer, E. J.: The saliva as it is related to the wearing of dentures, J. Prosthet. Dent. 4:312-318, 1954.

Michell, D. L., and Wilke, N. D.: Articulators through the years. I. Up to 1940, J. Prosthet. Dent. **39**:330-338, 1978. II. From 1940, **39**:451-458, 1978.

Miller, E. L.: Critical factors in selecting removable prostheses, J. Prosthet. Dent. 34:486-490, 1975.

Miller, E. L.: Clinical management of denture-induced inflammations, J. Prosthet. Dent. **38**:362-365, 1977.

Mohamed, S. E., Schmidt, J. R., and Harrison, J. D.: Articulators in dental education and practice, J. Prosthet. Dent. 36:319-325, 1976.

Morris, H. F., and Asgar, K.: Physical properties and microstructure of four new commercial partial denture alloys, J. Prosthet. Dent. 33:36-46, 1975.

Morse, P. K., and Boucher, L. J.: What a prosthodontist does, J. Prosthet. Dent. 21:402-408, 1969.

Mosteller, J. H.: Use of prednisolone in the elimination of postoperative thermal sensitivity, J. Prosthet. Dent. 12:1176-1179, 1962.

Neufeld, J. O.: Changes in the trabecular pattern of the mandible following the loss of teeth, J. Prosthet. Dent. 8:685-697, 1958.

Öatlund, S. G.: Saliva and denture retention, J. Prosthet. Dent. 10:658-663, 1960.

Osborne, J., and Lammie, G. A.: The bilateral free-end saddle lower denture, J. Prosthet. Dent. 4: 640-652, 1954.

Overton, R. G., and Bramblett, R. M.: Prosthodontic services: a study of need and availability in the United States, J. Prosthet. Dent. 27:329-339, 1972.

Pascoe, D. F., and Wimmer, J.: A radiographic technique for the detection of internal defects in dental castings, J. Prosthet. Dent. 39:150-157, 1978.

Phillips, R. W., and Leonard, L. J.: A study of enamel abrasion as related to partial denture clasps, J. Prosthet. Dent. 6:657-671, 1956.

Plainfield, S.: Communication distortion. The language of patients and practitioners of dentistry, J. Prosthet. Dent. 22:11-19, 1969.

Prieskel, H. W.: The distal extension prosthesis reappraised, J. Dent. 5:217-230, 1977.

Ramsey, W. O.: The relation of emotional factors to prosthodontic service, J. Prosthet. Dent. 23: 4-10, 1970.

Raybin, N. H.: The polished surface of complete dentures, J. Prosthet. Dent. 13:236-239, 1963.

Reynolds, J. M.: Crown construction for abutments of existing removable partial dentures, J. Am. Dent. Assoc. 69:423-426, 1964.

Rothman, R.: Phonetic considerations in denture prosthesis, J. Prosthet. Dent. 11:214-223, 1961.

Rudd, K. D., and Dunn, B. W.: Accurate removable partial dentures, J. Prosthet. Dent. 18:559-570, 1967.

Rushford, C. B.: A technique for precision removable partial denture construction, J. Prosthet. Dent. 31:377-383, 1974.

Ruyter, I. E., and Svendsen, S. A.: Flexural properties of denture base polymers, J. Prosthet. Dent. 43:95-104, 1980.

Savage, R. D., and MacGregor, A. R.: Behavior therapy in prosthodontics, J. Prosthet. Dent. 24: 126-132, 1970.

Schabel, R. W.: Dentist-patient communication—a major factor in treatment prognosis, J. Prosthet. Dent. 21:3-5, 1969.

Schabel, R. W.: The psychology of aging, J. Prosthet. Dent. 27:569-573, 1972.

Schole, M. L.: Management of the gagging patient, J. Prosthet. Dent. 9:578-583, 1959.

Schopper, A. F.: Removable appliances for the preservation of the teeth, J. Prosthet. Dent. 4:634-639, 1954.

Schopper, A. F.: Loss of vertical dimension: causes and effects: diagnosis and various recommended treatments, J. Prosthet. Dent. 9:428-431, 1959.

Schuyler, C. H.: Stress distribution as the prime requisite to the success of a partial denture, J. Am. Dent. Assoc. 20:2148-2154, 1963.

Schuyler, A. F.: Planning the removable partial denture to restore function and maintain oral health, N.Y. Dent. J. 13:4-10, 1947.

Schwarz, W. D., and Barsby, M. J.: Design of partial dentures in dental practice, J. Dent. 6:166-170, 1978.

Sears, V. H.: Comprehensive denture service, J. Am. Dent. Assoc. 64:531-552, 1962.

Skinner, E. W., and Gordon, C. C.: Some experiments on the surface hardness of dental stones, J. Prosthet. Dent. 6:94-100, 1956.

Skinner, E. W., and Jones, P. M.: Dimensional stability of self-curing denture base acrylic resin, J. Am. Dent. Assoc. 51:426-431, 1955.

Smith, B. H.: Changes in occlusal face height with removable partial prostheses, J. Prosthet. Dent. 34:278-285, 1975.

Smith, F. W., and Applegate, O. C.: Roentgenographic study of bone changes during exercise stimulation of edentulous areas, J. Prosthet. Dent. 11:1086-1097, 1961.

Stendahl, C. G., and Grob, D. J.: Detection of binding areas on removable partial denture frameworks, Dent. Clin. North Am. 23:101-106, 1979.

Sweeney, W. T., Myerson, R. L., Rose, E. E., and Semmelman, J. O.: Proposed specification for plastic teeth, J. Prosthet. Dent. 7:420-424, 1957.

Sykora, O.: Extracoronal removable partial denture service in Canada, J. Prosthet. Dent. 39:37-41, 1978.

Tallgren, A.: Alveolar bone loss in denture wearers as related to facial morphology, Acta Odontol. Scand. 28:251-270, 1970.

Teppo, K. W., and Smith, F. W.: A method of immediate clasp repair, J. Prosthet. Dent. 34:77-80, 1975.

Tomlin, H. R., and Osborne, J.: Cobalt-chromium partial dentures; a clinical survey, Br. Dent. J. 110:307-310, 1961.

Trainor, J. E., and Elliott, R. W., Jr.: Removable partial dentures designed by dentists before and after graduate level instruction: a comparative study, J. Prosthet. Dent. 27:509-514, 1972.

Wagner, A. G.: Maintenance of the partially edentulous mouth and care of the denture, Dent. Clin. North Am. 17:755-768, 1973.

Wagner, A. G., and Forgue, E. G.: A study of four methods of recording the path of insertion of removable partial dentures, J. Prosthet. Dent. 35: 267-272, 1976.

Wallace, D. H.: The use of gold occlusal surfaces in complete and partial dentures, J. Prosthet. Dent. 14:326-333, 1964.

Walter, J. D.: Partial denture technique. I. Introduction, Br. Dent. J. 147:241-243, 1979. II. The purpose of the denture: choice of material, 147: 302-304, 1979. III. Supporting the denture, 148: 13-16, 1980. IV. Guide planes, 148:70-72, 1980.

Weaver, R. E., and Goebel, W. M.: Reactions to acrylic resin dental prostheses, J. Prosthet. Dent. 43:138-142, 1980.

Wilson, J. H.: Some clinical and technical aspects of partial dentures, Dent. J. Aust. 26:176-183, 1954.

Wise, H. B., and Kaiser, D. A.: A radiographic technique for examination of internal defects in metal frameworks, J. Prosthet. Dent. 42:594-595, 1979.

Young, H. A.: Factors contributory to success in prosthodontic practice, J. Prosthet. Dent. **5:**354-360, 1955.

Zach, G. A.: Advantages of mesial rests for removable partial dentures, J. Prosthet. Dent. **33:**32-35, 1975.

Zerosi, C.: A new type of removable splint: its indications and function, Dent. Abstr. **1:**451-452, 1956.

MOUTH PREPARATIONS

Alexander, J. M., and Van Sickels, J. E.: Posterior maxillary osteotomies: an aid for a difficult prosthodontic problem, J. Prosthet. Dent. **41:**614-617, 1979.

Atwood, D. A.: Reduction of residual ridges in the partially edentulous patient, Dent. Clin. North Am. **17:**747-754, 1973.

Axinn, S.: Preparation of retentive areas for clasps in enamel, J. Prosthet. Dent. **34:**405-407, 1975.

Belinfante, L. S., and Abney, J. M., Jr.: A teamwork approach to correct a severe prosthodontic problem, J. Am. Dent. Assoc. **91:**357-359, 1975.

Boitel, R. H.: The parallelometer, a precision instrument for the prosthetic laboratory, J. Prosthet. Dent. **12:**732-736, 1962.

Gaston, G. W.: Rest area preparations for removable partial dentures, J. Prosthet. Dent. **10:**124-134, 1960.

Glann, G. W., and Appleby, R. C.: Mouth preparations for removable partial dentures, J. Prosthet. Dent. **10:**698-706, 1960.

Johnston, J. F.: Preparation of mouths for fixed and removable partial dentures, J. Prosthet. Dent. **11:**456-462, 1961.

Kahn, A. E.: Partial versus full coverage, J. Prosthet. Dent. **10:**167-178, 1960.

Laney, W. R., and Desjardins, R. P.: Comparison of base metal alloys and Type IV gold alloys for removable partial denture framework, Dent. Clin. North Am. **17:**611-630, 1973.

Lorey, R. E.: Abutment considerations, Dent. Clin. North Am. **24:**63-79, 1980.

Marquardt, G. L.: Dolder bar joint mandibular overdenture: a technique for nonparallel abutment teeth, J. Prosthet. Dent. **36:**101-111, 1976.

McArthur, D. R., and Turvey, T. A.: Maxillary segmental osteotomies for mandibular removable partial denture patients, J. Prosthet. Dent. **41:**381-387, 1979.

McCracken, W. L.: Mouth preparations for partial dentures, J. Prosthet. Dent. **6:**39-52, 1956.

Mills, M.: Mouth preparation for removable partial denture, J. Am. Dent. Assoc. **60:**154-159, 1960.

Mopsik, E. R., Buck, R. P., Connors, J. O., and Watts, L. N.: Surgical intervention to reestablish adequate intermaxillary space before fixed or removable prosthodontics, J. Am. Dent. Assoc. **95:**957-960, 1977.

Phillips, R. W.: Report of the Committee on Scientific Investigation of the Academy of Restorative Dentistry, J. Prosthet. Dent. **13:**515-535, 1963.

Schorr, L., and Clayman, L. H.: Reshaping abutment teeth for reception of partial denture clasps, J. Prosthet. Dent. **4:**625-633, 1954.

Sollé, W.: The parallelo-facere: a parallel drilling machine for use in the oral cavity, J. Am. Dent. Assoc. **63:**344-352, 1961.

Stamps, J. T., and Tanquist, R. A.: Restoration of removable partial denture rest seats using dental amalgam, J. Prosthet. Dent. **41:**224-227, 1979.

Stern, W. J.: Guiding planes in clasp reciprocation and retention, J. Prosthet. Dent. **34:**408-414, 1975.

Tucker, K. M., and Heget, H. S.: The incidence of inflammatory papillary hyperplasia, J. Am. Dent. Assoc. **93:**610-613, 1976.

OCCLUSION; JAW RELATION RECORDS; TRANSFER METHODS

Applegate, O. C.: Loss of posterior occlusion, J. Prosthet. Dent. **4:**197-199, 1954.

Baraban, D. J.: Establishing centric relation and vertical dimension in occlusal rehabilitation, J. Prosthet. Dent. **12:**1157-1165, 1962.

Bauman, R.: Minimizing postinsertion problems: a procedure for removable partial denture placement, J. Prosthet. Dent. **42:**381-385, 1979.

Beck, H. O.: A clinical evaluation of the arcon concept of articulation, J. Prosthet. Dent. **9:**409-421, 1959.

Beck, H. O.: Selection of an articulator and jaw registration, J. Prosthet. Dent. **10:**878-886, 1960.

Beck, H. O.: Choosing the articulator, J. Am. Dent. Assoc. **64:**468-475, 1962.

Beckett, L. S.: Accurate occlusal relations in partial denture construction, J. Prosthet. Dent. **4:**487-495, 1954.

Berke, J. D., and Moleres, I.: A removable appliance for the correction of maxillomandibular disproportion, J. Prosthet. Dent. **17:**172-177, 1967.

Berman, M. H.: Accurate interocclusal records, J. Prosthet. Dent. **10:**620-630, 1960.

Beyron, H. L.: Occlusal relationship, Int. Dent. J. **2:**467-496, 1952.

Beyron, H. L.: Characteristics of functionally optimal occlusion and principles of occlusal rehabilitation, J. Am. Dent. Assoc. **48:**648-656, 1954.

Beyron, H. L.: Occlusal changes in adult dentition, J. Am. Dent. Assoc. **48:**674-686, 1954.

Block, L. S.: Preparing and conditioning the patient for intermaxillary relations, J. Prosthet. Dent. **2:**599-603, 1952.

Block, L. S.: Tensions and intermaxillary relations, J. Prosthet. Dent. **4:**204-207, 1954.

Boos, R. H.: Occlusion from rest position, J. Prosthet. Dent. **2:**575-588, 1952.

Boos, R. H.: Basic anatomic factors of jaw position, J. Prosthet. Dent. **4:**200-203, 1954.

Boos, R. H.: Maxillomandibular relations, occlusion, and the temporomandibular joint, Dent. Clin. North Am., pp. 19-35, March, 1962.

Borgh, O., and Posselt, U.: Hinge axis registration: experiments on the articulator, J. Prosthet. Dent. **8:**35-40, 1958.

Boucher, C. O.: Occlusion in prosthodontics, J. Prosthet. Dent. **3:**633-656, 1953.

Braly, B. V.: Occlusal analysis and treatment planning for restorative dentistry, J. Prosthet. Dent. **27:**168-171, 1972.

Cerveris, A. R.: Vibracentric equilibration of centric occlusion, J. Am. Dent. Assoc. **63:**476-483, 1961.

Christensen, P. B.: Accurate casts and positional relation records, J. Prosthet. Dent. **8:**475-482, 1958.

Clayton, J. A., et al.: Pantographic tracings of mandibular movements and occlusion, J. Prosthet. Dent. **25:**389-396, 1971.

Cohn, L. A.: Factors of dental occlusion pertinent to the restorative and prosthetic problem, J. Prosthet. Dent. **9:**256-277, 1959.

Collett, H. A.: Balancing the occlusion of partial dentures, J. Am. Dent. Assoc. **42:**162-168, 1951.

Colman, A. J.: Occlusal requirements for removable partial dentures, J. Prosthet. Dent. **17**:155-162, 1967.

D'Amico, A.: Functional occlusion of the natural teeth of man, J. Prosthet. Dent. **11**:899-915, 1961.

Draper, D. H.: Forward trends in occlusion, J. Prosthet. Dent. **13**:724-731, 1963.

Emmert, J. H.: A method for registering occlusion in semiedentulous mouths, J. Prosthet. Dent. **8**:94-99, 1958.

Fedi, P. F.: Cardinal differences in occlusion of natural teeth and that of artificial teeth, J. Am. Dent. Assoc. **62**:482-485, 1962.

Fountain, H. W.: Seating the condyles for centric relation records, J. Prosthet. Dent. **11**:1050-1058, 1961.

Gilson, T. D.: Theory of centric correction in natural teeth, J. Prosthet. Dent. **8**:468-474, 1958.

Goodfriend, D. J.: New facebow for dentist-laboratory cooperation, J. Am. Dent. Assoc. **68**:866-872, 1964.

Granger, E. R.: The articulator and the patient, Dent. Clin. North Am., pp. 527-539, Nov., 1960.

Hausman, M.: Interceptive and pivotal occlusal contacts, J. Am. Dent. Assoc. **66**:165-171, 1963.

Henderson, D.: Occlusion in removable partial prosthodontics, J. Prosthet. Dent. **27**:151-159, 1971.

Hindels, G. W.: Occlusion in removable partial denture prosthesis, Dent. Clin. North Am., pp. 137-146, March, 1962.

Hughes, G. A., and Regli, C. P.: What is centric relation? J. Prosthet. Dent. **11**:16-22, 1961.

Jaffe, V. N.: The functionally generated path in full denture construction, J. Prosthet. Dent. **4**:214-221, 1954.

Jankelson, B.: Considerations of occlusion on fixed partial dentures, Dent. Clin. North Am., pp. 187-203, March, 1959.

Jeffreys, F. E., and Platner, R. L.: Occlusion in removable partial dentures, J. Prosthet. Dent. **10**:912-920, 1960.

Kapur, K. K.: The comparison of different methods of recording centric relation, 1956, Tufts Univ. Dent. Abstr. **2**:508, 1957.

Lauritzen, A. G., and Bodner, G. H.: Variations in location of arbitrary and true hinge axis points, J. Prosthet. Dent. **11**:224-229, 1961.

Lindblom, G.: Balanced occlusion with partial reconstructions, Int. Dent. J. **1**:84-98, 1951.

Lindblom, G.: The value of bite analysis, J. Am. Dent. Assoc. **48**:657-664, 1954.

Long, J. H., Jr.: Location of the terminal hinge axis by intraoral means, J. Prosthet. Dent. **23**:11-24, 1970.

Lucia, V. O.: Centric relation—theory and practice, J. Prosthet. Dent. **10**:849-956, 1960.

Lucia, V. O.: The gnathological concept of articulation, Dent. Clin. North Am., pp. 183-197, March, 1962.

Lundquist, D. O., and Fiebiger, G. E.: Registration for relating the mandibular cast to the maxillary cast based on Kennedy's classification system, J. Prosthet. Dent. **35**:371-375, 1976.

Mann, A. W., and Pankey, L. D.: The P. M. philosophy of occlusal rehabilitation, Dent. Clin. North Am., pp. 621-636, Nov., 1963.

McCollum, B. B.: The mandibular hinge axis and a method of locating it, J. Prosthet. Dent. **10**:428-435, 1960.

McCracken, W. L.: Functional occlusion in removable partial denture construction, J. Prosthet. Dent. **8**:955-963, 1958.

McCracken, W. L.: Impression materials in prosthetic dentistry, Dent. Clin. North Am., pp. 671-684, Nov., 1958.

McCracken, W. L.: Occlusion in partial denture prosthesis, Dent. Clin. North Am., pp. 109-119, March, 1962.

Mehta, J. D., and Joglekar, A. P.: Vertical jaw relations as a factor in partial dentures, J. Prosthet. Dent. **21**:618-625, 1969.

Meyer, F. S.: The generated path technique in reconstruction dentistry. I and II. J. Prosthet. Dent. **9**:354-366, 432-440, 1959.

Millstein, P. L., et al.: Determination of the accuracy of wax interocclusal registrations, J. Prosthet. Dent. **25**:189-196, 1971.

Moore, A. W.: Ideal versus adequate dental occlusion, J. Am. Dent. Assoc. **55**:51-56, 1957.

Moulton, G. H.: The importance of centric occlusion in diagnosis and treatment planning, J. Prosthet. Dent. **10**:921-926, 1960.

Nuttall, E. B.: Establishing posterior functional occlusion for fixed partial dentures, J. Am. Dent. Assoc. **66**:341-348, 1963.

O'Leary, T. J., et al.: Tooth mobility in cuspid-protected and group-function occlusions, J. Prosthet. Dent. **27**:21-25, 1972.

Olsson, A., and Posselt, U.: Relationship of various skull reference lines, J. Prosthet. Dent. **11**:1045-1049, 1961.

Reitz, P. V.: Technique for mounting removable partial dentures on an articulator, J. Prosthet. Dent. **22**:490-494, 1969.

Reynolds, J. M.: Occlusal wear facets, J. Prosthet. Dent. **24**:367-372, 1970.

Ricketts, R. M.: Occlusion—the medium of dentistry, J. Prosthet. Dent. **21**:39-60, 1969.

Robinson, M. J.: Centric position, J. Prosthet. Dent. **1**:384-386, 1951.

Scaife, R. R., Jr., and Holt, J. E.: Natural occurrence of cuspid guidance, J. Prosthet. Dent. **22**:225-229, 1969.

Scandrett, F. R., and Hanson, J. G.: Technique for attaching the master cast to its split mounting index, J. Prosthet. Dent. **40**:467-469, 1978.

Schireson, S.: Grinding teeth for masticatory efficiency and gingival health, J. Prosthet. Dent. **13**:337-345, 1963.

Schuyler, C. H.: Fundamental principles in the correction of occlusal disharmony—natural and artificial (grinding), J. Am. Dent. Assoc. **22**:1193-1202, 1935.

Schuyler, C. H.: Correction of occlusal disharmony of the natural dentition, N.Y. Dent. J. **13**:445-462, 1947.

Schuyler, C. H.: Factors of occlusion applicable to restorative dentistry, J. Prosthet. Dent. **3**:772-782, 1953.

Schuyler, C. H.: An evaluation of incisal guidance and its influence in restorative dentistry, J. Prosthet. Dent. **9**:374-378, 1959.

Schuyler, C. H.: Factors contributing to traumatic occlusion, J. Prosthet. Dent. **11**:708-715, 1961.

Sears, V. H.: Occlusion: the common meeting ground in dentistry, J. Prosthet. Dent. **2**:15-21, 1952.

Sears, V. H.: Occlusal pivots, J. Prosthet. Dent. **6**:332-338, 1956.

Sears, V. H.: Centric and eccentric occlusions, J. Prosthet. Dent. **10**:1029-1036, 1960.

Sears, V. H.: Mandibular equilibration, J. Am. Dent. Assoc. **65**:45-55, 1962.

Shanahan, T. E. J., and Leff, A.: Interocclusal records, J. Prosthet. Dent. 10:842-848, 1960.

Silverman, M. M.: Determination of vertical dimension by phonetics, J. Prosthet. Dent. 6:465-471, 1956; Dent. Abstr. 2:221, 1957.

Skurnik, H.: Accurate interocclusal records, J. Prosthet. Dent. 21:154-165, 1969.

Stuart, C. E.: Accuracy in measuring functional dimensions and relations in oral prosthesis, J. Prosthet. Dent. 9:220-236, 1959.

Teteruck, W. R., and Lundeen, H. C.: The accuracy of an ear face-bow, J. Prosthet. Dent. 16:1039-1046, 1966.

Wagner, A. G.: A technique to record jaw relations for distally edentulous dental arches, J. Prosthet. Dent. 29:405-407, 1973.

Weinberg, L. A.: The transverse hinge axis: real or imaginary, J. Prosthet. Dent. 9:775-787, 1959.

Weinberg, L. A.: An evaluation of the face-bow mounting, J. Prosthet. Dent. 11:32-42, 1961.

Weinberg, L. A.: Arcon principle in the condylar mechanism of adjustable articulators, J. Prosthet. Dent. 13:263-268, 1963.

Weinberg, L. A.: An evaluation of basic articulators and their concepts. I and II. J. Prosthet. Dent. 13:622-663, 1963.

Wilson, J. H.: The use of partial dentures in the restoration of occlusal standards, Aust. Dent. J. 1:93-101, 1956.

PARTIAL DENTURE DESIGN

Antos, E. W., Jr., Tenner, R. P., and Foerth, D.: The swing-lock partial denture: an alternative approach to conventional removable partial denture service, J. Prosthet. Dent. 40:257-262, 1978.

Askinas, S. W.: Facings in removable partial dentures, J. Prosthet. Dent. 33:633-636, 1975.

Avant, E. W.: Indirect retention in partial denture design, J. Prosthet. Dent. 16:1103-1110, 1966.

Axinn, S., O'Connor, R. P., Jr., and Kopp, E. N.: Immediate removable partial denture frameworks, J. Am. Dent. Assoc. 95:583-585, 1977.

Berg, T., Jr.: I-Bar: myth and countermyth, Dent. Clin. North Am. 23:65-75, 1979.

Berg, T., Jr., and Caputo, A. A.: Anterior rests for maxillary removable partial dentures, J. Prosthet. Dent. 39:139-146, 1978.

Blatterfein, L.: A systematic method of designing upper partial denture bases, J. Am. Dent. Assoc. 46:510-525, 1953.

Blatterfein, L.: The use of the semiprecision rest in removable partial dentures, J. Prosthet. Dent. 22:301-306, 1969.

Bolouri, A.: Removable partial denture design for a few remaining natural teeth, J. Prosthet. Dent. 39:346-348, 1978.

Campbell, L. D.: Subjective reactions to major connector designs for removable partial dentures, J. Prosthet. Dent. 36:507-516, 1977.

Casey, D. M., and Lauciello, F. R.: A method for marking the functional depth of the floor of the mouth, J. Prosthet. Dent. 43:108-111, 1980.

Cecconi, B. T.: Lingual bar design, J. Prosthet. Dent. 29:635-639, 1973.

Chick, A. O.: Correct location of clasps and rests on dentures without stress-breakers, Br. Dent. J. 95:303-309, 1953.

Collett, H. A.: Biologic approach to clasp partial dentures, Dent. Dig. 61:309-313, 1955.

Demer, W. J.: An analysis of mesial rest-I-bar clasps designs, J. Prosthet. Dent. 36:243-253, 1976.

Dunny, J. A., and King, G. E.: Minor connector designs for anterior acrylic resin bases: a preliminary study, J. Prosthet. Dent. 34:496-497, 1975.

Firtell, D. N.: Effect of clasp design upon retention of removable partial dentures, J. Prosthet. Dent. 20:43-52, 1968.

Firtell, D. N., Herzberg, T. W., and Walsh, J. F.: Root retention and removable partial denture design, J. Prosthet. Dent. 42:131-134, 1979.

Fisher, R. L., and Jaslow, C.: The efficiency of an indirect retainer, J. Prosthet. Dent. 33:24-30, 1975.

Frank, R. P.: An investigation of the effectiveness of indirect retainers, J. Prosthet. Dent. 38:494-506, 1977.

Frantz, W. R.: Variations in a removable maxillary partial denture design by dentists, J. Prosthet. Dent. 34:625-633, 1975.

Frechette, A. R.: Partial denture planning with special reference to stress distribution, J. Ont. Dent. Assoc. 30:318-329, 1953.

Giradot, R. L.: History and development of partial denture design, J. Am. Dent. Assoc. 28:1399-1408, 1941.

Henderson, D.: Major connectors for mandibular removable partial dentures, J. Prosthet. Dent. 30:532-548, 1973.

Henderson, D.: Major connectors—united it stands, Dent. Clin. North Am. 17:661-668, 1973.

Jordan, L. G.: Designing removable partial dentures with external attachments (clasps), J. Prosthet. Dent. 2:716-722, 1952.

Kelly, E. K.: The physiologic approach to partial denture design, J. Prosthet. Dent. 3:699-710, 1953.

King, G. E.: Dual-path design for removable partial dentures, J. Prosthet. Dent. 39:392-395, 1978.

King, G. E., Barco, M. T., and Olson, R. J.: Inconspicuous retention for removable partial dentures, J. Prosthet. Dent. 39:505-507, 1978.

Knodle, J. M.: Experimental overlay and pin partial denture, J. Prosthet. Dent. 17:472-478, 1967.

Krikos, A. A.: Preparing guide planes for removable partial dentures, J. Prosthet. Dent. 34:152-155, 1975.

Krikos, A. A.: Artificial undercuts for teeth which have unfavorable shapes for clasping, J. Prosthet. Dent. 22:301-306, 1969.

LaVere, A. M., and Freda, A. L.: A simplified procedure for survey and design of diagnostic casts, J. Prosthet. Dent. 37:680-683, 1977.

LaVere, A. M., and Krol, A. J.: Selection of a major connector for the extension base removable partial denture, J. Prosthet. Dent. 30:102-105, 1973.

Lorencki, S. F.: Planning precision attachment restorations, J. Prosthet. Dent. 21:506-508, 1969.

MacKinnon, K. P.: Indirect retention in partial denture construction, Dent. J. Aust. 27:221-225, 1955.

Maxfield, J. B., Nicholls, J. E., and Smith, D. E.: The measurement of forces transmitted to abutment teeth of removable partial dentures, J. Prosthet. Dent. 41:134-142, 1979.

McCartney, J. W.: Lingual plating for reciprocation, J. Prosthet. Dent. 42:624-625, 1979.

McCracken, W. L.: Contemporary partial denture designs, J. Prosthet. Dent. 8:71-84, 1958.

McCracken, W. L.: Survey of partial denture designs by commercial dental laboratories, J. Prosthet. Dent. 12:1089-1110, 1962.

Moore, D. S.: Some fundamentals of partial denture design to conserve the supporting structures, J. Ont. Dent. Assoc. **32**:238-240, 1955.

Nairn, R. I.: The problem of free-end denture bases, J. Prosthet. Dent. **16**:522-532, 1966.

Perry, C.: Philosophy of partial denture design, J. Prosthet. Dent. **6**:775-784, 1956.

Pipko, D. J.: Combinations in fixed-removable prostheses, J. Prosthet. Dent. **26**:481-490, 1971.

Potter, R. B., Appleby, R. C., and Adams, C. D.: Removable partial denture design: a review and a challenge, J. Prosthet. Dent. **17**:63-68, 1967.

Ryan, J.: Technique of design in partial denture construction, J. Dent. Assoc. S. Afr. **9**:123-133, 1954.

Rybeck, S. A., Jr.: Simplicity in a distal extension partial denture, J. Prosthet. Dent. **4**:87-92, 1954.

Schmidt, A. H.: Planning and designing removable partial dentures, J. Prosthet. Dent. **3**:783-806, 1953.

Schuyler, C. H.: The partial denture as a means of stabilizing abutment teeth, J. Am. Dent. Assoc. **28**:1121-1125, 1941.

Scott, D. C.: Suggested designs for metal partial dentures, Dent. Tech. **2**:21, 26, 1954.

Shohet, H.: Relative magnitudes of stress on abutment teeth with different retainers, J. Prosthet. Dent. **21**:267-282, 1969.

Steffel, V. L.: Simplified clasp partial dentures designed for maximum function, J. Am. Dent. Assoc. **32**:1093-1100, 1945.

Steffel, V. L.: Fundamental principles involved in partial denture design, J. Am. Dent. Assoc. **42**:534-544, 1951.

Steffel, V. L.: Fundamental principles involved in partial denture designs—with special reference to equalization of tooth and tissue support, Aust. J. Dent. **54**:328-333, 1950; Dent. J. Aust. **23**:68-77, 1951.

Sykora, O., and Calikkocaoglu, S.: Maxillary removable partial denture designs by commercial dental laboratories, J. Prosthet. Dent. **22**:633-640, 1970.

Thompson, W. D., Kratochvil, F. J., and Caputo, A. A.: Evaluation of photoelastic stress patterns produced by various designs of bilateral distal-extension removable partial dentures, J. Prosthet. Dent. **38**:261-273, 1977.

Tsao, D. H.: Designing occlusal rests using mathematical principles, J. Prosthet. Dent. **23**:154-163, 1970.

Waller, N. I.: The root rest and the removable partial denture, J. Prosthet. Dent. **33**:16-23, 1975.

Warren, A. B., and Caputo, A. A.: Load transfer to alveolar bone as influenced by abutment design for tooth-supported dentures, J. Prosthet. Dent. **33**:137-148, 1975.

Weinberg, L. A.: Lateral force in relation to the denture base and clasp design, J. Prosthet. Dent. **6**:785-800, 1956.

Zach, G. A.: Advantages of mesial rests for removable partial dentures, J. Prosthet. Dent. **33**:32-35, 1975.

PERIODONTAL CONSIDERATIONS

Amsterdam, M., and Fox, L.: Provisional splinting—principles and technics, Dent. Clin. North Am., pp. 73-99, March, 1959.

App, G. R.: Periodontal treatment for the removable partial prosthesis patient. Another half century? Dent. Clin. North Am. **17**:601-610, 1973.

Applegate, O. C.: The interdependence of periodontics and removable partial denture prosthesis, J. Prosthet. Dent. **8**:269-281, 1958.

Bates, J. F., and Addy, M.: Partial dentures and plaque accumulation, J. Dent. **6**:285-293, 1978.

Brill, N., et al.: Ecologic changes in the oral cavity caused by removable partial dentures, J. Prosthet. Dent. **38**:138-148, 1977.

Clarke, N. G.: Treatment planning for fixed and removable partial dentures: a periodontal view, J. Prosthet. Dent. **36**:44-50, 1976.

Gilson, C. M.: Periodontal considerations, Dent. Clin. North Am. **24**:31-44, 1980.

Ivancie, G. P.: Interrelationship between restorative dentistry and periodontics, J. Prosthet. Dent. **8**:819-830, 1958.

Jordan, L. G.: Treatment of advanced periodontal disease by prosthodontic procedures, J. Prosthet. Dent. **10**:908-911, 1960.

Kimball, H. D.: The role of periodontia in prosthetic dentistry, J. Prosthet. Dent. **1**:286-294, 1951.

Krogh-Poulsen, W.: Partial denture design in relation to occlusal trauma in periodontal breakdown, Int. Dent. J. **4**:847-867, 1954; also Acad. Rev. **3**:18-23, 1955.

McCall, J. O.: The periodontal element in prosthodontics, J. Prosthet. Dent. **16**:585-588, 1966.

McKenzie, J. S.: Mutual problems of the periodontist and prosthodontist, J. Prosthet. Dent. **5**:37-42, 1955.

Morris, M. L.: Artificial crown contours and gingival health, J. Prosthet. Dent. **12**:1146-1155, 1962.

Nevin, R. B.: Periodontal aspects of partial denture prosthesis, J. Prosthet. Dent. **5**:215-219, 1955.

Orban, B. S.: Biologic principles in correction of occlusal disharmonies, J. Prosthet. Dent. **6**:637-641, 1956.

Overby, G. E.: Esthetic splinting of mobile periodontally involved teeth by vertical pinning, J. Prosthet. Dent. **11**:112-118, 1961.

Perel, M. L.: Periodontal consideration of crown contours, J. Prosthet. Dent. **26**:627-630, 1971.

Picton, D. C. A., and Wills, D. J.: Viscoelastic properties of the periodontal ligament and mucous membrane, J. Prosthet. Dent. **40**:263-272, 1978.

Rissin, L., et al.: Effect of age and removable partial dentures on gingivitis and periodontal disease, J. Prosthet. Dent. **42**:217-223, 1979.

Rudd, K. D., and O'Leary, T. J.: Stabilizing periodontally weakened teeth by using guide plane removable partial dentures: a preliminary report, J. Prosthet. Dent. **16**:721-727, 1966.

Schuyler, C. H.: The partial denture and a means of stabilizing abutment teeth, J. Am. Dent. Assoc. **28**:1121-1125, 1941.

Schwalm, C. A., Smith, D. E., and Erickson, J. D.: A clinical study of patients 1 to 2 years after placement of removable partial dentures, J. Prosthet. Dent. **38**:380-391, 1977.

Sternlicht, H. C.: Prosthetic treatment planning for the periodontal patient, Dent. Abstr. **2**:81-82, 1957.

Stipho, H. D. K., Murphy, W. M., and Adams, D.: Effect of oral prostheses on plaque accumulation, Br. Dent. J. **145**:47-50, 1978.

Talkov, L.: Survey for complete periodontal prosthesis, J. Prosthet. Dent. **11**:124-131, 1961.

Tebrock, O. C., et al.: The effect of various clasping systems on the mobility of abutment teeth for distal-extension removable partial dentures, J. Prosthet. Dent. **41**:511-516, 1979.

Thomas, B. O. A., and Gallager, J. W.: Practical management of occlusal dysfunctions in periodontal therapy, J. Am. Dent. Assoc. **46**:18-31, 1953.

Trapozzano, V. R., and Winter, G. R.: Periodontal aspects of partial denture design, J. Prosthet. Dent. **2:** 101-107, 1952.

Waerhaug, J.: Justification for splinting in periodontal therapy, J. Prosthet. Dent. **22:**201-208, 1969.

Ward, H. L., and Weinberg, L. A.: An evaluation of periodontal splinting, J. Am. Dent. Assoc. **63:**48-54, 1961.

White, J. T.: Abutment stress in overdenture, J. Prosthet. Dent. **40:**13-17, 1978.

PHYSIOLOGY; MANDIBULAR MOVEMENT

Brekke, C. A.: Jaw function. I. Hinge rotation, J. Prosthet. Dent. **9:**600-606, 1959. II. Hinge axis, hinge axes, **9:**936-940, 1959. III. Condylar placement and condylar retrusion, **10:**78-85, 1960.

Brotman, D. N.: Contemporary concepts of articulation, J. Prosthet. Dent. **10:**221-230, 1960.

Emig, G. E.: The physiology of the muscles of mastication, J. Prosthet. Dent. **1:**700-707, 1951.

Fountain, H. W.: The temporomandibular joints—a fulcrum, J. Prosthet. Dent. **25:**78-84, 1971.

Gibbs, C. H., et al.: Functional movements of the mandible, J. Prosthet. Dent. **26:**604-620, 1971.

Jankelson, B.: Physiology of human dental occlusion, J. Am. Dent. Assoc. **50:**664-680, 1955.

Kurth, L. E.: Mandibular movement and articulator occlusion, J. Am. Dent. Assoc. **39:**37-46, 1949.

Kurth, L. E.: Centric relation and mandibular movement, J. Am. Dent. Assoc. **50:**309-315, 1955.

McMillen, L. B.: Border movements of the human mandible, J. Prosthet. Dent. **27:**524-532, 1972.

Messerman, T.: A concept of jaw function with a related clinical application, J. Prosthet. Dent. **13:**130-140, 1963.

Naylor, J. G.: Role of the external pterygoid muscles in temporomandibular articulation, J. Prosthet. Dent. **10:**1037-1042, 1960.

Plotnick, I. J., Beresin, V. E., and Simkins, A. B.: The effects of variations in the opposing dentition on changes in the partially edentulous mandible. I. Bone changes observed in serial radiographs, J. Prosthet. Dent. **33:**278-286, 1975.

Plotnick, I. J., Beresin, V., and Simkins, A. B.: The effects of variations in the opposing dentition on changes in the partially edentulous mandible. III. Tooth mobility and chewing efficiency with various maxillary dentitions, J. Prosthet. Dent. **33:**529-534, 1975.

Posselt, U.: Studies in the mobility of the human mandible, Acta Odontol. Scand. **10**(supp. 10):19-160, 1952.

Posselt, U.: Movement areas of the mandible, J. Prosthet. Dent. **7:**375-385, 1957.

Posselt, U.: Terminal hinge movement of the mandible, J. Prosthet. Dent. **7:**787-797, 1957.

Saizar, P.: Centric relation and condylar movement, J. Prosthet. Dent. **26:**581-591, 1971.

Schweitzer, J. M.: Masticatory function in man, J. Prosthet. Dent. **11:**625-647, 1961.

Shanahan, T. E. J.: Dental physiology for dentures: the direct application of the masticatory cycle to denture occlusion, J. Prosthet. Dent. **2:**3, 1952.

Shore, N. A.: Educational program for patients with temporomandibular joint dysfunction (ligaments), J. Prosthet. Dent. **23:**691-695, 1970.

Sicher, H.: Positions and movements of the mandible, J. Am. Dent. Assoc. **48:**620-625, 1954.

Skinner, C. N.: Physiology of the occlusal coordination of natural teeth, complete dentures, and partial dentures, J. Prosthet. Dent. **17:**559-565, 1967.

Söstenbö, H. R.: C. E. Luce's recordings of mandibular movement, J. Prosthet. Dent. **11:**1068-1073, 1961.

Ulrich, J.: The human temporomandibular joint: kinematics and actions of the masticatory muscles, J. Prosthet. Dent. **9:**399-406, 1959.

Vaughan, H. C.: The external pterygoid mechanism, J. Prosthet. Dent. **5:**80-92, 1955.

REBASING AND RELINING

Beckett, L. S.: Partial denture. The rebasing of tissue borne saddles; theory and practice, Aust. Dent. J. **16:** 340-346, 1971.

Blatterfein, L.: Rebasing procedures for removable partial dentures, J. Prosthet. Dent. **8:**441-467, 1958.

Steffel, V. L.: Relining removable partial dentures for fit and function, J. Prosthet. Dent. **4:**496-509, 1954.

Wilson, J. H.: Partial dentures—rebasing the saddle supported by the mucosa and alveolar bone, Dent. J. Aust. **24:**185-188, 1952.

Wilson, J. H.: Partial dentures—relining the saddle supported by the mucosa and alveolar bone, J. Prosthet. Dent. **3:**807-813, 1953.

STRESSBREAKER DESIGNS

Bartlett, A. A.: Duplication of precision attachment partial dentures, J. Prosthet. Dent. **16:**1111-1115, 1966.

Bickley, R. W.: Combined splint-stress breaker removable partial denture, J. Prosthet. Dent. **21:**509, 512, 1969.

Cecconi, B. T., Kaiser, G., and Rahe, A.: Stress-breakers and the removable partial denture, J. Prosthet. Dent. **34:**145-151, 1975.

Hirschtritt, E.: Removable partial dentures with stress-broken extension bases, J. Prosthet. Dent. **7:**318-324, 1957.

James, A. G.: Stress breakers which automatically return the saddle to rest position following displacement. Mandibular distal extension partial dentures, J. Prosthet. Dent. **4:**73-81, 1954.

Kabcenell, J. L.: Stress breaking for partial dentures, J. Am. Dent. Assoc. **63:**593-602, 1961.

Kane, B. E.: Buoyant stress equalizer, J. Prosthet. Dent. **14:**698-704, 1964.

Kane, B. E.: Improved buoyant stress equalizer, J. Prosthet. Dent. **17:**365-371, 1967.

Levin, B.: Stressbreakers: a practical approach, Dent. Clin. North Am. **23:**77-86, 1979.

Levitch, H. C.: Physiologic stress-equalizer, J. Prosthet. Dent. **3:**232-238, 1953.

Marris, F. N.: The precision dowel rest attachment, J. Prosthet. Dent. **5:**43-48, 1955.

Neill, D. J.: The problem of the lower free-end removable partial denture, J. Prosthet. Dent. **8:**623-634, 1958.

Parker, H. M.: Impact reduction in complete and partial dentures, a pilot study, J. Prosthet. Dent. **16:**227-245, 1966.

Plotnik, I. J.: Stress regulator for complete and partial dentures, J. Prosthet. Dent. **17:**166-171, 1967.

Simpson, D. H.: Considerations for abutments, J. Prosthet. Dent. **5:**375-384, 1955.

Terrell, W. H.: Split bar technic applicable to both precision attachment and clasp cases, J. South. Calif. Dent. Assoc. **9:**10-14, 1942.

SURVEYING

Applegate, O. C.: USe of paralleling surveyor in modern partial denture construction, J. Am. Dent. Assoc. **27**:1317-1407, 1940.

Atkinson, H. F.: Partial denture problems: surveyors and surveying, Aust. J. Dent. **59**:28-31, 1955.

Chestner, S. G.: A methodical approach to the analysis of study cases, J. Prosthet. Dent. **4**:622-624, 1954.

Hanson, J. G.: Surveying, J. Am. Dent. Assoc. **91**:826-828, 1975.

Katulski, E. M., and Appleyard, W. N.: Biological concepts of the use of the mechanical cast surveyor, J. Prosthet. Dent. **9**:629-634, 1959.

Knapp, J. G., Shotwell, J. L., and Kotowicz, W. E.: Technique for recording dental cast–surveyor relations, J. Prosthet. Dent. **41**:352-354, 1979.

Sollé, W.: An improved dental surveyor, J. Am. Dent. Assoc. **60**:727-731, 1960.

Wagner, A. G., and Forque, E. G.: A study of four methods of recording the path of insertion of removable partial dentures, J. Prosthet. Dent. **35**:267-272, 1976.

Yilmaz, G.: Optical surveying of casts for removable partial dentures, J. Prosthet. Dent. **34**:292-296, 1975.

WORK AUTHORIZATIONS

Brown, E. T.: The dentist, the laboratory technician, and the prescription law, J. Prosthet. Dent. **15**:1132-1138, 1965.

Dutton, D. A.: Standard abbreviations (and definitions) for use in dental laboratory work authorizations, J. Prosthet. Dent. **27**:94-95, 1972.

Gehl, D. H.: Investment in the future, J. Prosthet. Dent. **18**:190-201, 1968.

Henderson, D.: Writing work authorizations for removable partial dentures, J. Prosthet. Dent. **16**:696-707, 1966.

Henderson, D., and Frazier, Q.: Communicating with dental laboratory technicians, Dent. Clin. North Am., pp. 603-615, July, 1970.

Leeper, S. H.: Dentist and laboratory: a "love-hate" relationship, Dent. Clin. North Am. **23**:87-99, 1979.

Quinn, I.: Status of the dental laboratory work authorization, J. Am. Dent. Assoc. **79**:1189-1190, 1969.

Travaglini, E. A., and Jannetto, L. B.: A work authorization format for removable partial dentures, J. Am. Dent. Assoc. **96**:429-431, 1978.

INDEX

A

Abutment teeth
  alveolar support for, 132, 175
  axial surface of, in design of minor connector, 35
  bone quality around, 175-178
  caries in, 228
  classification of, 231-232
  in cleft palate prostheses, 430
  consideration of, in choosing fixed vs removable partial denture, 198
  definition of, 3
  disking of, 229, 232
    use of surveyor for, 148
  effect of minor connector on, 34
  effect of occlusal rests on, 46
  effect of rigid denture design on, 118
  effect of treatment partial denture on, 421
  for fixed partial dentures, 195
  height of contour of, 3, 9
    lowering of, 232
    with respect to path of placement, 65
    survey of, 148-150, 159
  influence of, on clasp design, 72-73
  isolated, use of, 243-244
  lamina dura of, 178
  loss of, repair of denture with, 414
  multiple support from, 242
  occlusal or vertical forces on, 97, 122
  overlay, 139-141
  periodontal disease to, 405
  placement of clasp arms along, 73
  posterior, rotation of distal extension partial denture through, 49-51
  preparation of, for partial denture, 227-229, 231-254
    sequence of, 232-233
    using cast crowns, 236-241
    using cast inlays, 233
    using veneer crowns, 241-242
  protection of, 231
  reduction of excessive contours of, 232
  rest seats of, 228-229
    outline form of, 44-46
  restoration of, 194, 227-229
    contouring wax patterns for, 228
    including rest seats in, 228-229
    full cast gold crowns, 228
    inlay, gold, 228
    veneer crowns, 228
  retentive areas of, survey of, 155

Abutment teeth—cont'd
  roentgenographic interpretation of, 178
  root morphology of, 178
  with sound enamel, 321
  splinting of, 242-243
  stressbreaker between, and denture base, 113
  as support for partial denture, 136
  suprabulge and infrabulge of, 65
  surveying of, in treatment planning, 172
  torque to, 53, 128, 175-176
  transfer of stress to
    in distal extension partial denture, 44, 46, 175-176
    through rests, 44
    in tooth-supported partial dentures, 44, 175
  vulnerable areas of, 228, 233
Acrylic resin; *see* Resin, acrylic
Adaptol impression materials, 257
Adhesion, 62
Adjustments to partial denture, 395-405
  occlusal
    for distal extension partial denture, 397
    prior to denture fabrication, 299
    for tooth-borne partial denture, 397, 400
Agar hydrocolloid, 258, 259; *see also* Hydrocolloid, reversible
  differences between, and alginate hydrocolloid, 260
  disadvantages of, 260
  immersion of, in potassium sulfate, 260
Alginate hydrocolloid, 258, 269; *see also* Hydrocolloid, irreversible
  chemistry of, 260
  differences between, and agar hydrocolloid, 260
  disadvantages of, 260-261
  for impressions
    for cleft palate prostheses, 429-430
    for crowns, inlays to fit existing partial dentures, 250
    for diagnostic casts, 179
    functional, 279
    for making temporary crowns, 246, 247, 248
    for partial denture fabrication, 127
    trays for, 362
Alloys, metal
  chromium-cobalt; *see* Chromium-cobalt alloys
  gold; *see* Gold alloys
  for partial denture framework, factors in selecting, 200-207
  stellite, 201, 325

Aluminum crowns, 245, 248
  cementation of, 249
Alveolar bone, 120
  condensation of, 176, 177
  consideration of, in treatment planning, 176
  consideration of, in tooth extraction, 195
  height of, 176
  quality of, 176
  stress on, 176, 177
  trabecular pattern of, 176
Amalgam
  overhang margins of, 220
  as restoration for abutment teeth, 228
  in support of occlusal rests, 53, 232
Anatomic replica, 3
  patterns for, 349-351
    materials for, 350
    procedure, 350-351
Angle of cervical convergence, 65
  effect of, on placement of clasp arm, 67
  in establishing retention for partial denture, 152
  observation of, 155
Applegate's rules for applying Kennedy classification,
    16-17
Appliance, 2
Arches, partially edentulous
  classification of, 13-17
    Kennedy's, 13-16
      Applegate's rules for applying, 16-17
      in design of maxillary major connectors, 30
    requirements for method of, 13
Arcon articulator, 181
Articulating paper, 397, 400
  in guiding arrangement of teeth to occluding tem-
    plate, 312
Articulation ribbon, 397, 400
Articulator, 371
  arcon, 181
  definition of, 181
  Dentatus, 181, 182, 190, 300
  Gysi, 181
  Hanau, 181, 182, 190, 300, 303
  hinge, 320-321
  limitations of, 299
  non-arcon, 181
  occlusal and jaw relation records in programming, 11
  for establishing occlusion on relined partial denture,
    409-410
  semiadjustable, 299, 303
  in simulation of jaw movement, 299
  Whip-Mix, 300
Artificial teeth
  adding to occlusal surfaces of, 408
  anterior, types of, 375-376
  arrangement of, 197
    to occluding template, 311-316
  attachment of, to metal bases, 109-111
  effect of, on occlusal load applied to denture, 280
  loss of, from partial denture, 414
  maxillary, placement of, in relation to ridge, 299, 300
  metal, 111

Artificial teeth—cont'd
  plastic; *see* Resin teeth
  porcelain
    for anterior spaces, 376
    attachment of, to metal bases, 109-111
    and facings cemented to metal bases, 110
    as posterior teeth, 373
    reshaping of occlusal surfaces of, 383
    against resin teeth, 309-311
    vs resin teeth, 309, 310, 311
    in waxing metal bases, consideration of, 346
  posterior
    arrangement of, 300, 372-375
      procedure, 374-375
    materials for, 309-311
    tooth forms of, 372
  reshaping of, after occlusal adjustment, 401-402
  resin
    abrasive surface of, 311
    for anterior spaces, 376
    attachment of, to metal bases, 109-111, 348
    and facings cemented to metal base, 110
    with gold occlusal surfaces, 309, 311, 373
    modification of, 311
    against porcelain teeth, 309-311
    vs porcelain teeth, 309-311
    for posterior teeth, 373
    pressing on, 110
    processed directly to metal base, 111
    reestablishment of occlusion in reline of, 409-
      410
    reshaping of occlusal surfaces of, 383, 384
Asbestos, 355
  in impression trays, 362
  purpose of, in casting, 354
ASC 52 attachment, 114
Atlas, 426
Atmospheric pressure in retention of denture base,
    62
Attachments
  ASC 52, 114
  Baker, 63
  Brown, 63
  C&M, 114
  Crismani, 114
  Dalbo, 114
  dowel rest, 91-95
  frictional, 3
  Hart-Dunn, 87-89
  internal, 3, 6, 63, 86
    disadvantages of, 64
    with distal extension partial denture, 93
    vs extracoronal attachment, 63
    vs internal rest, 49, 151
    limitations in use of, 64
    principle of, 63
    surveyor for placement of, 150
  internal clip, 139
  intracoronal, 222
  Neurohr spring-lock, 89-91
  Ney-Chayes, 63

Attachments—cont'd
  precision, 3
    vs internal occlusal rest, 49
    as intracoronal retainer, 63
  Stern-Goldsmith, 63
  Williams, 63
Austenal Micro Analyzer, 159

B

Back-action clasp, 77
Baker attachment, 63
Balanced occlusion, 5, 220, 298
Balancing contacts, 221, 300
Ball-and-socket stressbreakers, 114
Bar, palatal, 3
Bar clasp, 71, 127
  vs circumferential clasp, 74
  in Class II partial denture, 131
  in Class III partial denture, 128
  in combination clasp, 83
  contraindications for use of, 83
  definition of, 3
  depth of undercut for, 68
  for distal extension partial denture, 127, 132
  to eliminate interference in path of placement, 156
  with embrasure clasp, 79
  esthetics of, 157
  flexibility of, 68
  I, 81
  indications for use of, 81-83
  in infrabulge clasp, 86
  length of, 68
  T, 81
  for tooth-borne partial denture, 127, 134
  waxing of, 336, 344, 345
  Y, 81
Bar retainer, continuous, 3
Base, denture; *see* Denture base
Baseplate wax, 161
  in fabrication of acrylic temporary crowns, 246, 247
  for occlusion rims, 367
  as spacer in tray construction, 267, 269
Bennett movement, 299
Bite plane, acrylic resin, 421
Blockout
  arbitrary, 164, 165
  consideration of, in duplicating stone cast, 328
  duplicate casts for, 325
  of ledges, 161
  for malaligned teeth, 169
  on master cast, 161-162
    for major connectors, 39-41
      anterior-posterior strap palatal, 41
      full palatal coverage, 41
      lingual bar, 39
      linguoplate, 40
      single broad palatal, 40
      single strap palatal, 40
  material for, 161
  paralleling, 161, 162, 164, 165

Blockout—cont'd
  in preparation of retentive framework for resin base, 106-107
  vs relief, 162, 165
  shaped, 161, 164, 165
Blowtorch, 359
Boilout, 380
Bone, alveolar, 120
  condensation of, 176, 177
  consideration of, in extractions, 194
  consideration of, in treatment planning, 176
  height of, 176
  quality of, 176
  stress on, 176, 177
  trabecular pattern of, 176
Borax-type flux, 206, 416
Border molding
  with metallic oxide paste, 256
  with modeling plastic, 256-257
  with rubber base, 259
Brown attachment, 63
Buccal shelf, 10, 275
Buccinator muscle, 214
Burnout, 357-359
  for framework casting, 359
  purpose of, 357
  temperature for, 359
Button of casting, 327

C

C & M attachment, 114
Calcium alginate, 260
Calcium sulfate, 260
  in soaking stone casts, 329
Calculus, 218, 220
Canine, 4
  extensions on, from occlusal rests, 101-102
  incisal rests on, 58, 102
  indirect retention on, 100, 102, 137
  lingual rests on, 56-58
  with premolar, splinting of, 243
Canine guidance, 304
Cantilever, 122, 196
  retention arms as, 206
Caries, 168, 193, 198
Cast
  altered, technique for, 258
  apposition of, direct, as occlusal relationship, 301
  arranging artificial teeth to, 372-375
  definition of, 4
  diagnostic; *see* Diagnostic cast
  duplicating, 325-333, 334, 336
    materials and flasks for, 326-328
    procedure, 328-333
    purpose of, 325
  from hydrocolloid impression, making, 262, 263
    inaccuracies in, 263-264
    pouring of, 270-271
  investment
    abrasion of, 325, 326
    for anatomic replica pattern, 351

Cast—cont'd
  investment—cont'd
    preparation of, 325
    purpose of, 325
    spraying of, with plastic model spray, 333
    trimming of, 333
    for waxing framework, 334, 336
  master; *see* Master cast
  for maxillofacial prosthesis, 436
  metal, 248
  mounting of, 181
    centric relation in, 190-192
    jaw relation records for, 185-190
    with respect to axis-orbital plane, 181-185
  from plaster of Paris impression, 259
  recording relation of, to surveyor, 158
  refractory, 4, 336
  remounting, 384, 409
  from rubber base impression, 258
  split stone, 383
  tripoding of, 158
  for waxing framework, 334
  working, for fabrication of abutment restorations, 265-266
Casting, 4
  button of, 327
  cooling of, 359
  electropolished, 359
  factors influencing excellence of, 351-352
  faulty, due to gas entrapment, 352
  pickling of, 360
  porosity of, 327, 352
  removal of, from investment, 359
  shrinkage of, 352, 355
Casting machine, 359
Casting rings, 356-357
Cement
  effect of, on gingiva, 249
  semipermanent, 253
  temporary, 252-253
  zinc oxide and eugenol, 252-253
Cementum, 220
Central bearing devices, intraoral, 303, 322, 369
Centric occlusion, 300
  adjustments into, occlusal, 220, 221, 401
  coinciding with centric relation, 300
  vs centric relation, 185, 189
  correction of, intraorally, 382
  definition of, 2
  for fixed restorations, 316
  mounting diagnostic casts in, 189
  in partial denture fabrication, 299
Centric relation, 300-301
  vs centric occlusion, 185
  definition of, 2, 189
  mounting diagnostic casts in, 189
  in occlusal adjustments, 220, 221
  in partial denture fabrication, 11, 299
  recording of
    materials for, 190
    methods for, 190-192

Centric relation—cont'd
  recording of—cont'd
    with occlusion rims, 303
    in wax, 301-302
  verification of, 189
Cerrosafe metal, 266
Chromium-cobalt alloys
  casting shrinkage of, 355
  density of, 201
  flexibility of, 201
  vs gold alloy, 200
  hardness of, 201
  heat hardening of, 361
  investment for, 355
  modulus of elasticity of, 200-201
  for partial denture framework, 200
  solder for, 416
  soldering of, 206
  for splint bars, 138
  in stressbreaker fabrication, 114
  work hardening of, 201
  wrought-wire retainer arms of, 202
  yield strength of, 200
Circumferential clasp, 74-81
  adjustments of, 71
  basic form of, 74
  vs bar clasp, 74
  in Class II partial denture, 131
  in Class III partial denture, 128
  in combination clasp, 83
  cross sectional form of, 69
  definition of, 3
  depth of undercut for, 68
  for distal extension partial denture, 127, 128, 132
  disadvantages of, 74
  esthetics of, 157
  flexibility of, 68
  indications for use of, 74
  interference to, 156
  in interim partial dentures, 418
  length of, 67
  lowering height of contour for, 232
  modifications of, into
    back-action clasp, 77
    embrasure clasp, 77-79
    half-and-half clasp, 79-80
    multiple clasp, 79
    reverse-action or hairpin clasp, 80-81
    ring-type clasp, 75-77
  shape of, 128
  for tooth-borne partial denture, 134
  waxing of, 336
Clasps, 3
  back-action, 77
  bar; *see* Bar clasp
  combination, 83-85, 128
  circumferential; *see* Circumferential clasp
  for cleft palate prosthesis, 430
  Crozat-type, 418
  designs of
    consideration for esthetics in, 156-157

Clasps—cont'd
  designs of—cont'd
    reshaping teeth to, 169
  disadvantages of, 6
  embrasure, 77-79
  hairpin, 80-81
  half-and-half, 79-80
  infrabulge, 86, 127
  and minor connectors, 34
  movable-arm, 86-87
  multiple, 79
  reverse-action, 80-81
  ring-type, 75-77
  wrought-wire; *see* Wrought-wire clasp
Clasp arms
  advantages and disadvantages of, 70-71
  broken
    precautions against, 412-413
    reasons for, 412, 413
    repair of, 412, 413, 415
  cross-sectional form of, 69
  design of, 70
  diameter of, 68-69
  effect of, on design of minor connector, 35
  flexibility of, 67-70, 151, 152-153
  interference to placement of, 156
  length of, 67-68
  location of, 8-9, 134
  material used for, 69
  movement of, 72
  reciprocal and stabilizing, 3, 69-70
    in clasp assembly, 71
    continuity of, with crown ledge, 241
    diameter of, 69-70
    functions of, 73-74, 237
    as indirect retainer, 74
    lingual apron to, 71-72
    path of, in placement and removal of partial denture, 65, 73, 156
    in principles of clasp design, 72
    in relation to height of contour, 232
    in resisting partial denture movement, 52
    vs retentive arms, 69, 70
    in stabilization against horizontal movement, 73
    tooth surfaces of, 8
    waxing of, 340, 341
  retention with, 64
  retentive, 3, 63
    cast vs wrought wire, 113
    in clasp assembly, 71
    contour of, 206
    degree of retention from, 67
    effect of, on dislodging vertical forces, 44
    effect of guiding plane on, 152
    effect of rest on, 44
    flexibility of, 67
    lowering height of contour for, 232
    metal alloys for, 201
    as orthodontic force, 72, 73
    passivity of, 127

Clasp arms—cont'd
  retentive—cont'd
    placement of, along tooth, 65, 73
      in relation to undercut, 67
      on veneer crowns, 241, 242
    in principles of clasp design, 72
    in relation to angle of cervical convergence, 67
    in resistance of dislodging vertical forces, 51
    tapering of, 206
    undercut for, measurement of, 159
    use of surveyor for placing, 148, 150
    waxing of, 340, 344
  selection of, 70-71
  as stressbreaker, 134
Clasp assembly
  combinations in, 71
  components of, 71
  definition of, 3
  design of, 72
Cleft lip, 423
Cleft palate
  anatomy of, 424-427
  Class I, 423, 424, 429
  Class II, 423, 424, 429
  Class III, 423, 424, 429, 435
  Class IV, 423, 424, 429
  classification of, 423, 424
  with cleft lip, 423
  etiology of, 423
  pathology of, 427
  and personality evaluation, 423-424
  in physiology of speech, 427
  prosthetic treatment of, 429
  surgical treatment of, 427-429
Cleft palate prostheses, 429-435
  framework for, 430
  impression with alginate for, 429-430
    pharyngeal, 431-433
  obturator
    design of, 430-431
    meatus, 433-434
  pharyngeal portion of, 432
  psychologic effect of, 435
Cohesion, 62
Combination clasp, 83-85, 134
  advantages of, 83-84
  in Class II partial denture, 131
  in Class III partial denture, 128
  disadvantages of, 84
  waxing of, 336, 344
Compression molding, 381
Condylar path, 181
Connectors, 18-42
  major, 18-34
    characteristics of, 21
    definition of, 3
    design of, 39
    distortion and breakage of, 413-414
      repair of, 413
    divided, 114, 116
      disadvantages of, 117

Connectors—cont'd
  major—cont'd
    effect of indirect retainers on, 102, 107, 137, 161
    in failure of partial denture, 18
    height of floor of mouth to, 173
    interference to, 155-156
    joining of, to minor connector, 35, 36
    location of, 18, 39, 133
      with respect to gingival tissue, 18, 20, 39
    mandibular
      borders of, 22, 25
      continuous bar retainer, 22-24, 25, 26, 102, 133
      form of, 21
      labial bar, 22
      lingual bar; *see* Lingual bar
      linguoplate; *see* Linguoplate
      location of, 21
      need for determining type of, 169
      selection of, in treatment planning, 194-195
    maxillary, 20, 26-34
      combination anterior and posterior palatal strap, 26
      design of, 32-34
      margins of, 20
      palatal, 3
      palatal plate, 26, 30, 32, 41
      single palatal bar or strap, 26-27, 34, 40
      U-shaped palatal, 26, 27-28, 41-42
    in resisting partial denture movement, 51, 53
    in retention of partial denture, 62
    rigidity of, 18, 39, 113, 133
  minor, 18, 34-38
    against inlays, 233
    in clasp assembly, 3, 71
    definition of, 34
    distortion and breakage of, 413-414
      repair of, 413
    effect of, on indirect retainer, 100, 102
    effect of stressbreakers on, 117
    form and location of, 34-38
    function of, 34
    interference to, 156
    in joining to direct retainer arms, 38
    in joining to occlusal seat, 46
    in joining to major connector, 21, 35, 36
    for mandibular distal extension partial dentures, 36
    in resisting partial denture movement, 52
    in retention of partial denture, 62
    rigidity of, 113
    as stabilizing components, 134
    waxing of, 339, 340, 341
  wrought wire, 114
Constrictor muscle, superior, 425, 426, 427
Copings
  in making crowns and inlays, 250
  in waxing metal bases, 346
Copper bands, 245-247
  impressions with, 250
  for temporary coverage of crown preparations, 245
Crismani attachment, 114

Crown, 2
  for abutment teeth, 236-242
    ledges on, 237-241
  aluminum, 245, 248, 249
  cementation of, 252
  with embrasure clasps, 77
  establishing functional occlusion on, 316, 317-322
  to fit existing partial dentures, 250-252
  for fixed partial dentures, 195
  full cast, 228
    indication for, 228
    ledge on, 239
    preparation of, 236
    temporary coverage for, 245
  machining of, with surveyor, 151
  overhang margins of, 220
  polycarbonate, 245
  rest seats in, 55, 56
  as support for rests, 53
  survey of, 150
  temporary, 245
    cementation of, 249-250
    with partial denture, 248-250
  three-quarter, 234
    ledge on, 239
    preparation for, 234, 245
  vs tooth reduction, 170
  veneer, 228
    for abutment teeth, 241-242
    preparations for, 236
    shaping of, for clasp arms, 242
Crozat-type clasp, 418
Crucible, 352, 356
Crucible former, 356, 357
Curette, 220
Cysts, 212

D

Dalbo attachment, 114
Dentatus articulator, 181, 190, 300
  facebow transfer to, 182
Dentist
  responsibility of, in denture service, 393
  role of, in partial denture design, 9, 70
Dentofacial deformity, 215
Dentures, complete, 2
  occlusion in, 298
  posterior palatal seal in, 32
  in recording occlusal relations, 303, 304, 323, 324
  vs removable partial dentures, 198-200
  retention of, 5, 62
  support of, 1, 10
Dentures, partial, fixed, 1, 2, 6, 137, 138, 245-248
  cementation of, 252
  with dowel rest attachment, 93
  functional registration of occlusal surfaces, 316-322
  indications for use of, 195-196
  with isolated abutment, 244
  for missing anterior teeth, 244
  for missing molars, 196
  for modification spaces, 195-196

Dentures, partial, fixed—cont'd
  pontic of, 197
  splinting effect of, 243, 244
  for tooth-bounded edentulous regions, 195
  in treatment planning, 194
Dentures, partial, removable
  adjustments to, 395-405
  cast gold, 69
  clasp-retained, 6
  Class I, 13, 16, 30
    design of, 129-131
    fulcrum line of, 97
    impressions for, 129-131
    indirect retainers in, 101, 102, 103, 104
    support of, 97, 126, 129
    survey of, 155
  Class II, 13, 16, 30
    clasps for, 131
    denture base for, 132
    design of, 131-132
    framework for, 336-346
    fulcrum line of, 97
    modification 1, 102-103
    retainers for, 131
      indirect, 101, 102
    support of, 97, 126
    survey of, 155
  Class III
    components of, 132
    denture base for, 129
    design of, 128-129
    fulcrum line of, 99, 100
    impressions for, 128
    interocclusal records for, 301, 302
    in periodontal treatment, 129
    rebasing of, 126
    retainers for, 128
    retention of, 126
    support of, 126
    survey of, 155
  Class IV, 16, 30
    fulcrum line of, 99, 100
    occlusion of, 300
  classification of, 13
  cleanliness of, 38, 402
  vs complete dentures, 198-200
  opposing complete dentures, 303, 304, 323, 324
  components of, 18, 132-137
  definition of, 1
  dentist, role of, in fabrication of, 9
  design of, 118, 120-142
    biomechanical considerations, 120-125
    components of, 132-137
    essentials of, 128-132
    factors influencing, 125-126, 137-141
    with missing teeth, 245
    types of, differentiation between, 126-128
      differences in clasp design, 127-128
      differences in support, 126
      impression registration, 127

Dentures, partial, removable—cont'd
  distal extension, 1
    balancing contacts in, 300
    denture base of, 105-108
      function of, 105-106
      space available for, 105
      stresses transferred to ridge by, 275
      support for, 9-10, 106, 274-281
    direct retainers for, 127-128, 134
    displacement of, 97
    framework for, 380-381
    Hart-Dunn attachment for, 87-89
    with internal attachments, 64, 93
    with internal rests, 151
    mandibular vs maxillary, 10
    movements of, 49-52
      rotation about axis through posterior abutment, 49-51
      rotation along longitudinal axis, 51-52
      rotation about vertical axis, 52
    occlusal adjustment of, 397
    relining of, 112, 468-469
      method, 469
      reason for, 468-469
    retention of, 126, 132
    retentive clasp for, 369
    stressbreakers for, 6
    support for, 9-10, 97, 126, 132, 274-280
      loss of, 112
    transfer of stresses in, 44
    treatment partial denture in preparation for, 421
    treatment planning of, 8
    working side contacts of, 300
  fabrication and service of, phases of, 6-11
    establishment of occlusal relations, 7, 10-11
    initial placement procedures, 7, 11
    patient education, 6, 7-8
    periodic recall, 7, 11
    support for distal extension base, 7, 9-10
    treatment planning and design, 6, 8-9
  failure of, reasons for, 11-12, 18
  framework for; *see* Framework
  fulcrum line of, 97
  impression materials and procedures; *see* Impressions
  indications for, 196-198
    economic considerations of, 198
    esthetics, 197
    excessive loss of residual bone, 197
    distal extension situations, 196
    for long span, 197
    need for bilateral stabilization, 197
    after recent extractions, 196-197
    sound abutment teeth, 196
  initial placement of, 395-405
  interim, 418-419
  investing of, 378-381
  mouth preparations for, 8, 11
    on abutment teeth, 227-229
      contouring wax patterns for, 228
      rest seats, 228-229
      restorations for, 227-228

Dentures, partial, removable—cont'd
  mouth preparations for—cont'd
    oral surgical, 210-215
      bony spines and knife edge ridges, 215
      cysts and odontogenic tumors, 212
      dentofacial deformity, 215
      exostoses and tori, 212-214
      extractions, 211
      hyperkeratoses, erythroplasia, ulcerations, 215
      hyperplastic tissue, 214
      impacted teeth, 212
      malposed teeth, 212
      muscle attachments and freni, 214-215
      polyps, papilloma, and traumatic hemangiomas,
        215
      removal of residual roots, 211
    periodontal, 215-227
      advantages of periodontal therapy, 226-227
      diagnosis and treatment planning, 217-218
      general therapy, 223-226
      initial disease control therapy, 218-223
      objectives of periodontal therapy, 216-217
      recall maintenance, 226
  movement of, 73, 134
  occlusal relationships in, 298-323
    desirable, 299-300
    establishing, 10-11
    methods, 300-316
      arranging teeth to occluding template, 311-
        316
      direct apposition of casts, 301
      interocclusal records with posterior teeth remain-
        ing, 301-302
      materials for artificial posterior teeth, 309-310
      with occlusion rims only, 303
      with occlusion rims on record bases, 302-303
      by recording occlusal pathways, 308-309
    opposing complete dentures, 299, 322-323
  occlusion in
    adjustment of, 299
    balanced, 298
    centric occlusion; *see* Centric occlusion
    centric relation; *see* Centric relation
    influence of existing teeth on, 298
  path of placement of, 64
    consideration of, in treatment planning, 171
    effect of, on location of clasp arms, 65
    factors determining, 148, 152-153
      esthetics, 153
      guiding planes, 152
      interference, 153
      retentive areas, 152-153
    recording of, 171-172
    and removal, 148, 152-153
    use of surveyor in establishing, 157-158
  patient education of, 7-8, 12
  polishing, 384-386
    borders, 384-385
    facial surfaces, 385
    gingival and interproximal areas, 385-386
  pressure from, 38

Dentures, partial, removable—cont'd
  processing of, 381-382
    errors in, 381, 382
    occlusal discrepancies with, 299
  relining; *see* Relining
  removal of, at night, 403
  repairs and additions to; *see* Repairs and additions
    to partial denture
  retainers of; *see* Retainers
  retention of, 5, 62
  rocking of, 404
  servicing of, 395-405
  with splint bar, 137-139
  success of, 12
  support of, 1, 44, 62
  technician, role of, in fabrication of, 9
  temporary crowns to fit, 248-250
  tooth-borne
    circumferential clasp arm for, 74
    denture base for, 105, 406-408
    design for, clasp, 127
    impression for, 274
    with internal rests, 151
    movement of, 52-53, 97
    occlusal adjustments of, 397, 400
    occlusion in, 299
    relining of, 406-408
    retainers for, 133-134
    retention of, 126
    retentive clasp arm for, 69
    support for, 274
    transfer of stresses in, 44, 53
    transitional, 419
    treatment, 419-422
    treatment planning for, 8-9, 11, 157
  work authorization for, 389-393
    content, 389
    characteristics, 389
    definition of, 389
    definitive instructions by, 392
    delineation of responsibilities by, 393
    function of, 389
    legal aspects of, 392-393
Denture base, 18
  accuracy of, 136, 280
  adjustments to bearing surfaces of, 396
  for arranging posterior teeth, 372
  characterization of, 379-381
  for Class II partial dentures, 132
  for Class III partial dentures, 129
  cosmetic effect of, 105
  definition of, 2
  dimensional changes in, 381
  in distal extension partial dentures, 105-108
    function of, 105-106
    space available for, 105
    stresses transferred from, to ridge, 275
    support for, 9-10, 106
      accuracy of denture base, effect of, on, 280
      design of framework, effect of, on, 280
      extent of coverage of ridge, effect of, on, 275-276

Denture base—cont'd
 in distal extension partial dentures—cont'd
  support for—cont'd
   factors influencing, 274-281
   impression registration, effect of, on, 276-280
   loss of, 112
   methods for obtaining, 282
   ridges, quality of, in, 275
   total occlusal load, effect of, on, 280-281
 function of, 105-108
 fabrication of, from functional vs anatomic impressions, 136-137
 functional contours of, 109
 horizontal shifting of, 52
 ideal, 108
 materials for, 2, 106-108
  development of, 382
 metal
  accuracy and permanence of form of, 108
  adding of, to partial denture, 294-296
  advantages of, 108-109
  attaching artificial teeth to, 109-111
  cleanliness of, 108-109
  reline of, 406-408
  thermal conductivity of, 108
  waxing of, 346-349
  weight and bulk of, 109
 movement of, to ridge, 51
 overlay abutments in support of, 139-141
 polishing of, 384-385
 and primary bearing areas, 32
 for recording jaw relations, 361-367
  acrylic, 362
  attaching of, to framework, 363
  contact of, with tissues, 362-363
  making of, 361
  metal, 362
 for recording occlusal relations, 302, 305
  of partial to complete dentures, 322
 relining of
  as consideration in design, 126
  for distal extension partial denture, 408-409
   method, 409
   reason, 408
  impressions for
   with Iowa wax, 257
   with metallic oxide paste, 256
   with modeling plaster, 257
  for tooth-borne partial denture, 406-408
   method, 407-408
   reason for, 406
 resin, acrylic, 293, 294
  attachment of, to framework, 106-107
   retention for, 342, 414
  accuracy and permanence of form of, 108
   cleanliness of, 108
  finishing line for, 343
  functional contours of, 109
  and minor connectors, 35-36
  preference of, 112
  processing errors in, 282

Denture base—cont'd
 resin, acrylic—cont'd
  reline of, 372, 406-408
  repair of broken, 414
  thermal conductivity of, 108
  weight and bulk of, 109
 in retention of partial denture, 62
 stability of, 112
 stimulation of tissues of residual ridge with, 105
 stressbreaker between, and abutment teeth, 413
 tinting of, 379-380
 for tooth-borne partial denture, 105, 406-408
 waxing of, 336, 339-340, 376-379
Denturism, 393
Diagnosis and treatment planning, 168-209
 for complete vs partial dentures, 198-200
 dental cast surveyor, use of, in, 170-172
 diagnostic casts in, 179-193
 examination data for, 193-195
 factors in selecting metal alloys for framework, 200-207
 for fixed vs removable partial dentures, 195-198
 oral examination in, 172-175
 periodontal, 217-218
 roentgenographic interpretation of, x rays in, 175-179
 visual examination in, 168-170
Diagnostic casts, 179-193
 in centric relation, 190-192
 for definitive treatment plan, 168
 in design of major connectors, 32-34
 design of mouth preparations on, 9, 11
 in design of partial dentures, 125, 128
 impressions for making, 179
  use of alginate for, 258
 for making individual acrylic resin tray, 267
 marks on, 157-158
 mounting of, 181
  jaw relation records for, 185-190
  maxillary cast to axis-orbital plane in, 181-185
  for occlusal adjustment in periodontal treatment, 226
 occlusal analysis of, 192-193
 as patient record, 181
 purpose of, 179-181
 stone for, 179
 survey of, 148-150, 179
  steps in, 153-157
   determining anterior-posterior tilt, 154, 155
   determining lateral tilt, 154, 155
   esthetics, consideration of, 156-157
   guiding planes, consideration of, 153-155
   interferences, consideration of, 151-156
   retentive areas, location of, 155
  treatment planning, use of, in, 8, 157
Diagnostic waxing, 179
Dial gauge, 159
Dialoy, 248, 266
Diastemas, 24, 26
Die stone, 179
Dies, 317
 dowel pin for, 265

Dies—cont'd
    electroformed, 265-266, 313
    trimming of, 266
    from working cast, 265
Diet control, 404-405
Disclosing wafers, 218
Disuse atrophy, 105, 293
Dowel rest attachment, 91-95
Drill press, 150
Duroc, 371

E

Eccentric occlusion, 299
Education, patient, 6, 7-8, 12
Electroforming
    of dies, 265-266, 313
    of occluding template, 313
Electroplating, 313
Electropolishing, 359
Embrasure clasp, 77-79
Enamel, 53
Endodontic treatment, 194, 231
Epoxy resin, 382
Erythroplasia, 215
Ethyl silicate, 355
Examination of patient
    data in, 193-195
        caries activity, 193
        health status, 193
        hygiene habits, 193
        need for endodontic treatment, 194
        need for occlusal corrections, 194
        need for orthodontic treatment, 194
        need for periodontic treatment, 194
        need for restorations, 194
        need for surgery or extractions, 193-194
        periodontal status, 193
        selection of mandibular major connector, 194-195
    exploration of teeth and investing structures in, 173
    objectives of, 172
    oral, 172-175
    placement of temporaries for, 172
    prophylaxis in, 172
    sequence for, 172-175
    visual, 168-170
    vitality tests in, 173
    x rays in, 173
Exostoses, 39, 169, 212-214

F

Face-bow
    definition of, 181
    development of, 81-82
    ear, 185
    elevation of, on patient, 184
    function of, 181
    positioning of, on articulator, 185
Face-bow fork, 183
    cast support for, 185

Face-bow transfer, 11, 299, 300, 303, 322
    arbitrary axis in, 182-183
    kinematic axis in, 183
    occlusion rims for, 183
    radius aspect of, 184-185
Finishing lines
    for anterior-posterior strap palatal major connector, 41
    for full coverage palatal major connector, 41
    at junction of major and minor connector, 36-38
    for linguoplate major connector, 40
    between major connector and retention ladder, 342-343
    for single broad palatal major connector, 40
    for single strap palatal major connector, 40
Fixed partial denture; *see* Denture, partial, fixed
Fixed-type obturator, 430-431
Flap surgery, periodontal, 223-226
Flask
    duplicating, 326-327, 332
    effect of, on cooling of casting, 359
Flasking, layered silicone rubber, 381-382
Floss, 218
Fluoride-type flux, 206, 416
Flux, 417
    borax, 206, 416
    fluoride, 206, 416
Formica, 326
Framework
    attachment of artificial anterior teeth to, 376
    attachment of resin base to, 106-107, 414
    burnout of, 357-359
    casting of, 359
        removal of, from investment, 359-360
    for cleft palate prosthesis, 429, 430, 433
    design of, 8-9, 280
    distal extension, 380-381
    for distributed stress, 280
    finishing of, 361
        heat hardening, 361
        heat soaking, 361
    investing of, 354-357
        procedure, 355-357
    for maxillofacial prosthesis, 435-436
    metal alloys for
        comparative physical properties of, 200-202
        factors in selecting, 200
    occlusal interferences from, 396
    polishing, 361
    reduction of unfavorable tooth contours for, 170
    specifications for waxing, 352
    spruing, 352-354
    waxing of, 333-349
Freni, 214-215, 226
    use of linguoplate with, 25
Fulcrum line, 51, 120, 128
    in Class I partial denture, 97, 99
    in Class II partial denture, 97, 99, 103
    in Class III partial denture, 99, 100
    in Class IV partial denture, 99, 100
    definition of, 97
    distance of, from indirect retainers, 101, 102, 103

Fulcrum line—cont'd
   rotation around, with need for relining, 112
Functional form of residual ridge, 278, 279, 280
Functional impression, 4, 136
   definition of, 278
   objective of, 280
   relining, 282-285
   technique for, 278-279
Functionally generated path, 299

G

Gag reflex, 424
Genioglossus muscle, 214
Gingival areas
   polishing of, on partial denture, 385-386
   waxing of, 377, 385
Gingivectomy, 223
Gingivoplasty, 223
Gold alloys
   vs chromium-cobalt alloys, 200
   cooling of, 327, 359
   density of, 201
   for denture bases, 108
   dimensional changes in, 355
   flexibility of, 201
   grain structure of, 202
   hardness of, 201
   heat hardening of, 361
   investment for, 325
   modulus of elasticity of, 200-201
   in partial denture framework, 200
   solder for, 416
   soldering of, 206
   work hardening of, 201
   with wrought-wire retainer arms, 202
   yield strength of, 200
Gold foil
   to eliminate defects in rest seats, 54, 55
   rest seats in, 53
Gold solder, 416
Gold teeth, 348
Grafts
   free gingival, 226
   mucosal, 215
   pedicle, 226
   skin, 215
Gravity, 62
Grinding, selective, 220, 221, 222
Guideline, 65
Guiding planes, 101
   auxiliary, 101
   contact of, to partial denture, 135
   of crowns, 240
   definition of, 4, 134
   design of, 8
   disking tooth surfaces for, 54, 232
   effect of, on clasp arms, 9
   effect of, on clasp retention, 64
   effect of, on design of minor connectors, 35
   as factor in determining path of placement,
      152

Guiding planes—cont'd
   function of, 135, 152
   of inlays, 235
   reciprocal clasp arms parallel to, 237
   reshaping teeth for, 169
   size of, 135
   use of surveyor for, 148, 153-155, 240-241
Gypsum, 5
Gypsum investment, 325
Gysi articulator, 181

H

Hagman Balancer, 309, 321, 371
Hairpin clasp, 80-81
Half-and-half clasp, 79-80
Hanau articulator, 181, 190, 300, 303
   in face-bow transfer, 182
Hart-Dunn attachment, 87-89
Heat hardening, 361, 417
Heat soaking, 359, 361
Height of contour
   definition of, 3
   in design of partial denture, 9
   lowering of, 232
   with respect to path of placement, 65
   survey of, 148-150, 159
Hemangioma, traumatic, 215
Hinge articulator, 320-321
Hinge stressbreakers, 114
Hinge-type obturator, 430, 431
Hydrochloric acid, 360
Hydrocolloid
   agar, 258, 259, 260
   alginate; *see* Alginate hydrocolloid
   dimensional stability of, 260
   handling of, precautions in, 261
   imbibition of, 261
   irreversible, 258, 260
      chemistry of, 260
      differences between, and agar hydrocolloid,
         260
      uses of, 258
   reversible, 127, 258
      base for, 259
      differences between, and alginate, 260
      gelation of, 259
      sol state of, 259
   shrinkage of, 261
   syneresis, 260
Hydrocolloid duplicating materials, 329, 332
Hydrocolloid impressions
   of anatomic ridge, 276
   distortion of, 263
   procedure for, 261-262
Hypochlorite solution, 403
Hydrocortisone acetate, 250
Hygiene, oral, 403, 405
   instructions on, 218
   in treatment planning, 54, 193
Hyperkeratoses, 215
Hyperplastic tissue, 214

I

Impressions
  altered cast, 258
  anatomic, 136-137, 274, 276
  for anatomic replica pattern, 350, 351
  for cleft palate prostheses, 429-430
  correction, 289
  for diagnostic casts, 173
  in differentiation of partial denture types, 126, 127
  for distal extension partial dentures, 136, 276-280
  fluid-wax functional, 289-292, 363
    objectives of, 291
  final, 8, 272
  functional, 4, 136
    definition of, 278
    objective of, 280
    relining of, 282-285
    technique for, 278-279
  hydrocolloid, 263, 276
    procedure for making, 261-262
    stone cast from, procedure for making, 262
  for making acrylic temporary crowns, 246, 247, 248
    to fit partial dentures, 248
  for making crowns and inlays to fit partial dentures, 250
  for making denture repairs and additions, 414-415
  materials used for, 255
    elastic, 255, 258, 259
      irreversible hydrocolloids, 258, 259, 260
      mercaptan rubber base, 258-259
      reversible hydrocolloid, 258, 259
      silicone, 259
    rigid
      metallic oxide pastes, 256
      plaster of Paris, 255-256, 259
    thermoplastic, 255, 256-258
      modeling plastic, 256-257, 259
      waxes and resins, 257-258
  of partially edentulous arch, 259-266
  pharyngeal, 431-433
  preliminary, 8
  pressure, 278, 280
  primary, 256
  for relining and rebasing, 406
  requirements for, 127
  secondary, 10, 256, 257, 258, 278, 282
  selective tissue placement, method, 285-289
  static, 278
  of teeth, after mouth preparations, 233
  wax, 10
Impression trays; *see* Trays, impression
Incisal guidance, 304
Incisal rest, 3
Incisors
  effect of, on design of palatal strap connector, 28
  indirect retainers on, 100, 101, 137
  lingual rests on, 56-58
  and use of linguoplate, 25-26
Inclined plane, 120
Infrabulge clasp, 86, 127
Injection molding, 381

Inlay
  on abutment teeth, 228, 233-236
    preparation of, 233-235
  with embrasure clasps, 77
  to fit existing partial dentures, 250-252
  for fixed partial dentures, 195
  machining of, with surveyor, 151
  occlusal coverage by, 233
  overhang margins of, 220
  on resin teeth, 111
  rest seats in, 55, 56, 234
  temporary filling of tooth preparations for, 245
  vs tooth reduction, 170
Inlay wax, 257, 410
  for blockout, 161, 165
  for functional occlusal records, 369, 370
  Kerr Ivory, 289
  for recording occlusal pathways, 304, 305
Interim partial denture, 418-419
Interocclusal records
  with adjustable frame, 302
  centric occlusion; *see* Centric occlusion
  centric relation; *see* Centric relation
  of impression paste, 2
  in mounting diagnostic casts, 189
  with occlusion rims, 303
  with occlusion rims on record bases, 302-303
  protrusive, 11, 189, 300
  with occluding template, 303-309
Intracoronal retainer, 6
Investment
  for chromium-cobalt alloy, 355
  for gold alloys, 325
  gypsum, 325
  purposes of, 355
  quartz, 325, 355
  refractory, 4
  removing casting from, 359
  silica, plaster-bound, 325, 355
  spatulation and mixing of, 333, 355, 356
  for stellite alloys, 325
  for Ticonium, 325
Investment cast
  abrasion of, 325, 326
  for anatomic replica patterns, 351
  properties of, 325
  purpose of, 325
  spraying of, with plastic model spray, 333
  trimming of, 333
  for waxing framework, 334-336
Iowa wax, 289
  for functional relining method, 257, 284, 285
  as secondary impression material, 257

J

Jel-Pac, 360
Jelenko surveyor, 144
  vs Ney surveyor, 143
  principal parts of, 143
  undercut gauge of, 159

K

Kennedy's classification, 13-17
    Applegate's rules for applying, 16-17
Kerr occlusal indicator, 400
Korecta wax, 257, 289

L

Laboratory procedures, 325-388
    anatomic replica patterns, 349-351
        procedure for making, 350-351
    anterior teeth, types of, for, 375-376
    arranging posterior teeth to an opposing cast or template, 372-375
    burnout procedures, 357-359
    casting framework, 359
    duplicating a stone cast, 325-333
        materials and flasks for, 326-329
        procedures, 328-333
    finishing and polishing framework, 360-361
        heat hardening, 361
        heat soaking, 361
    impression trays, making of, 361-367
        attached to framework, 367
    investing framework, 354-357
    investing partial denture, 378-381
    making occlusal corrections to opposing template, 382-384
    making stone occlusal template from functional occlusal records, 370-372
    occlusion rims, making, 367-370
    polishing partial denture, 384-386
        borders, 384-385
        facial surfaces, 385
        gingival and interproximal areas, 385-386
    processing partial denture, 381-382
        with layered silicone rubber flasking, 381-382
    record bases, making of, 361-367
    remounting partial denture, 382-384
    removal of casting from investment, 359-360
    spruing framework, 352-354
    waxing framework, 333-349
        for Class II partial denture, mandibular, 336-346
    waxing partial denture, 376-378
Lamina dura
    consideration of, in treatment planning, 178
    definition of, 178
    in determining bone height, 176
    effect of stress of abutment teeth on, 178
    function of, 178
Levator veli palatini muscle, 424, 427
Lever, 120, 122
Lingual bar
    blockout and relief of master cast for, 39
    characteristics and location of, 39
    contour of, 21, 22
    criteria for use of, 169
    effect of indirect retainer on, 101
    finishing lines of, 39
    food traps under, 170
    indications for use of, 39

Lingual bar—cont'd
    inferior border of, 22
    interference to, 155
    margins of, 20
    relief for, 133, 162, 163
    rigidity of, 133
    shape of, 133
    superior border of, 22
    wax and plaster patterns for, 21, 22
    waxing of, 336, 338-339
        specifications of, 39
    of wrought metal, 114-116
Lingual rests, 3, 56-58
Linguoplate
    blockout and relief of master cast for, 40
    borders of, 24
    characteristics and location of, 40
    contour of, 24
    contraindications for use of, 24
    definition of, 24
    finishing lines of, 40
    indications for use of, 25-26, 39-40, 133, 169
    with indirect retainers, 102, 137
    margins of, 20
    and minor connector, 34
    thickness of, 24
    waxing specifications for, 40
Logopedist, 433

M

Machines, 120
Major connectors; *see* Connectors, major
Master cast
    adaptation of record bases to, 303
    blockout areas of, 158, 160-162
        for anterior-posterior strap palatal connector, 41
        for full palatal coverage, 41
        for lingual bar, 39
        for linguoplate, 40
        for single broad palatal connector, 40
        for single strap-type palatal connector, 41
    correcting, method for, 289, 291
    in design of framework, 8-9
    in design of partial denture, 128
    drawing final design on, 159
    duplication of, 325
    establishing posterior palatal seal on, 32
    impressions for, 8
        use of alginate for, 258
    keying of, 370
    relationship of, to surveyor, 9, 158
    relieving, 162-165
    survey of, 8, 9, 151-152, 158-159
    tripoding of, 9, 158
Maxillofacial prosthesis, 435-437
Meatus obturator, 433
Mentalis muscle, 214
Metal
    occluding template of, 313-316
    reaction of tissues to, 38
    used in functional reline method, 282

Metal denture base, 293-296
  accuracy and permanence of form of, 168
  advantages of, 108-109
  attaching artificial teeth to, 109-111
  cleanliness of, 108-109
  reline of, 406-407
  thermal conductivity of, 108
  use of, vs resin bases, 112, 113
  waxing of, 346-349
  weight and bulk of, 109
Metal die, 248
Metal teeth, 111
Metallic oxide impression pastes
  border molding with, 256
  dispensation and mixing of, 256
  for impressions of anatomic ridge, 276
  for impressions of supporting form of ridge, 131
  for interocclusal records, 302
  for recording centric relation, 190
  for reline impressions, 256, 406
  for secondary impressions, 256
Methyl methacrylate resin, 382
  for denture bases, 106
Mica, 116
Minor connector; *see* Connector, minor
Model, 4
Modeling clay, 161
Modeling plastic
  border molding with, 256-257
  in fabrication of meatus obturator, 433
  forms of, 257
  for functional relining method, 283-284
  handling of, 256
  for occlusion rims, 367-369
  overheating of, 256
  for pharyngeal impressions, 431
  for recording centric relation, 190
  as reline impression material, 257
  as secondary impression material, 257
Modification spaces, 13, 16
  fixed partial dentures for, 195-196
  in placement of indirect retainers, 102
Modulus of elasticity, 200
Molars
  reduction of unfavorable contours of, 170
  replacement of, with fixed partial dentures, 196
  rests on, 44
  rest seats of, form of, 44-46
  second
    in classification of arches, 16
    replacement of, in metal, 111
  splinting of, 243
  third
    in classification of arches, 16
    consideration of, in treatment planning, 179
Muffle, electric, 359
Muscle attachments, 214-215, 224
Mylohyoid muscle, 214
Mylohyoid ridge, 396

N

Nailheads, 343, 349
  formation of, 343-344
Nasal cavity, 427
Nasopharynx, 424
Neurohr spring-lock attachment, 89-91
Neurohr-Williams rest shoe, 89-91
Ney blockout wax, 328
Ney-Chayes attachment, 63
Ney surveyor, 144
  handpiece holder with, 147, 148
  vs Jelenko surveyor, 143-148
  principal parts of, 143
  undercut gauge of, 159
Night guard, 222
Nonbearing areas, 32-34

O

Oblique ridge, external, 396
Obturator, 2, 423, 429
  design of, 430-431
  fixed-type, 430-431
  function of, 423, 427
  hinge-type, 430, 431
  meatus, 430, 433
Occlusal pathways, registering of, 303-305
  method, 305-309
Occlusal plane, 184
Occlusal rest, 3, 44, 132, 133
  auxiliary, 79, 80
    advantages of, 75
    as indirect retainers, 101
    vs reciprocal clasp arm, 71
  canine extensions from, 101-102
  design of, 8
  for distributed stress denture, 280
  effect of stressbreakers on, 117
  form of, 44, 53
  fractured, 413
  function of, 53
  internal, 49, 53
  interproximal, 46
  in joining minor connector, 34, 46
  location of, 44
  in principles of clasp design, 72
  secondary, 46, 55
  shape of, in restorations, 229
Occlusal rest seats
  form of, 44-46
  interproximal, 46-49
Occlusal wax, 400
Occlusion
  adjustment of
    on articulator, 397
    at delivery of denture, 397-403
    guide to, 220-221
    intraoral, 382, 397
    in preparation for partial denture, 194, 301
    after reline, 282
  alteration of, for partial denture, 185-189
  analysis of, in treatment planning, 179, 192-193

Occlusion—cont'd
   when attaching artificial teeth to metal base, 110, 111
   balanced, 5, 220, 298
   centric; *see* Centric occlusion
   of complete dentures, 298
   errors in, remounting to correct, 378
   establishment of, to occlusal template, 382-384
   examination of, in treatment planning, 169
   in fabrication of acrylic temporary crowns, 249
   functional records of, 4
      making occlusal templates from, 370-372
      occlusion rims for, 369
   interference in
      elimination of, 220
      from framework, 396
   loss of, with changes in residual ridge, 112
   in maxillofacial prosthesis, 437
   of partial dentures; *see* Dentures, partial, removable, occlusal relationships in
   periodic recheck of, 401
   after relining, reestablishing, 409-410
Occlusion rims
   in face-bow transfer, 183
   materials for making, 367-369
   for recording occlusal relations, 303
      on record bases, 302-303
   for registering occlusal pathways, 304, 305, 306-307
   resin, 419
Odontogenic tumors, 212
Oral cavity, 427
Orthodontic treatment, 194, 212, 222
   in cleft palate patients, 429, 432
Osteoporosis, 293

P

Palatal bar, 3
Palatal major connector, 3
   bar, 21, 26-27, 34, 40
   combination anterior and posterior strap, 26, 28-30
   designing of, method of, 32-34
   margins of, 21
   plate, 21, 26, 30-32, 41
   rigidity of, 133
   single broad, 40
   U-shaped, 26, 27-28, 41-42
Palatal median suture line, 18, 39
Palatal raphe, median, 21, 169, 275
   as nonbearing area, 32-34
Palatal rugae, 21
Palatal seal, posterior
   with complete dentures, 32
   with metal bases, 108
   with palatal plate, 31, 32
   tissues in area of, 285
Palatal tori, 18, 27, 29, 34, 133
Palate
   anatomic replica of, 349-350
      irregular contour of, 350
   closure of, 428
   lengthening of, 428
   hemisection of, 435

Palate—cont'd
   soft, 424
      function of, 427
      muscle attachments to, 424-427
Palatoglossus muscle, 427
Palatopharyngeus muscle, 425, 427
Papilla, interdental, 377
Papilloma, 215
Papillomatosis, 214
Partial denture; *see* Denture, partial
Passavant's pad, 426, 430, 431
Patient
   education of, 6, 7-8, 12
   examination of
      data for, 193-195
      exploration of teeth and investing structures, 173
      objectives of, 172
      oral, 172-175
      placement of temporaries for, 172
      prophylaxis in, 172
      sequence for, 172-175
      visual, 168-170
      vitality tests, 173
      x rays, 173
   instructions to, 402-403, 412
   periodic recall of, 11, 404
   presentation of treatment plan to, 179-180
   and previous experience with dentures, 125
Periodontal diagnosis, 217-218
Periodontal disease
   around abutment teeth, 405
   in considering removable partial denture, 197
   examination for, 193
   in loss of abutment teeth, 414
   in treatment planning, 168, 198
Periodontal flap surgery, 223-226
Periodontal pocket
   elimination of, 217
      surgically, 223
Periodontal probe, 217
Periodontal space, 176
Periodontal surgery, 223-226
   adjunctive procedures, 226
   flap, 223-226
   gingivectomy, 223
Periodontal therapy, 194
   advantages of, 226-227
   general, 223-226
      adjunctive surgical procedures, 226
      flap surgery, 223-226
      gingivectomy, 223
   initial, 218-223
      elimination of gross occlusal interferences, 220
      elimination of local irritating factors, 220
      guide to occlusal adjustment, 220-221
      for minor tooth movement, 222-223
      nightguard, 222
      oral hygiene instructions, 218
      scaling and root planing, 218-220
      splinting, 221-222

Periodontal therapy—cont'd
  objectives of, 216-217
  planning for, 217, 218
  recall maintenance, 226
Pharyngeal flap operation, 428
Pharyngeal impressions, 431-433
Pharynx, 425
  musculature of, bunching of, 426
Phonation, 426
Phonetics, 402
Pickling, 359, 360
Pickling solution, 360
Plaque, 218, 220
Plaster, impression, 190
Plaster of Paris
  fracture of impressions of, 255
  in impressions of anatomic ridges, 276
  setting and flow characteristics of, 255
  use of, 255-256
Plastic, 2
Plastic, modeling
  border molding with, 256-257
  in fabrication of meatus obturator, 433
  forms of, 257
  for functional reline method, 283-284
  handling of, 256
  for occlusion rims, 367-369
  overheating of, 256
  for pharyngeal impressions, 431
  for recording centric relation, 190
  as reline impression material, 257
  as secondary impression material, 257
Plastic teeth; *see* Resin teeth
Polycarbonate crowns, 245
Polyps, 215
Pontics, 348
Porcelain crowns, 236, 241-242
Porcelain teeth
  for anterior spaces, 376
  attachment of, to metal bases, 109-111
  and facings cemented to metal bases, 110
  as posterior teeth, 373
  reshaping of occlusal surfaces of, 383
  against resin teeth, 309-311
  vs resin teeth, 309, 310, 311
  in waxing metal bases, consideration of, 346
Potassium sulfate, 260
Precision attachments, 3
  vs internal occlusal rest, 49
  as intracoronal retainer, 63
Premolar, 4
  indirect retainer on, 100, 101, 137
  in multiple abutments, splinted, 243
  reduction of unfavorable contours of, 170
  rests on, 44
  rest seats of, 44-46
Pressure indicator paste, 396
Prevox, 360
Primary stress bearing areas, 32, 39
Prophylaxis, oral, 172
Proportional limit, 202, 203

Prosthesis
  articulated, 113
  cleft palate, 429-435
    framework for, 430
    impression with alginate for, 429-430, 431-433
    obturator, 430-431
      meatus, 433-434
      pharyngeal portion of, 432
      psychologic portion of, 435
  definition of, 1, 2
  fixed, 1
  maxillofacial, 435-437
Prosthetic dentistry, 1
Prosthetics, 1
Prosthodontics, 1
Prosthodontic treatment, 172
Protrusive occlusion, 11
  in partial denture fabrication, 300
  purpose of, 189
Pterygomaxillary notch, 396

Q

Quartz investment, 325
Quenching, 359, 417

R

Radiation, effect of, 436
Radiograph, 5
Rebasing, 406-411
  definition of, 2
  vs relining, 406
Refractory cast, 158, 336
Relief
  beneath major connectors, 18-20, 21, 28-29, 39, 40, 41
  inadequate, effect of, 38
Relining partial dentures
  definition of, 2
  dimensional changes during, 378
  distal extension, 408-409
  functional, 179, 180
    method, 282-285
    objectives of, 285
    problems with, 282
  impressions for
    with Iowa wax, 257
    with metallic oxide paste, 256
    with modeling plastic, 257
  need for, 112
  reasons for, 106
  vs rebasing, 406
  vs rebuilding occlusal surfaces, 111
  reestablishing occlusion with, 409-410
  with stressbreakers, 117, 118
  tooth-borne, 406-408
  use of tissue conditioners prior to, 410-411
Remounting cast, 384, 409
Remounting partial denture, 382-384
  precautions, 383-384
Repairs and additions to partial dentures
  classification of, 412-414
    broken clasp arms, 412

Repairs and additions to partial dentures—cont'd
  classification of—cont'd
    distortion and breakage of components, 413-414
    fractured, occlusal rests, 413
    loss of teeth, 414
    procedures, 414-415
    replacing broken clasp arms with wrought-wire retention arms, 415
    by soldering, 415-417
Resin, acrylic, 2
  for attaching metal bases to partial denture, 293
  for attaching porcelain and plastic teeth to metal bases, 346-348
  as bite plane, 421
  development of, 381-382
  dimensional changes in, 381
  in fabrication of denture base, 106, 126, 293, 294
    for arranging artificial posterior teeth, 372
    attachment of, retention for, 342
    finishing line for, 343
    and minor connectors, 35-36
    preference for, 112
    processing errors in, 282
    thermal conductivity of, 108
  in fabrication of impression trays, 267-272
    mixing of, 361
    packaging of, 361
  fluid, for tissue conditioning, 416
  impressions, 257-258
  interim partial denture of, 418
  for maxillofacial prostheses, 436
  packaging of, in flasks, 380
  for record bases, 302, 305
  as reline material, 407
  sprinkle on method of application, 363-367
  for temporary crowns, 245, 250
    cementation of, 249-250
    with existing partial dentures, 248
    fabrication of, 246-248
Resin teeth
  abrasive surfaces of, 311
  for anterior spaces, 376
  attachment of, to metal bases, 109-111, 348
  and facings cemented to metal base, 110
  with gold occlusal surfaces, 309, 311, 373
  modification of, 311
  against porcelain teeth, 309-311
  vs porcelain teeth, 309, 310, 311
  for posterior teeth, 373
  pressing on, of, 110
  processed directly to metal base, 111
  reestablishment of occlusion of, in reline, 409-410
  reshaping of occlusal surfaces of, 383-384
Resin veneer crowns, 241, 242, 252, 376
Resonation, 427
Respiration, 427
Rests, 18, 44-61
  auxiliary, 58, 101
  canine, 102
  in clasp assembly, 3, 71
  definition of, 3, 44

Rests—cont'd
  with anterior and posterior strap connectors, 28
  with continuous bar retainer, 25
  design of, 44
  on diagnostic casts, 157
  effect of, on partial denture movement, 97, 100
  function of, 44
  incisal, 3, 44, 58-60
    vs lingual, 56
    in splinting, 243
  as indirect retainers, 25, 100, 137
  internal
    vs internal attachment, 151
    lingual retention with, 85-86
  intracoronal, 53
  lingual, 44
    vs incisal, 56
    preparation for, 56-60
    in splinting, 243
  with linguoplate, 25
  location of, 44
  occlusal, 3, 44, 132, 133
    auxiliary, 79, 80
      advantages of, 75
      as indirect retainers, 101
      vs reciprocal clasp arms, 71
    canine extensions from, 101-102
    design of, 8
    for distributed stress denture, 280
    effect of stressbreakers on, 117
    form of, 44, 53
    fractured, 413
    function of, 53
    internal, 49, 53
    interproximal, 46
    in joining minor connector, 34, 46
    location of, 44
    in principles of clasp design, 72
    secondary, 46, 55
    shape of, in restorations, 229
  placement of, surveyor for, 150-151
  in resisting movement of tooth-supported partial denture, 52
  support for, 53-54
  topography of, 60
  with U-shaped palatal connector, 28
  waxing of, 340
Rest seats, 44-61
  in amalgam, 53
  in cast restorations, 53
  in crowns, 236-237
  in enamel, 53, 229
    preparation of, 54-55
  indication of, on diagnostic casts, 233
  incisal, 58-60
  in inlays, 234
  lingual, 56
  occlusal
    form of, 44-46
    interproximal, 46-49

Rest seats—cont'd
  preparation of, 169
  in restorations of abutment teeth, 228-229
Retainer
  bar, continuous, 3
  definition of, 3
  direct, 2, 3, 18, 62-96
    clasp, 64-67, 86-87
      bar; *see* Bar clasp
      circumferential; *see* Circumferential clasp
      combination, 83-85
      design of, 70-72
        principles of, 72-74
      flexibility of, 67-69
      relative uniformity of retention with, 67
    classification of, 127
    definition of, 63
    differences in design of, 127-128
    for distal extension partial denture, 134
    dowel rest attachment, 91-95
    effect of, on indirect retainers, 100
    extracoronal, 3, 127, 134
    in fulcrum line, 97
    Hart-Dunn attachment, 87-89
    internal attachment, 64, 86
    intracoronal, 3, 63, 127, 134
      placement of, surveyor for, 150
      with stressbreakers, 118
    and minor connectors, 34
    Neurohr spring-lock attachment, 89-91
    in resistance to partial denture movement, 52, 53
    for tooth-borne partial denture, 133-134
    types of, 63
    waxing of, 336, 344
    yield strength of, 202
  indirect, 18, 97-104, 128
    auxiliary functions of, 101
    in Class II partial denture, 97
    components of, 100
    definition of, 3, 100
    distance of, from fulcrum line, 101, 102, 103
    for distributed stress denture, 280
    effect of, on direct retainer, 100-101
    effect of, on fulcrum line, 97
    effect of stressbreaker on, 117, 118
    effectiveness of, factors influencing, 100-101
    forms of, 101-104
      auxiliary occlusal rest, 101
      canine extensions from occlusal rests, 101-102
      canine rests, 102
      with continuous bar retainers and linguoplates, 102
      coverage of rugae, 103-104
      direct-indirect retention from, 104
      in modification areas, 102-103
    function of, 137
    in functional relining method, 282
    incisal rests as, 58
    placement of, 100, 137
    reciprocal clasp arm as, 74
    in resistance to vertical forces, 51
    in rigid denture design, 118

Retromolar pad, 280, 300
Retromylohyoid space, 396
Reverse-action clasp, 80-81
Rhinolalia clausa, 433
Ridge, residual, 2
  anatomic form of, 4, 276, 279
    impressions of, 131
  changes in, with previous dentures, 113
  changes in form of, 112
  in design of major connector, 39
  disuse atrophy of, 105
  effect of stressbreaker on, 117, 118
  effect of treatment partial denture on, 421
  extent of coverage of, by denture base, 275-276
  functional form of, 4, 278, 279-280
    impressions of, 131
    vs static form, 4
  impressions of, 136
  knife-edge, 215
  mandibular, 275, 396
  massage of, by denture base, 105
  maxillary, 275
  movement of distal extension partial denture about,
    51-52
  quality of, 274
  in resistance of tissueward movement of denture base,
    51
  resorption of
    in consideration of removable vs fixed partial den-
      ture, 197
    use of linguoplate with, 25, 133
    use of palatal plate with, 32
    visual examination of, 168-169
  soft and flabby, 214
  stresses on, 275
  support for denture from, 105, 126, 136-137, 274
Ring-type clasp, 75-77
Roach clasp, 3, 81
Roentgenogram, 5
Roentgenographic survey
  interpretation of, 175-179
    alveolar lamina dura, 178
    bone density, 176-177
    index areas, 177-178
    root morphology, 178
    third molars, 179
  panoramic, 212
  in treatment planning, 173
Roentgenographic technique, 176
Root planing, 218-220
Rubber base impression materials, 258-259
  for impression of anatomic ridge, 276
  for impressions of supporting form of ridge, 131
  for partial denture impressions, 127
  for reline impressions, 406
Rugae, 21, 103-104

S

Saddle area, 2
Saddle Lock Retentoscope, 159
Salpingopharyngeus muscle, 426-427

Scaling, 218-220
Scarring, 436
Shellac bases, 302
Silica investment, 325
Silicone impression materials, 259
  electroplating of, 313
  in impression of anatomic ridge, 276
  in impression of supporting form of ridge, 131
  for partial denture impressions, 127
  for reline impressions, 406
Silicone rubber flasking, layered, 381-382
Sodium alginate, 260
Sodium silicate, 355
Soft palate, 424
  function of, 427
  musculature of, 424-427
Solder, 416
  gold, 206
Soldering
  electric, 415
    advantages of, 415-416
    procedure for, 416
    of wrought wire, 203, 206
  gold teeth to metal base, 348
  repairing by, 415-417
  torch, 206, 416
Space maintainers, 2
Speech, physiology of, 427
Splints, 2
  acrylic resin, 222
  cast removable, 222
  occlusal, fixed, 419-421
  treatment partial denture as, 419-421
Splint bar, 137-139, 245
  materials used for, 138
Splinting, 125, 195, 414
  of abutment teeth, 242-243
  form of, 222
  for mobile teeth, 218
  in partial denture design, 132
  removable partial denture, 197
  temporary, in periodontal treatment, 221
  in treatment plan, 193
Sprue channel, 352
Sprue pin, 356
Sprues, 352
Spruing of framework, 352-354
  multiple vs single, 352-353
  procedure for, 353-354
Spurs, interproximal, 418
Stability, 5
Stainless steel, 116
Stellite alloys, 201
  investment for, 325
Stern-Goldsmith attachment, 63
Stone, dental, 5
  for diagnostic casts, 179
  for making casts from hydrocolloid impressions, 262-263
  mixing of, 333
  for mounting casts, 185

Stone, die, 179
Stone cast
  duplicating, 325-333
    materials and flasks for, 326-328
    procedure, 328-333
  duplicate, 334, 336
  for waxing framework, 334, 336
Stone split cast, 383
Stone template, 313
Stress
  lateral, 52
  transfer of, to abutment teeth, 34, 44
Stress-bearing areas, primary
  impression registration of, 127
  in mandible
    buccal shelf, 275
    slopes of residual ridge, 275
  in maxilla, 275
Stress equalizer, 113
Stressbreakers, 6, 128, 113-118
  advantages of, 117
  clasp retainers as, 73
  definition of, 113
  direct retainers as, 134
  disadvantages of, 117-118
  for equalizing support in distal extension partial denture, 280
  function of, 117
  in maintenance of denture cleanliness, 116-117
  promotion of, 114
  repair and maintenance of, 118
  types of, 114-117
  with use of internal attachment, 64
Stylus tracings of occlusal relations, 303, 322
Styrene resins, 382
Surface tension, 108
Surgery
  need for, prior to prosthodontic treatment, 193
  periodontal, 223-226
    adjunctive procedures, 226
    flap, 223-226
    gingivectomy, 223
  in preparation for partial denture, 210-215
    on bony spines and knife-edge ridges, 215
    on cysts, 212
    on dentofacial deformity, 215
    extractions, 211
    freni, 214-215
    hemangiomas, 215
    hyperkeratoses, erythroplasia, and ulcerations, 215
    hyperplastic tissue, 214-215
    impacted teeth, 212
    on malposed teeth, 212
    on muscle attachments, 214-215
    on odontogenic tumors, 212
    on polyps, papilloma, 215
    removal of residual roots, 211
    on tori, 212-214
Surveyor
  for contouring wax pattern, 150

Surveyor—cont'd
in establishing height of contour of abutment teeth, 65-67
in fabrication of crown, 317
definition of, 143
description of, 143-148
as drill press, 150
handpiece holder, 150, 240
Jelenko, 143, 144
for machining cast restorations, 151
main parts of, 170-171
Ney, 143, 144
for placement of internal rests, 150-151
for placement of intracoronal retainers, 150
purposes of, 148-152
relation of cast to, recording of, 9, 158
for surveying ceramic veneer crowns, 150
for surveying diagnostic casts, 148-150
for surveying master casts, 151-152, 159
for treatment planning, 8, 11, 170-172
Williams, 143, 146
Syneresis, 260

T

Technician
in blocking out master cast, 161-162
in fabrication of partial denture, 133
responsibility of, in denture service, 393
role of, in partial denture fabrication, 9, 11
Teeth
abutment; *see* Abutment teeth
anterior
missing, 244-245
recording occlusal relations of, 304
artificial; *see* Artificial teeth
extractions of, 193-194, 211
temporary removable partial denture for, 197
impacted, 212
incisors
effect of, on design of palatal strap connector, 28
indirect retainers on, 100, 101, 137
lingual rests on, 56-58
and use of linguoplate, 25-26
malposed, 194, 212
reposition and retention of, 222-223
metal, 111
mobile
due to periodontal disease, 221-222
treatment of, 193
molar; *see* Molars
periodontally weakened, 25, 26
porcelain; *see* Porcelain teeth
posterior, 421
premolar, 4
indirect retainer on, 100, 101, 137
in multiple abutments splinted, 243
reduction of unfavorable contours of, 170
rests on, 44
rest seats of, 44-46
reduction of, in treatment planning, 170
resin; *see* Resin teeth

Teeth—cont'd
reshaping of, in treatment planning, 169-170
roots of
morphology of, 178
removal of, 211
tube, 110
Template, occluding, 303-304, 307-309
arranging teeth to, 311-316, 372-375
metal, 313-316
occlusal correction to, 382-383
for reestablishing occlusion in reline, 410
for registering fixed restoration occlusion, 319, 320, 321
stone, 313
making of, from functional occlusal records, 370-372
Tensor veli palatini muscle, 424-425, 427
Tensile strength
of Ticonium wire, 207
of wrought wire, 202
Thermotrol, 359
Thiokol impressions, 127, 258
electroplating, 313
Thompson Tru-Rugae technique, 349
Thyropalatal muscle, 427
Ticonium, 203, 206
hidden lock design with, 116
investment for, 325
for stressbreakers, 116
Ticonium Stress-o-graph, 159
Ticonium wire, 207
Tissue conditioners, 410-411
Toothbrush, 218
Tori
mandibular, 18, 22
palatal, 18, 27, 29, 34, 133
removal of, 193, 212-214
in treatment planning, 169
Transitional partial denture, 419
Trays, impression
acrylic resin, 266, 279, 361
advantages of, 266
denture base as, 294
perforations in, 270
technique for making, 267-272
attached to framework, 363, 367
with baseplate material, 361
for distal extension impressions, 10
embedding of, to minor connectors, 36
in establishing height of floor of mouth, 22
existing denture as, 406
for functional impression, 278, 279
for hydrocolloid impression, 261
for impression of cleft palate, 430
individual, 266-272
for impression for tooth-borne partial denture, 274
for selective tissue placement impression, 285-289
making of, 361-367
modeling plastic for, 361
relief for, 362, 363
for retention of alginate, 362
stock, 266, 272

Treatment partial denture, 419-422
Treatment planning, 8-9, 11, 157
  in design of major connector, 39
  diagnosis and, 168-209
    for complete vs partial denture, 198-200
    diagnostic casts for, 179-193
    examination data for, 193-195
    factors in selecting metal alloys for framework, 200-207
    for fixed vs removable partial denture, 195-198
    oral examination in, 172-175
    periodontal, 217-218
    presentation of, to patient, 179-180
    roentgenographic interpretation of, 175-179
    surveyor for, 170-172
    visual examination for, 168-170
  economic considerations of, 180
Tripoding, 9, 158, 171
Tube teeth, 110, 346
Tuberosity, maxillary
  effect of denture coverage on, 196
  fibrous, 169, 214
  with movement of denture base, 280
  as pressure area, 396
Tumors, odontogenic, 212
Twin-stage occluder, 320

U

Ulcerations, 215
Undercut
  of abutment tooth
    for bar clasp, 83
    for combination clasp, 84
  in determining clasps, 69
  effect of path of denture placement on degree of, 65
  for retentive clasp arm, 64, 150
  in crown made to fit partial denture, 252
  definition of, 3
  impression materials for, 259
  measurement of, 159
  in removable partial dentures, 39
  tissue, 162
Undercut gauge, 148, 159

V

Vacuum mixing, 333
Vel-Mix, 371
Velopharyngeal closure, 424
  through pharyngeal flap operation, 427, 428
Vertical dimension, 305, 306, 307, 367, 370, 371
  changing, treatment partial denture for, 419, 421
  changes in, during reline procedures, 407, 409
  increase in, through processing errors, 378
Verticulator, 320, 321
Vibrating line, 34
  palatal tissue of, displacability of, 285
Vibrator, 333
Vinyl resins, 382
Vitality tests, 173

W

Water bath, 256
Wax
  for blockout procedure, 161
  in fluid-wax functional impression method, 289
  for functional impression of ridge, 131
  for functional reline method, 283, 285
  for impression registration, 127, 228
  inlay; *see* Inlay wax
  interocclusal records of, 301
  Iowa, 257, 284, 285, 289
  Korecta, 257, 289
  occlusal indicator, 400
  for recording centric relation, 190
  for reestablishing occlusion in reline, 410
  for registering occlusal pathways, 304, 305, 306
  for relieving master cast, 163
  for reline impression, 406
Wax pattern, 4
  for Class II mandibular partial denture framework, 336-346
  contouring, surveyor for, 150, 235
  for crowns, 317
    creating ledge in, 239-240
    to fit existing partial denture, 250-252
  for fixed partial denture, 319, 320
  for framework, 346
    preformed, 326, 333, 334, 344
  smoothing of, 341-342
  of teeth, 348
Wax wash, 289
Waxing
  abrasion of investment cast with, 326
  in making framework, 333, 334
Wetting agent, 355-356
Whip Mix articulator, 300, 303
Williams attachment, 63
Williams surveyor, 143, 146
Wills sprue pin, 356
Wills undercut materials, 328
Wire loop, 418
WondrPak cement, 245
Work authorization, 389-393
  characteristics of, 389
  content of, 389
  definition of, 389
  definitive instructions by, 392
  delineation of responsibilities by, 393
  function of, 389
  legal aspects of, 392-393
  for repairs and additions to partial dentures, 414-415
Working cast, 265-266
Working side contacts, 221, 300
Wrought, 5
Wrought wire
  attachment of, to framework, 202, 203
  fusion temperature of, 202
  gold, 203, 206
  hardness of, 206
  percentage elongation of, 202
  proportional limit of, 202, 203, 206

Wrought wire—cont'd
  recrystallization of, 203
  selection and quality control of, 202-207
  soldering of, 203, 206
  tensile strength of, 202, 206
Wrought-wire clasp, 11, 69
  advantages and disadvantages of, 83-84, 128
  for better esthetics, 157
  broken, 412-413
  vs cast, 113
  in clasp assemblies, 71
  for Class II partial denture, 131
  in combination clasp, 83
  distortion of, 84, 85
  duplicate casts for, 325, 332
  formation of, 336-337, 346
  investing pattern for, 356
  in interim partial denture, 418
  readjustments of, 413
  replacement of broken clasp arm with, 415
  short vs long, 128
  soldering, 413
  as stressbreaker, 113, 118, 128

Wrought-wire clasp—cont'd
  waxing for, 345
  undercut needed for, 159
Wrought-wire connector, 114

X

X ray, 5
  in treatment planning, 173

Y

Yield strength
  in chromium-cobalt alloy, 200
  definition of, 200
  of gold alloy, 200
  of Ticonium, 207
  of wrought wire, 202

Z

Zinc oxide and eugenol cements, 252
Zinc oxide and eugenol impression paste, 256
  for centric relation recording, 302
  for functional impression, 279
  for impression registration, 127